Anatomy & Physiology

for Speech, Language, and Hearing

Third Edition

Anatomy & Physiology

for Speech, Language and Hearing

Third Edition

J. Anthony Seikel, Ph.D.
Department of Communication Sciences & Disorders,
and Education of the Deaf
Idaho State University
Pocatello, Idaho

Douglas W. King, Ph.D.
Basic Medical Science
Washington State University
Pullman, Washington

David G. Drumright, B.S.
Computer Programmer
Spokane, Washington

Illustrations by Sarah Moore
Photography by Sarah Moore and Susan Duncan

THOMSON
—™
DELMAR LEARNING

Australia   Canada   Mexico   Singapore   Spain   United Kingdom   United States

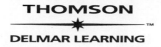

THOMSON
DELMAR LEARNING

Anatomy and Physiology for Speech, Language, and Hearing Third Edition
by J. Anthony Seikel, PhD, Douglas W. King, PhD, and David G. Drumright, BS

Vice President, Health Care Business Unit:
William Brottmiller

Editorial Director:
Cathy L. Esperti

Acquisitions Editor:
Kalen Conerly

Developmental Editor:
Juliet Steiner

Editorial Assistant:
Molly Belmont

Marketing Director:
Jennifer McAvey

Marketing Coordinator:
Chris Manion

Technology Project Specialist:
Mary Colleen Liburdi

Production Coordinator:
Mary Ellen Cox

Art and Design Coordinator:
Christi Dininni

Library of Congress Cataloging-in-Publication Data
Seikel, John A.
  Anatomy & physiology for speech, language, and hearing / John A. Seikel, Douglas W. King, David G. Drumright ; illustrations by Sarah Moore ; photography by Sarah Moore and Susan Duncan.—3rd ed.
      p. ; cm.
  Rev. ed. of: Anatomy and physiology for speech, language, and hearing / John A. Seikel, Douglas W. King, David G. Drumright. 2nd ed. 2000.
  Includes bibliographical references and index.
  ISBN 1-4018-2581-8
  1. Speech—Physiological aspects. 2. Human anatomy. 3. Human physiology. 4. Ear—Anatomy. 5. Ear—Physiology. 6. Neuroanatomy.
  [DNLM: 1. Speech—physiology. 2. Hearing— physiology. 3. Nervous System—anatomy & histology. 4. Respiratory Physiology. 5. Respiratory System—anatomy & histology. WV 501 S459a 2005] I. Title: Anatomy and physiology for speech, language, and hearing. II. King, Douglas W. III. Drumright, David G. IV. Title.
  QP306.S49 2005
  612.7'8--dc22

2004029224

NOTICE TO THE READER

Publisher does not warrant or guarantee any of the products described herein or perform any independent analysis in connection with any of the product information contained herein. Publisher does not assume, and expressly disclaims, any obligation to obtain and include information other than that provided to it by the manufacturer.

The reader is expressly warned to consider and adopt all safety precautions that might be indicated by the activities described herein and to avoid all potential hazards. By following the instructions contained herein, the reader willingly assumes all risks in connection with such instructions.

The publisher makes no representations or warranties of any kind, including but not limited to, the warranties of fitness for particular purpose or merchantability, nor are any such representations implied with respect to the material set forth herein, and the publisher takes no responsibility with respect to such material. The publisher shall not be liable for any special, consequential, or exemplary damages resulting, in whole or part, from the readers' use of, or reliance upon, this material.

Contents

Chapter 10   Anatomy of Hearing   435

Preface to the Third Edition

Introduction

This third edition of *Anatomy and Physiology for Speech, Language, and Hearing* is one of the most personally pleasing events of the authors' lives. Our fields of speech-language pathology and audiology are growing at a breathtaking pace, and this growth places exponentially increasing demands on students, particularly in the realm of the biological sciences. This text and its ancillary materials are designed to serve the upper division undergraduate or graduate student in the fields of speech-language pathology and audiology. Information on anatomical structures and their relationships is always subject to refinement and clarification. We can always improve the text's figures to make the material more accessible, and we must always strive to improve our descriptions so that the text is more readable. To this end we have added more than 60 figures to the text, as well as significant content revisions, clinical notes, a second color to the interior design, and a completely updated CD-ROM containing ANATESSE v. 2.0, which is an excellent study tool for students. We are very excited about these revisions.

We are convinced that we learn most what we are able to experience, and that learning is not a spectator sport. As instructors, we all know that if we are able to manipulate the material under study, or to view the material using different sensory modalities, we are better able to integrate that material into our knowledge base. We are committed to making the text and its ancillary materials as useful to twenty-first century students as possible. This revision not only provides students with a great interactive study tool in the ANATESSE v. 2.0 CD-ROM, but also makes available the *Electronic Classroom Manager to Accompany Anatomy and Physiology of Speech, Language, and Hearing, 3d Edition,* which provides a wealth of instructor resources to facilitate student learning.

Organization of Anatomy and Physiology for Speech, Language, and Hearing

This text is organized around the classical framework of systems of speech, language, and hearing. We separate out the anatomy and physiology components to facilitate learning. We introduce the student to the terminology of anatomy and physiology, and bring those terms to life in the anatomy and physiology chapters of the respiratory system. An investigation of the phonatory system follows, although in this third edition we have moved the discussion of the Bernoulli Principle and the material on acoustics to the chapter on phonatory physiology. Anatomy and physiology of the articulatory/resonatory system follows, but now the text includes an additional chapter on the physiology of swallowing, reflecting the vital importance of this function in the field of speech-language pathology. We follow this with the auditory system, a change from previous editions. Anatomy and physiology of the nervous system make up the final chapters of the revised text.

New to the Third Edition

With the third edition we acknowledge the importance of swallowing physiology with an entire chapter devoted only to that content. This is one of the more exciting areas of change in our profession, and we welcome the opportunity to address it in *Anatomy and Physiology for Speech, Language, and Hearing, 3d Edition.* We have also moved the hearing section to precede the neuroanatomy and neurophysiology sections. The presentation of all the content has been updated, with additional glossary terms appearing in the margins, a clean new design, and the addition of a second interior color to make the material more visually interesting and to highlight important structures in many of the figures.

We seek feedback from our students and others, and we make changes based on that feedback. One of the most consistent responses from students is that the study software is very useful for both preparation and review. We have taken that to heart, and have completely revised the software. ANATESSE is the fourth generation of anatomy software, and has marvelous and captivating graphics. David Drumright, co-author of the text, has brought his deep understanding of computers, instruction, and speech science to this task, and we hope you enjoy using the software as much as we have enjoyed developing it.

How to Use this Text

This text provides a sequential tour of the anatomy and physiology associated with speech, language, and hearing. It was designed with today's students in mind, and provides ancillary materials that greatly enhance learning. As you read the text, realize that you will be presented with the details of anatomy first, and that it is very important to master them to make these details your own. Use the companion software to support that learning and you will find that the quizzes and animations it provides will greatly reinforce your learning. We, as teachers of anatomy and physiology, have found that frequent quizzes really help a student learn the material. The software has these same frequent quizzes, and you will find that they will greatly enhance your understanding of the material. We want you to be the best therapist you can be, and sincerely hope that these materials move you along the path of your chosen career.

Supplements Accompanying the Third Edition

With the third edition we have developed an *Electronic Classroom Manager to Accompany Anatomy and Physiology of Speech, Language, and Hearing, 3d Edition* for instructors. This set of materials provides the instructor with a searchable Image Library containing high-quality scans of all figures in the text for use in individualized class presentations or testing. In addition, the *Electronic Classroom Manager* provides a downloadable and customizable *Instructor's Manual* containing a syllabus with materials and suggested activities for the lecture, and lab guides to facilitate learning outside of the classroom. Finally, the *Electronic Classroom Manager* offers a *Computerized Test Bank* with 1,000+ questions and answers for use in instructor-created quizzes and tests. The most important feature of all the components in the *Electronic Classroom Manager* is that everything is customizable. Just as the syllabus can be downloaded and reworked to meet an individual's personal instructional goals, the instructor can pick and choose the questions in the *Computerized Test Bank* that best fit the needs of a particular course or group of students. This comprehensive package provides something for all instructors, from those teaching anatomy and physiology for the first time to seasoned instructors who want something new.

About the Authors

J. Anthony (Tony) Seikel is on faculty at Idaho State University in Pocatello, Idaho. His research interests center around the relationship of pathology to acoustics and perception, but extend as well to the improvement of pedagogy through technology.

Douglas W. King was a professor within the Basic Medical program at Washington State University until the time of his death in 2001. He was greatly loved by his students and fellow faculty, and had set up a scholarship program in anatomy for students with diabetes.

David G. Drumright is a programmer and teacher in Spokane, Washington. He has taught electronics at numerous schools, and has a background in speech-language pathology and audiology. His software includes the original ANIMA programs of this text; the new ANATESSE application that you see in this third edition; AUDIN, which is software for instruction in audiology; and numerous smaller instructional tools.

J. Anthony (Tony) Seikel
David G. Drumright

Preface to the Second Edition

We are pleased to have the opportunity to update and improve upon *Anatomy and Physiology for Speech, Language, and Hearing*. We have enjoyed sharing our passion for this subject with you, and have listened carefully to the many people who have kindly provided us with corrections and suggestions to the text and software.

We maintain our primary goal of providing accessible instruction, and have taken many steps to improve that accessibility. Thanks to the insight of several readers we have added labeling to most of the photographs so that students may compare them with line drawings. We also redrew a number of the figures either to add new information or to make the information clear. We took this opportunity to add a number of figures throughout the book to illustrate information that is critical to the understanding of anatomy in communication.

We have made many changes throughout the text in an attempt to make the information more meaningful and relevant. Toward that goal we have added an appendix suggesting communication disorders related to the systems under discussion, and have added new clinical notes to provide a broader context for the information in the chapters. The most significant editorial changes came within the neuroanatomy and neurophysiology chapters: These two chapters were largely reorganized, based upon the suggestions of several generous reviewers, and rewritten to provide broader scope and deeper coverage of neuroanatomical structures and neurophysiological topics.

From feedback that we received from instructors and students, the ANIMA software has been a very useful study tool for anatomy and physiology. ANIMA has also undergone a major revision in response to suggestions of users in an attempt to make it an even better learning tool. We have eliminated the grading aspect to streamline installation and use of the software, and have modified the sequence of events upon termination from a lesson so that it is more logical and "user friendly." Many students and faculty noted that it would be helpful if students received more immediate and visual feedback of correctness in their responses, and you will see that we have incorporated this into the new design. We have also combined some lessons when it made conceptual sense to do so.

We hope that you will continue to provide your comments about the usefulness and effectiveness of these learning materials. We appreciate these, and look forward to incorporating them into future editions.

Preface to the First Edition

Anatomy and physiology provide the bedrock for communication. To understand human communication processes one must first know the structures that support those processes. Audiologists and speech-language pathologists are faced with assessing communication abilities that have been compromised by illness, trauma, or developmental anomaly. To be effective audiologists and speech-language pathologists, you must be able to relate the communication deficit to the structures on which communication depends. Armed with knowledge of the physical systems of speech, language, and hearing, you will be better equipped to serve those who depend on you for assessment, and your understanding of the physical systems will give you insights into treatment alternatives that might otherwise go unnoticed.

Our desire is to help you reach your goal of becoming a competent speech-language pathologist or audiologist. We recognize that there is a wide variety of learning styles, and that learning occurs best when instruction comes in many different forms. As you will see, the materials we have prepared include text, software, and videotaped lab activities. It is our hope that the text will provide your instructor with support for lectures, and we have found the software to be extremely helpful preparation for labs and tests. Our video experience provides you with the opportunity to examine the actual anatomical structures through a cadaver lab.

This expanded edition includes a number of changes over the original instructional materials. We are pleased to include units on the anatomy and physiology of hearing, the system that provides the input for oral communication. We have also significantly revised the software, making it an even stronger learning tool. There are eight new software lessons dedicated to audition, and we have developed a video for auditory anatomy as well. We are certain that you will share our awe of the auditory mechanism.

We hope that these materials help to solidify your knowledge. We join with your instructor in welcoming you to the world of anatomy and physiology for speech, language, and hearing, and trust that this marks only your first stop on a lifetime journey of learning.

Acknowledgments

Even though this revision appears to be the work of the authors, in reality an amazing number of people have made this third edition possible. Thomson Delmar Learning has a policy of seeking numerous reviews by faculty who work "in the trenches" before initiating a revision, and our first acknowledgment goes to those anonymous individuals who were willing to undertake that task. We read every word you wrote, and greatly appreciate your valuable suggestions and corrections. The authors also wish to thank the amazingly professional individuals at Thomson Delmar Learning, especially Juliet Steiner. Juliet is somehow able to remain upbeat during the most stressful and time-critical stages of this process. Thanks go out as well to the production and technology team members: Mary Ellen Cox, Christi DiNinni, Carolyn Fox, and Mary Colleen Liburdi. I wish everyone could meet Kalen Conerly, a person with amazing insight and vision who is an inspiration to the authors of Thomson Delmar Learning. Thanks to Marty Flanagan of Flanagan's Publishing Services, Inc., who has the patience of Job and the eye of an eagle.

We owe a tremendous debt to Sarah Moore of Pullman, Washington: Her masterful work on the drawings and photographs cannot be overstated. This text debuts the photographic work of Susan Duncan of Idaho State University Photographic Services, and we are deeply appreciative of her skill and abilities. We owe a special debt to Dr. Chad Ellis of Pocatello Family Dentistry, as well as to Tammy Grunig and Wendy Morgan of Portneuf Regional Medical Center. Special thanks go to Karlene Stefanakos, a truly dedicated therapist. Our friends Elda Voth, Tannis

Knopp, Matt and John Foster, Marilyn Russell, and Rachelle Ruffing were greatly helpful in the revision of this text. Finally, I (JAS) owe a deep debt of gratitude to my students in past and future classes. You continue to amaze me.

DEDICATION

We wish to dedicate this revision to the memory of our co-author, Douglas King

(JAS & DD)

The programmer (DD) dedicates this software to Professor Merle Phillips,
who taught him something about audiology and a lot about life.
The narrative author (JAS) wishes to dedicate the text to speech-language
pathologists, audiologists, and learners in training for their
dedication to the betterment of the lives of their clients.
You represent that which is the best of society.

CHAPTER 1

Overview of the Text

We continue to be impressed with the complexity and beauty of the systems of human communication. Humans use an extremely complex system for communication, requiring extraordinary coordination and control of an intensely interconnected sensorimotor system. It is our heartfelt desire that study of the physical system will lead you to an appreciation of the importance of your future work as a speech-language pathologist or audiologist.

We also know that the intensity of your study will work to the benefit of your future clients and that the knowledge you gain through your effort will be applied throughout your career. We appreciate the fact that the study of anatomy is difficult, but we also recognize that the effort you put forth now will provide you with the background for work with the medical community.

A deep understanding of the structure and function of the human body is critical to the individual who is charged with diagnosis and treatment of speech and language disorders. As beginning clinicians you are already aware of the awesome responsibility you bear in clinical management. It is our firm belief that knowledge of the human body and how it works will provide you with the background you need to make informed and wise decisions. We welcome you on your journey into the world of anatomy.

We have organized the text around the four "classic" systems of speech: the respiratory, phonatory, articulatory/resonatory, and nervous systems. The respiratory system (involving the lungs) provides the "energy source" for speech, while the phonatory system (involving the larynx) provides voicing. The articulatory/resonatory system modifies the acoustic source provided by voicing (or other gestures) to produce the sounds we acknowledge as speech. The nervous system lets us control musculature, receive information, and make sense of the information. Finally, the auditory mechanism processes those speech and nonspeech acoustic signals received by the listener who is trying to make sense of her or his world.

There are few areas of study where the potential for choking on detail is greater than in the discipline of anatomy. Our desire with this text and the accompanying software lessons is to provide a stable foundation upon which detail may be learned. In the text we have tried to provide you with an introductory section that sets the stage for the detail to follow, and we try to bring you back to a more global picture with summaries. We have also provided derivations of words where we thought it would help you to remember technical terms.

ANATESSE SOFTWARE LABS

We have created a series of software labs (Anatesse CD-ROM) that give you the opportunity to examine structures and function of the speech mechanism in the more flexible environment of the personal computer. The Anatesse software is keyed to the text, reinforcing identification of the structures presented during lecture, but more importantly illustrating the function of those structures. We've included an icon in the margin of the text as an indication that you'll find a lesson on the Anatesse software that supports the topic under discussion.

Whenever you see this icon in the text, you can go to your Anatesse CD-ROM to examine speech physiology through interactive manipulation of the structures under study, learning the relationship of the parts and how they function together. The Anatesse software labs are self-paced, and there are frequent quizzes to help you examine the effectiveness of your study habits. If you spend two or three half-hour sessions per week with the Anatesse software, you will get the greatest benefit from your class and readings. The Anatesse software will also provide a great refresher in preparation for quizzes and examinations. We continue to fine-tune Anatesse in response to the very relevant comments from learners, and hope that these materials serve you as well as they have served our students.

HOW TO USE THIS INSTRUCTIONAL PACKAGE

We feel that experience is the key to understanding. In the text, we will periodically take you on a guided tour of your own body and its functions. If you take advantage of these "tours," you will get a chance to experience the phenomena under study, setting the stage for a deeper understanding of the processes.

We have found that anatomy is not a "spectator sport"; learning is greatly enhanced through active participation. Your understanding of the anatomy and physiology of speech will be greatly enhanced through the interactive Anatesse software labs as you solidify the concepts of anatomy and physiology presented through the text.

As clinicians you want the insight of clinical details, and we have provided Clinical Notes within the text to broaden your appreciation of the importance of anatomy in your clinical practice. We have included tables of relevant pathologies that you will run across in your practice. We have also included an appendix with a sampling of the speech, language, and hearing disorders arising from physical malformation, illness, or trauma to the systems you will be studying. We hope that these elements of the text inspire you to a lifetime study of the organic components of your field.

We have attempted to facilitate your work with terminology. Anatomy has its own vocabulary, and you will make it yours before the course is through. As new terms are presented in text, they are highlighted in boldface type and defined on the same page. The glossary at the end of your text includes a pronunciation guide for some of the more challenging words.

If you supplement your reading with the relevant computer lessons, you will have provided yourself with the best opportunity to gain the insight you are seeking. We hope that this text and the accompanying Anatesse software serve you well in your career as speech-language pathologists and audiologists.

CHAPTER 2

Basic Elements of Anatomy

The study of the human body and its parts has a long and rich tradition. Although students of anatomy must still rely on their powers of observation, the task faced by the first anatomists was even more daunting. Modern study of anatomy and physiology is performed with myriad instruments and techniques, but our colleagues from earlier times were not so blessed. If you listen closely you will hear the echoes of the early anatomists' voices as you struggle with terminology that, at times, seems foreign and confusing. It is then that you should open your medical dictionary to see for yourself the roots of the words that seem confusing. The fact that the terminology remains in our lexicon indicates the accuracy with which your "academic ancestors" studied their field, despite extraordinarily limited resources.

In this chapter, we will provide some basic elements to prepare you for your study of the anatomy and physiology of speech, language, and hearing. To do this, we will provide a broad picture of the field of anatomy and then introduce you to the basic tissues that make up the human body. When tissues are combined to form structures, those structures must be bound together to form a functioning body, and we will discuss the means of connecting those parts. We will thus try to set the stage for your understanding of the new and foreign terminology of anatomy.

anatomy: *Gr., anatome, dissection*

dissect: *L., dissecare, to cut up*

physiology: *Gr., physis, nature + logos, study*

gross anatomy: *study of the body and its parts as visible without the aid of microscopy*

microscopic anatomy: *study of the structure of the body by means of microscopy*

surface anatomy: *study of the body and its surface markings as related to underlying structures*

developmental anatomy: *study of anatomy with reference to growth and development from conception to adulthood*

pathological: *Gr., pathos, disease + logos, study*

pathological anatomy: *study of parts of the body with respect to the pathological entity*

comparative anatomy: *study of homologous structures of different animals*

respiratory physiology: *the study of function in respiration*

ANATOMY AND PHYSIOLOGY

The term **anatomy** refers to the study of the structure of an organism. At one time it referred to the actual **dissection** or cutting of parts of the organism, but over time has evolved to encompass a field of study that involves much more than gross separation of body parts. **Physiology** is the study of the function of the living organism and its parts, as well as the chemical processes involved. As science and technology advanced, subspecializations of both anatomy and physiology arose. **Applied anatomy**, also known as **clinical anatomy**, entails application of anatomical study for diagnosis and treatment of disease, particularly as it relates to surgical procedures. **Descriptive anatomy**, also known as **systematic anatomy**, is involved in the description of individual parts of the body without reference to disease conditions. Descriptive anatomy views the body as a composite of systems that function together.

Gross anatomy studies structures visible without the aid of microscopy, while **microscopic anatomy** examines structures not visible to the unaided eye. **Surface anatomy** is the study of the form and structure of the surface of the body, especially with reference to the organs beneath the surface. **Developmental anatomy** deals with development of the organism from conception to adulthood.

When your study turns to the pathological entity, you will have entered the domain of **pathological anatomy**. Quite often in anatomy and physiology comparisons are made across species boundaries, because, among other things, knowledge of similarities and differences across the animal kingdom gives insight into the utility of different animal models of research. This study, **comparative anatomy**, provides that information.

Physiology has undergone similar change as technology has been refined. Examination of physiological processes may use a range of methods, from fairly simple methodologies, such as measuring the forces exerted by muscles, to highly refined **electrophysiological** techniques that measure the electrical activity of single cells or groups of cells, including muscle and nervous system tissue. Indeed, the audiologist will be particularly interested in auditory electrophysiological procedures measuring the electrical activity of the brain caused by auditory stimuli (**evoked auditory potentials**). **Respiratory physiology** is concerned with all processes involved in breathing.

You will sample the fruits of many of these areas during your study of anatomy. We rely heavily on descriptive anatomy to guide our understanding of the physical mechanisms of speech and to aid our discussion of its physiology as well. We will call on pathological anatomy as we deal with the results of conditions that change how systems work. Even as we discuss these changes, we will need to call on microscopic anatomy to reveal the impact of disease on structures invisible to the unaided eye.

Teratogens

A **teratogen** or **teratogenic agent** is anything causing **teratogenesis**, the development of a severely malformed fetus. For an agent to be teratogenic, its effect must occur during prenatal development.

Because development of the fetus involves the proliferation and differentiation of tissue, timing of the teratogen is particularly critical. The heart undergoes its most critical period of development from the third embryonic week to the eighth, while the critical period for the palate begins around the fifth week and ends around the twelfth week. The critical period for neural development stretches from the third embryonic week until birth. These critical periods for development mark the points at which the developing human is most susceptible to insult. An agent destined to have an effect on the development of an organ or system will have its greatest impact during that critical period.

Many teratogens have been identified, including organic mercury (which causes cerebral palsy, mental retardation, blindness, cerebral atrophy, and seizures), heroin and morphine (causing neonatal convulsions, tremors, death), alcohol (fetal alcohol syndrome, mental retardation, microcephaly, joint anomalies, maxillary anomalies), and tobacco (growth retardation) to name just a few.

We also must call on knowledge from related fields to support our understanding of anatomy and physiology. **Cytology** is the discipline that examines structure and function of cells; **histology** is the microscopic study of cells and tissues. **Osteology** is the study of structure and function of bones, while **myology** examines muscle form and function. **Arthrology** studies the joints that unite the bones, and **angiology** is the study of blood vessels and the lymph system. **Neurology** is the study of the nervous system. We will capitalize on all of these disciplines to explain the mechanisms involved in speech production.

To summarize:

- **Anatomy** is the study of the structure of an organism; **physiology** is the study of function.
- Several subspecializations of anatomy interact to provide the detail required for understanding the anatomy and physiology of speech, language, and hearing.
- **Descriptive anatomy** relates the individual parts of the body to functional systems.
- **Pathological anatomy** refers to changes in structure as they relate to disease.
- **Gross** and **microscopic anatomy** refer to levels of visibility of structures under study.
- **Developmental anatomy** studies the growth and development of the organism.

cytology: *Gr., kytos, cell + logos, study*

histology: *Gr., histos, web; tissue + logos, study*

osteology: *Gr., osteon, bone + logos, study*

myology: *Gr., mys, muscle + logos, study*

arthrology: *Gr., arthron, joint + logos, study*

angiology: *Gr., angio, blood vessels + logos, study*

neurology: *Gr., neuron, sinew; nerve + logos, study*

- Disciplines such as **cytology** and **histology** study cells and tissues, and **myology** examines muscle form and function.
- **Arthrology** refers to study of the joint system for bones, while **osteology** is the study of form and function of bones.
- **Neurology** refers to the study of the nervous system.

TERMINOLOGY OF ANATOMY

We talk about the structures in anatomy through modifying terms. Clarity of terminology lets us accurately represent structures, and is of the utmost importance in the study of anatomy. Terminology also links us to the roots of this field of study. To the budding scholar of Latin or Greek, learning the terms of anatomy will be an exciting reminder of our linguistic history. To the rest of us, the terms we are about to discuss may be less easily digested, but are nonetheless important.

As you prepare for your study of anatomy, please realize that this body of knowledge is extremely hierarchical. What you learn today will be the basis for what you learn tomorrow. Not only are the terms the bedrock for understanding anatomical structures, mastery of their usage will let you gain the maximum benefit from new material presented.

Parts of the Body

thorax: *the part of the body between the diaphragm and the seventh cervical vertebra*

abdomen: *L., belly*

The human body can be defined in terms of specific regions. The **thorax** is the chest region; the **abdomen** is the region represented externally as the anterior abdominal wall. Together, these two components make up the **trunk** or **torso**. The **dorsal trunk** is the region we commonly refer to as the *back*. The area of the hip bones is known as the **pelvis**. Resting atop the trunk is the head or **caput**. The **cranium** is the portion of the skull housing the brain.

The upper and lower extremities are appended to the trunk. The **upper extremity** consists of the arm (from the shoulder to the elbow), the forearm, wrist, and hand. The **lower extremity** is made up of the thigh, leg, ankle, and foot.

Terms of Orientation

Terminology in anatomy is very important, as it lets us communicate relevant information concerning location and orientation of various body parts and organs.

In the **anatomical position**, the body is erect and the palms, arms, and hands face forward, as shown in Figure 2-1. Discussion of terms of direction assumes this position. Intrinsic to this discussion is the concept

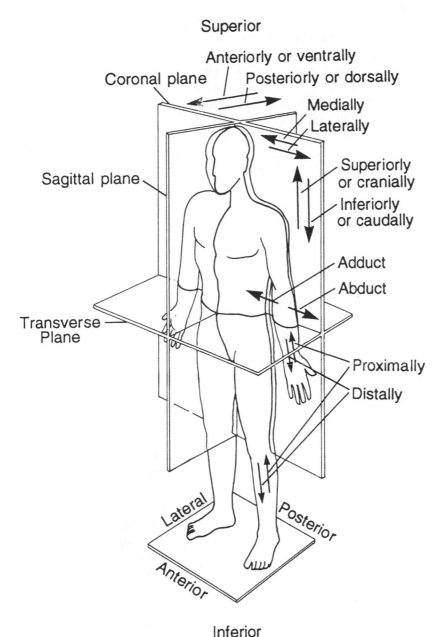

Superior

Anteriorly or ventrally

Coronal plane

Posteriorly or dorsally

Medially

Laterally

Sagittal plane

Superiorly or cranially

Inferiorly or caudally

Adduct

Abduct

Transverse Plane

Proximally

Distally

Lateral

Posterior

Anterior

Inferior

Figure 2-1. Terms of orientation and planes of reference.

of axis. The body and brain (and many other structures) are seen to have axes or midlines from which other structure arise. The **axial skeleton** is the head and trunk, with the spinal column being the axis, while the **appendicular skeleton** includes the lower and upper limbs. The **neuraxis** or axis of the brain is slightly less straightforward, due to morphological changes of the brain during development. The embryonic nervous system is essentially tubular, but as the cerebral cortex develops, a flexure occurs and the telencephalon (the region that will become the cerebrum) folds forward. As a result, the neuraxis takes a T-formation. The spinal cord and brain stem have dorsal and ventral surfaces corresponding to those of the surface of the body. Because the cerebrum folds forward, the dorsal surface is also the superior surface, and the ventral surface is the inferior surface. Most anatomists avoid this confusing state by referring to the superior and inferior surfaces.

Some terms are sensitive to the physical orientation of the body (such as *vertical* or *horizontal*). Other terms (such as *frontal*, *coronal*, and *longitudinal*) refer to planes or axes of the body, and are therefore insensitive to the position of the body.

With the anatomical position in mind, let us turn to planes of reference. You may think of the following planes as referring to sections of a standing body, but they are actually defined relative to imaginary axes of the body. If you were to divide the body into front and back sections you would have produced a frontal section or **frontal view**. (Realize that a frontal view is the product of a frontal section but, in practice, frontal section often refers to the view.) However, if you cut the body into left and right halves you would have **midsagittal sections**. A sagittal section is any cut that divides the body into left and right portions, and the cut is in the sagittal plane. A transverse section produces upper and lower halves of a body. Figure 2-1 illustrates these sections.

A **frontal** or coronal section results in front and back portions of a body, and is so called because the plane is parallel to the coronal suture of the skull, which roughly divides the body in half along that axis. Recognize that these are midline sections, which provide equal halves, but sections can also be made off midline. Armed with these basic planes of reference, you could rotate a structure in space and still discuss the orientation of its parts.

The term anterior refers to the front surface of a body. (Those of you who play cards may remember "ante up," meaning, "put your money up front!" You may remember the term *antebellum*, meaning "before the war.") Ventral and *anterior* are synonymous for the standing human, but have different meanings for a quadruped. The ventral aspect of a standing dog includes its abdominal wall, which happens to be directed toward the ground. The anterior of the same dog would be the portion including the face.

The opposite of anterior is posterior, meaning "toward the back," and the synonym for bipeds is dorsal. Again, the posterior of a four-footed animal differs from that of humans. Thus, you may refer to a muscle running toward the anterior surface, or a structure having a specific landmark in the posterior aspect. These terms are "body-specific": No matter what the position of the body is, anterior is "toward the front" of that body. The term rostral is often used to mean "toward the head." If the term is used to refer to structures within the cranium, *rostral* refers to a structure anterior to another.

frontal section: *divides body into front and back halves*

sagittal: *L., sagittalis, arrow-like*

sagittal section: *divides body or body part into right and left*

coronal section: *divides body into front and back halves*

anterior: *L., front*

ventral: *pertaining to the belly or anterior surface*

The term "quadruped" refers to four-footed animals. The term "biped" refers to two-footed animals.

posterior: *toward the rear*

dorsal: *pertaining to the back of the body or distal*

rostral: *L., rostralis, beak-like*

When discussing the course of a muscle, we often need to clarify its orientation with reference to the surface or level within the body. Thus, a structure may be referred to as peripheral (away from the center) to another. A structure is superficial if it is confined to the surface.

When we say one organ is " deep to another," we mean it is closer to the axis of the body. A structure may also be referred to as being external or internal, but these terms are generally reserved for cavities within the body. Likewise, you may refer to an aspect of an appendicular structure (such as arms and legs) as being **distal** (away from the midline) or **medial** (toward the midline).

A few terms refer to the actual present position of the body rather than a description based on the anatomical position. **Superior** (above, farther from the ground) and **inferior** (below, closer to the ground) are used in situations in which gravity is important. The terms prone (on the belly) and supine (on the back) are also commonly used in describing the present actual position.

Often we must describe the orientation of a structure relative to another structure, and subsequently disregard the anatomical position. Some terms that will assist you are lateral (related to the side, as in football's "lateral pass"), proximal (nearest to the point of attachment or some point of reference, as in "approximate"). These two terms are usually reserved for discussion of the relationship between limbs and trunk.

There are specialized terms associated with movement. Flexion refers to bending at a joint, usually toward the ventral surface. That is, flexion usually results in two ventral surfaces coming closer together. Thus, sit-ups would be an act of flexion, because you are bending at the waist. Extension is the opposite of flexion, being the act of pulling two ends farther apart. Again, having completed a sit-up, you return to the extended condition. Hyperextension, as in arching your back at the end of your sit-up, is sometimes referred to as dorsiflexion.

Use of flexion and extension with reference to feet and toes is a little more complex. Plantar refers to the sole of the foot, the flexor surface. If you rise on your toes, you are extending your foot, but the gesture is reasonably referred to as **plantar flexion**. A **plantar grasp reflex** would be one in which stimulation of the sole of the foot causes the toes of the feet to "grasp." The term **dorsiflexion** may be used to denote elevation of the dorsum (upper surface) of the foot. You may turn the sole of your foot inward, termed inversion. A foot turned out is in eversion.

The term palmar refers to the palm of the hand, that is, the ventral (flexor) surface. The side opposite the palmar side is the dorsal side. If the hand is rotated so that the palmar surface is directed inferiorly, it is pronated (remembering that in the prone position one is lying on his or her stomach or ventral surface). Supination refers to rotating the hand so that the palmar surface is directed superiorly. A **palmar grasp reflex** is elicited by lightly stimulating the palm of the hand. The response is to flex the fingers to grasp.

peripheral: *relative to the periphery or away from*

superficial: *on or near the surface*

deep: *further from the surface*

external: *L., externus, outside*

internal: *within the body*

prone: *body in horizontal position with face down*

supine: *body in horizontal position with face up*

lateral: *toward the side*

proximal: *L., proximus, next*

flexion: *L., flexio, bending*

extension: *Gr., ex, out + L., tendere, to stretch*

hyperextension: *extreme extension*

dorsiflexion: *flexion that brings dorsal surfaces into closer proximity (syn., hyperextension)*

plantar: *pertaining to the sole of the foot*

inversion: *L., in, in + versio, to turn*

eversion: *L., ex, from; out + versio, to turn*

palmar: *pertaining to the palm of the hand*

pronate: *to place in the prone position*

supinate: *to place in the supine position*

ipsi: *same*

These and other useful terms and their definitions may be found in Appendixes A and B at the end of the book, as well as in the Glossary. A good medical dictionary will be another invaluable aid in the process of sorting out anatomical terminology.

The names of muscles, bones, and other organs were mostly set down at a time in history when medical people spoke Latin and Greek as universal languages. The intention was to name parts unambiguously rather than to make things mysterious. Many of the morphemes left over from Latin and Greek are worth learning separately. When you come across a new term, you will often be able to determine its meaning from these components. For instance, when a text mentions an "**ipsilateral**" course for a nerve tract, you can see "ipsi" (same) and "**lateral**" (side) and conclude that the nerve tract is on the same side as something else. Your study of the anatomy and physiology of the human body will be greatly enhanced if it includes memorization of some of the basic word forms found in the appendixes.

While you are studying the nomenclature of the field, do not let the plurals get you down. Fortunately, Latin is a well-organized language with a few general rules that will assist you in sorting through terminology. If a singular word ends in "-a," the plural will most likely be "-ae" (pleura; pleurae). If the word ends in "-us" (such as "locus"), the plural will be "-i." When the singular form ends in "-um" (as in "datum" or "stratum"), the plural will have "-a" ("data" or "strata").

Often you can feel comfortable using the Anglicized version ("hiatuses," but never "datas"), but do not assume everyone will. Many combined forms involve a possessive form, denoting ownership (the genitive case, in linguistic jargon): "corpus"—body; "corporum"—of the body.

The English pronunciation of these forms is unfortunately less predictable; the dictionary often does not agree with the pronunciations common among medical personnel.

In summary:

- The **axial skeleton** consists of the trunk and head, whereas the **appendicular skeleton** comprises the upper and lower extremities.
- The **trunk** consists of the abdominal and thoracic regions.
- Anatomical terminology is the specialized set of terms used to define position and orientation of structures.
- A **frontal section** is one in which there are front and back halves, whereas a **sagittal section** divides the body into right and left halves.
- A **transverse section** divides the body into upper and lower portions.
- **Anterior** and **posterior** refer to the front and back surfaces of a body, as do **ventral** and **dorsal** for the erect human.
- **Superficial** refers to the surface of a body, while **peripheral** and **deep** refer to directions toward and away from the surface.

- **Distal** and **medial** refer to being away from or toward the midline of a free extremity, respectively.
- **Superior** refers to an elevated position, whereas **inferior** is closer to the ground.
- **Prone** and **supine** refer to being on the belly or back, respectively.
- **Lateral** refers to the side, **proximal** refers to a point near the point of attachment of a free extremity, and **distal** refers to a point away from the root of the extremity.
- **Flexion** and **extension** refer to bending at a joint. Flexion refers to bringing ventral surfaces closer together and extension is moving them farther apart.
- **Plantar** refers to the sole of the foot, while **palmar** refers to the palm of the hand. Both are ventral surfaces.

In the sections that follow, we will present the building blocks of the physical system you are preparing to study. These blocks include the basic tissues, organs, and structures made up of these tissues and the systems made up of the organs. Let us turn our attention to the basic elements of which all bodies are composed.

BUILDING BLOCKS OF ANATOMY: ORGANS, TISSUES, AND SYSTEMS

Organs

The body is composed of cells, living tissue that contains a nucleus and a variety of cellular material specialized to the particular function of the individual cell. Cells differ based on the type of **tissue** they comprise. Our study of anatomy will focus on muscle cells, nerve cells, and bone cells, as these cells combine to form the structures involved in speech and hearing. Four basic tissues constitute the human body, and variants of these combine to make up the structures of the body. These are epithelial, connective, muscular, and nervous tissue. These tissues have numerous subclasses, as shown in Table 2-1. Let us look at each tissue in turn.

tissue: *L., texere, to weave*

Table 2-1. Tissue types.

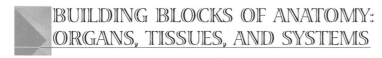

I. Epithelial

  A. Simple Epithelium: Single layer of cells.

    Squamous (pavement) epithelium: Single layer of flat cells; linings of blood vessels, heart, alveoli, lymph vessels.

    Cuboidal (cubical) epithelium: Cube-shaped; secretory function in some glands, such as thyroid.

(continues)

Table 2-1. *(continued)*

Columnar epithelium: Single layer, cylindrical cells; inner lining for stomach, intestines, gall bladder, bile ducts.

Ciliated epithelium: Cylindrical cells with cilia; lining of nasal cavity, larynx, trachea, bronchi.

B. Compound Epithelium: Different layers of cells.

Stratified epithelium: Flattened cells on bed of columnar cells; epidermis of skin, lining of mouth, pharynx, esophagus; conjunctiva.

Transitional epithelium: Pear-shaped cells; lining of bladder, etc.

C. Basement Membrane (baseplate)

Made predominantly of collagen; underlies epithelial tissue; serves stabilizing and other functions, including joining epithelial and connective tissues.

II. Connective

A. Areolar: Elastic; supports organs, between muscles.

B. Adipose: Cells with fat globules; between muscles and organs.

C. White Fibrous: Strong, closely packed; ligaments binding bones; periosteum covering bone; covering of organs; fascia over muscle.

D. Yellow Elastic: Elastic; in areas requiring recoil, such as trachea, cartilage, bronchi, lungs.

E. Lymphoid: Lymphocytes; make up lymphoid tissue of tonsils, adenoids, lymph nodes.

F. Cartilage: Firm and flexible.

1. Hyaline cartilage: Bluish white and smooth; found on articulating surfaces of bones, costal cartilage of ribs, larynx, trachea, and bronchial passageway.

2. Fibro-cartilage: Dense, white, flexible fibers; intervertebral disks, between surfaces of knee joints.

3. Yellow (elastic) cartilage: Firm elastic; pinna, epiglottis.

G. Blood: Corpuscles (cells: red, white), platelets, blood plasma.

H. Bone: Hardest connective tissue.

1. Compact bone: Has haversian canal, lamellar structure.

2. Cancellous (spongy) bone: Spongy appearance, larger haversian canal, red bone marrow producing red and white blood cells and plasma.

III. Muscular

A. Striated: Skeletal, voluntary.

B. Smooth: Muscle of internal organs, involuntary.

C. Cardiac: Combination of striated and smooth, involuntary.

IV. Nervous

A. Neurons: Transfer information; communicating tissue.

B. Glial cells: Nutrient transfer; blood-brain barrier.

Taxonomy from *Foundations of Anatomy and Physiology* by J. S. Ross & K. J. W. Wilson, 1966, pp. 1–32. Baltimore, MD: Williams & Wilkins.

Tissues

Epithelial Tissue

Epithelial tissue refers to the superficial (outer) layer of mucous membranes and the cells constituting the skin. The hallmark of epithelial tissue is its shortage of material between cells. This is in contrast to bone, cartilage, and blood, all of which have significant quantities of intercellular matter. The absence of intercellular material lets the epithelial cells form a tightly packed sheet, a protective quality. There may be many layers of epithelium. Some forms of epithelium are secretory (glandular epithelium) and others have **cilia** or hairlike protrusions that actively beat to remove contaminants from the epithelial surface (beating ciliated epithelia). We are most familiar with the surface covering of the human body, but epithelial tissue lines nearly all of the cavities of the body as well as the tubes that connect them.

A **baseplate** or **basement membrane** made predominantly of collagen underlies epithelial tissue, serving a number of functions, depending on the location of the epithelium. Basement membrane may act as a filter (for instance, in the kidneys), or stabilize the epithelial tissue (as in the juncture of connective tissue with epithelium). The basement membrane is important in the process of directing growth patterns for epithelial cells.

Connective Tissue

Connective tissue is perhaps the most complex of the categories, being specialized for the purpose of support. Unlike epithelium, connective tissue is composed predominantly of intercellular material, known as the **matrix**, within which the cells of connective tissue are bound. Connective tissue may be solid, liquid, or gel-like. The matrix is the defining property of a specific connective tissue.

Areolar tissue, also referred to as *loose connective tissue*, is supportive in nature. This elastic material is found between muscles and as a thin, membranous sheet between organs. It fills the **interstitial** space between organs, and its fibers form a mat or weave of flexible collagen. **Adipose** tissue is areolar tissue that is highly impregnated with fat cells. **Lymphoid tissue** is specialized connective tissue found in tonsils and adenoids.

> **interstitial:** *L., interstitium, space or gap in tissue*

Fibrous tissue binds structures together and may contain combinations of fiber types. **White fibrous** tissue is strong, dense, and highly organized. It is found in ligaments that bind bones together, as well as in the fascia that encase muscle, as will be described shortly. **Yellow elastic** tissue is found where connective tissue must return to its original shape after being distended, such as in the cartilage of the trachea or bronchial passageway. **Collagenous** and **reticular fibers** provide a flexible structure to fibrous connective tissue, while **elastic fibers** provide recoil to this tissue where needed.

Cartilage is a particularly important tissue because it has unique properties of strength and elasticity. The **tensile strength** of cartilage is the quality that keeps the fibers from being easily separated when pulled, while the **compressive strength** of cartilage lets it retain its form by being resistant to crushing, compressing forces. **Hyaline cartilage** is smooth and has a glassy, blue cast. It provides a smooth mating surface for the articulating surfaces of bones, as in the cartilaginous portion of the rib cage, constituting the larynx, trachea, and bronchial passageway. **Fibro-cartilage** contains collagenous fibers, providing the cushion between the vertebrae of the spinal column, as well as the mating surface for the temporomandibular joint between the lower jaw and the skull. Fibro-cartilage acts as a shock absorber and provides a relatively smooth surface for gliding. **Yellow (elastic) cartilage** has less collagen, endowed rather with elastic fibers. It is found in the pinna, nose, and epiglottis.

It might surprise you to know that **blood** is connective tissue. The fluid component of blood is called plasma, and blood cells (including red and white corpuscles) are suspended in this matrix. The blood cells arise from within the marrow of another type of connective tissue, bone.

Bone is the hardest of the connective tissues. The characteristic hardness of bone is a direct function of the inorganic salts that make up a large portion of bone. Bone is generally classified as being compact or spongy. **Compact** bone is characterized microscopically by its lamellar or sheetlike structure, whereas **spongy** bone looks porous. Spongy bone contains the marrow that produces red and white blood cells as well as the blood plasma matrix.

Muscle Tissue

Muscle is specialized contractile tissue. Although the connective tissues discussed previously have important supportive roles, they have no ability to contract. Muscle fibers are capable of being stimulated to contract.

Muscle function is described in Chapter 10.

striated: *L., stria, striped; streaked*

somatic: *Gr., soma, body*

autonomic: *Gr., autos, self + nomos, law; self-regulating*

Muscle is generally classified as being striated, smooth, or cardiac (see Figure 2-2). Striated muscle is so called because of its striped appearance on microscopic examination. Striated muscle is known as **skeletal muscle** as well, because it is the muscle used to move skeletal structures. Likewise, it is known as **voluntary** or somatic **muscle**, because it can be moved in response to conscious, voluntary processes. This is in contrast to **smooth** muscle, which includes the muscular tissue of the digestive tract and blood vessels. Smooth muscle is generally sheetlike, with spindle-shaped cells. **Cardiac muscle** is composed of cells that interconnect in a net-like fashion. Smooth and cardiac muscle are generally outside of voluntary control, relegated to the autonomic or involuntary nervous system, which will be discussed in Chapter 13.

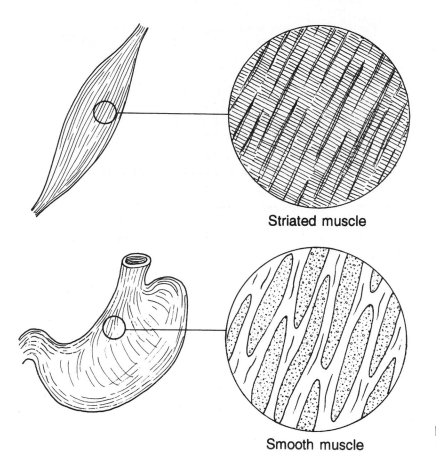

Striated muscle

Smooth muscle

Figure 2-2. Striated (upper) and smooth muscle (lower).

Nervous tissue structure is described in Chapter 12.

Nervous Tissue

Nervous tissue is highly specialized communicative tissue. Nervous tissue consists of **neurons** or nerve cells that take on a variety of forms. The function of nervous tissue is to transmit information from one neuron to another, from neuron to muscle, or from sensory receptors to other neural structures.

To summarize:
- Four **basic tissues** constitute the human body: epithelial, connective, muscular, and nervous.
- **Epithelial tissue** includes the surface covering of the body and linings of cavities and passageways.
- **Connective tissue** varies as a function of the intercellular material (matrix) surrounding it.
- **Areolar connective tissue** is loose and thin. **Adipose tissue** is areolar tissue with significant fat deposits.
- White **fibrous connective** and **yellow elastic tissue** is found in ligaments, tendons, and cartilage.

- **Cartilage** has both tensile and compressive strength and is elastic (fibers of cartilage resist being torn apart or crushed, and cartilage tends to return to its original shape upon being deformed).
- **Hyaline cartilage** is smooth, while fibro-cartilage provides a collagenous cushion between structures.
- **Yellow cartilage** is highly elastic.
- **Blood** is a fluid connective tissue, whereas **bone** is a highly dense connective tissue.
- **Muscle** is the third type of tissue, consisting of **voluntary** (striated), **involuntary** (smooth), and **cardiac** muscle.
- **Nervous tissue** is specialized for communication.

Tissue Aggregates

organs: *tissue of the body with functional utility*

The basic body tissues (epithelial, connective, muscular, nervous) are used to form larger structures. For instance, organs are aggregates of tissue with **functional unity**, by which we mean that the tissues of the organ all serve the same general purpose. In the same sense, we speak of **muscles** (such as the diaphragm) as being structures made up of muscular tissue, and the muscles must be attached to bone or cartilage in some fashion. Let us examine some of the larger organizational units.

fascia: *L., band*

Fascia. As mentioned in the previous section, fascia surrounds organs, being a sheetlike membrane that may be either dense or filmy, thin or thick. Striated muscle is surrounded by **perimysium**, fascia sufficiently thick that the muscle cannot be seen clearly through it.

ligament: *L., ligamentum, a band*

viscera: *L., body organs*

Ligaments. The term ligament refers specifically to "binding." **Visceral ligaments** bind organs together or hold structures in place. **Skeletal ligaments** must withstand great pressure, as they typically bind bone to bone. To achieve this, the connective tissue fibers course in the same direction, giving ligaments great tensile strength. Most ligaments have little stretch, although some (such as the posterior spinal cord ligaments) are endowed with elastic fibers to permit limited stretching. Ligaments that stretch appear yellow, while inelastic ligaments have a white cast.

morphology: *Gr., morphe, form + mys, muscle*

Tendons. **Tendons** provide a means of attaching muscle to bone or cartilage (see Figure 2-3). The fibers of tendons are arrayed longitudinally (as opposed to interwoven or matted), giving them great tensile strength but reduced compressive strength. Because tendon is actually part of the muscle, it always binds muscle to another structure (typically bone), attaching to the connective tissue of that skeletal structure. Tendons tend to have the morphology (or form) of the muscles they serve. Compact, tubular muscles tend to have long, thin tendons. Flat muscles, such as

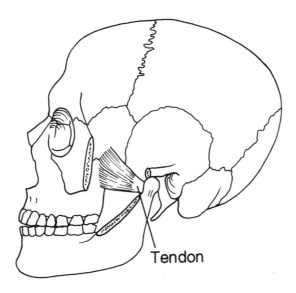

Tendon

Figure 2-3. Tendon attaching muscle to bone.

the diaphragm, will have flat tendons. The microscopic structure of a tendon makes it quite resistant to damage. Because the collagenous fibers intertwine, the forces placed on the tendon are distributed throughout the entire bundle of fibers.

When a tendon is sheetlike, it is called an **aponeurosis**. Aponeuroses greatly resemble fascia, but are much denser. In addition, an aponeurosis will retain the longitudinal orientation of the connective tissue fibers, whereas fascia are made up of matted fibers.

The dense packing of longitudinal fibers makes tendons quite strong. A tendon can withstand pulling of more than 8,000 times the stretching force that a muscle the same diameter can. In fact, the tendon for a given muscle will be able to withstand at least twice the pulling force of the muscle itself. That is to say, a sudden pull on a muscle will damage the muscle itself or the musculo-tendinous junction well before the tendon itself is actually damaged.

Bones. Bones and cartilage have an interesting relationship. Developing bone typically has a portion that is cartilage, and all bone begins as a cartilaginous mass. Many points of **articulation** or joining between bones are comprised of cartilage, because cartilaginous surfaces are smoother and will glide across each other more freely than surfaces of bone. Likewise, cartilage will replace bone where elasticity is beneficial. We will see this in the cartilaginous portion of the rib cage (Chapter 3), in the cartilage of the larynx (Chapter 5), and in the nasal cartilages (Chapter 7). As cartilage becomes impregnated with inorganic salts, it begins to harden, ultimately becoming bone.

aponeurosis: *Gr., apo, from + neuron, nerve; tendon*

Cartilage becomes quite important as we discuss the respiratory system (Chapter 3), the phonatory system (Chapter 5), and the articulatory/resonatory system (Chapter 7).

articulation: *the point of union between two structures*

Osteoporosis

Osteoporosis is a condition wherein bone becomes increasingly porous due to loss of calcium. The reduction in calcium may be the result of aging or may arise from vitamin D deficiency, as in **osteomalacia**. Loss of calcium may also arise from disuse, as found in individuals confined to bed during illness. Individuals with osteoporosis are particularly susceptible to bone fractures arising from what would be considered normal application of force. The elderly individual who has fallen and broken a hip may actually have broken the hip prior to the fall. An individual with osteoporosis may break ribs while coughing.

Osteoporosis may be localized, as seen in the bones of the skull in **Paget's disease** (osteitis deformans).

fibroblast: *L., fibra, fibrous + Gr., blastos, germ*

joint: *L., junctio, a joining*

diarthrodial: *the class of joints of the skeletal system that permits maximum mobility*

amphiarthrodial: *bony articulation in which bones are connected by cartilage*

synarthrodial: *the class of joints of the skeletal system that permit no movement*

fibrous joints: *joints that are connected by fibrous tissue*

cartilaginous joints: *joints in which cartilage serves to connect two bones*

synovial joints: *a type of diarthrodial joint that has encapsulated fluid as a cushion*

Bones provide rigid skeletal support and protect organs and soft tissue. Thirty percent of a bone is collagen, providing great tensile strength. The rigidity and compressive strength of bone tissue comes from the even greater proportion of calcium deposited within it. Indeed, bones of the aged become more susceptible to compression as a result of loss of calcium through aging.

Bones are broadly characterized by length (long or short) or shape (flat), or generally as having irregular morphology. The periosteum (fibrous membrane covering of a bone) extends along its entire surface, with the exception of regions endowed with cartilage. This outer periosteum layer is most tightly bound to the bone at the tendinous junctures. Although the outer periosteum layer is tough and fibrous, the inner layer of periosteum contains cells that facilitate bone repair, fibroblasts.

Bone growth and development stand as a classic example of "use it or lose it." The density of bone and its conformation are directly related to the amount of force placed on the bone. Use of muscles actually causes bone to strengthen and become more dense in regions stressed by that activity. Males tend to have greater muscle mass than females, and the bones of males will often have more readily identifiable landmarks.

Joints.   The union of bones with other bones, or cartilage with other cartilage, is achieved by means of joints (see Figure 2-4). Joints take a variety of forms. Generally, joints are classified based on the degree of movement they permit: high mobility (diarthrodial joints), limited mobility (amphiarthrodial), or no mobility (synarthrodial) (see Table 2-2). The joints are classified in parallel form based on the primary component involved in the union between bones. Synarthrodial joints are anatomically classified as fibrous joints, while amphiarthrodial joints are cartilaginous joints, and diarthrodial joints are synovial joints, or joints containing synovial fluid within a joint space.

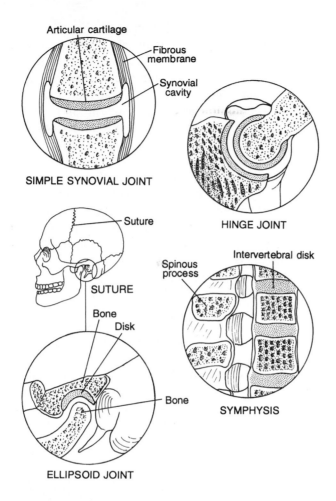

Articular cartilage

Fibrous membrane

Synovial cavity

SIMPLE SYNOVIAL JOINT

HINGE JOINT

Suture

SUTURE

Bone

Disk

Spinous process

Intervertebral disk

Bone

SYMPHYSIS

ELLIPSOID JOINT

Figure 2-4. Different types of joints.

Table 2-2. Types of joints.

I. Fibrous Joints (Immobile). *synarthrodial*
  A. Syndesmosis: Banded by ligament.
  B. Suture: Skull bone union.
  C. Gomphosis: Tooth in alveolus.
II. Cartilaginous Joints (Limited movement). *amphiarthrodial*
  A. Synchondrosis: Cartilage that ossifies through aging.
  B. Symphysis: Bone connected by fibro-cartilage.
III. Synovial Joints (Highly mobile). *diarthrodial*
  A. Plane joint (gliding joint; arthrodia): Shallow or flat surfaces.
  B. Spheroid (cotyloid).
  C. Condylar joint: Shallow ball-and-socket joints.
  D. Ellipsoid joint: "Football" shaped ball-and-socket joint.
  E. Trochoid joint (pivot).
  F. Sellar joint.
  G. Ginglymus (hinge) joint.

syndesmosis: *Gr.,
syndesmos, ligament + osis,
condition*

suture: *L., sutura, seam*

gomphosis: *Gr., bolting
together*

synchondrosis: *Gr., syn,
together + chondros,
cartilage + osis, condition*

symphysis: *Gr., growing
together*

articular capsule: *the
fibrous connective tissue
covering of a synovial joint*

cotyloid: *Gr., kotyloeides,
cup-shaped*

Fibrous Joints. There are three major types of fibrous or synarthrodial joints: syndesmosis, suture, and gomphosis. Syndesmosis joints are bound by fibrous ligaments but have little movement. Sutures are joints between bones of the skull that are not intended to move at all. The mating surfaces of the bones form a rough and jagged line that enhances the strength of the joint. A gomphosis is a type of joint in which a structure is bound within a cavity, as in the union of a tooth root to the hole that holds it, the alveolus.

Cartilaginous Joints. As the name implies, cartilaginous or amphiarthrodial joints are those in which cartilage provides the union between two bones. Considering that bone arises from cartilage during development, it makes sense that in some cases cartilage would persist. In synchondrosis, the cartilaginous union is maintained, as in the junction of the manubrium sterni and the corpus sterni, although it ossifies as the individual ages. The second type of cartilaginous joint is a symphysis, as found between the pubic bones (pubic symphysis) or between the disks of the vertebral column.

Synovial Joints. The distinguishing feature of synovial or diarthrodial joints is that they all include some form of joint cavity within which is found **synovial fluid**, a lubricating substance, and around which is an articular capsule. The articular capsule is made up of an outer fibrous membrane of collagenous tissue and ligament to which binds the bone and an inner synovial membrane lining. Hyaline cartilage covers the surface of each bone of the joint, providing a smooth, strong mating surface.

Synovial joints are either simple or composite, depending on whether two bone surfaces are being joined or more than two, respectively. **Plane synovial joints** (gliding joints; arthrodial) are those in which the mating surfaces of the bone are more or less flat. Bones joined in this manner are permitted some gliding movement. **Spheroid** (or cotyloid) **joints** are **reciprocal** in nature (as are all but plane joints), in

Craniosynostosis

As the infant develops, the sutures of the skull become ossified, a process called **synostosis**. Complete synostosis normally occurs well into childhood, but in some instances synostosis may occur prenatally. Continued normal growth of the brain, especially during the first postnatal year, places pressure on the skull. The effects of premature synostosis or **craniosynostosis** on skull development are quite profound. With **premature sagittal synostosis**, the child's head becomes peaked along the suture and elongated in back. In **Apert syndrome**, a genetic condition, the affected child's stereotypic "peaked head" is the result of premature closure of the coronal suture, resulting in pronounced bulging along that articulation.

that one member of the union has a convex portion that mates with a concave portion of the other member. The spheroid joint is a ball-and-socket joint, in which a convex ball or head fits into a cup or **cotylica**. This joint permits a wide range of movement, including rotation.

Condylar joints are more shallow versions of the ball-and-socket joint, and these joints permit more limited movement. Ellipsoid joints capitalize on an elliptical (football-shaped) member. These joints permit a wide range of movement, but obviously not rotation. A trochoid joint (**pivot joint**), in contrast, is designed for rotation, and little else. It consists of a bony process protruding into a space. A **saddle joint** (or sellar joint) is perhaps the most descriptive of the joint names. One member of the saddle joint is convex, like a saddle, while the other concave member "sits" on the saddle. A hinge joint (ginglymus) acts like the hinge of a cabinet door: One member rotates on that joint with a limited range, permitting only flexion and extension.

To summarize:

- Tissues combine to form larger structures.
- **Fascia** is a sheet-like membrane surrounding organs.
- **Ligaments** bind organs together or hold bones to bones or cartilage.
- **Tendons** attach muscle to bone or to cartilage; if the tendon is flat, it is referred to as an **aponeurosis**.
- Bones and cartilage provide the structure for the body, articulating by means of joints.
- **Diarthrodial** (synovial) **joints** are highly mobile, **amphiarthrodial** (cartilaginous) **joints** permit limited mobility, and **synarthrodial** (fibrous) **joints** are immobile.
- **Fibrous joints** bind immobile bodies together, **cartilaginous joints** are those in which cartilage serves the primary joining function, and **synovial joints** are those in which lubricating synovial fluid is contained within an articular capsule.
- Among synovial joints are **plane** (gliding) joints, **spheroid**, **condylar**, **trochoid**, **sellar**, and **ellipsoid** joints (all variants of ball-and-socket joints), as well as **hinge** joints.

Muscles. The combination of muscle fibers into a cohesive unit is both functionally and anatomically defined. Anatomically, muscles are bound groups of muscle fibers with functional unity. A fascia of connective tissue termed the epimysium surrounds muscles, and muscles are endowed with a tendon to permit attachment to skeletal structure. Muscles have a nerve supply to provide stimulation of the contracting bundle of tissue; muscles also have a vascular supply to meet their nutrient needs. Muscle morphology or form varies widely, depending on function. Fibers of wide, flat muscles tend to radiate from a broad point of origination to a

---

condylar: *Gr., kondylos, knuckle*

condylar joint: *a shallow ball-and-socket joint with limited mobility*

ellipsoid joint: *a shallow ball-and-socket joint in which the convex and concave elements are elliptical in shape*

trochoid joint: *a joint consisting of a process and fossa, permitting only rotation*

sellar: *L., sella, Turkish saddle*

sellar joint: *a ball-and-socket joint in which the concave member rests on an elongated convex member (syn., sellar joint)*

hinge joint: *a joint that acts like a hinge, permitting only flexion and extension*

ginglymus: *Gr., ginglymos, hinge*

epimysium: *Gr., epi, upon; over + mys, muscle*

morphology: *Gr., morphe, form + mys, muscle*

See Chapter 13 for a discussion of neuromuscular function.

agonist: *muscle contracted for purpose of a specific motor act (as contrasted to the antagonist)*

antagonist: *a muscle that opposes the contraction of another muscle (the agonist)*

more focused insertion. More cylindrical muscles will have unitary points of attachment on either end. In all cases, the orientation of the muscle fibers defines the region on which force will be applied, because muscle fiber can only actively shorten.

A muscle can contract to approximately one-half its original length, and thus long muscles can contract greater distances than short muscles. The diameter of a muscle is directly related to its strength, because that represents the number of muscle fibers allocated to perform the task.

The work performed by the body is widely varied between extremes of muscular effort (very little to great amounts) and extremes of muscle rate of contraction (very rapid to slow and sustained). Although muscle morphology accounts for much of the variation in function, the physical relationship between muscle and bone provides a great deal of flexibility in muscle use.

Muscles can exert force only by shortening the distance between two points and can contract only in a straight line (with the exception of sphincteric muscles). By convention, the point of attachment of the least mobile element is termed the **origin**, and the point of attachment that moves as a result of muscle contraction is termed the **insertion**. When referring to limbs, the insertion point is more distant from the body. Muscles that move a structure are referred to as **agonists** or prime movers, whereas those that oppose a given movement are called **antagonists**. Thus, an agonist for one movement may become an antagonist for the opposite movement. Muscles used to stabilize structures are termed **synergists**.

As you can see in Figure 2-5, the points of muscle attachment have a great deal to do with how much force can be exerted by muscle

Figure 2-5. Mechanical advantage derived from point of insertion. On the left, the muscle inserts closer to the point of rotation and the movable point will undergo a greater excursion on contraction of the muscle. On the right, the muscle is attached a greater distance from the point of rotation so that the bone will move a smaller distance, but the muscle is capable of exerting greater force in the direction of movement.

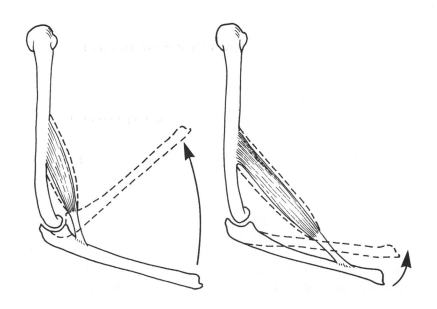

Neuromuscular Diseases

A host of neuromuscular conditions prey on the muscular system and the nerve components that supply it. **Amyotrophic lateral sclerosis** is a condition in which the myelin sheath surrounding the nerve axon is progressively destroyed, resulting in loss of muscle function. A similar but less predictable myelin destruction occurs in **multiple sclerosis**, although the course and severity of the disease are markedly different from amyotrophic lateral sclerosis. **Myasthenia gravis** is a condition in which the nerve-muscle junction is destroyed as a result of an immune system response. The result is weakness and loss of muscle range due to inability of the nerve and muscle to communicate.

contraction to achieve work. A muscle attached closer to a joint will move the bone farther and faster than one attached farther from the joint. In contrast, the muscle farther from the joint will be able to exert more force through its range, because of the leverage advantage. Thus, the more distally placed muscle will have an advantage for lifting, while the muscle closer to the joint will provide greater range to the bone to which it is attached.

Muscles are innervated or supplied by a single nerve. Innervation can be sensory (generally termed afferent) or excitatory (efferent) in nature. A **motor unit** consists of one efferent nerve fiber and the muscle fibers to which it attaches. Every muscle fiber will be innervated. In addition, muscles have sensory components providing information to the central nervous system concerning the state of the muscle.

> **innervation:** *stimulation by means of a nerve*

> **afferent:** *L., ad, to + ferre, carry*

> **efferent:** *L., ex, from + ferre, carry*

To summarize:

- **Muscle** is contractile tissue, with muscle bundles capable of shortening to about half their length.
- The point of attachment with the least movement is termed the **origin**, while the **insertion** is the point of attachment of relative mobility.
- Muscles that move a structure are **agonists** and those that oppose movement are called **antagonists**.
- Muscles that stabilize structures are termed **synergists**.
- Muscles are innervated by a single nerve.
- A **motor unit** is the efferent nerve fiber and muscle fibers it innervates.

Body Systems

In the same way that tissues combine to form organs, organs combine to form functional systems. Systems of the body are groups of organs with functional unity. That is, the combination of organs performs

> **system:** *a functionally defined group of organs*

muscular system:
the anatomical system that includes smooth, striated, and cardiac muscle

skeletal system:
the anatomical system that includes the bones and cartilages that make up the body

respiratory system:
the physical system involved in respiration, including the lungs, bronchial passageway, trachea, larynx, pharynx, oral cavity, and nasal cavity

phonatory system:
the system including the laryngeal structures through which phonation is achieved

articulatory system:
in speech science, the system of structures involved in shaping the oral cavity for production of the sounds of speech

resonatory system:
the portion of the vocal tract through which the acoustical product of vocal fold vibration resonates (usually the oral, pharyngeal, and nasal cavities combined; sometimes referring only to the nasal cavities and nasopharynx)

The logic of combining the articulatory and resonatory systems will become clear in Chapter 7.

a basic function, and failure or deficiency of an organ will result in a change in function of the system. Because systems are functionally defined, organs can belong to more than one system. Similarly, we can define the physical communication systems of the human organism through combinations of organs.

The basic systems of the body are fairly straightforward. The **muscular system** includes the smooth, striated, and cardiac muscle of the body. The **skeletal system** includes the bones and cartilages that form the structure of the body. The **respiratory system** includes the passageways and tissues involved in gas exchange with the environment, including the oral, nasal, and pharyngeal cavities, the trachea and bronchial passageway, and lungs. The **digestive system** also includes the oral cavity and pharynx, in addition to the esophagus, liver, intestines, and associated glands. The **reproductive system** includes the organs involved with reproduction (ovaries; testes), and the **urinary system** includes the kidneys, ureters, bladder, and urethra. The **endocrine system** involves production and dissemination of hormones, so it includes glands, such as the thyroid gland, testes, and ovaries. The **nervous system** includes the nerve tissue and structures of the central and peripheral nervous systems.

Systems of Speech

Speech is an extraordinarily complex process that capitalizes on these systems. The functionally defined systems of speech combine organs and structures in a unique fashion.

A classical categorization of the systems of speech includes respiratory, phonatory, articulatory, resonatory, and nervous systems. The **respiratory system** is a precise match with the anatomical respiratory system, including the respiratory passageway, lungs, trachea, and so forth. The **phonatory system** is the system involved in production of voiced sound and utilizes components of the respiratory system (the laryngeal structures). The **articulatory system** is the combination of structures that are used to alter the characteristics of the sounds of speech, including parts of the anatomically defined digestive and respiratory systems (the tongue, lips, teeth, soft palate, etc.). The **resonatory system** includes the nasal cavity and soft palate and portions of the anatomically defined respiratory and digestive systems. Although some speech scientists view the resonatory system as separate from the articulatory system, we take an alternate view in this text, combining them into the articulatory/resonatory system of speech production.

Our definition of systems of speech is truly a convenience. None of the systems operate in isolation. Speech requires the integrated action of all of the systems, and the level of coordination involved in this task is complicated (see Figure 2-6).

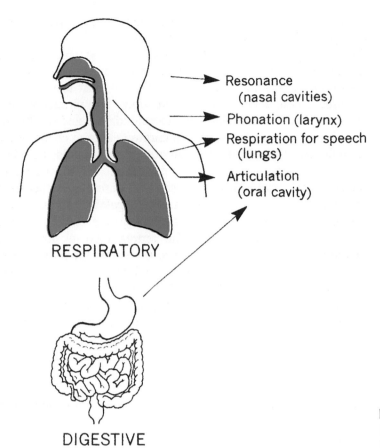

Resonance
(nasal cavities)

Phonation (larynx)

Respiration for speech
(lungs)

Articulation
(oral cavity)

RESPIRATORY

DIGESTIVE

Figure 2-6. Relationship of anatomical systems and overlaid speech systems.

To summarize:

- Organs combine to form **functional systems**, including the system concerned with muscles (**muscular system**), with the framework of the body (**skeletal system**), breathing (**respiratory system**), digestion (**digestive system**), reproduction (**reproductive system**), the **urinary** and **endocrine systems**, and **nervous system**.

- Within the discipline of speech pathology we have functionally defined four systems.

- The **respiratory system** is the system concerned with respiration, the **phonatory system** is made up of the components of the respiratory and digestive systems associated with production of voiced sounds (the larynx), the **articulatory/resonatory system** (including the structures of the face, mouth, and nose), and the **nervous system** (related to central and nervous system control of speech processes).

◤ CHAPTER SUMMARY

Anatomy and **physiology** are the study of structure and function of an organism. Subspecializations of anatomy interact to provide the detail required for understanding the anatomy and physiology of speech. **Descriptive anatomy** relates the individual parts of the body to functional systems and **pathological anatomy** relates to changes in structure from disease. Disciplines such as **cytology** and **histology** study cells and tissues, and **myology** examines muscle form and function. **Arthrology** refers to the study of the joint system for bones, while **osteology** is the study of form and function of bones. **Neurology** relates to the study of the nervous system.

The **axial skeleton** is that supporting the trunk and head, and the **appendicular skeleton** is related to the extremities. Anatomical terminology relates position and orientation of the body and its parts. A **frontal plane** is that involving a cut that produces front and back halves of a body, a **sagittal plane** is produced by a cut dividing the body into left and right halves, and a **transverse plane** is produced by dividing the body into upper and lower halves. **Anterior** and **posterior** refer to front and back of a body, as do **ventral** and **dorsal** for the human. **Peripheral** refers to a direction toward the surface or superficial region, while **deep** refers to direction away from the surface. **Distal** and **proximal** refer to away from and toward the root of a free extremity, respectively. **Superior** and **inferior** refer to upper and lower regions. **Lateral** and **medial** refer to the side and midline, respectively. **Flexion** refers to bending ventral surfaces toward each other at a joint, and **extension** is moving those surfaces farther apart. **Plantar** and **palmar** refer to ventral surfaces of the feet and hands, respectively.

The four basic tissues of the human body are **epithelial, connective, muscular**, and **nervous. Epithelial tissue** provides the surface covering of the body and linings of cavities and passageways. **Connective tissue** provides the variety of tissue linking structures together, those comprising **ligaments, tendons, cartilage, bone**, and **blood. Muscular tissue** is contractile in nature, comprised of **striated, smooth**, and **cardiac. Nervous tissue** is specialized for communication.

Tissues combine to form structures and organs. **Fascia** surrounds organs, **ligaments** bind bones or cartilage, **tendons** attach muscle to bone or to cartilage, and **bones** and **cartilage** provide the structure for the body. **Joints** between skeletal components may be **diarthrodial (synovial**; highly mobile), **amphiarthrodial (cartilaginous**; slightly mobile), and **synarthrodial (fibrous**; immobile). **Fibrous joints** bind immobile bodies together, **cartilaginous joints** are those in which cartilage serves the primary joining function, and **synovial joints** are those in which lubricating synovial fluid is contained within an articular capsule.

Muscle bundles are capable of shortening to about half their length. The **origin** is the point of attachment with the least movement, and the **insertion** is the relatively mobile point of attachment. **Agonists** are muscles that move a structure, **antagonists** oppose movement, and **synergists** stabilize a structure. Muscles are **innervated** by a single nerve, and innervation can be **afferent** or **efferent**. A **motor unit** is the efferent nerve fiber and muscle fibers it innervates.

Systems of the body include the **muscular, skeletal, respiratory, digestive, reproductive, urinary, endocrine**, and **nervous** systems. Systems of speech production include the **respiratory, phonatory, articulatory/resonatory**, and **nervous systems**.

STUDY QUESTIONS

1. _____ is the study of the structure of an organism.

2. _____ is the study of the function of a living organism and its parts.

3. _____ anatomy is anatomical study for diagnosis and treatment of disease.

4. _____ anatomy is involved in the description of individual parts of the body without reference to disease conditions, viewing the body as a composite of systems that function together.

5. _____ is the study of structure and function of cells.

6. _____ is the study of structure and function of bones.

7. _____ is the study of form and function of muscle.

8. _____ is the study of the nervous system.

9. Skin and mucous membrane are made up of _____ tissue.

10. _____ is a particularly important connective tissue because it is both strong and elastic.

11. _____ is contractile tissue.

12. _____ bind organs together or hold bones to bone or cartilage.

13. _____ is a sheetlike membrane surrounding organs.

14. _____ attach muscle to bone or to cartilage.

15. The relatively immobile point of attachment of a muscle is termed the _____ .

16. The relatively mobile point of attachment of a muscle is termed the
    _____ .

17. Identify the systems defined below:
    a. _____ This system includes smooth, striated, and cardiac muscle of the body.
    b. _____ This system includes the bones and cartilages that form the structure of the body.
    c. _____ This system includes the passageways and tissues involved in gas exchange with the environment, including the oral, nasal, and pharyngeal cavities, the trachea and bronchial passageway, and lungs.
    d. _____ This system includes the esophagus, liver, intestines, and associated glands.
    e. _____ This system includes the nerve tissue and structures of the central and peripheral nervous system.

18. Identify the systems of speech defined below:
    a. _____ This system includes the passageways and tissues involved in gas exchange with the environment, including the oral, nasal, and pharyngeal cavities, the trachea and bronchial passageway, and lungs.
    b. _____ This system is involved in production of voiced sound and utilizes components of the respiratory system (the laryngeal structures).
    c. _____ This system is the combination of structures used to alter the characteristics of the sounds of speech, including parts of the anatomically defined digestive and respiratory systems (the tongue, lips, teeth, soft palate, etc.).
    d. _____ This system includes the nasal cavity and soft palate and portions of the anatomically defined respiratory and digestive systems.

19. Terms of orientation: On the figure below, identify the descriptive terms indicated.
    a. _____ plane
    b. _____ plane
    c. _____ plane
    d. _____ aspect
    e. _____ aspect
    f. _____ (movement away from midline)
    g. _____ (movement toward midline)
    h. _____ (located away from midline)

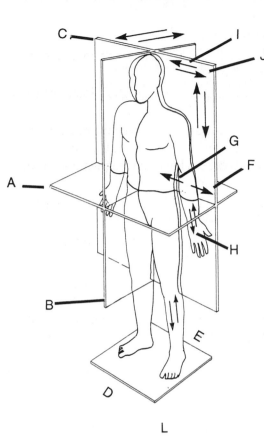

i. _____ (located near midline)

j. _____ (related to the side)

k. _____ (above)

l. _____ (below)

20. As our field has developed, the professionals working with speech and language became known as "speech-language pathologists." Reflecting on the terminology you have just reviewed, to what does the term "pathologist" refer?

STUDY QUESTION ANSWERS

1. ANATOMY is the study of the structure of an organism.
2. PHYSIOLOGY is the study of the function of a living organism and its parts.
3. CLINICAL OR APPLIED anatomy is anatomical study for diagnosis and treatment of disease.
4. SYSTEMIC ANATOMY is involved in the description of individual parts of the body without reference to disease conditions, viewing the body as a composite of systems that function together.
5. CYTOLOGY is the study of structure and function of cells.
6. OSTEOLOGY is the study of structure and function of bones.
7. MYOLOGY is the study of form and function of muscle.
8. NEUROLOGY is the study of the nervous system.
9. Skin and mucous membrane are made up of EPITHELIAL tissue.
10. CARTILAGE is a particularly important connective tissue because it is both strong and elastic.
11. MUSCLE is contractile tissue.
12. LIGAMENTS bind organs together or hold bones to bone or cartilage.
13. FASCIA is a sheetlike membrane surrounding organs.
14. TENDONS attach muscle to bone or to cartilage.
15. The relatively immobile point of attachment of a muscle is termed the ORIGIN .
16. The relatively mobile point of attachment of a muscle is termed the INSERTION .
17. Identify the systems defined below:
    a. MUSCULAR SYSTEM This system includes smooth, striated, and cardiac muscle of the body.
    b. SKELETAL SYSTEM This system includes the bones and cartilages that form the structure of the body.
    c. RESPIRATORY SYSTEM This system includes the passageways and tissues involved in gas exchange with the environment, including the oral, nasal, and pharyngeal cavities, the trachea and bronchial passageway, and lungs.
    d. DIGESTIVE SYSTEM This system includes the esophagus, liver, intestines, and associated glands.
    e. NERVOUS SYSTEM This system includes the nerve tissue and structures of the central and peripheral nervous system.
18. Identify the systems of speech defined below.
    a. RESPIRATORY SYSTEM This system includes the passageways and tissues involved in gas exchange with the environment, including the oral, nasal, and pharyngeal cavities, the trachea and bronchial passageway, and lungs.
    b. PHONATORY SYSTEM This system is involved in production of voiced sound and utilizes components of the respiratory system (the laryngeal structures).
    c. ARTICULATORY SYSTEM This system is the combination of structures used to alter the characteristics of the sounds of speech, including parts of the anatomically defined digestive and respiratory systems (the tongue, lips, teeth, soft palate, etc.).
    d. RESONATORY SYSTEM This system includes the nasal cavity and soft palate and portions of the anatomically defined respiratory and digestive systems.
19. Terms of orientation: On the figure below, identify the descriptive terms indicated.
    a. TRANSVERSE plane

   b. <u>SAGITTAL</u> plane

   c. <u>CORONAL OR FRONTAL</u> plane

   d. <u>ANTERIOR OR VENTRAL</u> aspect

   e. <u>POSTERIOR OR DORSAL</u> aspect

   f. <u>ABDUCT</u> (movement away from midline)

   g. <u>ADDUCT</u> (movement toward midline)

   h. <u>DISTAL</u> (located away from midline)

   i. <u>MEDIAL</u> (located near midline)

   j. <u>LATERAL</u> (related to the side)

   k. <u>SUPERIOR</u> (above)

   l. <u>INFERIOR</u> (below)

20. Pathology is the study of diseased tissue. By extension, a speech-language pathologist is one who studies the "pathology" of our field, communication disorders.

 # REFERENCES

Barnett, H. L. (1972). *Pediatrics.* New York: Appleton-Century-Crofts.

Basmajian, J. V. (1975). *Grant's method of anatomy.* Baltimore: The Williams & Wilkins Company.

Bateman, H. E. (1977). *A clinical approach to speech anatomy and physiology.* Springfield, IL: Charles C. Thomas.

Bateman, H. E., & Mason, R. M. (1984). *Applied anatomy and physiology of the speech and hearing mechanism.* Springfield, IL: Charles C. Thomas.

Duffy, J. R. (1995). *Motor speech disorders.* St. Louis, MO: Mosby.

Fink, B. R., & Demarest, R. J. (1978). *Laryngeal biomechanics.* Cambridge, MA: Harvard University Press.

Gosling, J. A., Harris, P. F., Humpherson, J. R., Whitmore, I., Willan, P. L. T. (1985). *Atlas of human anatomy.* Philadelphia: J. B. Lippincott.

Gray, H., Bannister, L. H., Berry, M. M., & Williams, P. L. (Eds.) (1995). *Gray's anatomy.* London: Churchill Livingstone.

Grobler, N. J. (1977). *Textbook of clinical anatomy* (Vol. 1). Amsterdam: Elsevier Scientific.

Kaplan, H. (1960). *Anatomy and physiology of speech.* New York: McGraw-Hill.

Kuehn, D. P., Lemme, M. L., & Baumgartner, J. M. (1989). *Neural bases of speech, hearing, and language.* Boston: Little, Brown.

Moore, K. L., Persaud, T. V. N., & Chabner, D.-E. B. (2003). *The developing human.* Philadelphia: W. B. Saunders.

Rahn, H., Otis, A., Chadwick, L. E., & Fenn, W. (1946). The pressure-volume diagram of the thorax. *American Journal of Physiology, 146,* 161–178.

Ross, J. S., & Wilson, K. J. W. (1966). *Foundations of anatomy and physiology.* Baltimore: Williams & Wilkins.

Williams, P., & Warrick, R. (1980). *Gray's anatomy* (36th Brit. ed.). Philadelphia: W. B. Saunders.

Zemlin, W. R. (1998). *Speech and hearing science: Anatomy and physiology* (4th ed.). Needham Heights, MA: Allyn & Bacon.

CHAPTER 3

Anatomy of Respiration

"Breathe! You are alive!"

—Thich Nhat Hanh, Zen Master

We *must* breathe with great regularity to maintain bodies that are dependent on efficient oxygen exchange. In parallel with this process we, as humans, have "hijacked" the respiratory system to provide the energy source for oral communication. As you will see in our discussion of respiratory physiology, we exercise a great deal of external control over the respiratory mechanism while still working within the bounds of the biological requirements for life. First, let us discuss respiration as it is needed to sustain life.

Respiration is defined as the exchange of gas between an organism and its environment. We bring oxygen to the cells of the body to sustain life by breathing in, the process of inspiration, and eliminate waste products by breathing out, or **expiration**.

Gas exchange happens within the minute air sacs known as the alveoli, only after gas has been drawn into the system. The process of bringing air into the lungs is muscular. It capitalizes on the fact that all forces in nature seek balance and equilibrium. The basic mechanism for inspiration may be likened to a hypodermic needle. If the plunger on the hypodermic needle in Figure 3-1 is pulled down, whatever is near the opening will enter the tube and be drawn into the awaiting chamber. If you envision the respiratory system as a syringe, with your mouth

inspiration: *Gr., spiro, breath*

alveolus: *L., small hollow or cavity*

35

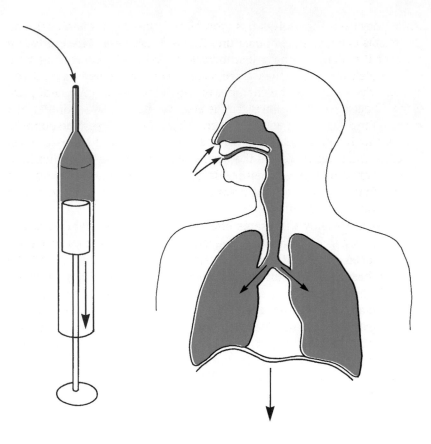

Figure 3-1. Comparison of the action of the diaphragm with that of a plunger on a syringe. As the diaphragm pulls down, air enters the lungs, just as it enters the chamber of the syringe when the plunger is pulled down.

or nose as the tip, you will realize that pulling on the plunger (your diaphragm) causes air to enter the chamber (your lungs). If you were to hold your finger over the opening as you pulled back the plunger, you would feel the suction of the device on your finger. This suction is the product of *lowering the relative air pressure within the chamber*, producing an imbalance in relation to atmospheric pressure. Let us examine the physical principles involved a little more deeply.

Before we can talk about the forces driving respiration, you need an intuitive feel for what air pressure really is. **Air pressure** is the force exerted on walls of a chamber by molecules of air. Because of the molecular charge, air molecules tend to keep their distance from other air molecules. If the chamber is opened to the atmosphere, the pressure exerted on the inner walls of the chamber will be the same as that exerted on the outer walls.

The action starts when you close off the chamber and change the volume. Making the chamber smaller does not change the forces that keep molecules apart, but rather lets those forces be manifest on the walls of the chamber. Although the forces have not changed, the area on

air pressure: *the force exerted on a surface by air molecules*

which they exert themselves has (you made it smaller, remember?), and that results in an increase in pressure. That is, **Pressure** is *Force* exerted on *Area*, or **P = F/A**. You have just increased pressure by decreasing area.

Boyle's law states that, given a gas of constant temperature, if you increase the volume of the chamber in which the gas is contained, pressure will decrease. If you increase the size (volume) of the chamber of a syringe, the air pressure within that chamber will decrease. The opposite also is true: If you decrease the volume of the chamber, the pressure will increase. Once again we see that forces seek stability and equilibrium. When volume increases, pressure decreases, and natural law says that air will flow to equalize that pressure. Thus, air flows into the chamber—in our case, the lungs.

Figure 3-2 shows the same effect graphically. The chamber has 11 molecules in it in both cases. On the left, the volume of the chamber has been reduced, so the 11 molecules are much closer together and the pressure has increased (known as **positive pressure**). Likewise, when you pull the plunger back so the molecules are farther apart than the forces dictate, the pressure decreases, and the pressure is now referred to as **negative pressure**. The beauty of this arrangement is that it provides all the principle we need to discuss respiratory physiology at the macro- or microscopic level. The forces that draw air into the lungs also are responsible for drawing carbon dioxide out.

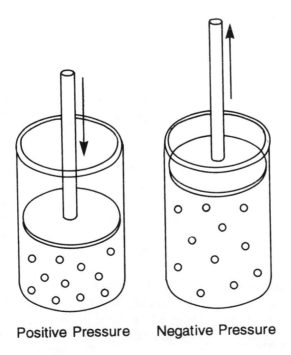

Positive Pressure   **Negative Pressure**

Figure 3-2. The piston on the left has been depressed, compressing the air in the chamber and increasing the air pressure. On the right, the piston has been retracted, increasing the space between the molecules and creating a relatively negative pressure.

In summary:

- **Pressure** is defined as force distributed over area.
- **Boyle's law** tells us that as the volume of a container increases, the air pressure within the container will decrease.
- This relatively **negative pressure** will cause air to enter the container until the pressure is equalized.
- If volume is decreased, pressure increases and air flows out until the pressures inside and outside are equal.
- This principle forms the basis for movement of air into and out of the lungs.

 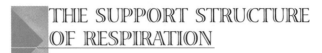

THE SUPPORT STRUCTURE OF RESPIRATION

Overview

The respiratory system consists of a gas-exchanging mechanism supported and protected by a bony cage (see Table 3-1). Gas exchange is carried out by the lungs, while the rib cage performs a protective function.

Table 3–1. Structures of respiration.

Bony Thorax
    Vertebrae and vertebral column
    Ribs and their attachment to vertebral column
    Pectoral girdle
      scapula and clavicle
    Sternum
    Pelvic girdle
      ischium
      pubic bone
      sacrum
      ilium

Visceral Thorax
    Respiratory passageway
      mouth and nose
      trachea and bronchi
    Lungs
    Mediastinum

Muscles of Respiration
    Diaphragm
    Accessory muscles of inspiration
    Accessory muscles of expiration
    Muscles of postural control

Let us take a guided tour of the respiratory system. To begin, pay attention to your own breathing. Try the following. Sit up straight and close your eyes while taking 10 quiet breaths through your nose. First, concentrate attention on your nose, feeling the air entering and leaving your nostrils. Then feel your abdominal region stretch out a little with each inspiration, and then become aware that your thorax (rib cage) is expanding a little with each inhalation. Now take a good, deep breath (still through your nose) and feel your whole chest rise and your shoulders straighten out a little.

Besides relaxing you, attending to your breathing has given you a sense of the parts of your body that are activated for inspiration and expiration. At first you attended to your nostrils, the part of the respiratory passageway that warms and moistens air going into the lungs. Then you noticed your abdomen protruding, which is a natural process associated with inspiration, because the diaphragm is pushing against the abdomen when it contracts to bring air in. Then you noticed that your thorax was expanding a little as you breathed in quietly, and then you noted that your thorax expanded markedly as you breathed in deeply. If you missed any of these things happening, take a minute and breathe a little more. This will set the stage for understanding what is going on with the bones and muscles of respiration.

Developing an understanding of respiratory function requires knowledge of the skeletal system. The lungs are housed within the thorax, an area bounded in the superior aspect by the **first rib** and **clavicle**, and in the inferior by the twelfth rib (see Figure 3-3). The lateral

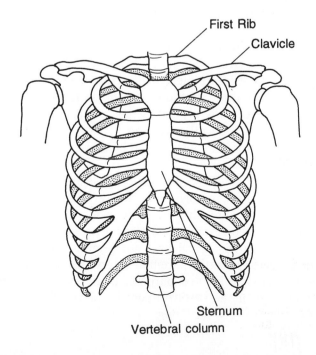

Figure 3-3. Anterior view of the thorax.

Palpation

Palpation, or the process of examining structures with the hands, can be a very useful tool to understanding anatomy. When you perform an oral peripheral examination as a clinician you will need to be comfortable with the process of palpating, because it is one means of gathering information about your client's physical condition that may help you in your diagnosis and remediation of speech problems. For instance, palpation of the temporo-mandibular joint (the joint forming the articulation of the mandible and the temporal bone) while your client moves his or her jaw will provide you with insight into the integrity of the joint, as well as the degree of muscular control your client is able to exert.

Throughout these chapters we will provide you with palpation activities that you can perform on yourself. Identifying these landmarks will help you understand the structures with which we deal in speech-language pathology.

sternum: *L., sternum, breastplate*

vertebral column: *the bony structure made of vertebrae*

spinal cord: *the nerve tracts and cell bodies within the spinal column*

and anterior aspects are composed of the **ribs** and **sternum**. The entire thorax is suspended from the **vertebral column** (spinal column), a structure that doubles as the conduit for the **spinal cord**, the nervous system supply for the body and extremities.

Vertebral Column

The functional unit of the vertebral column is the **vertebra** (plural, vertebrae) or vertebral column segment. The vertebral column has five divisions: cervical, thoracic, lumbar, sacral, and coccygeal (see Figure 3-4). The anatomical shorthand associated with the vertebral column and spinal nerves is as follows. The vertebrae are numbered sequentially from superior to inferior by section, so that the uppermost **cervical vertebra** is C1, the second is C2, and so forth to C7. Likewise, the first **thoracic vertebra** is T1, and the last is T12. **Lumbar vertebrae** include L1 through L5, **sacral vertebrae** include S1 through S5, and the **coccygeal vertebrae** are considered to be a fused unit, known as the **coccyx**.

The vertebral column is composed of 33 segments of bone with a rich set of fossa and protuberances clearly designed for function. Although vertebrae have roughly the same shape, their form and landmarks vary depending on location and area they serve, their attachments (such as ribs), and their neural payload. The area serving the head requires more security for the vertebral artery, so there are protected **foramina** (or openings) for that purpose. In lower regions, there is a great deal more bone in the **corpus** or body of the vertebra, reflecting the power of the muscles used for lifting.

foramina, foramen: *L., opening*

corpus: *L., body*

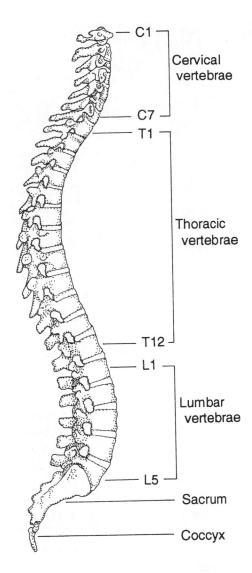

Figure 3-4. A. Components of the vertebral column. *(continues)*

Cervical Vertebrae

Major landmarks of the vertebrae include a prominent **spinous process** (the collection of which can be felt by rubbing the spine of your friend's back) and **transverse processes** on both sides (see Figure 3-5). The corpus of the vertebra makes up the anterior portion, with a prominent hole or **vertebral foramen** just posterior to that. It is through this foramen that the tracts of the spinal cord pass. The spinal nerves must somehow exit and enter the spinal cord; the **intervertebral foramina** on either side of the vertebra permits this. Vertebral segments ride one atop another to form the vertebral column. This articulation is completed by means of the

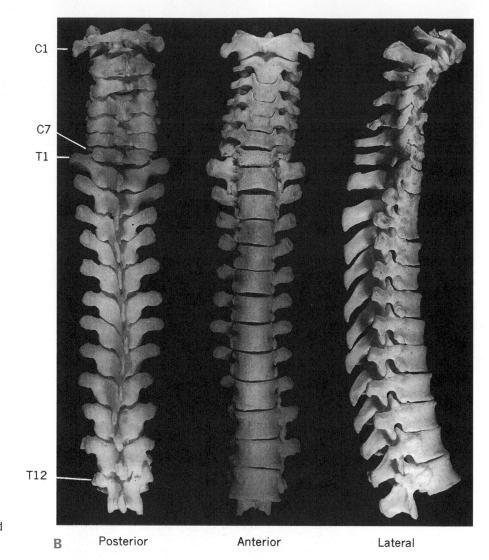

C1

C7

T1

T12

Figure 3-4. *(continued)*
B. Articulated cervical and thoracic vertebrae.

B   Posterior   Anterior   Lateral

superior and **inferior articular facets**. These facets provide the mating surfaces for two adjacent vertebrae, limiting movement in the anterior-posterior dimension, thus protecting the spinal cord and allowing limited rotatory and rocking motion. We must be able to move freely, but not *too* freely, considering the importance of the spinal cord within that column.

The uppermost cervical vertebra, C1, is the **atlas**, so named for its singular role in supporting the skull for rotation (after the mythical figure supporting the earth). Articulating with the inferior surface of the atlas is C2, the **axis**, on which the skull pivots (see Figure 3-6). C1 and C2 differ markedly from C3 through C7. The posterior of C1 has a reduced prominence, here called the **posterior** tubercle. The **superior articular** facet is larger than those of C3 through C7, providing increased

tubercle: *L., tuberculum, little swelling*

facet: *Fr., facette, small face*

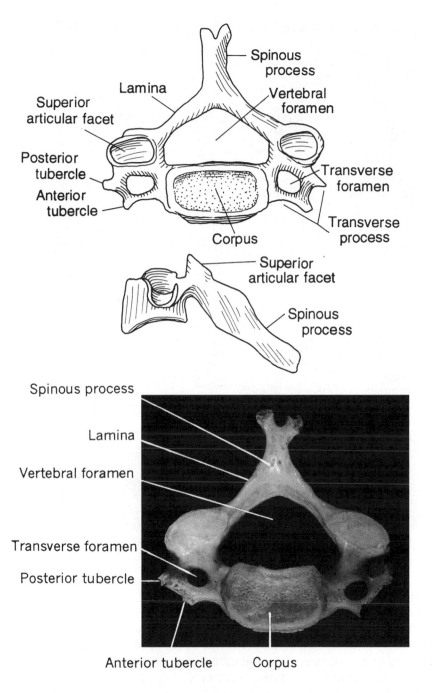

Figure 3-5. Superior and lateral views of cervical vertebra.

surface area for vertebra-skull articulation. Similarly, the vertebral foramen is larger than those in the lower cervical vertebrae, reflecting the transition from spinal cord to brainstem that begins at that level. The **dens process** of the axis (also known as the **odontoid process**) protrudes through it. This loose lock-and-key arrangement is protective,

dens: *L., tooth*

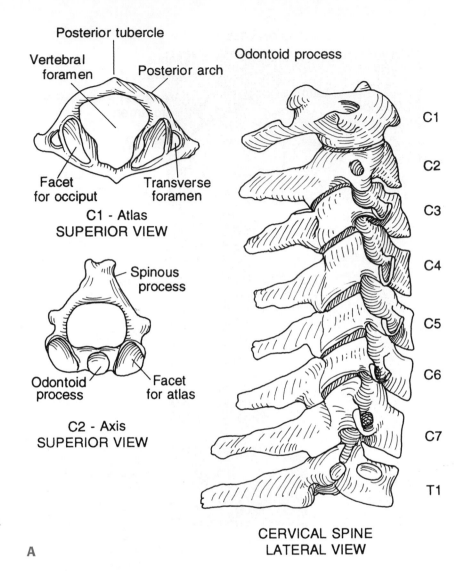

Posterior tubercle

Vertebral foramen

Posterior arch

Odontoid process

Facet for occiput

Transverse foramen

**C1 - Atlas
SUPERIOR VIEW**

Spinous process

Odontoid process

Facet for atlas

**C2 - Axis
SUPERIOR VIEW**

C1
C2
C3
C4
C5
C6
C7
T1

**CERVICAL SPINE
LATERAL VIEW**

Figure 3-6. A. Cervical vertebrae. On the left are atlas (C1, upper) and axis (C2, lower). On the right are the articulated cervical vertebrae. *(continues)*

A

because unchecked movement could result in damage to the spinal cord at this level, which would be life-threatening. You might notice that the axis (C2) has a rudimentary spinous process, although the atlas does not. The articulation of C1 and C2 is shown in Figure 3-6.

As you can see in Figure 3-5, a typical cervical vertebra has a number of landmarks. The corpus and spinous process provide a clue to orientation, because the corpus is in the anterior aspect and the posterior spinous process will slant downward.

Examination of Figure 3-5 also reveals lateral wings known as the **transverse processes**, which are directed in a posterolateral (*postero* =

Spinous process

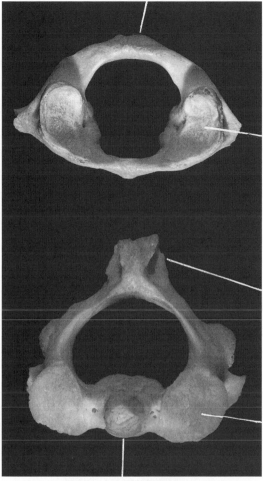

C1-Atlas
SUPERIOR VIEW

Facet for occiput

C2-Axis
SUPERIOR VIEW

Spinous process

Facet for atlas

Odontoid process

B

Figure 3-6. *(continued)* **B.** Superior view of atlas and axis.

back; *lateral* = side) direction. The superior surface is marked by a **superior articular facet**, which rests atop the **pedicle**. The inferior surface retains an **inferior articular facet**. In the articulated vertebral column, these facets mate. The paired transverse foramina shown in Figure 3-5 are found only in the cervical vertebrae and may even be absent in C7. Figure 3-7 shows that the vertebral artery passes through this foramen. You can palpate the seventh cervical vertebra by bending your head forward so that your chin touches your chest. The first prominent spinous process you feel on your neck is C7. You can also palpate the large transverse processes of the atlas, inferior to the mastoid process of the temporal bone.

pedicle: *L., pedalis, foot*

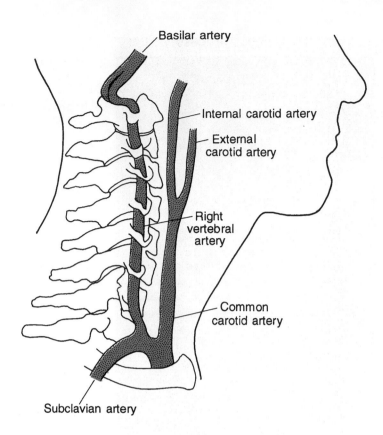

Figure 3-7. Course of vertebral artery through the transverse foramina of cervical vertebrae.

Thoracic Vertebrae

The 12 thoracic vertebrae (T1 to T12) provide the basis for the respiratory framework, because they form the posterior point of attachment for the ribs of the bony thorax. As seen in Figure 3-8, the thoracic vertebrae have larger spinous and transverse processes. Between vertebrae is the

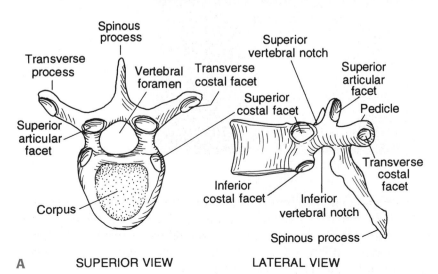

Figure 3-8 A. Superior and lateral views of thoracic vertebrae. *(continues)*

A   SUPERIOR VIEW   LATERAL VIEW

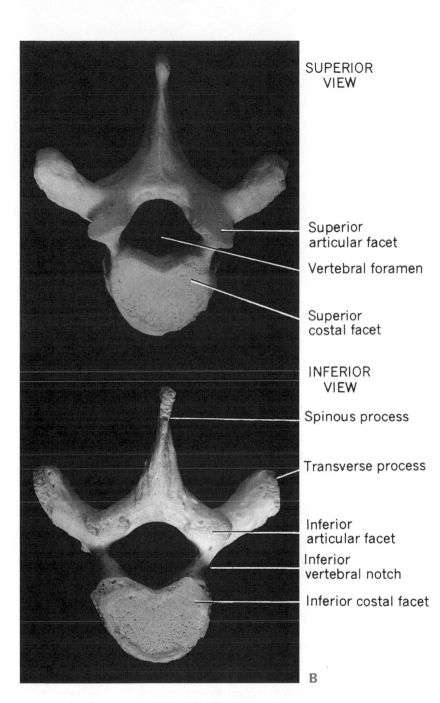

SUPERIOR
VIEW

Superior
articular facet

Vertebral foramen

Superior
costal facet

INFERIOR
VIEW

Spinous process

Transverse process

Inferior
articular facet

Inferior
vertebral notch

Inferior costal facet

B

Figure 3-8. *(continued)* **B.** Superior (upper) and inferior (lower) view of thoracic vertebra.

intervertebral foramen, the product of the inferior and superior **vertebral notches** of articulating vertebrae, through which spinal nerves communicate with the spinal cord in life. You should pay particular attention to the superior and inferior costal facets, because these are the points of attachment for the ribs, as seen in Figure 3-9.

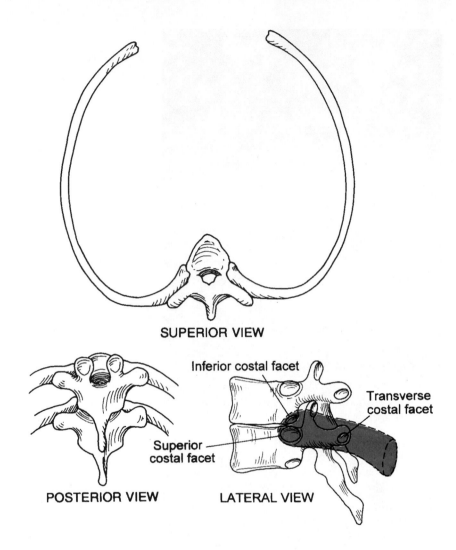

SUPERIOR VIEW

Inferior costal facet

Transverse costal facet

Superior costal facet

POSTERIOR VIEW · LATERAL VIEW

Figure 3-9. Articulation of rib and vertebrae.

The articulation of rib and thoracic vertebrae is complicated. Although it would have been simpler for us had the second rib been attached to the second vertebra, had the third rib been attached to the third vertebra, and so forth, only the first rib and the last three ribs (1, 10, 11, 12) have this nice one-to-one arrangement. Each of the remaining ribs (2 through 9) attaches to the transverse process and corpus of the same-numbered vertebra and also attaches to the body of the rib above it (e.g., rib 2 attaches to transverse process of T2 and body of T1 and T2). The utility of this articulation will become apparent as we discuss movement of the rib cage for respiration.

Lumbar Vertebrae

The five lumbar vertebrae are quite large in comparison to those of the thoracic or cervical region, reflecting the stresses placed on them during

Spinal Cord Injury

The spinal cord is well protected by the osseous vertebral column, in that the vertebrae fit together in a partial lock-and-key fashion to inhibit motion. The vertebral column is richly bound together by ligaments and surrounded by muscles of the back.

Despite this degree of redundant protection, the spinal cord is frequently traumatized. The most frequent cause of spinal cord injury is vehicle accidents, especially those in which the occupant is not properly restrained. When a person is ejected from a vehicle, the vertebral column can undergo rotatory stresses that can tear the spinal cord, and impact can compress the vertebral column, resulting in distention of the spinal cord. (Typically the compression occurs in the corpus, implying hyperflexion of the neck.) Significant transverse forces can cause a shearing of the spinal cord as well.

The result of spinal cord injury is frequently loss of motor and sensory function to the area below the spinal cord injury, with subsequent paraplegia (legs paralyzed) or quadriplegia (both arms and legs paralyzed). For an exhaustive review of spinal cord injury, see Mackay, Chapman, and Morgan (1997).

---

lifting and **ambulation** (walking). They provide direct or indirect attachment for a host of back and abdominal muscles, as well as for the posterior fibers of the diaphragm. The transverse and spinous processes are relatively smaller, and the corpus is much larger than in the thoracic and cervical vertebrae.

Sacrum and Coccyx

The five sacral vertebrae are actually a fused mass known as the **sacrum**. The sacrum and its ossified intervertebral discs retain vestiges of the vertebrae from which they are formed, with remnants of spinous and transverse processes. The sacral foramina perform the function of the intervertebral foramina, providing a passage for the sacral nerves (see Figure 3-10).

sacrum: *L., sacralis, sacred*

The **coccyx** is composed of the fused coccygeal vertebrae. It is so named because of its beaklike appearance, and it articulates with the inferior sacrum by means of a small disc.

coccyx: *Gr., kokkus, cuckoo (shaped like a cuckoo's beak)*

To summarize:
* The **vertebral column** is composed of vertebral segments that combine to form a strong but flexible column.
* **Vertebrae** are identified based on their level: C1 to C7 (**cervical**), T1 to T12 (**thoracic**), L1 to L5 (**lumbar**), S1 to S5 (**sacral**).
* The fused **coccygeal** vertebrae are referred to as the *coccyx*.
* This spinal column provides the points of attachment for numerous muscles by means of the **spinous** and **transverse processes**.

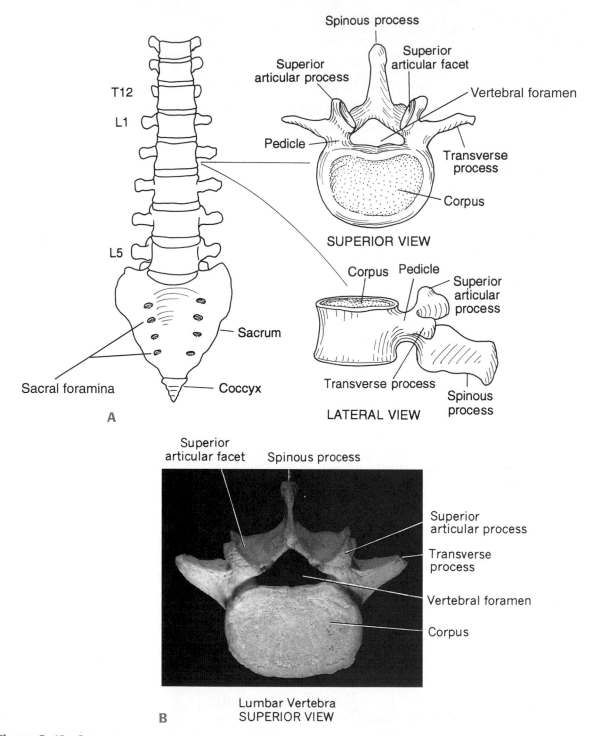

Figure 3-10. A. Lumbar vertebrae articulated with sacrum and coccyx (left). Upper right shows superior view of lumbar vertebra, and lower right shows lateral view. **B.** Superior view of lumbar vertebra.

- It also houses the **spinal cord**, with **spinal nerves** emerging and entering the spinal cord through spaces between the vertebrae.

- The ribs of the rib cage articulate with the spinal column in a fashion that permits the rib cage some limited movement for respiration.

Pelvic and Pectoral Girdles

The vertebral column is central to the body, and if we are to interact physically with our environment we must attach appendages to this column. The lower extremities are attached to this axis by means of the **pelvic girdle**, and the upper extremities are attached through the **pectoral girdle**.

The pelvic girdle is comprised of the ilium, sacrum, pubic bone, and ischium (see Figure 3-11). The combination provides an extremely strong structure capable of bearing a great deal of translated weight from use of the legs.

The pectoral girdle is the superior counterpart to the pelvic girdle. This structure permits attachment of the upper extremities to the vertebral column.

Pelvic Girdle

The pelvic girdle provides a strong structure for attaching the legs to the vertebral column (see Figure 3-11). By means of this structure, forces generated through movement of the legs are distributed across a mass of bone which, in turn, is attached to the vertebral column.

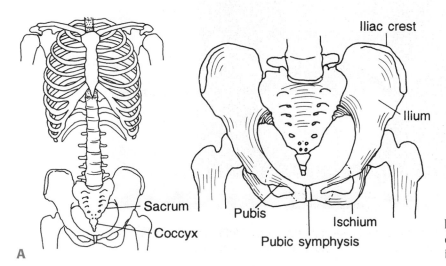

Figure 3-11. A. Pelvic girdle, consisting of the ilium, pubis, and ischium. *(continues)*

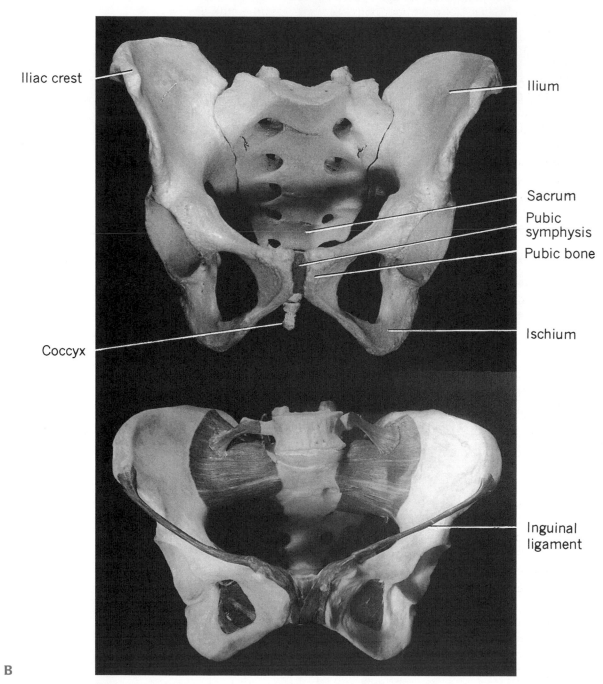

Iliac crest

Ilium

Sacrum

Pubic symphysis

Pubic bone

Ischium

Coccyx

Inguinal ligament

B

Figure 3-11. *(continued)* **B.** Anterior view of pelvis. Lower view shows location of the inguinal ligament.

The pelvic girdle is made up of the ilium, sacrum, pubic bone, and ischium. The **ilium** is a large, winglike bone (similar in this way to the **scapula** or shoulder blade of the upper body) that provides the bulk of the support for the abdominal musculature and the prominent hip bone on which many parents carry their children. The iliac crest of the superior-lateral surface is an important landmark as the superior point of attachment for the inguinal ligament, which runs from the crest of the iliac to the joining of the two pubic bones at the **pubic** symphysis. Deep to this bone is the massive medial structure, the sacrum. As may be seen in Figure 3-11, the sacrum articulates with the fifth lumbar vertebra. The iliac bones articulate with the sacrum laterally, forming the sacroiliac joints. (The structure comprised of the iliac, ischium, and pubis bones is referred to as the *innominate* or *hip bone*: "innominate" means, literally, "unnamed.") The coccyx is the inferior-most segment of the spinal column, consisting of four fused vertebrae articulating at the inferior aspect of the sacrum.

symphysis: *Gr., growing together*

Pectoral Girdle

The **pectoral** or **shoulder girdle** includes the **scapula** and **clavicle**, bones that support the upper extremities. The clavicle, also known as the collarbone, is attached to the superior sternum, running laterally to join with the winglike scapula. The clavicle provides the anterior support for the shoulder (see Figure 3-12). The scapula has its only skeletal attachment via the clavicle, which in turn has its only skeletal attachment at the sternum. From the scapula are slung several muscles that hold it in a dynamic tension that facilitates flexible upper body movement while not compromising strength in the balance. The down side of this "smoke and mirrors" arrangement is the vulnerability of the junction of the scapula and clavicle. Disarticulation of these two bones will cause a collapse of the structure so that the shoulder rotates forward and in.

pectoral, pectoralis: *L., pertaining to the chest*

clavicle: *L., clavicula, little key*

The physical arrangement of the pectoral girdle provides an "A-frame" of support to distribute force through relatively solid articulation at the scapula and muscular attachment in the form of the massive muscles of the thorax and back.

When taken together, one can view the human skeleton as a tube with two A-frames attached at the ends. The tube provides flexible yet strong support for the trunk, even as the A-frames give that trunk the opportunity to explore its environment by means of the arms and legs. The A-frame design provides maximum strength for these extremities with a minimum of bone mass.

To summarize:

- The bony support structure of the respiratory system is composed of the **rib cage** and **vertebral column**.

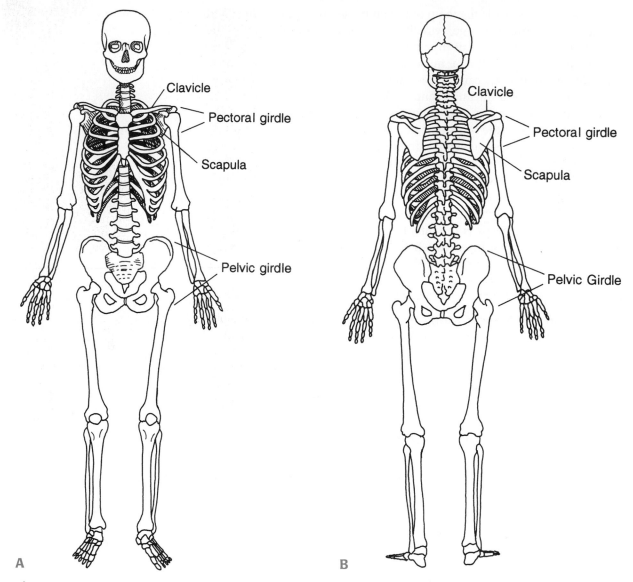

Figure 3-12. A. Anterior view of skeleton, showing components of pelvic and pectoral girdles. **B.** Posterior view.
(continues)

- At the base of the vertebral column is the **pelvic girdle**, composed of the **ilium**, **sacrum**, **pubic bone**, and **ischium**.
- The **pectoral girdle** is comprised of the **scapula** and **clavicle**, which attach to the **sternum**.
- These structures provide the points of attachment for the lower and upper extremities.

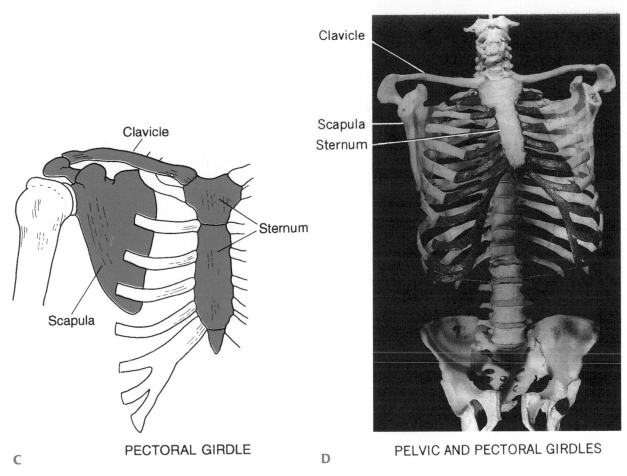

Clavicle

Sternum

Scapula

PECTORAL GIRDLE

C

Clavicle

Scapula

Sternum

PELVIC AND PECTORAL GIRDLES

D

Figure 3-12. *(continued)* **C.** Isolated pectoral girdle. **D.** Photograph of articulated thorax with pelvic and pectoral girdles.

Ribs and Rib Cage

Ribs are capable of a degree of movement, so that the rib cage can rock up in front and flare out via lateral rotation, hinged on the vertebral articulation with the rib cage. The rib cage is made up of 12 ribs, with all but the lowest two attached by means of cartilage to the sternum in the front aspect. Figure 3-13 shows that the sternum provides a focal point for the rib cage, and the sternum turns out to be a significant structure in respiration.

Another thing you might notice in Figure 3-13 is that the rib cage tends to slant down in front. With the mobility of the rib cage granted by the articulation of the vertebrae and ribs, the rib cage is quite capable of elevating during inspiration to increase the size of the thorax.

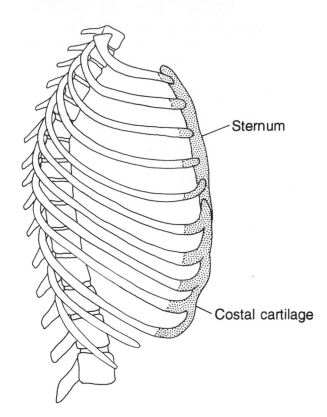

Figure 3-13. Lateral view of rib cage showing relationship among ribs and sternum. Note that the rib cage slants down in the front.

Ribs

There are 12 pairs of **ribs** in the human **thorax**, with each rib consisting generally of four components; the **head**, **neck**, **shaft**, and **angle** (see Figure 3-14). The head provides the articulating surfaces with the spinal column, and the angle represents the point at which the rib begins the significant curve in its course forward. The barrel shape of the thorax is

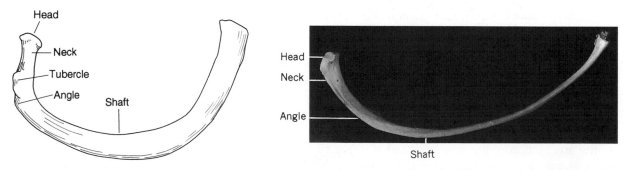

Figure 3-14. Schematic of second rib with landmarks.

created by the relatively small superior and inferior ribs as compared with the longer middle ribs. The rib cage provides attachment for numerous muscles that provide strength, rigidity, continuity, and mobility to the rib cage.

Ribs are of three general classes: **true ribs**, **false ribs**, and **floating ribs**. The true (or vertebrosternal) ribs consist of the upper ribs (1 through 7), all of which form more or less direct attachment with the sternum. Their actual attachment is by means of a cartilaginous union through the chondral (i.e., cartilaginous) portion of the rib (see Figure 3-15). The false, or vertebrochondral, ribs (ribs 8, 9, and 10) also are attached to the sternum through cartilage, although this chondral portion must run superiorly to attach to the sternum. The floating or vertebral ribs (ribs 11 and 12) articulate only with the vertebral column.

The elastic properties of cartilage permit the ribs to be twisted on the long axis (torqued) without breaking. Thus, the rib cage is quite strong (being made up predominantly of bone), but capable of movement (being well-endowed with resilient cartilage).

The rib cage also gives significant protection to the heart and lungs. The rib cage also provides the basis for respiration, and the general structure of the "barrel" deserves some attention at this juncture.

chondral: *Gr., chondros, cartilaginous*

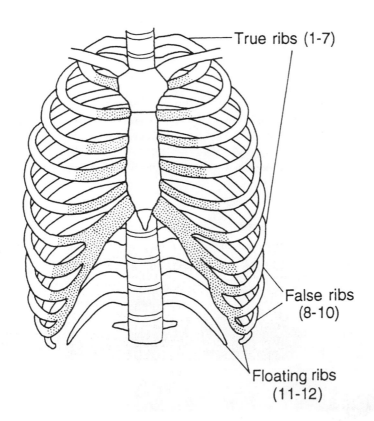

Figure 3-15. Schematic of relationships among true, false, and floating ribs.

As you can see in Figure 3-16, the ribs make their posterior attachment along the vertebral column. If a fly were to walk along the superior surface of a rib, starting from the tip of the head and walking to the point of attachment at the sternum, it would start out by walking in a postero-lateral direction, but would quickly round a curve that would aim it toward the front. Its hike would be along a great, sweeping arc ending when it reached the cartilaginous portion of the sternal attachment. In short, the rib's course—running postero-lateral and then arching around to the anterior aspect of the body—provides the bony structure for most of the posterior, lateral, and anterior aspects of the thorax. In addition, the fly would have hiked downhill, because the ribs slope downward when the rib cage is inactive and at equilibrium. The beauty of the rib cage, the vertebral attachments, and the chondral (cartilaginous) portion of the sternal attachment is that the rib cage can elevate, providing an increase in lung capacity for respiration.

The posterior attachment of the rib is made through a gliding (arthrodial) articulation with the thoracic vertebrae, thus permitting the rib to rock up in both lateral and anterior aspects during inspiration. As mentioned, most of the ribs actually attach to two vertebrae.

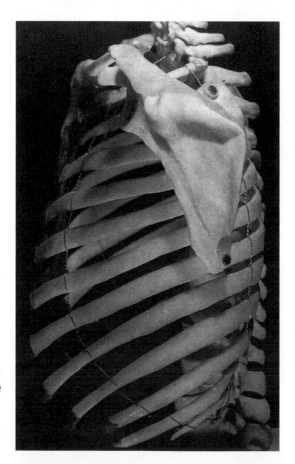

Figure 3-16. Lateral view of the rib cage. The downward tilt of the rib cage in front provides one of the mechanisms for increasing the volume of the thorax during respiration.

Sternum

The sternum has three components: the **manubrium sterni**, the **corpus** (body), and the **xiphoid** or **ensiform process** (see Figure 3-17). The sternum has articular cavities for costal attachment, with the manubrium sterni providing the attachment for the **clavicle** and first rib, and the second rib articulating at the juncture of the manubrium and corpus, known as the **manubrosternal angle**. The corpus provides articulation for five more ribs by means of relatively direct costal cartilage, and the remaining (false) ribs 8, 9, and 10 are attached by means of more indirect costal cartilage.

The sternum provides an excellent opportunity to investigate anatomy with your own hands. As you look at Figure 3-17 of the sternum, you can palpate your own sternal structures. First, find your "Adam's apple" (actually, the thyroid cartilage of the larynx), then bring your finger downward until you reach the significant plateau at about

> **manubrium sterni:** *L., handle of sternum*

> **xiphoid:** *Gr., sword*

> **ensiform:** *L., swordlike*

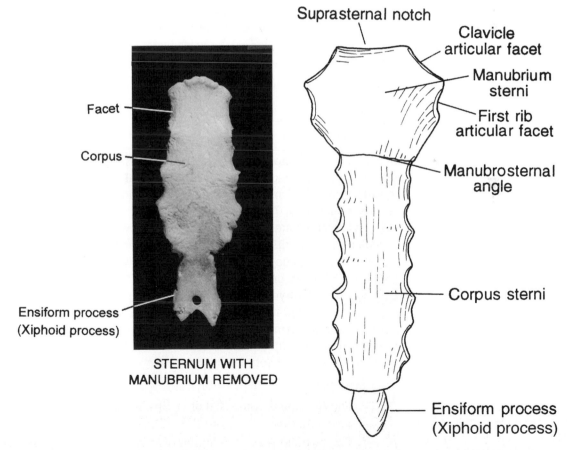

Facet

Corpus

Ensiform process
(Xiphoid process)

**STERNUM WITH
MANUBRIUM REMOVED**

Suprasternal notch

Clavicle
articular facet

Manubrium
sterni

First rib
articular facet

Manubrosternal
angle

Corpus sterni

Ensiform process
(Xiphoid process)

Figure 3-17. Schematic and photo of sternum. Note that the manubrium has been removed from the sternum on the left.

Congenital Thorax Deformities

A number of congenital (present at birth) problems may occur within the thoracic wall. *Pectus excavatum* is a condition in which the sternum and costal cartilages are depressed relative to the rib cage. This depression may be bilateral or asymmetrical, providing the individual with costal flaring, a broad-but-thin chest and hook-shoulder deformity. The deformity can be repaired surgically, but may reoccur, especially during the period of rapid growth in puberty. The opposite deformity, *pectus carinatum*, involves protrusion of the sternum anteriorly. Surgical repair is typically successful.

Poland's syndrome is a congenital condition in which the pectoralis major and minor muscles are both absent, and the child has fusion of the fingers or toes (syndactyly). The muscles may be partially or completely absent, and the breast is typically involved. In significantly affected individuals, the anterior portions of ribs 2 through 5 and their cartilaginous portions may be absent as well. Although the muscle cannot be restored, surgery can correct the defect of the rib cage to establish thoracic symmetry.

Cleft sternum is a rare congenital deformity that can have devastating consequences. In the simple and more benign case, the sternum has a simple cleft as a result of failure of the sternal bars during gestation. The cleft is covered with skin, and the heart and diaphragm are normal. *Ectopia cordis* is a life-threatening form of cleft sternum, in which the infant is born with the heart exposed extrathoracically. Repair of this condition is extremely difficult.

You may wish to examine the thorough discussion of these disorders in Schamberger (2000).

the level of your shoulders. This is the superior surface of the manubrium sterni, and is known as the **suprasternal** or **sternal notch**. Ignoring the tendon which you can feel on either side, palpate the bone that is directed laterally. This is the clavicle. If you can feel the place where the clavicle articulates with the manubrium, you can probably find the articulation of the first rib immediately inferior to it. If you once again find the sternal notch and draw your finger downward about two inches you may feel a very prominent bump, which is the manubrosternal angle or junction. Now if you draw your finger downward another four or five inches, you can find the point at which the sternum and xiphoid process articulate, an important landmark for individuals performing cardiopulmonary resuscitation (CPR). You have also found the anterior-most attachment of your diaphragm.

In summary:

- The **rib cage** is composed of 12 ribs (7 true ribs, 3 false ribs, and 2 floating ribs).
- The **cartilaginous attachment** of the ribs to the sternum permits the ribs to rotate slightly during respiration, allowing the rib cage to elevate.

- The construction of the rib provides the characteristic curved barrel shape of the rib cage.
- At rest the ribs slope downward, but they **elevate** during inspiration.

Soft Tissue of the Thorax and Respiratory Passageway

Deep to the rib cage lies the core of respiration. Gas exchange for life occurs within the lungs—spongy, elastic tissue that is richly perfused with vascular supply and air sacs. Healthy, young lungs are pink, whereas older lungs that have undergone the stresses of modern, polluted life are distinctly gray. Communication from the lungs with the external environment is by means of the respiratory passageway, which includes the oral and nasal cavities, larynx, trachea, and bronchial tubes.

The trachea is a flexible tube, approximately 11 cm in length and composed of a series of 16 to 20 hyaline cartilage rings that are open in the posterior aspect. This tube runs from the inferior border of the larynx for about 11 cm, where it bifurcates (divides) at a point known as the carina **trachea** to become the left and right **mainstem** bronchi (or **bronchial tubes**), which serve the left and right lungs respectively (see Figure 3-18).

The tracheal rings are 2 to 2.5 cm in diameter, and .4 to .5 cm wide. They are connected by a continuous mucous membrane lining, which provides both continuity and flexibility. The ring is discontinuous in the posterior aspect, allowing for expansion and contraction of the diameter of the ring, an action largely controlled by the trachealis muscle. The gap between the rings is spanned by smooth muscle that is in a steady state of contraction until oxygen needs of the individual increase, at which time the muscle relaxes. That is, the tube is in a state of slight constriction until oxygen needs are sufficiently great that the muscle action is inhibited, at which time the diameter of the trachea increases to improve air delivery to the lungs. The inner mucosal lining of the trachea is infused with submucosal glands that assist in cleaning the trachea.

The cartilaginous rings of the trachea are particularly well suited for the task of air transport. Because the process involves drawing air into the lungs and expelling it, pressures (negative and positive) must be generated to get that gas moving, but pressure tends to collapse or expand tissue that is not reinforced for strength. However, a strictly rigid tube would not permit the degree of flexibility dictated by an active life (i.e., differential head and thorax movement). Thus, the trachea must be both rigid and flexible. In response to this need, the trachea is built of hyaline cartilage rings connected by fibroelastic membrane. The cartilage provides support, while the membrane permits freedom of movement.

Posterior to the trachea is the **esophagus**. The esophagus is a long, collapsed tube running behind and adjacent to the trachea and providing

trachea: *Gr., tracheia, rough*

carina: *L., keel of boat*

bronchi: *Gr., bronchos, windpipe*

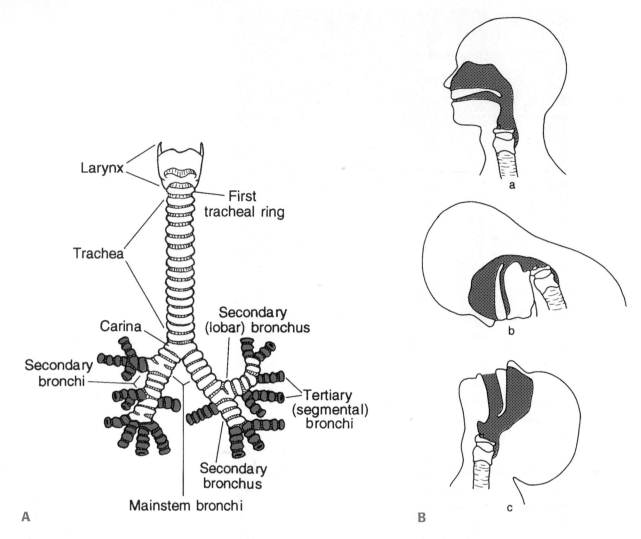

Figure 3-18. A. Bronchial passageway, including trachea, mainstem bronchi, secondary (lobar) bronchi, and tertiary (segmental) bronchi. **B.** Effect of head posture on airway patency (modified from data and view of Moser and Spragg, 1982). *(continues)*

bolus: *L., lump*

the conduit to the digestive system. It retains its collapsed condition except when occupied with a bolus of food being propelled by gravity and peristaltic contractions to the waiting stomach.

The trachea bifurcates to form right and left **mainstem** (or main) bronchi. The right side forms a 20–30° angle relative to the trachea, and the left forms a 45–55° angle. (This explains why the right lung is most often the landing site for the errant peanut that makes it past the protective laryngeal structure!)

The lungs are a composite of blood, arterial and venous network, connective tissue, respiratory pathway, and tissue specialized for gas exchange.

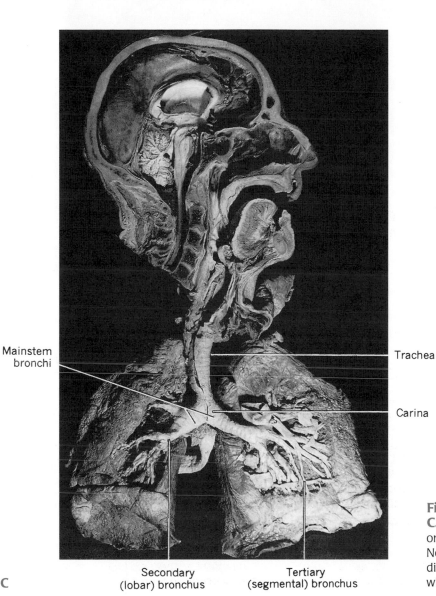

Mainstem
bronchi

Trachea

Carina

Secondary
(lobar) bronchus

Tertiary
(segmental) bronchus

C

Figure 3-18. *(continued)*
C. Respiratory passageway from
oral cavity to segmental bronchi.
Note that lungs have been
dissected to reveal the bronchi
within.

The **bronchial tree** is characterized by increasingly smaller tubes
as one progresses into the depths of the lungs, but the total surface area
at any given level of the tree is greater than the level before it. There are
14 generations of the bronchial tree in the left lung, and 28 generations
in the right lung, beginning with the single trachea. The mainstem
bronchi bifurcate off of the trachea to serve the left and right lungs, while
lobar (intermediate) bronchi supply the lobes of the lungs. Further
branchings occur, down to the final **terminal respiratory bronchioles**.
This division process is shown in Table 3-2 and Figure 3-19. Within the
cartilaginous passageway, there are 1 trachea, 5 lobar bronchi, 19 segmental bronchi, and so forth.

Table 3-2. Divisions of the bronchial tree.

| | GENERATION FROM | | | | | |
	TRACHEA	SEGMENTAL BRONCHUS	TERMINAL BRONCHIOLE	NUMBER	DIAMETER	CROSS-SECTION
Trachea	0			1	2.5 cm	5.0 cm^2
Main bronchi	1			2	11–19 mm	3.2 cm^2
Lobar bronchi	2–3			5	4.5–13.5	2.7 cm^2
Segmental	3–6	0		19	4.5–6.5 mm	3.2 cm^2
Subsegmental bronchi	4–7	1		38	3–6 mm	6.6 cm^2
Bronchi		2–6		variable	variable	variable
Terminal bronchi		3–7		1000	1.0 mm	7.9 cm^2
Bronchioles		5–14		variable	variable	variable
Terminal bronchioles		6–15	0	35,000	0.65 mm	116 cm^2
Respiratory bronchioles			1–8	variable	variable	variable
Terminal respiratory bronchioles			2–9	630,000	0.45 mm	1,000 cm^2
Alveolar ducts and sacs			4–12	14×10^6	0.40 mm	1.71 m^2
Alveoli				300×10^6	0.24–.3 mm	70 m^2

Source: From *Respiratory Emergencies* by K. M. Moser & R. G. Spragg, 1982, p. 15. St. Louis, MO: C. V. Mosby. Copyright 1982 C. V. Mosby Co. Reprinted with permission.

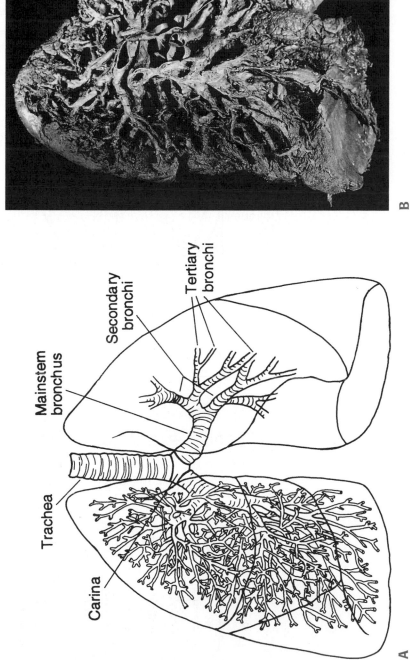

Figure 3-19. A. Bronchial tree (modified from data and view of Des Jardins and Burton, 2001). **B.** Lung dissected to reveal bronchial passageway.

65

The lobar or secondary divisions serve the lobes of the lungs. The right lung is composed of three lobes, separated by fissures. The left lung has only two lobes (see Figure 3-19). Space on the left is taken up by the heart and **mediastinal** or "middle space" structures. The right mainstem bronchus divides to supply the superior, middle, and inferior lobes of the right lung. The left mainstem bronchus bifurcates to serve the superior and inferior lobes of the left lung, although there is a vestigial middle lobe (called the *lingula*). The space of the missing lobe is taken up by the heart on the left side (see Figure 3-20).

mediastinum: *L., medius, middle*

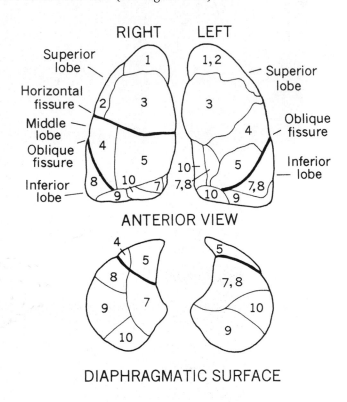

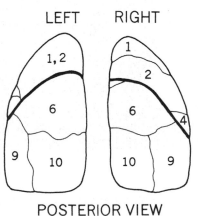

Figure 3-20. A. Schematic representation of lungs, showing lobes and segments. *(continues)*

A

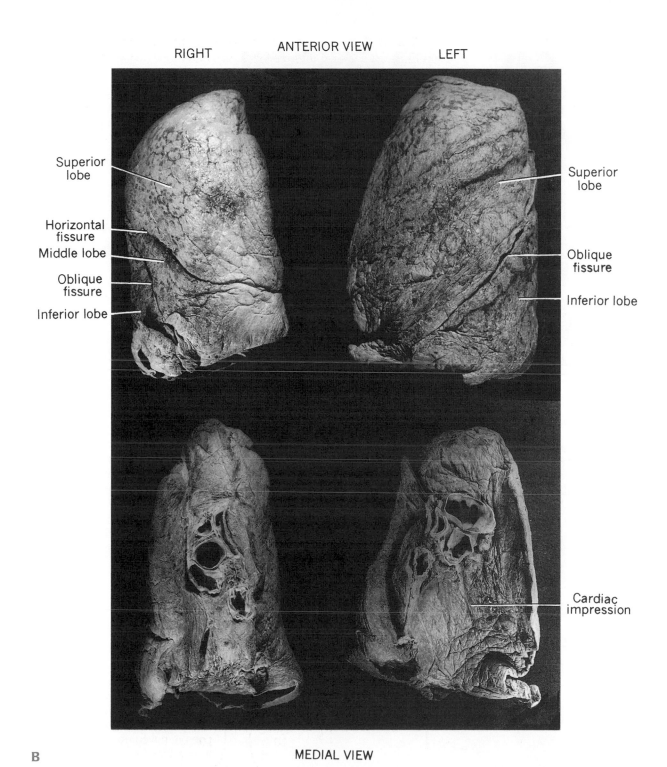

RIGHT ANTERIOR VIEW LEFT

Superior lobe

Horizontal fissure

Middle lobe

Oblique fissure

Inferior lobe

Superior lobe

Oblique fissure

Inferior lobe

Cardiac impression

B

MEDIAL VIEW

Figure 3-20. *(continued)* **B.** Anterior and medial view of lungs. *(continues)*

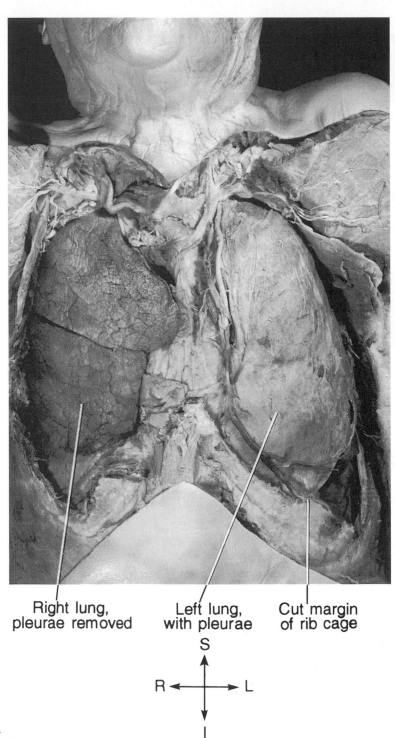

Right lung,
pleurae removed

Left lung,
with pleurae

Cut margin
of rib cage

S

R ← → L

I

Figure 3-20. *(continued)*
C. Anterior view of lungs *in situ*.
Note that the pleural lining has
been removed from the right
lung, while it remains on the left
lung.

C

The third level of branching serves the segments of each lobe. At this third level of division, the bronchi divide repeatedly into smaller and smaller cartilaginous tubes, with the final tube being the **terminal** (end) **bronchiole** (see Figure 3-21).

This repeated branching has an important effect on respiratory function. Examination of Table 3-2 reveals that there are 28 generations of subdivisions in the respiratory tree, providing a truly amazing amount of surface area for respiration. Although the cross-sectional area of the

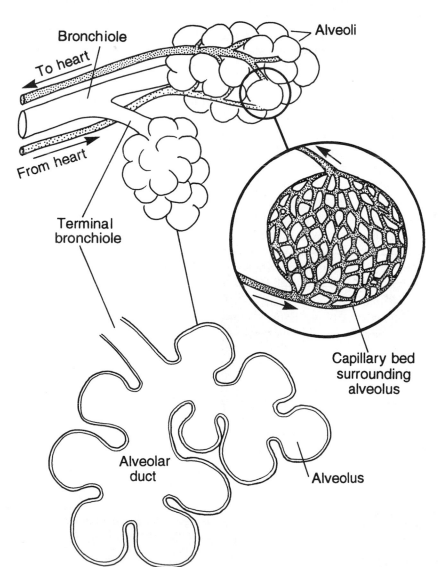

Figure 3-21. Schematic representation of cluster of alveoli with capillary bed. Lower portion shows a cross-section through alveoli and terminal bronchiole.

trachea is about 5 cm² (about the diameter of a quarter), the cross-sectional area of the 300,000,000 alveoli would equal 70 m², or the area of a throw rug large enough to cover a 10' × 24' room!

The first nine divisions of the bronchial tree are strictly conductive and cartilaginous, being designed only to transport gas between environment and lungs. Successive divisions of the noncartilaginous airway reach a minimal diameter of 1 mm. This conducting zone, which includes the conducting regions of both the upper and lower respiratory tracts and terminates with the terminal bronchioles, makes up approximately 150 ml in the adult, a volume known as *dead air* because air that does not descend below the space cannot undergo gas exchange with the blood.

The final seven divisions are actual respiratory zones comprised of the respiratory bronchioles, alveolar ducts, and alveoli. The respiratory bronchioles ("little bronchi") are the terminal bronchioles, serving the alveoli.

The terminal bronchiole is small (about 1 mm in diameter) and at its end becomes the alveolar duct, which in turn communicates with the alveolus. The alveoli are extremely small (approximately 1/4 mm in diameter) but extremely plentiful, with approximately 300 million in the mature lungs.

You might think of the final respiratory exchange region as a series of apartment houses. As you can see in Figure 3-20, the respiratory bronchioles are the entryways for each apartment building, and the alveolar duct is the passageway to the individual "apartment," the alveolus. Each of these alveoli is between 200 and 300 microns in diameter, which is quite small because a micron is one thousandth of a millimeter. Put another way, you could place five alveoli in the space between the millimeter marks on your ruler.

This "apartment house" analogy will serve you as you read about the devastating effects of emphysema on respiration. Among other things,

Keeping the Airway Open in Respiratory Emergency

In times of respiratory emergency, it sometimes becomes necessary to ensure that the respiratory pathway remains patent (open). In a conscious patient, the normal head and neck orientation places the mouth at a 90° angle from the airway above the larynx (pharynx). If an unconscious individual's head drops forward (see Figure 3–18B) the airway may become occluded and limit respiration.

In some cases there may be concern that the vocal folds or airway above that level will not remain open, so an emergency tracheostomy will be performed (*tracheo* = trachea; *stoma* = mouth). This medical procedure involves opening an artificial passageway into the trachea, typically 1–3 cm below the cricoid cartilage.

emphysema removes the "walls" within individual "apartments," greatly reducing the surface area available for participation in gas exchange.

The alveoli at this terminal point do the real work of respiration by virtue of their architecture and relationship with the vascular supply (see Figure 3-21). The alveolar lining is made up of two types of cells, Type I and Type II pneumocytes. Type I pneumocytes (membranous pneumocytes) are flat cells that are directly involved in gas exchange. Type II cells (cuboidal cells) are the source of the surfactant, a substance that reduces surface tension, that is released into the alveolus and alters the surface tension to keep the alveoli from collapsing during respiration. When Type I cells are damaged, Type II cells will proliferate, becoming Type I cells in a regenerative process. The rich investment with alveoli makes the lungs spongy, because the surfactant at that level promotes inflation of the alveoli.

The alveolar wall is extraordinarily thin, ranging from 0.35 to 2.5 microns (by comparison, a red blood cell is 7 microns in diameter), and this quality promotes rapid transfer of gas across the membrane. The capillaries in the lungs are the most dense in the body, being approximately

Gastroesophageal Reflux

The esophageal orifice is situated in the inferior laryngopharynx and is enveloped by the musculature of the inferior pharyngeal constrictors. The cricopharyngeus muscle, which is actually part of the inferior constrictor, controls the size of the orifice by contracting to constrict the opening.

Gastroesophageal reflux refers to the reintroduction of gastrointestinal contents into the esophagus and respiratory passageway. This condition may be found in the newborn and very young child who has a weak esophageal sphincter or hypersensitivity of the esophageal sphincter, resulting in reflux, inability to retain nourishment, and life-threatening malnutrition. It is not uncommon among children with cerebral palsy, typically resulting in frequent vomiting, loss of nutrition, and aspiration pneumonia (see clinical note on aspiration).

The size of the esophageal opening may be reduced surgically through a procedure known as Nissen fundoplication ("sling"), thereby inhibiting regurgitation of stomach contents. Nissen fundoplication involves surgical narrowing of the esophageal opening by releasing a flap of tissue from the stomach, followed by elevation and suturing of the flap to the esophageal orifice. The child may receive nutrition through a tube run through the nasal cavity into the esophagus (nasogastric tube; naso = nose; gastric = stomach) or through orogastric (oral feeding tube; a.k.a. "gavage") feeding, again via tube.

Surgical placement of a gastronomy tube may be required if reflux cannot be controlled adequately to guarantee nutrition. This procedure, referred to as "gastronomy," results in surgical placement of a feeding tube into the stomach wall. Similarly, "jejunostomy" is placement of a feeding tube into the small intestine. For a more detailed discussion, see Langley and Lombardino (1991).

Aspiration

Although not directly related to respiratory anatomy or physiology, aspiration *is* an issue in maintaining respiratory function. *Aspiration* refers to entry of liquid or solid materials into the lungs. Fluid or solids may enter the lungs as a result of some failure in strength, coordination, sensation, or awareness. Patients who are intubated to support respiration during crisis are *also* at risk for aspiration because the airway is artificially kept open: Vomitus or reflux from the stomach (logically via the esophageal opening at the level of the larynx) readily enters the unprotected lungs through the larynx. Aspiration of foreign matter into the lungs is a very real danger in cases of neurological deficit, and the individual who has had a stroke, or who has cerebral palsy or another compromising condition, is particularly vulnerable. The patient may demonstrate diminished or ineffective (nonproductive) cough, as well as reduced muscular strength and control of the muscles of deglutition, and perhaps diminished ability to recognize the threat involved. In children with cerebral palsy, reduction in coordinated movement ability may also arise from the neurological deficit.

Because the client with neurological deficit may not be aware or competent to seek help, it is wise to know the symptoms of aspiration. If the client's voice sounds wet or gurgly, or if the client has a history of respiratory illnesses, the client is at risk for aspiration pneumonia. Likewise, the client may have a weak, breathy vocalization or cry, indicating laryngeal muscle weakness and the potential for lack of adequate protective function.

pulmonary: *L., pulmonarius, pertaining to the lungs*

10 microns long and 7 microns wide. Their extremely small size and prolific presence permit 100 to 300 ml of blood to be spread over 70 square meters of surface. Moser and Spragg (1982) note that this is the equivalent of spreading one teaspoon of blood over a square meter of surface.

Each alveolus is richly supplied with blood for gas exchange from more than 2,000 capillaries. A little multiplication will reveal that there are more than 600,000,000,000 (600 billion) capillaries involved in gas exchange, reminding us of the amount of vascular tissue in the lungs. The lungs also have an intricate lacework of cartilage, because the bronchial tree is invested with this supportive tissue, and because most of the levels of branching of this tree contain cartilage.

During normal quiet respiration, the blood spends only about half a second in the capillaries, with gas exchange occurring within the first quarter of its transit through the pulmonary system. The **pulmonary artery** branches to follow the bronchial tree, ultimately serving the gas exchange process at the alveolar level. There is a parallel vascular supply to oxygenate the lung tissue (the bronchial arteries). The maintenance of lung tissue via the bronchial arteries requires only about 50 ml per minute, whereas the pulmonary system will process approximately 5,000 ml per minute.

The bronchial tree and trachea are obvious conduits for contaminants as well as air. The nasal and oral passageways provide some protection from respiratory contamination, but nature has not caught up

Protection against Trauma

The lungs are obviously important for life function, and are designed with damage control in mind. The two lungs are encased in separate pleural linings, so that if one lung is penetrated by an object (such as happens when a lung is punctured by a broken rib), the other lung will continue to function. Likewise, the segmented nature of lungs is a protective device. If a lung is punctured, the extremely rich vascular bed will cause significant and dangerous bleeding. The segmented nature of the lungs provides some protection against total lung failure: Bleeding in one segment is isolated to that segment, at least until the bronchial tree is filled with blood.

with the heavily polluted modern society. The respiratory pathway has multiple filtering functions to safeguard the lungs against pollutants. The nostril hairs provide a first line of defense, catching most particulate matter greater than 10 microns (a micron is one millionth of a meter) before it enters the trachea. The moist mucous membrane of the upper respiratory system provides another receptacle for foreign matter. Goblet cells within the mucosal lining and submucosal glands secrete lubricant into the respiratory tract to trap pollutants as they enter the trachea and larynx. The respiratory passageway from the nose to the beginning of the bronchi is lined with tall columnar epithelium covered by **cilia** (hairlike processes) that beat more than 1,000 times per minute. In the lower pathway, the beating action drives pollutants upward, and beating drives nasal passage contaminants posteriorly.

The beating epithelia progressively move the material up the bronchi to the level of the vocal folds in the larynx, at which time the individual feels the stimulation of secretion at the vocal folds and "clears the throat." That "ahem" is just enough force to blow the mucus off the folds (**mucus** is the dense fluid product of mucous membrane tissue), where it can be swallowed without further ado. Unfortunately, these beating epithelia may be damaged by pollutants such as cigarette smoke, resulting in failure of this system. Particles in the 2 to 10 micron range will settle on the walls of the bronchi, where they are eliminated by these beating epithelia. If a particle is less than 2 microns it will generally reach the alveolus.

The lymphatic system provides a final cleaning stage for the respiratory tissue. Particles not eliminated by the beating epithelia are removed by means of the lymphatic system, which serves down to the level of the terminal bronchiole. Pollutants are suspended in mucus and migrate to the bronchioles through coughing, where they can be eliminated by the lymphatics and macrophages.

The respiratory passageway also protects the lungs by warming and humidifying the air as it enters. The mucous membrane is highly vascularized, permitting rapid transfer of heat from blood to air.

Emphysema

Emphysema is generally considered to be a product of a modern society that has not solved its pollution problems. Often the disease results from tobacco smoking, but it may also arise from living in an industrial environment. Its progression is slow and may be arrested to some degree by altering the respiratory environment.

The mechanism for emphysema appears to be as follows. You will recall that the bronchial passageway is richly infused with ciliated epithelia that beat continuously to remove contaminants from the respiratory tract. This continuous waste removal process is seriously hampered by pollutants that, in the early stages of emphysema, destroy the epithelia.

The absence of epithelia greatly reduces the cleaning ability of the respiratory system and hampers the removal of waste products, promoting deposition of pollutants within the alveoli. The alveoli undergo a significant morphological (form) change: The walls of the alveoli break down and alveoli recombine so that clusters of alveoli become a single sac. Although this may seem benign, it has a devastating effect in that the surface area for gas exchange is greatly reduced as a result.

A second morphological change arises as a compensation for the first. The individual with emphysema is faced with an ongoing shortage of oxygen and is forced to attempt continually deeper inspirations to accommodate, and a characteristic "barrel chest" results from these efforts. (The thorax must be greatly expanded to accommodate the compromised alveolar surface area.)

This second morphological change causes a third pathological response. You will recall that the lower margin of the rib cage marks the point of attachment of the diaphragm. Because the rib cage is flared out due to emphysema, contraction of the diaphragm (which pulls on the rib cage) causes the rib cage to pull down and in medially, which actually *reduces* the size of thorax rather than increases it.

The final morphological change arising from this trilogy of tragedy is respiratory failure. The respiratory mechanism is highly compromised, leaving the individual susceptible to respiratory diseases such as pneumonia.

To summarize:
- The respiratory system is composed of right and left **lungs** having three and two **lobes,** respectively.
- Communication between the external and internal environments is by means of the **trachea** and **bronchial tree.**
- Repeated subdivisions of this bronchial tree end with the **alveoli,** the site of gas exchange.
- These highly vascularized alveoli provide the mechanism by which oxygen enters the bloodstream and carbon dioxide is removed.
- Pollutants entering the respiratory tract will be removed through the cleansing action of the **beating epithelia** that line the bronchial passageway.

MOVEMENT OF AIR THROUGH THE SYSTEM

The lung tissue is particularly prepared to process the gases of life by nature of their construction. Such great design, however, would be useless without a mechanism for bringing air into and out of those lungs.

We have already discussed the mechanics of the system, so you should be familiar with the idea that the lungs expand as a result of enlargement of the structure surrounding them. We contract the diaphragm to enlarge the **vertical dimension** (superior-inferior dimension), and elevate the rib cage to enlarge the **transverse dimension** (antero-posterior and lateral dimensions). You might be curious about *how* these changes cause the lungs to expand. The key is having a closed system.

You will recall that the cavity holding the lungs is supported by muscle and bone that cover every centimeter of the thoracic wall. Likewise, the bottom of the thoracic cavity is completely sealed by the diaphragm, making the thorax almost impervious to the outside world, were it not for the respiratory passageway. The only way air can enter or leave the lungs is by means of the tubes connected to them (the bronchial tree, continuous with the upper respiratory passageway).

Now comes the tricky part. The lungs are simply placed inside this cavity, not held to the walls by ligaments or cartilage. It is as if you placed a too-small sponge in a too-large bottle, because the thoracic volume is *greater* than that of the lungs at rest.

The lungs and inner thoracic wall are each completely covered with a **pleural** lining (Figure 3-22) that provides a means of smooth contact for rough tissue, as well as a mechanism for translating the force of thorax enlargement into inspiration. The lungs are encased in linings referred to as the **visceral pleurae**, and the thoracic linings are the **parietal pleurae**. The regions of the parietal pleurae are identified by location: mediastinal, pericardial, diaphragmatic, parietal, and apical pleurae. The **mediastinal pleura** covers the mediastinum and the **diaphragmatic pleura** covers the diaphragm. The **costal** pleurae cover the inner surface

pleural: *Gr., pleura, a side*

costal: *L., costae, coast*

Pleurisy

Pleurisy is a condition in which the pleural linings of the thoracic cavity are inflamed. When the inflammation results in "dry pleurisy," the patient will experience extreme pain upon breathing as a result of the loss of lubricating quality of the intrapleural fluid. "Adhesions" may result, in which portions of the parietal pleurae adhere to the visceral pleurae. (The patient may experience "breaking up" of these adhesions for quite some time following his or her bout with pleurisy.) Pleurisy may be unilateral or bilateral and may result in excessive fluid (potentially purulent) in the pleural space.

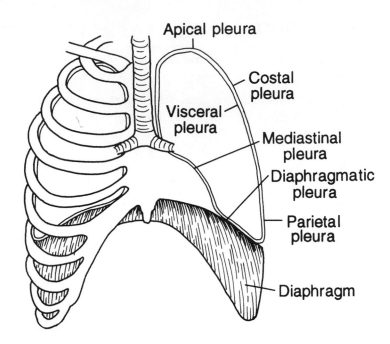

Figure 3-22. Pleural linings of the lungs and thorax. Parietal pleurae include costal, diaphragmatic, mediastinal, and apical pleurae. Visceral pleurae line the surface of the lungs.

venules: *L., venula, tiny veins*

of the rib cage. The **apical pleurae** cover the superior-most region of the rib cage.

The pleural membranes are composed of elastic and fibrous tissue and are endowed with **venules** and lymphocytes. Although it is convenient to think of the pleural linings as being separate entities, the visceral and parietal pleurae are actually continuous with each other. These wrappings completely encase both the lungs and the inner thorax, with the reflection point being the hilum (root of lung, at about the level of T4 or T5). This continuous sheet provides the airtight seal required to permit the lungs to follow the movement of the thorax.

To understand how these pleura help us breathe will take a little thought. You have probably experienced the difficulty involved in separating two pieces of plastic food wrap, especially if there is fluid between the two sheets. There is a degree of surface tension arising from the presence of fluid and highly conforming surfaces that helps keep the sheets together. Cuboidal cells within the pleural lining produce a mucous solution that is released in the space between the parietal and visceral pleurae. This surfactant reduces the surface tension in the lungs and provides a slippery interface between the lungs and the thoracic wall, permitting easy, low-friction gliding of the lungs within the thorax. The presence of surfactant keeps the two sheets from clinging to each other. If you were to wrap the lungs in sheets of similar quality (we will call them pleurae) and line the thoracic cavity with the same, you would have an analogous situation. The two surfaces conform to each other as a result of the fluid bond between them, and a negative pressure is maintained by lack of contact with the outside atmosphere. (If you puncture a lung, the bond is broken.)

When you contract the **diaphragm**, the pleural lining of the diaphragm maintains its contact with the visceral pleurae of the two lungs above it, and the lungs expand. Likewise, if you expand the thorax transversely by elevating the rib cage, you will find that the lungs will follow faithfully. In this manner, the lungs are able to follow the action of the muscles without actually being attached to them.

The pleural linings serve another function as well. Because the mating surfaces of the two linings are infused with a liquid serous secretion, the friction of movement of the two linings is greatly reduced, making respiration much more efficient. When this fluid is lost or reduced, as in the disorder known as *dry pleurisy*, the friction is greatly increased and pain results. As a protection, each lung is separately endowed with pleural lining. If the lining of one lung is damaged through disease or trauma, we still have the other lung in reserve.

We have discussed the lungs and hinted at the second most important muscle of the body (the diaphragm), but have glossed over the fact that the most important muscle of the body (the heart) is located deep within the thorax, in a region known as the **mediastinum**. The heart is encased in the mediastinal pleurae, along with nerves, blood vessels, the esophagus, and lymph vessels (see Figure 3-23).

The mediastinum is the most protected region of the body. This space is occupied primarily by the heart, as well as the trachea, major blood vessels, nerves, thymus gland, lymph nodes, and the conducting portion of the gastrointestinal tract known as the esophagus.

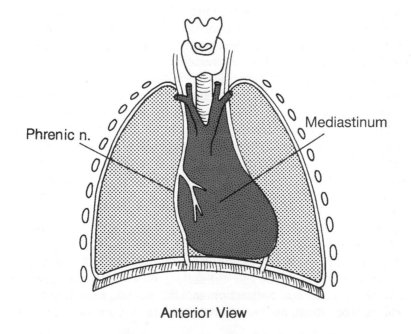

Anterior View

Figure 3-23. Relationship among mediastinum, diaphragm, and lungs. Note the phrenic nerve innervation of the diaphragm.

The mediastinum lies deep to the bony thorax and its muscular coverings and is nestled deep to the lungs. Its central location in the body belies its importance to all regions, and its critical placement surrounded by lung tissue guarantees efficient transfer of gas to (and from) the blood pumped by the heart.

Because the heart is such an important muscle, it is located deep within several layers of thick muscle and bone. In the posterior are the vertebrae and massive muscles of the back, and the anterolateral aspect of the thorax is a strong wall of bone and muscle. The heart is well protected against most trauma, with the exception of romantic disappointment!

The organs and structures of the mediastinum are encased by a continuation of the parietal pleurae. This lining provides a low-friction mating surface between the lungs and the middle space. The visceral pleural lining of the lungs adjacent to the mediastinum is termed the *mediastinal pleurae.*

The left and right phrenic nerves serving the diaphragm pass anterior to the root structures of the lungs, coursing along the lateral surfaces of the pericardium (the membranous sac enclosing the heart) to innervate the diaphragm. The two vagi enter the posterior mediastinum to innervate the heart, first passing behind the root structures of the lung, coursing inferiorly to the anterior and posterior surfaces of the esophagus. They descend through the diaphragm adjacent to the esophagus through the esophageal **hiatus** to innervate the abdominal viscera. The vagal pulmonary branches provide a parasympathetic nerve supply for the lungs, with nerve fibers found even in the smallest bronchioles. The vagus mediates the cough reflex and control of airway diameter.

hiatus: *L., an opening*

Movement of the rib cage for inspiration requires muscular effort. Muscles of respiration may be divided into muscles of inspiration and expiration (see Table 3-3). Before delving into these muscles, we should give you a word of caution. The primary muscles of respiration are relatively easy to identify, but we will inevitably make some assumptions about function of secondary muscle groups based on muscle attachment. It also is wise to explain at the start that expiration can be either forced or passive and is much more often a passive process. Thus, the muscles of expiration are not always active and depend on some other forces to help us eliminate carbon dioxide-laden air.

In summary:
- The lungs are covered with **pleural linings** which, in conjunction with the lungs, provide the mechanism for air movement through muscular action.
- When the diaphragm contracts, the lungs are pulled down because of the association between the pleurae and the diaphragm.
- **Diaphragmatic contraction** expands the lungs, drawing air into them through the bronchial passageway.

Table 3–3. Muscles of respiration.

INSPIRATION	EXPIRATION
Muscles of Trunk	**Muscles of Trunk**
Primary of Thorax Diaphragm	**Muscles of Thorax, Back, and Upper Limb** **Anterior** Internal intercostal (interosseous portion) Transversus thoracis
Accessory of Thorax **Anterior** External intercostal Interchondral portion, internal intercostal **Posterior** Levatores costarum (brevis and longis) Serratus posterior superior	**Posterior** Subcostal Serratus posterior inferior Innermost intercostal Latissimus dorsi
Muscles of Neck Sternocleidomastoid (superficial neck) Scalenus (anterior, middle, posterior) Trapezius	**Abdominal Muscles** **Anterolateral** Transversus abdominis Internal oblique abdominis External oblique abdominis Rectus abdominis
Muscles of Thorax, Back, and Upper Limb Pectoralis major Pectoralis minor Serratus anterior Subclavius Levator scapulae Rhomboideus major Rhomboideus minor	**Posterior** Quadratus lumborum

MUSCLES OF INSPIRATION

As with many voluntary bodily functions, inspiration is a graded activity. Depending on the needs of your body, you are capable of **quiet inspiration**, which requires only one muscle, and **forced inspiration**, which calls on many more muscles. We enlist the help of increasingly larger numbers of muscles as our respiratory needs increase. You may wish to refer to Appendix C for a summary of the muscles of respiration.

If the lungs are to expand and fill with air, the thorax must increase in size as well. As mentioned, there are only two ways this can happen. The first way to expand the thorax is to increase its **vertical** (superior-inferior) dimension, a process that will occur for both quiet and forced inspiration. First, picture the lungs encased in bone around the barrel-shaped midsection of the rib cage, and bounded above by the clavicle and first rib. Remember that the rib cage is open at the bottom.

A thin but strong muscle placed across the bottom margin of the rib cage, configured like a drum-head, would be an economical means of expanding the size of the rib cage without having to manipulate the bony portion at all. The thorax and abdominal cavity below are separated by one of the most important muscles of the body, the diaphragm.

The diaphragm takes the form of an inverted bowl, with its attachments along the lower margin of the rib cage, sternum, and vertebral column. It forms a complete separation between the upper (thoracic) and lower (abdominal) chambers, and when it contracts the force of contraction is directed downward toward the abdominal viscera. This contraction results in elongation of the cavity formed by the ribs, so that the lungs expand and air enters through the respiratory passageway.

Primary Inspiratory Muscle of Thorax

Diaphragm

The primary muscle of inspiration is the diaphragm. As seen in Figure 3-24, the diaphragm completely separates the abdominal and thoracic cavities (with the exception of vascular and esophageal hiatuses). The edges attach along the inferior boundary of the rib cage, to the xiphoid process, and to the vertebral column in the posterior aspect. The intermediate region is made up of a large, leafy aponeurosis called the **central tendon**. When the muscle contracts, muscle fibers shorten and the diaphragm pulls the central tendon down and forward. Let us look at this extremely important muscle in detail.

The muscle fibers of the diaphragm radiate out from the central tendon, forming the sternal, costal, and vertebral attachments. The anterior-most sternal attachment is made at the xiphoid process, with fibers coursing up and back to insert into the anterior central tendon. Lateral to the xiphoid, the fibers of the diaphragm attach to the inner border of ribs 7 through 12 and to the costal cartilages to form the costal attachment. In the posterior aspect, the vertebral diaphragmatic attachment is made with the corpus of L1 through L4 and transverse processes L1.

The fibers from these attachments course upward and inward to insert into the central tendon (see Figure 3-25). The posterior vertebral attachment also provides support for the esophageal hiatus. The vertebral attachment is accomplished by means of two **crura**. The right crus arises from attachment at L1 through L4, wherein the fibers ascend and separate to encircle the esophageal hiatus. Fibers of the left crus support this endeavor by passing to the left of the hiatus.

Although the diaphragm separates the thorax from the abdomen, the need for nutrients dictates that there be communication between the oral cavity and abdominal region. The region below the diaphragm also has vascular needs, and these require supply routes through the diaphragm.

crura: *L., crosses*

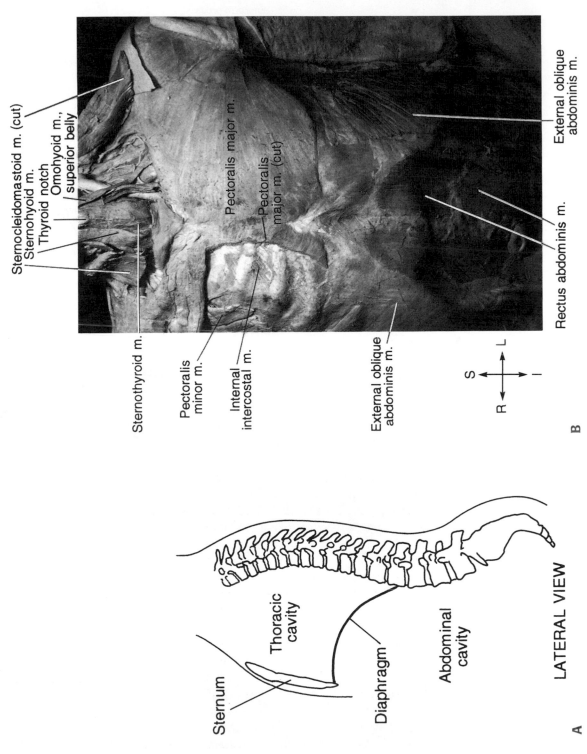

Sternocleidomastoid m. (cut)
Sternohyoid m.
Thyroid notch
Omohyoid m.,
superior belly

Sternothyroid m.

Pectoralis
minor m.

Internal
intercostal m.

External oblique
abdominis m.

Pectoralis major m.

Pectoralis
major m. (cut)

Rectus abdominis m.

External oblique
abdominis m.

B. Anterior view of rib cage.

S

R

L

I

B

Sternum

Thoracic
cavity

Diaphragm

Abdominal
cavity

A

LATERAL VIEW

Figure 3-24. A. Lateral-view schematic of the diaphragm and thorax. Notice that the diaphragm courses markedly down from the sternum to the vertebral attachment, completely separating the thorax from the abdomen. **B.** Anterior view of rib cage.

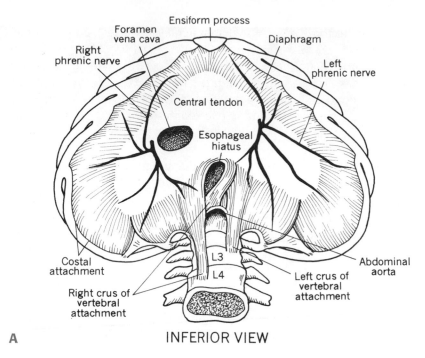

A   INFERIOR VIEW

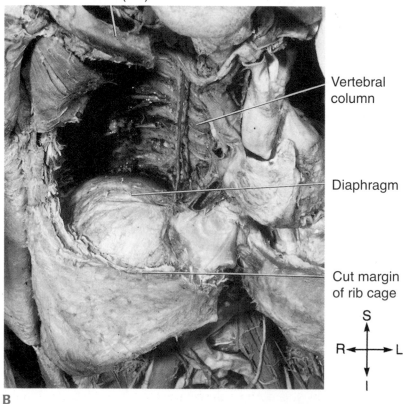

Figure 3-25. A. Inferior-view schematic of diaphragm, as seen from the abdominal cavity. B. Photograph of superior view of diaphragm.

B

There are three openings (diaphragmatic hiatuses) through which structures pass. As seen in Figure 3-25, the *descending abdominal aorta* passes through the aortic hiatus located adjacent and lateral to the vertebral column. The *esophageal hiatus*, through which the esophagus passes, is found immediately anterior to the aortic hiatus, while the *inferior vena cava* traverses these two cavities by means of the foramen vena cava (which is in the right-central aspect of the diaphragm as viewed from above).

The actual muscle fibers of the diaphragm radiate out from the imperfect center formed by the central tendon. Careful examination of the forces of muscular contraction will be most helpful in later discussion of muscular contraction and action. Realize, again, that muscle can perform only one task, and that is to shorten. If a muscle is attached to two points, shortening will tend to bring those two points closer together, or simply tense the muscle if neither point is capable of moving. The diaphragm will stretch your understanding of this basic muscle function somewhat. Although the principles of muscle action and result still hold, movement of the diaphragm will not make a great deal of sense until you realize where the points of attachment really are.

Figure 3-26 is a schematic drawing of the diaphragm and central tendon. First, look at the upper portion of the figure. If you choose some subset of those fibers and shorten them, the end result will be that the central tendon moves toward the point of firm attachment, the origin. But when the diaphragm contracts, all fibers contract together, which means that all fibers will pull equally on the central tendon. Now look at the second part of the figure, and trace the same effect. If you contract (shorten) one fiber, the central tendon will move down toward the origin for the fiber. If you contract the entire diaphragm, the net result will be that the diaphragm is pulled down as a unit. Notice that the fibers in the front are longer than those in the back. *Contraction of the diaphragm has the result of pulling the central tendon down and forward.* It is directly analogous to placing someone in the middle of a blanket while a host of his or her friends pull on all of the corners of the blanket. When the friends pull together, the person in the middle flies up. Because the diaphragm has the shape of an inverted bowl, pulling on the edges (muscular contraction) draws the center down, but (gravity notwithstanding) the analogy holds.

The prominent **central tendon** is the last element of the diaphragm that we need to consider. Look again at Figure 3-26 and notice that the central tendon is a crescent-shaped aponeurosis that is white and translucent. The tendon tends to conform to the prominence of the vertebral column in the thoracic cavity, so its shape mimics the curvature of the transverse thoracic cavity. It has the flexibility of an aponeurosis, but has no contractile qualities. It depends on the radiating fibers of the diaphragm to account for movement. Above the central tendon is the heart, and this tendon provides a strong and secure floor for that mediastinal organ.

Innervation of the diaphragm is by means of the **phrenic nerves** (see Figure 3-23). The diaphragm can be placed under voluntary control (you can hold your breath), but it is under primary control of the autonomic system (you have no choice but to breathe eventually). Nature has provided bilateral innervation of the diaphragm, supporting the notion that this is an exceptionally important unpaired muscle. The phrenic nerves originate in the **cervical plexus** (a *plexus* is a group of nerves coming together for a common purpose) from spinal nerves C3, C4, and C5 of both sides of the spinal cord.

The phrenic nerve descends deep to the omohyoid and sternoclei-

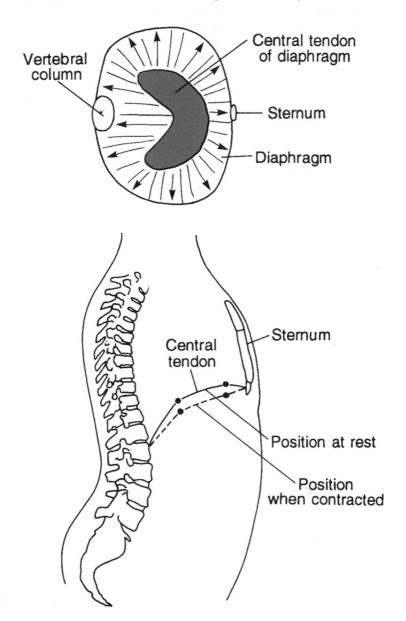

Figure 3-26. Top: Schematic of transverse view of the diaphragm with central tendon. The arrows depict the direction of force upon contraction of the diaphragm. Bottom: This lateral view of the diaphragm shows that contractions of the diaphragm pull the central tendon down.

domastoid muscles and superficial to the anterior scalenus muscle, into the mediastinal space on the left and right sides of the heart. The fibers descend and divide to innervate the superior surface of the diaphragm. One branch (the left and right phrenicoabdominal) descends deep to innervate the inferior surface. The left branch is longer than the right, because it has a greater distance to travel around the mediastinum. The phrenic nerve mediates both motor and sensory information. The lower intercostal nerve serves the inferior-most boundary of the diaphragm.

One final comment is warranted on the diaphragm and its action. Throughout this description we have ignored the abdominal viscera, but beneath the diaphragm are numerous organs that undergo continual cycles of compression during respiration, a fact that will work to the advantage of anyone wishing to forcefully exhale (or perform the Heimlich maneuver, as we shall see).

To summarize:

- The primary muscle of inspiration is the **diaphragm**, the dividing point between the thorax and the abdomen.
- The fibers of the diaphragm pull on the **central tendon**, resulting in downward motion of the diaphragm during inspiration, and this movement expands the lungs in the **vertical dimension**.

Muscle:	Diaphragm, Sternal head
Origin:	Xiphoid process of sternum
Course:	Superiorly and medially
Insertion:	Central tendon
Innervation:	Phrenic nerve arising from cervical plexus of spinal nerves C3, C4, C5
Function:	Depresses central tendon of diaphragm; enlarges vertical dimension of thorax; distends abdomen

Muscle:	Diaphragm, Costal head
Origin:	Inferior margin of ribs 7–12
Course:	Superiorly and medially
Insertion:	Central tendon
Innervation:	Phrenic nerve arising from cervical plexus of spinal nerves C3, C4, C5
Function:	Depresses central tendon of diaphragm; enlarges vertical dimension of thorax; distends abdomen

Muscle:	Diaphragm, Vertebral head
Origin:	Corpus of L1, transverse processes of L1–L5
Course:	Superiorly and medially
Insertion:	Central tendon
Innervation:	Phrenic nerve arising from cervical plexus of spinal nerves C3, C4, C5
Function:	Depresses central tendon of diaphragm; enlarges vertical dimension of thorax; distends abdomen

Accessory Muscles of Inspiration

Although the diaphragm is the major contributor to inspiration, it needs help to meet the needs of your body for **forced inspiration**. If you take a look at Figure 3-27 you will see the rib cage from the side. Direct your attention first to the way the ribs run: They are directed distinctly downward as they make their path to the front of the skeleton. Next, imagine raising the ribs in front, and realize that when you do that, the front of the rib cage expands as a result. Swinging those ribs up means that they will swing out a bit in both anterior and lateral aspects, thereby increasing the volume of the rib cage.

To put this function in everyday terms, look at Figure 3-27 showing venetian blinds from the side. When they are closed they are similar to the rib cage at rest, and when they are tilted so that you can see through them it is similar to the point of elevation of the ribs. That elevation brings the ribs more nearly horizontal, just like the blinds, and that increases the overall front-back dimension.

Because the goal is to raise all of the ribs and *all* parts of the ribs, we must have muscles attached to broad areas of the ribs to achieve this. The **external intercostal** muscles (see Figure 3-28) are positioned so that when they contract, the entire rib cage elevates, with most of the distance moved being in the front aspect.

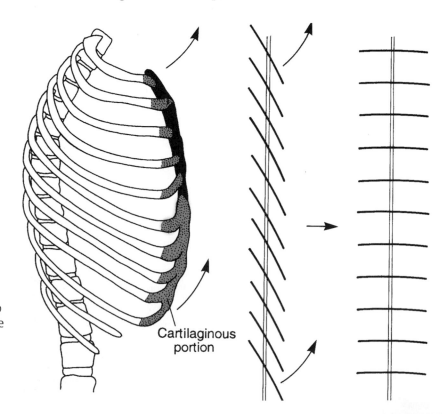

Figure 3-27. Schematic of rib cage from the side. Notice that the ribs slant down as they run forward. During inspiration the rib cage will elevate, as shown by the arrows. On the right side, the Venetian blinds shown from the side demonstrate the change in volume achieved by elevation of the rib cage.

Cartilaginous portion

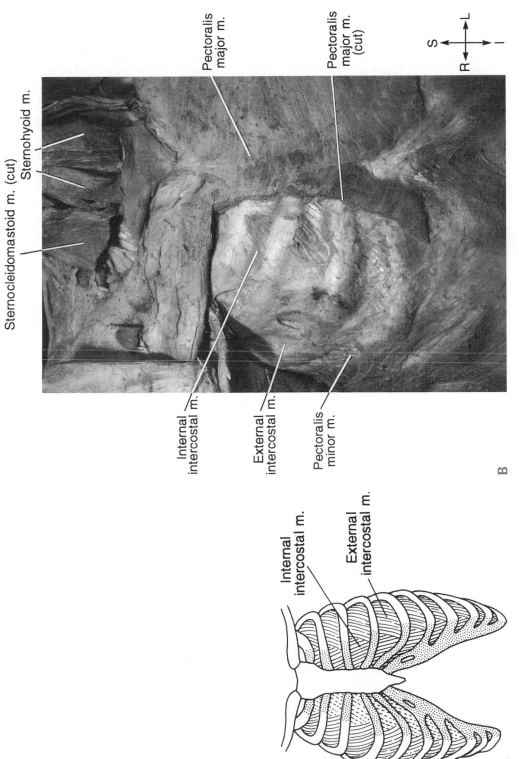

Sternocleidomastoid m. (cut)

Sternohyoid m.

Pectoralis major m.

Pectoralis major m. (cut)

Internal intercostal m.

External intercostal m.

Pectoralis minor m.

B

S
R — L
I

Internal intercostal m.

External intercostal m.

A

Figure 3-28. A. Rib cage with external and internal intercostal muscles. Note that on the left rib cage the fascia covering the internal intercostals has been removed, whereas it remains present and translucent on the right. External intercostals are absent near the sternum, and thus one can see the deeper internal intercostals within that region. **B.** Photograph showing some accessory muscles of inspiration and expiration.

By labeling these muscles as "accessory muscles" of inspiration, we are acknowledging the simple fact that you could perform the respiratory act without them. They provide a significant increase in the amount of air we are able to process, but one is capable of surviving on diaphragmatic support in absence of the accessory muscles. You most likely are not using the accessory muscles as you quietly read this text, but you would probably invoke them to help you discuss this chapter in front of the class. We will differentiate these based on region of the body: anterior and posterior thoracic muscles, neck muscles, and muscles of the arm and shoulder.

Anterior Thoracic Muscles of Inspiration

- **External Intercostal**
- **Interchondral Portion, Internal Intercostal**

External Intercostal and Interchondral Portion, Internal Intercostal Muscles. The external intercostal muscles are among the most significant respiratory muscles for speech. They not only provide a significant proportion of the total respiratory capacity, but they also perform functions that are uniquely speech-related.

As you can see in Figure 3-28, the 11 external intercostal muscles reside between the 12 ribs of the thorax, providing the ribs with both unity and mobility. The external intercostal muscles originate on the lower surface of each rib (except rib 12), and course downward and inward to insert into the upper surface of the rib immediately below. These muscles provide a unified surface of diagonally slanting striated muscle on all costal surfaces of the rib cage *with the exception of the region near the sternum*, because contraction of external intercostal fibers in that region would provide little benefit (and perhaps some negative effect) to the job of increasing cavity size.

The external intercostal muscles are covered with the translucent intercostal membrane that separates them from the internal intercostal muscles.

The internal intercostal muscles (to be discussed) are predominantly muscles of expiration, with the exception of the chondral portion. The **parasternal** (near the sternum) portion of the internal intercostal muscles encompassing the chondral aspect of the ribs has been shown to be active during forced inspiration. The musculature is quite capable of segmental activation, so that one portion of this muscle can contract while contraction of the rest of the muscle is inhibited. The cross-laced effect of external and internal intercostal muscles forms a strong protective barrier for the lungs and heart and an impervious cavity for the forces of gas exchange.

Functionally, the external intercostal muscles elevate the rib cage. When the rib cage is elevated, the flexible coupling of the costo-sternal attachment permits the chondral portion of the ribs to rotate as they elevate. The net result is that the sternum remains relatively parallel to the vertebral column even as the rib cage expands, increasing the anterior dimension and thus the volume of the lungs (see Figure 3-27). The effort involved in raising the ribs twists (torques) the elastic cartilaginous portion of the ribs, and when that force is relaxed, the cartilage returns to its original form. Inspiration is an active process: Expiration can simply involve letting nature take its course, but it may be active as well.

Innervation of the external intercostal muscles is achieved by the anterior divisions of the 12 pairs of thoracic spinal nerves, identified by the location of the region they innervate. The thoracic intercostal nerves arise from T1 through T6, and the thoracoabdominal intercostal nerves that pass into the abdominal wall arise from T7 through T11. These intercostal nerves supply not only the intercostal muscles but also a number of other muscles of respiration located in the anterior abdominal wall (see Figure 3-29).

Although the external intercostals account for most of the second dimensional change (the anterior-posterior dimension), there are other muscles which, by virtue of their arrangement, are assumed to be of help. Any muscle that attaches to the rib cage or sternum, and could feasibly elevate either, could assist in the process of inspiration.

Muscle:	External intercostal muscles
Origin:	Inferior surface of ribs 1–11
Course:	Down and obliquely in
Insertion:	Upper surface of rib immediately below
Innervation:	Intercostal nerves: thoracic intercostal nerves arising from T2–T6 and thoracoabdominal intercostal nerves from T7–T11
Function:	Elevate rib

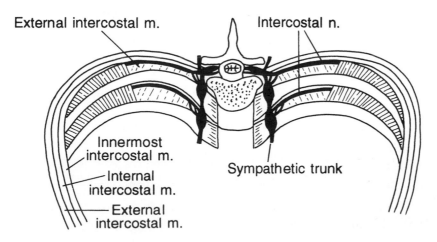

Figure 3-29. Schematic of intercostal nerves as seen from within the thoracic cavity.

Muscle:	Internal intercostal muscles, interchondral portion
Origin:	Inferior margin of ribs 1–11
Course:	Down and lateral
Insertion:	Superior surface of the rib below
Innervation:	Intercostal nerves: thoracic intercostal nerves arising from T2–T6 and thoracoabdominal intercostal nerves from T7–T11
Function:	Elevate ribs 1–11

Some other possible assistants in respiration are the **levatores costarum** (brevis and longis), and **serratus posterior superior**, shown in Figure 3-30. They would elevate the rib cage on contraction.

Posterior Thoracic Muscles of Inspiration

- **Levatores Costarum (Brevis and Longis)**
- **Serratus Posterior Superior**

Levator Costarum (Brevis and Longis). If you examine the course of the levator costarum (elevators of the ribs) shown in Figure 3-30, you will see that shortening these muscles tends to elevate the rib cage. Although these muscles may appear to be muscles of the back, they are considered to be thoracic muscles. The **brevis** (brief) portions of the levator costarum originate on the transverse processes of vertebrae C7 through T11, for a total of 12 levator costarum brevis muscles. Fibers course obliquely down and out to insert into the tubercle of the rib below.

Muscle:	Levator costarum, longis
Origin:	Transverse processes of T7–T10
Course:	Down and obliquely out
Insertion:	Bypass the rib below the point of origin, inserting into the next rib
Innervation:	Dorsal rami (branches) of the intercostal nerves arising from spinal nerves T2–T12
Function:	Elevate ribs 9–12

Muscle:	Levator costarum, brevis
Origin:	Transverse processes of vertebrae C7–T11
Course:	Obliquely down and out
Insertion:	Tubercle of the rib below
Innervation:	Dorsal rami (branches) of the intercostal nerves arising from spinal nerves T2–T12
Function:	Elevate ribs 1–12

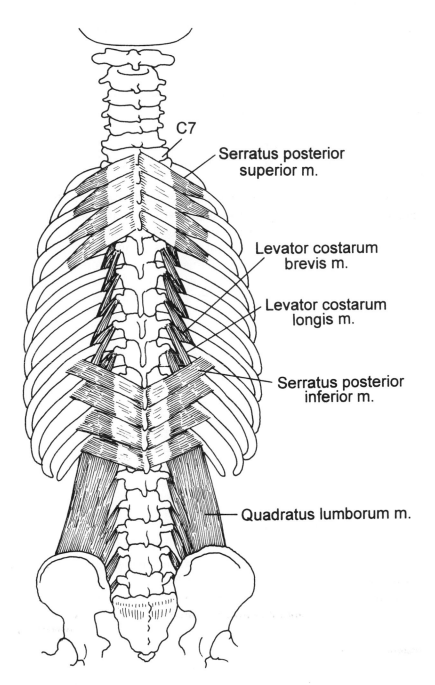

C7

Serratus posterior
superior m.

Levator costarum
brevis m.

Levator costarum
longis m.

Serratus posterior
inferior m.

Quadratus lumborum m.

Figure 3-30. Posterior thoracic muscles of inspiration. Note that the levatores costarum are present on all ribs, but in the superior aspect they are deep to the serratus posterior muscles.

The **longis** portions originate on the transverse processes of T7 through T10, with fibers coursing down and obliquely out. The fibers bypass the rib below the point of origin, inserting rather into the next rib. You can see that the longis portion will have a greater effect on elevation of the rib cage.

Much like the intercostal muscles, the levatores costarum take their innervation from the dorsal rami (branches) of the intercostal nerves arising from spinal nerves T2 through T12. Upon exiting the spinal column, the dorsal rami course abruptly back, dividing into medial and lateral branches. The lateral branch of the dorsal ramus provides innervation of the levatores costarum.

Serratus Posterior Superior. In Figure 3-30, you can see that, given their course, contraction of the serratus posterior superior muscles could easily contribute to elevation of the rib cage.

The serratus posterior superior muscles take their origins on the spinous processes of C7 and T1 through T3. Fibers from these muscles course down and laterally to insert just beyond the angles of ribs 2 through 5. This more lateral insertion provides significant enhancement of the mechanical advantage afforded this muscle, as compared with the levatores costarum brevis or longis. Innervation of the serratus posterior superior is completed by means of the ventral intercostal portion of the spinal nerves T1 through T4 or T5.

Muscle:	Serratus posterior superior
Origin:	Spinous processes of C7 and T1–T3
Course:	Down and laterally
Insertion:	Just beyond the angles of ribs 2–5
Innervation:	Ventral intercostal portion of the spinal nerves T1–T4 or T5
Function:	Elevate ribs 2–5

Accessory Muscles of Neck

- **Sternocleidomastoid**
- **Scalenes (Anterior, Middle, Posterior)**

Several neck muscles assist in inspiration (see Figure 3-31). The **sternocleidomastoid** muscle makes a direct attachment to the sternum and elevates that structure and the rib cage with it. Other potential muscles of inspiration are the **scalenus anterior, medius,** and **posterior** muscles, which are muscles of the neck. When they contract, they elevate the first and second ribs.

scalenus: *L., uneven*

As with virtually all anatomical structures involved in speech, the muscles of the neck serve double duty. Although the muscles that will be discussed in this section are important for respiration, they are also sources of stability and control of neck flexion and extension. As an infant develops, it is the early control of neck musculature that marks the shift from the neonatal flexion position to one of balance between flexion and extension. When flexion and extension are balanced, the infant is well on the road toward the whole-body stability required for speech.

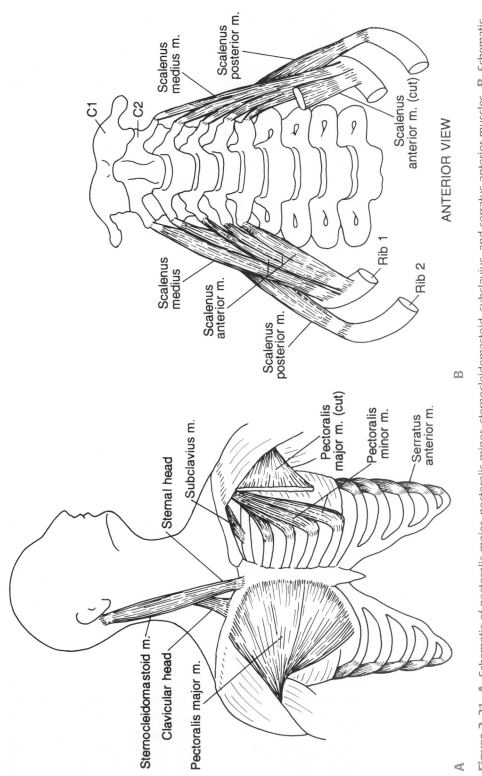

Figure 3-31. A. Schematic of pectoralis major, pectoralis minor, sternocleidomastoid, subclavius, and serratus anterior muscles. **B.** Schematic of scalenus anterior, medius, and posterior muscles.

Sternocleidomastoid. The sternocleidomastoid courses from origin on the mastoid process of the temporal bone to its insertion at the sternum (sterno) and clavicle (cleido) (see Figure 3-31). This muscle is prominent and its outline is easily visible on an individual, especially when the head is turned toward one side. When contracted separately, the sternocleidomastoid will rotate the head toward the side of contraction. When both left and right sternocleidomastoid muscles are simultaneously contracted, the sternum and the anterior rib cage will elevate.

The sternocleidomastoid and trapezius muscles derive their innervation from the eleventh cranial nerve, spinal branch (XI) accessory. The spinal portions of the accessory nerves originate from rootlets that arise from the side of the spinal cord in the regions of C2 through C4 or C5. These fibers join to become the spinal root, ascending within the vertebral column behind the denticulate ligament. The spinal root enters the skull via the foramen magnum, where it joins with the cranial root to exit the skull through the jugular foramen. The spinal and cranial branches separate, with the spinal branch coursing to innervate the sternocleidomastoid. It is supported in this by interconnection with C2 spinal nerve, which also innervates the muscle. This branch continues, descending deep to the trapezius muscle and above the clavicle, finally communicating with C3 and C4 to form a pseudoplexus, subsequently innervating the trapezius. The fibers of the cranial parts of the accessory nerve join the vagi to be distributed to skeletal muscles as vagal fibers.

Muscle:	Sternocleidomastoid (sternomastoid)
Origin:	Mastoid process of temporal bone
Course:	Down
Insertion:	Sternal head: superior manubrium sterni Clavicular head: superior surface of clavicle
Innervation:	XI accessory, spinal branch arising from spinal cord in the regions of C2–C4 or C5
Function:	Elevates sternum and, by association, rib cage

Scaleni Anterior, Middle, Posterior. The scaleni (or "scalenes," as they also are called) are muscles of the neck that provide stability to the head and facilitate rotation. By virtue of their attachment on the first and second ribs, they have the potential of increasing the vertical dimension of the thorax (see Figure 3-31).

The anterior scaleni originate on the transverse processes of vertebrae C3 through C6, with fibers coursing down to insert into the superior surface of the first rib. The middle scaleni take their origin on transverse processes of vertebrae C2 through C7, also inserting into the

Clavicular Breathing

Clavicular breathing is a form of respiration in which thorax expansion arises primarily from elevation of the rib cage via contraction of the accessory muscles of inspiration, most notably the sternocleidomastoid. Clavicular breathing often is an adaptive response by an individual to some previous or present pathological condition, such as chronic obstructive pulmonary disease, which prohibits use of other means to expand the thorax. Because elevation of the sternum results in only a small increase in thorax size, clavicular breathing is a less-than-perfect solution to the problem of respiration.

Use of accessory muscles of inspiration to augment diminished respiratory support most typically includes the anterior, middle, and posterior scalene muscles (to elevate the first and second ribs) and the sternocleidomastoid (to elevate the sternum and increase the antero-posterior dimension of the rib cage). You may have seen patients with severe respiratory difficulties stretch out their arms and hold onto the back of a chair to breathe: When they do this, they give the pectoralis major muscles something to work against, thus allowing these muscles to increase the antero-posterior dimension. You may have also seen "shrugging" action by these patients, a sure sign that the trapezius muscle is in use to raise the rib cage.

first rib. The posterior scaleni insert into the second rib, having coursed from the transverse processes of C5 through C7.

The scaleni anterior are innervated by spinal nerves C4 through C6. The middle scalenes are innervated primarily by the cervical plexus derived from C3 and C4 (although spinal nerves C5 through C8 also are involved in their innervation). Spinal nerves C5 through C8 innervate the posterior scalenes.

Muscle:	Scalenus anterior
Origin:	Transverse processes of vertebrae C3–C6
Course:	Down
Insertion:	Superior surface of rib 1
Innervation:	C4–C6
Function:	Elevates rib 1

Muscle:	Scalenus medius
Origin:	Transverse processes of vertebrae C2–C7
Course:	Down
Insertion:	Superior surface of the first rib
Innervation:	Cervical plexus derived from C3 and C4 and spinal nerves C5–C8
Function:	Elevates rib 1

Muscle:	Scalenus posterior
Origin:	Transverse processes of C5–C7
Course:	Down
Insertion:	Second rib
Innervation:	Spinal nerves C5–C8
Function:	Elevates rib 2

Muscles of Upper Arm and Shoulder

The accessory muscles of the arm may assist the external intercostal in elevation of the thorax by virtue of their attachment to the sternum and ribs. Although not all have been confirmed through physiological study, the action of each of the following muscles has the potential to increase the anterior-posterior dimension of the thorax.

- **Pectoralis Major**
- **Pectoralis Minor**
- **Serratus Anterior**
- **Subclavius**
- **Levator Scapulae**
- **Rhomboideus Major**
- **Rhomboideus Minor**
- **Trapezius**

Pectoralis Major and Minor. The pectoralis major is a large, fan-shaped muscle that originates from two heads (see Figure 3-31). The sternal head attaches along the length of the sternum at the costal cartilages, while the clavicular head arises from the anterior surface of the clavicle. The muscle converges at the crest of the greater tubercle of the humerus. In respiration, the pectoralis major elevates the sternum and thus increases the transverse dimension of the rib cage.

The pectoralis minor originates on the anterior surface of ribs 2 through 5, with fibers coursing up to converge on the coracoid process of the scapula. As with the pectoralis major, respiratory function could

Muscle:	Pectoralis major
Origin:	Sternal head: length of sternum at costal cartilages
	Clavicular head: anterior clavicle
Course:	Fan-like laterally, converging at humerus
Insertion:	Greater tubercle of humerus
Innervation:	Superior branch of the brachial plexus (spinal nerves C4–C7 and T1)
Function:	Elevates sternum, and subsequently increases transverse dimension of rib cage

Muscle:	Pectoralis minor
Origin:	Anterior surface of ribs 2–5 near chondral margin
Course:	Up and laterally
Insertion:	Coracoid process of scapula
Innervation:	Superior branch of the brachial plexus (spinal nerves C4–C7 and T1)
Function:	Increases transverse dimension of rib cage

involve elevation of the rib cage, although this function has not been verified for either muscle.

Innervation of the pectoralis major and pectoralis minor is by the pectoral nerves arising from the medial and lateral cords of the brachial plexus, a formation of C5 through C8 and T1 spinal nerves (see Figure 3-32).

Serratus Anterior. Fibers of the **serratus anterior** arise from ribs 1 through 9 along the side of the thorax, coursing up to converge on the inner vertebral border of the scapula. The sawlike fingers of this muscle give it its name ("serratus" as in "serrated knife"), and contraction of the muscle may elevate the ribs to which it is attached and subsequently the rib cage (see Figure 3-31).

serratus: *L., serratus, toothed; notched*

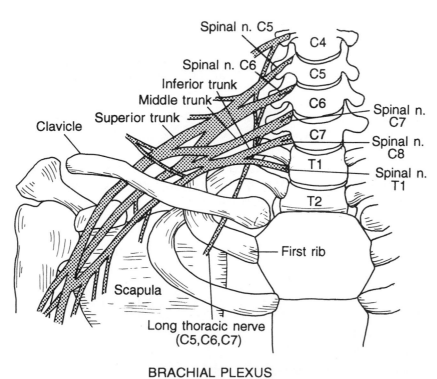

BRACHIAL PLEXUS

Figure 3-32. Schematic of brachial plexus arising from C5 through C8 and T1 spinal nerves. (Modified from data and view of Twietmeyer and McCracken, 1992.)

Muscle: Serratus anterior
Origin: Ribs 1–9, lateral surface of thorax
Course: Up and back
Insertion: Inner vertebral border of scapula
Innervation: Brachial plexus, long thoracic nerve from C5–C7
Function: Elevates ribs 1–9

As with the pectoralis major and minor, the serratus anterior receives innervation from the brachial plexus. The long thoracic nerve arises from C5 through C7 and passes between the middle and posterior scalene neck muscles to descend to the level of the serratus anterior.

Subclavius. As the name implies, the subclavius muscle courses under the clavicle, originating from the inferior margin of the clavicle and taking an oblique and medial course to insert into the superior surface of the first rib at the chondral margin. It is a small muscle that may elevate the first rib during inspiration (see Figure 3-31). The subclavius muscle is innervated by branches from the brachial plexus, with fibers originating in the fifth and sixth spinal nerves.

Levator Scapulae. The levator scapulae provides neck support secondarily as a result of its function as an elevator of the scapula. This muscle originates from the transverse processes of C1 through C4, and courses down to insert into the medial border of the scapula (see Figure 3-33). As with the scaleni anterior, middle, and posterior, the levator scapulae derives its innervation from C3 through C5 of the cervical plexus.

Muscle: Subclavius
Origin: Inferior surface of clavicle
Course: Oblique and medial
Insertion: Superior surface of rib 1 at chondral margin
Innervation: Brachial plexus, lateral branch, from spinal nerves 5 and 6
Function: Elevates rib 1

Muscle: Levator scapulae
Origin: Transverse processes of C1–C4
Course: Down
Insertion: Medial border of scapula
Innervation: C3–C5 of cervical plexus
Function: Neck support; elevates scapula

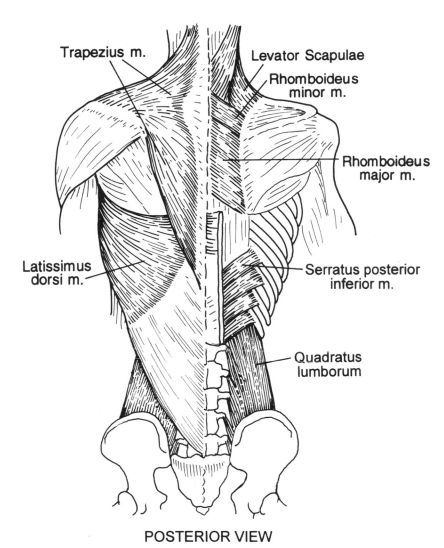

Trapezius m.

Levator Scapulae

Rhomboideus
minor m.

Rhomboideus
major m.

Latissimus
dorsi m.

Serratus posterior
inferior m.

Quadratus
lumborum

POSTERIOR VIEW

Figure 3-33. Accessory muscles
of respiration: Trapezius, levator
scapulae, rhomboideus minor,
rhomboideus major, serratus
posterior inferior, latissimus dorsi,
and quadratus lumborum.

Rhomboideus Major and Minor. The rhomboids (major and minor) lie
deep to the trapezius, originating on the spinous processes of T2 through
T5 (**rhomboideus** major) and from C7 and T1. The muscle courses
down and laterally to insert into the medial border of the scapula.

rhomboideus: L., rhombus,
parallelogram + oid, like

Muscle:	Rhomboideus major
Origin:	Spinous processes of T2–T5
Course:	Down and laterally in
Insertion:	Scapula
Innervation:	Spinal C5 from the dorsal scapular nerve of upper root of brachial plexus
Function:	Stabilizes shoulder girdle

Muscle: Rhomboideus minor
Origin: Spinous processes of C7 and T1
Course: Down and laterally in
Insertion: Medial border of scapula
Innervation: Spinal C5 from the dorsal scapular nerve of upper root of brachial plexus
Function: Stabilizes shoulder girdle

Primary speech function of the rhomboids is the support they provide for the upper body, and especially for the stability of the shoulder girdle.

The rhomboids receive their innervation from the dorsal scapular nerves off the upper roots of the brachial plexus (C5). The dorsal scapular nerves pass through the scaleni medius muscles in their course to the rhomboids.

Trapezius. The trapezius muscle (see Figure 3-33) is a massive muscle making up the superficial upper back and neck, originating along the spinous processes of C2 to T12 by means of fascial connection. (The trapezius is alternately considered a muscle of the arm.) Fibers of this muscle fan laterally to insert into the acromion of the scapula and the superior surface of the clavicle. Contraction of this muscle clearly plays a significant role in elongation of the neck and head control.

For respiration, support is the primary function of the back muscles, although there are distinct respiratory actions, as we shall see. Back muscles provide a dense, multilayered mass of tissue that supports and protects (see Figure 3-33). Perhaps the most important function of these muscles is maintenance of the delicate balance of upper body mobility in the face of required stability. To experience this firsthand, place both feet firmly on the ground while sitting erect, and then with one arm reach straight ahead as if you were about to grasp an object beyond your reach. You will need to overextend when you do this, but if you attend to the musculature of your head, shoulders, and back you will feel them tighten to support your efforts. Your shoulders rotated while the rest of your trunk remained relatively stable.

In the "big picture" of trunk control, the following back muscles are key players. The trapezius and levator scapulae muscles serve clear

Muscle: Trapezius
Origin: Spinous processes of C2 to T12
Course: Fan laterally
Insertion: Acromion of scapula and superior surface of clavicle
Innervation: XI accessory, spinal branch arising from spinal cord in the regions of C2–C4 or C5
Function: Elongates neck; controls head

roles in neck elongation and head stability. Support for the vertebral column is provided by the trapezius muscle and the rhomboideus major and minor muscles, and this support serves respiration in a stabilizing manner. The clinical note on development of motor coordination emphasizes the importance of trunk and back muscle development from an oral motor perspective.

In summary:

- The **diaphragm** is an exceptionally important muscle of inspiration, but there are many **accessory muscles** of inspiration and expiration that also serve respiration.
- Generally, muscles of the thorax and neck that elevate the rib cage serve some accessory function for inspiration.

In the next section we shall see that muscles that compress the abdomen or pull down on the rib cage also assist in expiration.

 ## MUSCLES OF FORCED EXPIRATION

Active expiration requires that musculature act on the lungs indirectly to "squeeze" the air out of them. This is achieved in two ways. Because the rib cage expands in two dimensions, it makes sense that it will contract in two dimensions as well. The front-to-back dimension was expanded by elevating the rib cage, so active expiration should reduce that dimension.

Trunk Stability and Upper Body Mobility

Infant motor development is a process of increasing control of motor function; control of speech musculature depends in large part on development of trunk control. It is truly a "for want of a nail" situation: If the infant fails to develop neck extension, he or she will not develop the ability to balance neck extensors and flexors. Once the normal extension begins development, the back muscles begin to come under control, again becoming dynamically opposed by anterior trunk muscles. Through this interplay of antagonist and agonist trunk muscles, the infant develops the ability to rotate the trunk, stabilize the hips (and, of course, walk), and elevate the head in preparation for speech. Once controlled, the infant can rotate his or her head, differentiate mandible movement from head movement, and tongue from mandible. All the while, the infant is developing the dynamic aspects of laryngeal control that permit the larynx to descend and the tongue to become controlled.

This is a long-winded way of saying that, although the respiratory function of the back muscles is open to question, absence of controlled use of the back muscles most certainly would result in loss of head control for speech, reduced differentiation of facial muscle control, and lack of laryngeal control due to the tonic imbalance of the torso. The indirect effects of muscle imbalance within the trunk are innumerable.

The rib cage can be pulled down by the **internal intercostal muscles**, the **innermost intercostal muscles**, and the **transversus thoracis muscles**. The second means of expanding the volume of the thorax is by increasing the vertical dimension through contraction of the diaphragm. If you examine Figure 3-34, you will realize that relaxing the diaphragm will return it to its original position, and no farther. If you note the viscera of the abdomen below the diaphragm, you can now see the second means of active expiration. If I could somehow squeeze my abdominal viscera, I could push my diaphragm higher into the thorax and remove more air from my lungs. (If you want to verify this, have one of your friends perform a gentle version of the Heimlich maneuver on you and feel what happens with your respiration. Do you inhale or exhale?)

We can forcefully expire by contracting the muscles of the abdominal region which, in turn, squeeze the abdomen and force the viscera upward, reducing the size of the thorax. This is half of the reason you "get the wind knocked out of you" when someone punches you in the abdomen. See the clinical note for the other half of that story.

If you examine the abdominal muscles of expiration (see Figure 3-35), you will see that they are very much like a cummerbund, wrapping the abdomen into a neat package in the front, side, and back. The major players in the anterior abdomen are the **internal** and **external oblique abdominis**, **transversus abdominis**, and the **rectus abdominis** muscles.

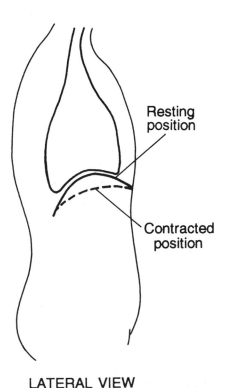

Resting position

Contracted position

LATERAL VIEW

Figure 3-34. Lateral-view schematic of diaphragm showing relative position during inspiration and passive expiration.

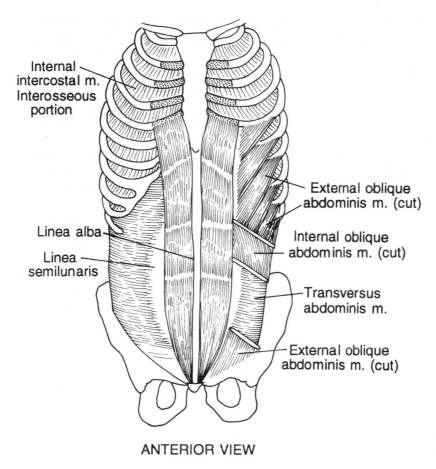

Internal intercostal m. Interosseous portion

Linea alba

Linea semilunaris

External oblique abdominis m. (cut)

Internal oblique abdominis m. (cut)

Transversus abdominis m.

External oblique abdominis m. (cut)

ANTERIOR VIEW

Figure 3-35. Accessory muscles of expiration and landmarks of the abdominal aponeurosis.

In the posterior abdomen, the **quadratus lumborum**, **iliacus**, and **psoas major** and **minor** muscles serve this function. If you look at the drawing in Figure 3-33, you will see that the **latissimus dorsi** muscles also could support expiratory efforts, although studies on function of this muscle are contradictory.

The layers of abdominal muscles provide excellent support for the rib cage during lifting and other body gestures. These gestures virtually demand fixing the thorax by inflating the lungs and closing off the vocal folds, and the abdominal muscles help to compress the viscera while simultaneously stabilizing the thorax.

Muscles of Thorax: Anterior/Lateral Thoracic Muscles

- **Internal Intercostal (Interosseous Portion)**
- **Transversus Thoracis**
- **Innermost Intercostals**

Internal Intercostal, Interosseous Portion

The interosseous portion of the internal intercostal muscles are significant contributors to forced expiration. As seen earlier in Figure 3-28, the internal intercostal muscles are pervasive throughout the thorax, originating on the superior margin of each rib (except the first) and running up and medially to insert into the inferior surface of the rib above. They are conspicuously absent in the posterior aspect of the rib cage near the vertebral column. Because the external intercostal muscles run at nearly right angles to the internals, these two sets of muscles provide significant support for the rib cage and protection of the ribs within, as well as maintenance of rib spacing.

The course of the muscle fibers is constant from front to side to back of rib cage. That is, while the fibers run up and medially in front, that translates to running up and laterally in the dorsal aspect.

Muscle:	Internal intercostal, interosseous portion
Origin:	Inferior margin of ribs 1–11
Course:	Down and lateral
Insertion:	Superior surface of the rib below
Innervation:	Intercostal nerves: thoracic intercostal nerves arising from T2–T6 and thoracoabdominal intercostal nerves from T7–T11
Function:	Depresses ribs 1–11

"Getting the Wind Knocked Out of You"

Why *does* a blow to the abdomen result in your losing your breath? Logic would dictate that you would lose your breath from being hit in the chest. You'll want to take a look at the explanation of reflexive responses in the clinical note entitled "paradoxical respiration," because that will go a long way toward explaining this response as well.

Try to recall what happened the last time you had the wind knocked out of you. First, something hit you in the abdominal region. From what you now know, forced expiration depends in large part on contraction of the abdominal muscles which, in turn, causes the abdominal viscera to push the diaphragm upward and pull the thorax down. Both of these gestures remove air forcefully from the lungs.

This doesn't explain the agony you experience trying to regain respiratory control, however. When those muscles are passively moved (stretched), a stretch reflex is triggered which causes the muscle to contract involuntarily. This contraction only serves to increase the effect of being hit in the abdomen, because it is essentially doing the same thing the blunt force did. To cap it all off, your attempts to contract your diaphragm add a third dimension to the problem, because that will once again stretch the abdominal muscles and promote further reflexive contraction.

Use of Abdominal Muscles for Childbirth and Other Biological Functions

Nature has a way of getting the most use out of structures, and the abdominal muscles are a great example. Clearly, we use the abdominal muscles to force air out of the lungs, but they serve several other worthwhile (even vital) functions. The act of vomiting requires evacuation of the gastric or even intestinal contents, and to do so necessitates forceful action from the abdominal muscles.

A less obvious function has to do with thoracic fixation. For the muscles of the upper body to gain maximum benefit, they need to pull against a relatively rigid structure. The thorax can be made rigid by inhaling and then capturing the respiratory charge by closing off the vocal folds. To demonstrate this process, take a very deep breath and hold it: To do this you must close off the folds.

This thoracic fixing gives leverage for lifting (notice that you "grunt" when you lift because some air is escaping past the vocal folds, having been compressed by your muscular effort), but it also gives leverage in the other direction. Defecation requires compression of the abdomen and an increase in abdominal pressure, and that process also demands thoracic fixation for efficiency.

Another not immediately obvious use for abdominal muscle contraction is childbirth. Although you may not have experienced this directly, you are probably familiar with midwives, nurses, or partners whose job it was to remind the mother-to-be to "breathe." It shouldn't surprise you to realize that the mother has not forgotten this basic biological process, but rather she has an overwhelming, deep biological urge to "push." The person who is doing the cheerleading is doing so to keep her from closing the vocal folds (you can't breathe through closed folds), because if she does, she will start pushing the baby to its new home before the time has come.

Besides their support function, the internal intercostal muscles also provide a mechanism for depressing the rib cage. As you can see from the schematic of Figure 3-36, when the interosseous portion of the internal intercostals contracts and shortens, the direction of movement is down, and the expanded rib cage will become smaller.

Innermost Intercostal (Intercostales Intimi)

The innermost intercostal muscles are the deepest of the intercostal muscles, with fibers coursing between the inner costal surfaces of adjacent ribs. The innermost intercostals have a course parallel to those of the internal intercostal muscles, with fibers originating on the surface of the lower rib and coursing obliquely up to insert into the rib above. As with the external intercostals, the innermost intercostals are absent in the chondral portion of the ribs, becoming apparent first in the lateral aspect of the inner rib cage. The innermost intercostals are absent near the vertebral and sternal borders, are sparse in the upper thorax, and parallel

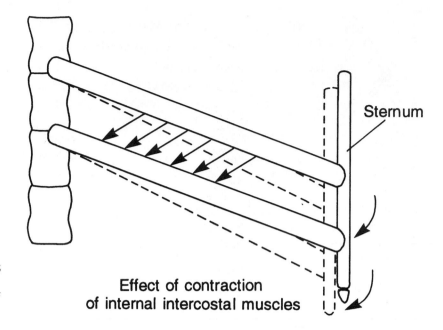

Figure 3-36. Effects of contraction of the interosseous portion of the internal intercostals is to pull the rib cage down, thereby decreasing the volume of the lungs.

Sternum

Effect of contraction
of internal intercostal muscles

Muscle:	Innermost intercostal
Origin:	Inferior margin of ribs 1–11; sparse or absent in superior thorax
Course:	Down and lateral
Insertion:	Superior surface of the rib below
Innervation:	Intercostal nerves: thoracic intercostal nerves arising from T2–T6 and thoracoabdominal intercostal nerves from T7–T11
Function:	Depresses ribs 1–11

the morphology of the internal intercostals. The innermost intercostals interdigitate with the subcostal muscles (see Figure 3-29).

Transversus Thoracis

As the name implies, the transversus thoracis (transverse muscles of thorax) muscles are found on the inner surface of the rib cage. The muscles originate on the margin of the sternum, with fibers coursing to the inner chondral surface of ribs 2 through 6. As seen in Figure 3-37, contraction of the muscles would tend to resist elevation of the rib cage and decrease the volume of the thoracic cavity.

Considering the proximity of the transversus thoracis to the internal intercostal muscles, it should not be surprising that the transversus thoracis takes its innervation from the same source (the thoracic intercostal nerves), as well as from the thoracoabdominal intercostal nerves and subcostal nerves derived from T2 through T1 spinal nerves.

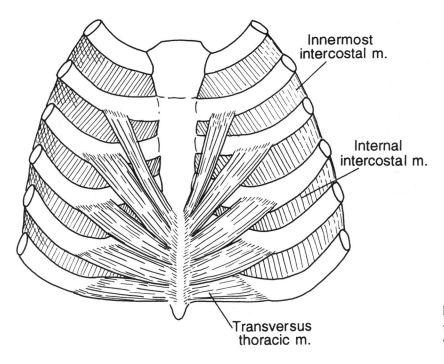

Innermost intercostal m.

Internal intercostal m.

Transversus thoracic m.

Figure 3-37. Transversus thoracis muscles, as viewed from within the thoracic cavity.

Muscle:	Transversus thoracis
Origin:	Inner thoracic lateral margin of sternum
Course:	Laterally
Insertion:	Inner chondral surface of ribs 2–6
Innervation:	Thoracic intercostal nerves and thoracoabdominal intercostal nerves and subcostal nerves derived from T2–T12 spinal nerves
Function:	Depresses rib cage

Posterior Thoracic Muscles

- **Subcostals**
- **Serratus Posterior Inferior**

Subcostals. The subcostals are widely variable, but generally take a course parallel to the internal intercostals and thus have the potential of serving expiration. The subcostals are found on the inner posterior wall of the thorax. Unlike the intercostal muscles, the subcostals may span more than one rib. The subcostals are innervated by the intercostal nerves of the thorax, arising from the ventral rami of the spinal nerves.

Serratus Posterior Inferior. The serratus posterior inferior muscles originate on the spinous processes of the T11, T12, and L1 through L3 and course up and laterally to insert into the lower margin of the lower five

Muscle:	Subcostal
Origin:	Inner posterior thorax; sparse in upper thorax; from inner surface of rib near angle
Course:	Down and lateral
Insertion:	Inner surface of second or third rib below
Innervation:	Intercostal nerves of thorax, arising from the ventral rami of the spinal nerves
Function:	Depresses thorax

Muscle:	Serratus posterior inferior
Origin:	Spinous processes of T11, T12, L1–L3
Course:	Up and laterally
Insertion:	Lower margin of ribs 7–12
Innervation:	Intercostal nerves from T9–T11 and subcostal nerve from T12
Function:	Contraction of these muscles tends to pull the rib cage down, supporting expiratory effort

ribs. Contraction of these muscles would tend to pull the rib cage down, supporting expiratory effort (see Figure 3-33). The serratus posterior inferiors derive their innervation from the intercostal nerves arising from T9 through T11 and subcostal nerve from T12.

Abdominal Muscles of Expiration

If you examine once again the skeleton in Figure 3-3 and imagine placing muscles in the region between the rib cage and the pelvis, you will realize that there are few places from which muscles can originate. Clearly one could attach muscles to the rib cage, vertebral column, and the pelvic girdle to give some structure, but that leaves a great deal of territory to cover in the anterior aspect. To deal with this, nature has provided a tendinous structure, the **abdominal aponeurosis**. Let us examine how it is constructed and then attach some muscles to that structure.

Figure 3-38 shows a schematic representation of the abdominal aponeurosis from the front, as well as in transverse section.

linea alba: *L., white line*

The **linea alba** (white line) runs from the xiphoid process to the pubic symphysis, forming the midline structure for muscular attachment. As the linea alba progresses laterally, it differentiates into two sheets of aponeurosis, between which is placed the rectus abdominis. This aponeurotic wrapping comes back together to form another band of tendon, the linea semilunaris. This tendon once again divides, but this time into three sheets of aponeurosis, which will provide us with a way to attach three more muscles to this structure.

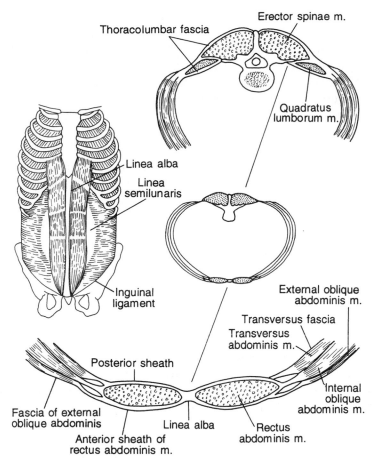

Thoracolumbar fascia

Erector spinae m.

Quadratus lumborum m.

Linea alba

Linea semilunaris

Inguinal ligament

External oblique abdominis m.

Transversus fascia

Transversus abdominis m.

Posterior sheath

Internal oblique abdominis m.

Fascia of external oblique abdominis

Linea alba

Rectus abdominis m.

Anterior sheath of rectus abdominis m.

TRANSVERSE VIEW

A

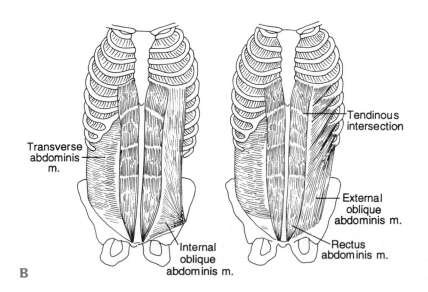

Transverse abdominis m.

Tendinous intersection

Internal oblique abdominis m.

External oblique abdominis m.

Rectus abdominis m.

B

Figure 3-38. A. Schematic of abdominal aponeurosis as related to the abdominal muscles of expiration. **B.** Transversus abdominis, rectus abdominis, external and internal oblique abdominis muscles.

In the posterior aspect, the fascia of the abdominal muscles join to form the lumbodorsal fascia. This structure provides the union of three abdominal muscles (**transversus abdominis**, **internal** and **external oblique abdominis**) with the vertebral column.

The external oblique aponeurosis communicates directly with the fascia covering the rectus **abdominis**, forming a continuous layer of connective tissue from the linea alba to the external oblique muscle.

▶ **rectus:** *L., straight (not crooked)*

Anterolateral Abdominal Muscles

The abdominal muscles of expiration function by compression of the abdominal viscera. This compression function is not only useful in respiration, but also aids in defecation, vomiting, and childbirth (with vocal folds tightly adducted).

- **Transversus Abdominis**
- **Internal Oblique Abdominis**
- **External Oblique Abdominis**
- **Rectus Abdominis**

Transversus Abdominis. Lateral to the rectus abdominis is the transversus abdominis, the deepest of the anterior abdominal muscles (Figure 3-38). The transversus abdominis runs laterally (that is, horizontally; hence the name "transversus"), originating in the posterior aspect at the vertebral column via the thoracolumbar fascia of the abdominal aponeurosis. Its anterior attachment is to the transversus abdominis aponeurosis, as well as to the inner surface of ribs 6 through 12, interdigitating at that point with the fibers of the diaphragm. Its inferior-most attachment is at the pubis. Contraction of the transversus will significantly reduce the volume of the abdomen.

Palpation of Rib Cage

Although you cannot palpate your diaphragm, you can identify its margins easily enough. First, find your xiphoid process. This point marks part of the origin of the rectus abdominis, but the diaphragm attaches on the inner surface. Place your fingers on the xiphoid process and the muscle below, and breathe deeply in and out once. You can feel the rectus abdominis being stretched during inspiration. Now place the fingers of both hands at the bottom of the rib cage on either side of the sternum, so that your fingers are pressing into your abdominal muscles. Breathe out as deeply as you can and hold that posture while you bend slightly forward. Your fingers are marking the margin of the diaphragm, although you are palpating abdominal muscles.

Bring your fingers up to feel your ribs. Place your fingers between the ribs, with your little finger of each hand on the abdominal muscles below the rib cage. Breathe in a couple of times and feel the abdominal muscles first draw in and then tighten up as you reach maximum inspiration. Feel your rib cage elevate as you do this.

Muscle:	Transversus abdominis
Origin:	Posterior abdominal wall at the vertebral column via the thoracolumbar fascia of the abdominal aponeurosis
Course:	Lateral
Insertion:	Transversus abdominis aponeurosis and inner surface of ribs 6–12, interdigitating at that point with the fibers of the diaphragm; inferior-most attachment is at the pubis
Innervation:	Thoracic and lumbar nerves from the lower spinal intercostal nerves (derived from T7–T12) and first lumbar nerve, iliohypogastric and ilioinguinal branches
Function:	Compresses abdomen

Innervation of the transversus abdominis is via the thoracic and lumbar nerves, specifically from the lower thoracoabdominal nerves (derived from T7 to T12) and first lumbar nerve, iliohypogastric and ilioinguinal branches.

Internal Oblique Abdominis. The internal oblique abdominis is located between the external oblique abdominis and the transversus abdominis. As seen in Figure 3-38, this muscle fans out from its origin on the inguinal ligament and iliac crest to the cartilaginous portion of the lower ribs and the portion of the abdominal aponeurosis lateral to the rectus abdominis, and thus, by association, inserts into the linea alba. Contraction of the internal oblique abdominis assists in rotation of the trunk, if unilaterally contracted, or flexion of the trunk, when bilaterally contracted.

External Oblique Abdominis. The external oblique abdominis are the most superficial of the abdominal muscles, as well as the largest of this group. These muscles originate along the osseous portion of the lower seven ribs, and fan downward to insert into the iliac crest, inguinal ligament, and abdominal aponeurosis (lateral to rectus abdominis). Bilateral contraction of these muscles will flex the vertebral column, while unilateral contraction results in trunk rotation. This muscle receives innervation from the thoracoabdominal nerve arising from T7 through T11 and subcostal nerve from T12.

Muscle:	Internal oblique abdominis
Origin:	Inguinal ligament and iliac crest
Course:	Fans medially
Insertion:	Cartilaginous portion of lower ribs and the portion of the abdominal aponeurosis lateral to the rectus abdominis
Innervation:	Thoracic and lumbar nerves from the lower spinal intercostal nerves (derived from T7–T12) and first lumbar nerve, iliohypogastric and ilioinguinal branches
Function:	Rotates trunk; flexes trunk; compresses abdomen

Muscle: External oblique abdominis

Origin: Osseous portion of the lower seven ribs

Course: Fan downward

Insertion: Iliac crest, inguinal ligament, and abdominal aponeurosis lateral to rectus abdominis

Innervation: Thoracoabdominal nerve arising from T7–T11 and subcostal nerve from T12

Function: Bilateral contraction flexes vertebral column and compresses abdomen; unilateral contraction results in trunk rotation

Rectus Abdominis. The rectus abdominis muscles are the prominent midline muscles of the abdominal region with origin at the pubis inferiorly (see Figure 3-35). The superior attachment is at the xiphoid process of sternum and the cartilage of the last true rib (rib 7) and the false ribs.

These "rectangular" (i.e., rectus) muscles are manifest in a series of four or five segments connected (and separated) by tendinous slips known as *tendinous intersections*. Use of this muscle is a "must" if you are to succeed at your sit-ups, because contraction will draw the chest closer to the knees, and the only way to do this is to bend. Contraction of the rectus abdominis also compresses the abdominal contents.

Innervation derives from T7 through T11 intercostal nerves (thoracoabdominal) and subcostal nerve from T12. This segmented muscle is segmentally innervated as well: T7 supplies the uppermost segment, T8 supplies the next section, and the remaining portions are supplied by T9.

Muscle: Rectus abdominis

Origin: Originates as four or five segments at pubis inferiorly

Course: Up to segment border

Insertion: Xiphoid process of sternum and the cartilage of ribs 5–7, lower ribs

Innervation: T7–T11 intercostal nerves (thoracoabdominal), subcostal nerve from T12 (T7 supplies upper segment, T8 supplies the second, T9 supplies remainder)

Function: Flexion of vertebral column

Posterior Abdominal Muscles

- **Quadratus Lumborum**

Quadratus Lumborum. As seen in Figure 3-38A, the quadratus lumborum is located in the dorsal aspect of the abdominal wall. These muscles

Muscle:	Quadratus lumborum
Origin:	Iliac crest
Course:	Fan up and in
Insertion:	Transverse processes of the lumbar vertebrae and inferior border of rib 12
Innervation:	Thoracic nerve T12 and L1–L4 lumbar nerves
Function:	Bilateral contraction fixes abdominal wall in support of abdominal compression

originate along the iliac crest and fan up and in to insert into the transverse processes of the lumbar vertebrae and inferior border of the twelfth rib. Unilateral contraction of the quadratus lumborum would assist lateral movement of the trunk, whereas bilateral contraction would fix the abdominal wall in support of abdominal compression. This muscle is innervated by the lowest thoracic nerve T12 and the first four lumbar nerves.

There are other abdominal muscles supporting abdominal wall fixation. The psoas major and minor muscles and the iliacus may provide abdominal support for forced expiration.

Muscles of Upper Limb
- **Latissimus Dorsi**

Latissimus Dorsi. The **latissimus** dorsi muscle (see Figure 3-33) originates from the lumbar, sacral, and lower thoracic vertebrae, with fibers rising fanlike to insert into the humerus. Its primary role is in movement of the upper extremity, but it clearly plays a role in chest stability, and perhaps expiration. With the arm immobilized, contraction of the latissimus dorsi would stabilize the posterior abdominal wall, performing a function similar to that of quadratus lumborum.

latissimus: *L., widest*

Innervation for this muscle arises from the posterior branch of the brachial plexus. Fibers from the regions C6 through C8 of this plexus form the long subscapular nerve to supply the latissimus dorsi.

Muscle:	Latissimus dorsi
Origin:	Lumbar, sacral, and lower thoracic vertebrae
Course:	Up fanlike
Insertion:	Humerus
Innervation:	Brachial plexus, posterior branch; fibers from the regions C6–C8 form the long subscapular nerve
Function:	For respiration, stabilizes posterior abdominal wall for expiration

In summary:

- To inflate the lungs, you need to expand the cavity that holds them so air can rush in.
- To do this, you can either increase the long dimension fairly easily by contracting the **diaphragm**, or you can elevate the rib cage with just a little bit more effort.
- **Forced expiration** reverses this process by pulling the thorax down and in and by forcing the diaphragm higher into the thorax.
- The next chapter will provide insight into these processes.

 ## CHAPTER SUMMARY

Respiration is the process of gas exchange between an organism and its environment. The **rib cage**, made up of the **spinal column** and **ribs**, houses the lungs, which are the primary mechanisms of respiration. By means of the cartilaginous **trachea** and **bronchial tree**, air is brought into the lungs for gas exchange within the minute **alveolar sacs**. Oxygen enters the blood and carbon dioxide is removed, to be expired.

Air is drawn into the lungs through muscular effort. The **diaphragm**, placed between the thorax and abdomen, contracts during inspiration. The **lungs** expand when the diaphragm contracts, drawn by **pleurae** linked through surface tension and negative pressure. When lungs expand, the air pressure within the lungs becomes negative with respect to the outside atmosphere, and **Boyle's law** dictates that air will flow from the region of higher pressure to fill the lungs. **Accessory muscles** also provide added expansion of the rib cage for further inspiration.

Expiration may occur passively, through the forces of **torque**, **elasticity**, and **gravity** acting on the ribs and rib cage. It also may be **forced**, utilizing muscles of the abdomen and those that depress the rib cage to evacuate the lungs.

STUDY QUESTIONS

1. _____ is defined as force distributed over area.

2. _____ pressure causes air to enter a chamber that has expanded until the pressure is equalized.

3. How many of each of the following vertebrae are there?

_____ cervical vertebrae

_____ thoracic vertebrae

_____ lumbar vertebrae

_____ sacral vertebrae (fused)

4. On the figure below, identify the landmarks indicated.

a. _____ process

b. _____ process

c. _____

d. _____ facet

e. _____ facet

f. _____ facet

g. _____ foramen

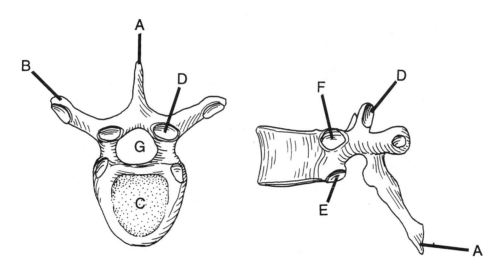

5. The _____ passes through the vertebral foramen.

6. On the figure below, identify the landmarks indicated.

a. _____ (bone)

b. _____ (bone)

c. _____ (bone)

d. _____

e. _____

f. _____

g. _____

h. _____ (bone)

i. _____ (bone)

j. _____

k. _____

l. _____

m. _____

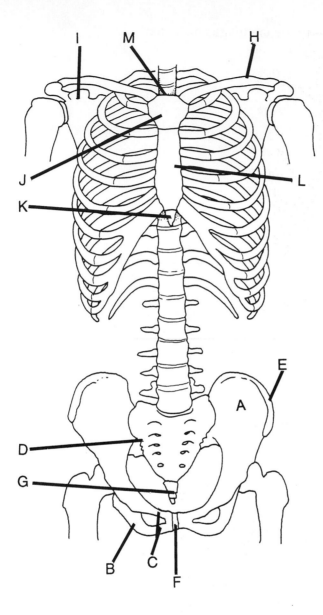

7. On the figure below, identify the landmarks indicated.

a. _____

b. _____

c. _____

d. _____

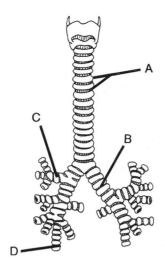

8. On the figure below, identify the muscles and structures indicated.

a. _____

b. _____

c. _____

d. _____

e. _____

f. _____ ligament

g. _____

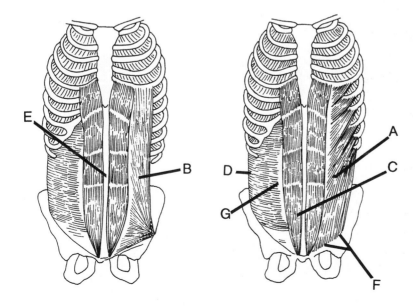

9. On the figure below, identify the muscles indicated.

a. _____

b. _____

c. _____

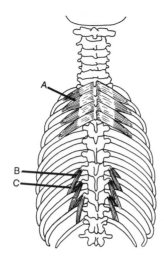

10. Identify the muscles indicated below.

a. _____

b. _____

c. _____

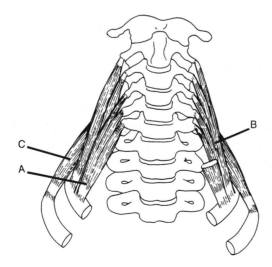

11. Identify the muscles and portions of muscles indicated below.

    a. _____

    b. _____ head

    c. _____ head

    d. _____

    e. _____

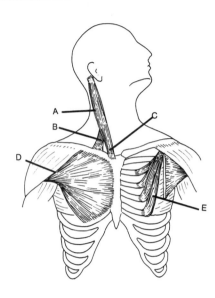

12. Contraction of the diaphragm increases the _____ dimension of the thorax.

13. Contraction of the accessory muscles of inspiration increases the _____ dimension of the thorax.

14. Contraction of the muscles of expiration _____ the volume of the thorax.

15. Emphysema results in a breakdown of the alveolar wall, resulting in enlargement of alveolar clusters and consequent enlargement of the thorax known as "barrel chest." The result of this is that the diaphragm is pulled down at rest. Discuss the implications of the muscular action of inspiration and expiration for this altered system.

STUDY QUESTION ANSWERS

1. <u>PRESSURE</u> is defined as force distributed over area.

2. <u>NEGATIVE</u> pressure causes air to enter a chamber that has expanded until the pressure is equalized.

3. How many of each of the following vertebrae are there?

<u>7</u> cervical vertebrae

<u>12</u> thoracic vertebrae

<u>5</u> lumbar vertebrae

<u>5</u> sacral vertebrae (fused)

4. On the figure below, identify the landmarks indicated.

   a. <u>SPINOUS</u> process
   b. <u>TRANSVERSE</u> process
   c. <u>CORPUS</u>
   d. <u>SUPERIOR ARTICULAR</u> facet
   e. <u>INFERIOR COSTAL</u> facet
   f. <u>SUPERIOR COSTAL</u> facet
   g. <u>VERTEBRAL</u> foramen

5. The <u>SPINAL CORD</u> passes through the vertebral foramen.

6. On the figure below, identify the landmarks indicated.

   a. <u>ILIUM</u>
   b. <u>ISCHIUM</u>
   c. <u>PUBIC BONE</u>
   d. <u>SACRUM</u>
   e. <u>ILIAC CREST</u>
   f. <u>PUBIC SYMPHYSIS</u>
   g. <u>COCCYX</u>
   h. <u>CLAVICLE</u>
   i. <u>SCAPULA</u>
   j. <u>MANUBRIUM STERNI</u>
   k. <u>XIPHOID</u> or <u>ENSIFORM PROCESS</u>
   l. <u>CORPUS STERNI</u>
   m. <u>STERNAL NOTCH</u>

7. On the figure below, identify the landmarks indicated.

   a. <u>TRACHEA</u>
   b. <u>MAINSTEM BRONCHUS</u>
   c. <u>SECONDARY BRONCHUS</u>
   d. <u>TERTIARY BRONCHUS</u>

8. On the figure below, identify the muscles and structures indicated.

   a. <u>EXTERNAL OBLIQUE ABDOMINIS</u>
   b. <u>INTERNAL OBLIQUE ABDOMINIS</u>
   c. <u>RECTUS ABDOMINIS</u>
   d. <u>TRANSVERSUS ABDOMINIS</u>
   e. <u>LINEA ALBA</u>

    f. INGUINAL LIGAMENT

    g. LINEA SEMILUNARIS

9. On the figure below, identify the muscles indicated.

    a. SERRATUS POSTERIOR SUPERIOR

    b. LEVATOR COSTARUM BREVIS

    c. LEVATOR COSTARUM LONGIS

10. Identify the muscles indicated below.

    a. SCALENUS ANTERIOR

    b. SCALENUS MEDIUS

    c. SCALENUS POSTERIOR

11. Identify the muscles and portions of muscles indicated below.

    a. STERNOCLEIDOMASTOID

    b. CLAVICULAR head

    c. STERNAL head

    d. PECTORALIS MAJOR

    e. PECTORALIS MINOR

12. Contraction of the diaphragm increases the VERTICAL dimension of the thorax.

13. Contraction of the accessory muscles of inspiration increases the TRANSVERSE dimension of the thorax.

14. Contraction of the muscles of expiration DECREASES the volume of the thorax.

15. In advanced emphysema, the diaphragm is pulled down and stretched relatively flat by the flaring of the rib cage. In normal inspiration, contraction of the diaphragm causes the central tendon to pull down, causing air to enter the lungs (Boyle's law dictates that a drop in alveolar pressure will cause air to flow into the lungs). When the diaphragm of an individual with advanced emphysema contracts, it pulls the ribs closer together because they were distended by the "barrel chest." As a result, the alveoli are compressed, causing an increase in alveolar pressure and causing air to leave the lungs. Thus, the inspiratory gesture of the diaphragm causes expiration. The single inspiratory avenue left to the individual is to elevate the sternum and clavicle using clavicular breathing.

REFERENCES

Arnott, W. M. (1973). *Disorders of the respiratory system.* Oxford, England: Blackwell Scientific Publications.

Baken, R., & Cavallo, S. (1981). Prephonatory chest wall posturing. *Folia phoniatrica, 33,* 193–202.

Baken, R. J., & Orlikoff, R. F. (1999). *Clinical measurement of speech and voice* (2nd ed.). San Diego, CA: Singular Publishing Group.

Basmajian, J. V. (1975). *Grant's method of anatomy.* Baltimore: Williams & Wilkins.

Bateman, H. E., & Mason, R. M. (1984). *Applied anatomy and physiology of the speech and hearing mechanism.* Springfield, IL: Charles C. Thomas.

Beck, E. W. (1982). *Mosby's atlas of functional human anatomy.* St. Louis, MO: C. V. Mosby Company.

Bergman, R., Thompson, S., & Afifi, A. (1984). *A catalog of human variation.* Baltimore: Urban & Schwarzenberg.

Bly, L. (1994). *Motor skills acquisition in the first year.* Tucson, AZ: Therapy Skill Builders.

Burrows, B., Knudson, R. J., & Kettel, L. J. (1975). *Respiratory insufficiency.* Chicago: Year Book Medical Publishers.

Campbell, E., Agostoni, E., & Davis, J. (1970). *The respiratory muscles, mechanics, and neural control.* Philadelphia: W. B. Saunders.

Chusid, J. G. (1985). *Correlative neuroanatomy and functional neurology* (17th ed.). Los Altos, CA: Lange Medical Publications.

Des Jardins, T., & Burton, G. G. (2001). *Clinical manifestation and assessment of respiratory disease.* Chicago: Mosby, Inc.

Fenn, W. O., & Rahn, H. O. (Eds.). (1964). *Handbook of physiology, respiration* (Vol. 1, §3, pp. 387–409). Washington, DC: American Physiological Society; Baltimore: Williams & Wilkins.

Ganong, W. F. (2003). *Review of medical physiology* (21st ed.). New York: McGraw-Hill/Appleton & Lange.

Gordon, M. S. (1972). *Animal physiology: Principles and adaptations.* New York: Macmillan.

Gosling, J. A., Harris, P. F., Humpherson, J. R., Whitmore, I., & Willan, P. L. T. (1985). *Atlas of human anatomy.* Philadelphia: J. B. Lippincott.

Gray, H., Bannister, L. H., Berry, M. M., & Williams, P. L. (Eds.). (1995). *Gray's anatomy.* London: Churchill Livingstone.

Grobler, N. J. (1977). *Textbook of clinical anatomy* (Vol. 1). Amsterdam: Elsevier Scientific.

Hlastala, M. P., & Berger, A. J. (1996). *Physiology of respiration.* New York: Oxford University Press.

Kahane, J. (1982). Anatomy and physiology of the organs of the peripheral speech mechanism. In N. Lass, L. McReynolds, J. Northern, & D. Yoder (Eds.), *Speech, language, and hearing. Vol. 1: Normal processes* (pp. 109–155). Philadelphia: W. B. Saunders.

Kahane, J. C., & Folkins, J. F. (1984). *Atlas of speech and hearing anatomy.* Columbus, OH: Charles E. Merrill.

Kao, F. F. (1972). *An introduction to respiratory physiology.* Amsterdam: Exerpta Medica.

Kaplan, H. (1960). *Anatomy and physiology of speech.* New York: McGraw-Hill.

Kent, R. D. (1997). *The speech sciences.* San Diego, CA: Singular Publishing Group.

Kuehn, D. P., Lemme, M. L., & Baumgartner, J. M. (1989). *Neural bases of speech, hearing, and language.* Boston: Little, Brown.

Langley, M. B., & Lombardino, L. J. (1991). *Neurodevelopmental strategies for managing communication disorders in children with severe motor dysfunction.* Austin, TX: Pro-Ed.

Lee, D. H. K. (1972). *Environmental factors in respiratory disease.* New York: Academic Press.

Logemann, J. (1998). *Evaluation and treatment of swallowing disorders* (2nd ed.). Austin, TX: Pro-Ed.

MacKay, L. E., Chapman, P. E., & Morgan, A. S. (1997). *Maximizing brain injury recovery.* Gaithersburg, MD: Aspen Publishers.

McMinn, R. M. H., Hutchings, R. T., & Logan, B. M. (1994). *Color atlas of head and neck anatomy.* London: Mosby-Wolfe.

Miller, A. D., Bianchi, A. L., & Bishop, B. P. (1997). *Neural control of the respiratory muscles.* Boca Raton, FL: CRC Press.

Mohr, J. P. (1989). *Manual of clinical problems in neurology.* Boston: Little, Brown.

Moser, K. M., & Spragg, R. G. (1982). *Respiratory emergencies.* St. Louis, MO: C. V. Mosby.

Murray, J. F. (1976). *The normal lung: The basis for diagnosis and treatment of pulmonary disease.* Philadelphia: W. B. Saunders.

Netter, F. H. (1983a). *The CIBA collection of medical illustrations. Vol. 1. Nervous system: Part I. Anatomy and physiology.* West Caldwell, NJ: CIBA Pharmaceutical Company.

Netter, F. H. (1983b). *The CIBA Collection of medical illustrations. Vol. 1. Nervous system: Part II. Neurologic and neuromuscular disorders.* West Caldwell, NJ: CIBA Pharmaceutical Company.

Netter, F. H. (1997). *Atlas of human anatomy.* Los Angeles: Icon Learning Systems.

Pace, W. R. (1970). *Pulmonary physiology.* Philadelphia: F. A. Davis.

Peters, R. M. (1969). *The mechanical basis of respiration.* Boston: Little, Brown.

Rohen, J. W., Yokochi, C., Lutjen-Drecoll, E., & Romrell, L. J. (2002). *Color atlas of anatomy* (5th ed.). Philadelphia: Williams & Wilkins.

Rosse, C., Gaddum-Rosse, P., & Rosse, G. (1997). *Hollinshead's textbook of anatomy.* Philadelphia: Lippincott-Raven.

Schamberger, R. C. (2000). Chest wall deformities. In T. W. Shields, J. LoCicero, III, & R. B. Ponn (Eds.). *General thoracic surgery* (5th ed., pp. 535–569). Philadelphia: Lippincott/ Williams & Wilkins.

Scott, J. R., Disaia, P. J., Hammond, C. B., & Spellacy, W. N. (1994). *Danforth's obstetrics and gynecology* (7th ed.). Philadelphia: J. B. Lippincott.

Snell, R. S. (1978). *Gross anatomy dissector.* Boston: Little, Brown.

Spector, W. S. (1956). *Handbook of biological data.* Philadelphia: W. B. Saunders Company.

Taylor, A. (1960). The contribution of the intercostal muscles to the effort of respiration in man. *Journal of Physiology, 151,* 390.

Tokizane, T., Kawamata, K., & Tokizane, H. (1952). Electromyographic studies on the human respiratory muscles. *Japan Journal of Physiology, 2,* 232.

Twietmeyer, A., & McCracken, T. D., (1992). *Coloring Guide to regional human anatomy* (2nd ed.). Philadelphia: Lea & Febiger.

Williams, P., & Warrick, R. (1980). *Gray's anatomy* (36th British ed.). Philadelphia: W. B. Saunders.

Zemlin, W. R. (1988). *Speech and hearing science. Anatomy and physiology.* Englewood Cliffs, NJ: Prentice-Hall.

CHAPTER 4

Physiology of Respiration

Respiration requires muscular effort, and the degree to which an individual can successfully control that musculature determines, in large part, the efficiency of respiration itself. Respiratory function (physiology) changes as we exercise, age, or suffer setbacks in health. Considering its importance in speech, it is no wonder that as the respiratory system goes, so goes communication.

We are capable of both quiet and forced inspiration. There is a parallel to this in expiration, because we are capable of **passive** and **active expiration**. In passive expiration, we let the forces inherent to the tissues restore the system to a resting position after inspiration. In active expiration, we use muscular effort to push just a little farther. Let us examine these forces.

The process of expiration is one of eliminating the waste products of respiration. Attend to your own respiratory cycle to learn an important aspect of quiet expiration. Close your eyes while you breathe in and out 10 times, quietly and in a relaxed manner. Pay particular attention to the area of your body around your diaphragm, including your rib cage and your abdomen.

What you experienced is the active contraction of the diaphragm, followed by a simple relaxing of the musculature. You actively contract to breathe in, and then simply let nature take its course for expiration. It is a little like blowing up a balloon, because the balloon will deflate as soon as you let go of your grip. The forces on the balloon that cause it to lose its air are among those that cause your lungs to deflate. The forces we need to talk about are torque, elasticity, and gravity.

Torquing refers to twisting of a shaft while not permitting one end to move. Take hold of a wooden or plastic ruler by the end in one hand, and grasp the other end of the ruler and twist it around its long axis (see Figure 4-1). When you perform this task, you will feel the ruler return to its original state, the product of a restoring force contributed by the elastic qualities of the material from which the ruler is made.

Think of the "shafts" we could twist in the rib cage. If you thought "rib," you thought right. Unfortunately, bone is quite inelastic. There is

torque: *rotary twisting*

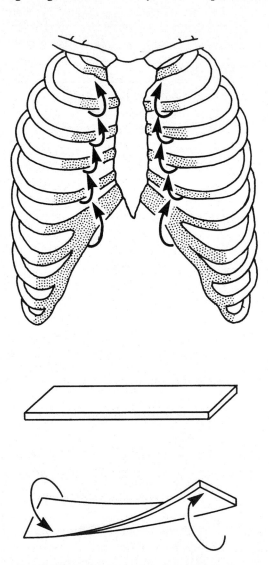

Figure 4-1. When the rib cage is elevated, the cartilage of the ribs is torqued or twisted. Because cartilage is highly elastic, it tends to return to its original condition after being torqued.

an elastic element, however, in the chondral portion of the rib cage, and we do take advantage of that.

Return to our earlier discussion of the elevation of the rib cage by the external intercostals and the accessory muscles of inspiration to recognize that, when those muscles pull the rib cage up and out, the anterior cartilage comes under some torquing strain. As soon as you stop pulling on the rib cage, it will return to its original shape, thanks to restoring forces of the elastic cartilage, and that will cause the rib cage to drop back down to its resting state. Restoring forces are those that tend to return a body to its original position.

You will recall that the lungs are highly elastic, porous tissue. They are spongelike, and when they are compressed will tend to expand as soon as the compression is released. Likewise, if you were to grab a sponge by its edges and stretch it, the sponge would tend to return to its original shape and size when you release it.

You can think of the lungs as small sponges in a large bottle. The lungs truly will not fill up that "bottle" of the chest cavity when they are left to their own devices (i.e., permitted to deflate to their natural resting condition). In the adult body, the lungs are actually stretched beyond their resting position, but this is not so with the infant.

During early development, the lungs completely fill the thorax, so that they are not stretched to fit the relaxed rib cage. As the child develops, the rib cage grows faster than the lungs, and the pleural linings and increased negative intrapleural pressure provide a means for the lungs to be stretched out to fill that space.

The result of this stretching is greatly increased capacity and reserve in adults, but not in infants. Because the thorax and lungs are the same size, infants must breathe two to three times as often as an adult for adequate respiration. The adult's lungs are stretched out and never are completely compressed, so there is always a reserve of air within them that is not at the moment undergoing gas exchange.

Upon increasing the thorax size, the lungs expand just as if you had grabbed them and stretched them out. When the muscles that are expanding the rib cage relax, the lungs tend to return to their original shape and size. In addition, when you inhale and your abdomen protrudes, you are stretching the abdominal muscles. Relaxing the inspiratory process will let those muscles return to their original length. That is, the abdominal muscles will tend to push your abdominal viscera back in and force the diaphragm up.

A final force acting in support of passive expiration is gravity. When standing or sitting erect, gravity acts on the ribs to pull them back after they have been expanded through the effort of the accessory muscles of inspiration. Gravity also works in favor of maximizing your overall capacity, because it pulls the abdominal viscera down, leaving more room for the lungs. We will talk about this more because body position becomes a significant issue in the efficiency of respiration.

To summarize:

- We are capable of quiet respiration as well as forced inspiration and expiration.
- Expiration may be passive, driven by the forces of **torque**, **elasticity**, and **gravity**.
- We also may use muscles that reduce the size of the thorax by compressing the **abdomen** or pulling the rib cage down, and this will force air out of the lungs beyond that which is expired in passive expiration.

THE MEASUREMENT OF RESPIRATION

The quantity of air processed through respiration is dictated primarily by bodily needs, and speech physiology operates within these limits. We will discuss respiration in terms of rate of flow in respiration, volume and lung capacities, and pressure.

Respiratory flow, volumes, and capacities are measured using a spirometer (see Figure 4-2). The classical wet spirometer consists of a

spirometer: *device used to measure respiratory volume*

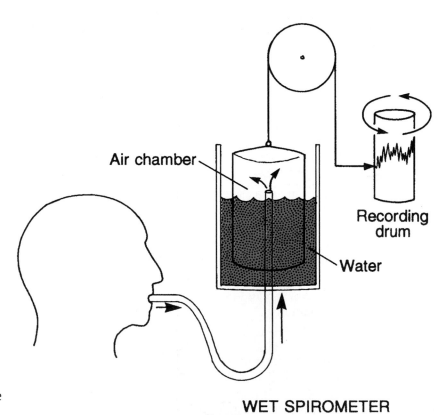

Figure 4-2. Wet spirometer used to measure lung volumes. When the individual exhales into the tube, gas entering the air chamber displaces the water, causing the chamber to rise. These changes are charted on the recording drum.

Air chamber

Recording drum

Water

WET SPIROMETER

tube connected to a container opened at the bottom. This container is placed inside another container that is full of water.

To measure lung volume, an individual breathes into the tube, causing a volume of water to be displaced. The amount of water displaced gives an accurate estimate of the air that was required to displace it. (We are ignoring the *pressure* required to raise the container and the effort involved in this process.)

The classic U-tube manometer is one means of measuring pressure, as shown in Figure 4-3. A subject is asked to place the tube in his or her mouth and to blow. The force of the subject's expiration is exerted on a column of water that rises as a result. The more force the person uses, the higher the column rises. We can measure the effects of that force in inches or in centimeters of water (barometric pressure is often reported in millimeters of mercury, which refers to how many millimeters of mercury were elevated by the pressure). Because water is considerably less dense than mercury, the same amount of pressure will elevate a column of water much higher than a similar column of mercury. For this reason we measure the rather small pressures of respiration with the water standard, although mechanical and electronic techniques are eliminating the water-filled tube.

Breathing requires that gas be exchanged on an ongoing basis. The body has specific needs that must be met continually, so we will need to discuss respiration in terms of the **rate of flow** of air in and out of the

manometer: *device for measuring air pressure differences*

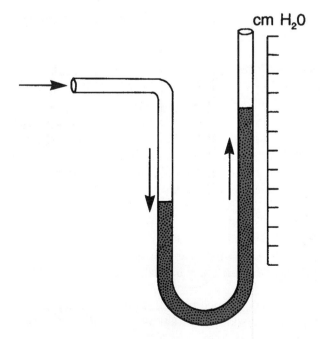

Figure 4-3. U-tube manometer for measurement of respiratory pressure.

lungs (measured as cubic centimeters per second or minute). We also need to speak of the quantities or **volumes** that are involved in this gas exchange (measured in liters [L], milliliters [ml], cubic centimeters [cc], or on occasion, cubic inches).

RESPIRATION FOR LIFE

What is obvious is that respiration is vital. If you are a swimmer, you probably remember staying under water a little too long, discovering the limits of your respiratory system and the panic you felt when you reached those limits. Let us examine why those limits are reached and how we work within those limits for speech.

When you breathe in, you are engaged in a simple gesture with very complex results. The goal of respiration, of course, is oxygenation of blood and elimination of carbon dioxide.

The basic process of gas exchange has four stages: ventilation, distribution, perfusion, and diffusion. **Ventilation** refers to the actual movement of air in the conducting respiratory pathway. This air is distributed to the 300 million alveoli where the oxygen-poor vascular supply from the right pulmonary artery is **perfused** to the 6 billion capillaries that supply those alveoli. The actual gas exchange across the alveolar-capillary membrane is referred to as **diffusion**.

The ventilation process is a direct function of the action of the diaphragm and muscles of respiration. As discussed earlier, contraction of muscles of inspiration causes expansion of the alveoli that results in a negative alveolar pressure and air being drawn into the lungs. Understanding the pressure changes in this process is critical.

ventilation: *air inhaled per unit time*

perfusion: *migration of fluid through a barrier*

diffusion: *migration or mixing of one material (e.g., liquid) through another*

Effects of Turbulence on Respiration

When lungs expand, pressure throughout the system drops as a result of expansion of the alveoli. Air courses through the large-diameter conducting bronchi, which, being comprised of cartilage, resist the negative pressure to collapse. In healthy lungs this results in relatively low resistance and laminar flow of air. Some slight turbulence occurs at bifurcations such as where the trachea splits to become the right and left mainstem bronchi, but generally the flow is unimpeded. This is not a trivial notion, because even a small irregularity in the airway (such as mucus) greatly increases the resistance to airflow and also the difficulty of respiration.

The expiratory act is performed by decreasing the thoracic volume, thus eliminating carbon dioxide. Gas that was previously captive in the blood has migrated across the alveolar-capillary membrane and is expelled into the atmosphere.

Respiratory Cycle

During quiet respiration, adults will complete between 12 and 18 cycles of respiration per minute (see Figure 4-4). A cycle of respiration is defined as one inspiration and one expiration. This quiet breathing pattern, known as **quiet tidal respiration** (because it can be visualized as a tidal flow of air into and out of the lungs) involves about 500 ml (1/2 liter) of air with each cycle. (You can visualize this by imagining a two-liter bottle of soda being one quarter full.) A quick calculation will reveal that we process something on the order of 6,000 to 8,000 ml (6–8 liters) of air every minute. (The volume of air involved in one minute of respiration is referred to as the minute volume.)

Because these values are based on quiet, sedentary breathing, it will not surprise you to learn that they increase during strenuous work.

> **minute volume:** *the volume of air exchanged by an organism in one minute*

Turbulence and Respiration

The respiratory passageway offers relatively low resistance to airflow, a fact that works in favor of efficient respiration with little effort. As resistance to airflow increases, the effort required to draw air into the lungs increases as well, which causes rapid fatigue. You may remember the exhaustion you felt the last time you had a respiratory infection that caused excessive secretions in your respiratory passageway. Part of the fatigue you felt was the product of the turbulence produced by the mucus within the passageway. The extra drag caused by these elements has to be overcome to keep the body oxygenated, and the muscles of respiration have to work overtime to do the task.

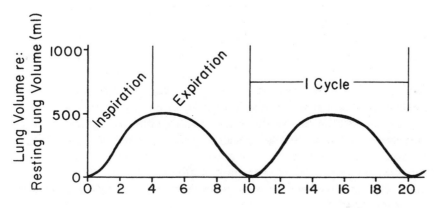

Figure 4-4. Volume display of two cycles of quiet respiration.

Table 4-1. Respiratory volume as a function of work intensity.

	WORK INTENSITY (Kg m/min)	VENTILATION (ml)
Female	600	3470
	900	5060
Male	900	4190
	1200	5520
	1500	7090

Source: Data from *Handbook of Biological Data* by W. S. Spector, 1956, p. 352. Philadelphia: W. B. Saunders.

An adult male will increase his oxygen requirements by a factor of 20 on increasing work output. As you can see in Table 4-1, as work increases the ventilation requirements are met by increased respiratory flow.

Developmental Processes in Respiration

There are developmental effects on respiration as well. The lungs undergo a great deal of prenatal development, as seen in Figure 4-5. By the time the infant is born, the cartilaginous conducting airway is complete, although the number of alveoli will increase from about 25 million at birth to more than 300 million by 8 years of age. We retain that number throughout life.

The conducting airways will grow steadily in diameter and length until thorax growth is complete, although the thorax will expand to a greater degree than the lungs. As the thorax expands, the lungs are stretched to fill the cavity, a fact that helps to explain two differences between adults and children. As we mentioned earlier, adults breathe between 12 and 18 times per minute while at rest, but the newborn will breathe an average of 40 to 70 cycles per minute. By 5 years, the child is down to about 25 breaths per minute (bpm), and that number drops to about 20 bpm at 15 years of age (see Table 4-2). The adult has a considerable volume of air that is never expelled, but the infant does not have this reserve. In essence, the thorax expands during growth and development and stretches the lungs beyond their natural volume.

As a result of this expansion, there is a volume of air in the adult lung that cannot be expelled (residual volume), and this volume helps to account for the reserve capacity of adults relative to infants. Infant lungs have yet to undergo the proliferation of the alveoli seen during childhood, and infants thus must breathe more frequently to meet their metabolic needs.

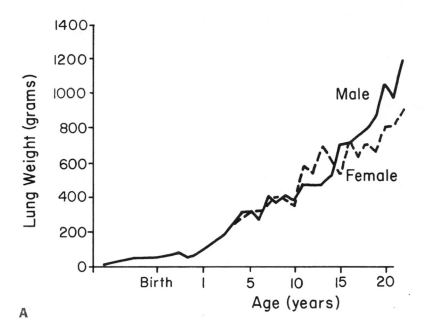

A

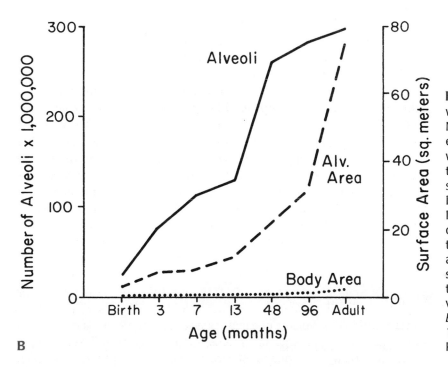

B

Figure 4-5. **A.** Changes in lung weight as a function of age. Notice that males and females are essentially equivalent in lung weight until puberty, at which time the increased thoracic cavity size of the male is reflected in larger lung weight. **B.** Changes in lung tissue with age. The number of alveoli increases radically through the fourth year of life, and the total alveolar area stabilizes around puberty when the thorax approximates its volume. (Data from *Handbook of Biological Data* by W. S. Spector, 1956, pp. 162, 176–180, 353. Philadelphia: W. B. Saunders.)

Table 4-2. Respiration rate in breaths per minute (BPM) as a function of age.

AGE	RESPIRATION RATE
Newborn	60 bpm
1 year	30 bpm
2 years	25 bpm
3 years	24 bpm
5 years	20 bpm
10 years	18 bpm
15 years	18 bpm
20 years	17 bpm

Source: Data from *Physical Growth and Development* by J. Valadian & D. Porter, 1977. p. 311. Boston: Little, Brown, & Co.

VOLUMES AND CAPACITIES

Respiration is the product of a number of forces and structures, and for us to make sense of them, we need to define some volumes and capacities of the lungs. When we refer to volumes, we are partitioning off the respiratory system so that we may get an accurate estimate of the amount of air each compartment can hold. (For instance, we could conceivably talk about the volume of a single alveolus, which is about 250 microns in diameter, or about 250 millionths of a meter, although this might not produce a very useful number.) We also might speak of **capacities**, which are more functional units. Capacities refer to combinations of volumes that express physiological limits. Volumes are discrete, whereas capacities represent functional combinations of volumes.

Both volumes and capacities are measured in milliliters (ml, which are thousandths of a liter) or cubic centimeters (cc, which is another name for the same thing). To get an idea of what these volumes and capacities really amount to, look at a two-liter soda bottle for a reference. One liter is 1,000 ml, which is also 1,000 cc.

There are five volumes that we should consider. Refer to Tables 4-3 and 4-4, as well as Figure 4-6 as we discuss these.

Table 4-3. Respiratory volumes and capacities.

VOLUMES
Tidal Volume (TV): Volume of air exchanged in one cycle of respiration.
Inspiratory Reserve Volume (IRV): Volume of air that can be inhaled after a tidal inspiration.

(continues)

Table 4-3. *(continued)*

Expiratory Reserve Volume (ERV): Volume of air that can be expired following passive, tidal expiration. Also known as **resting lung volume**.

Residual Volume (RV): Volume of air remaining in the lungs after a maximum exhalation.

Dead Air: Volume of air within the conducting passageways that cannot be involved in gas exchange (included as a component of residual volume).

CAPACITIES

Vital Capacity (VC): The volume of air that can be inhaled following a maximal exhalation; includes inspiratory reserve volume, tidal volume, and expiratory reserve volume (VC = IRV + TV + ERV).

Functional Residual Capacity (FRC): The volume of air in the body at the end of passive exhalation; includes expiratory reserve and residual volumes (FRC = ERV + RV).

Total Lung Capacity (TLC): The sum of inspiratory reserve volume, tidal volume, expiratory reserve volume, and residual volume (TLC = IC + FRC).

Inspiratory Capacity (IC): The maximum inspiratory volume possible after tidal expiration (IC = TV + IRV).

Table 4-4. Typical respiratory volumes and capacities in adults.

VOLUME/CAPACITY	MALES (in cc)	FEMALES (in cc)	AVERAGE (in cc)
Resting tidal volume	600	450	525
Inspiratory reserve volume	3000	1950	2475
Expiratory reserve volume	1200	800	1000
Residual volume	1200	1000	1100
Vital capacity	4800	3200	4000
Functional residual capacity	2400	2700	2550
Inspiratory capacity	3600	2400	3000
Total lung capacity	6000	4200	5100

Note: Volumes and capacities vary as a function of body size, gender, age, and body height. These volumes represent approximate values for healthy adults between 20 and 30 years of age. Vital capacity is estimated by accounting for age (in years) and height (in cm):

Males:
VC in ml = [27.63 − (0.112 @ age in yrs.)] @ ht. in cm

Females:
VC in ml = [21.78 − (0.101 @ age in yrs.)] @ ht. in cm

Source: Data from Baldwin, Cournand, and Richards (1948) as cited in *An Introduction to Respiratory Physiology* by F. F. Kao, 1972, p. 39. Amsterdam: Excerpta Medica; and *The Mechanical Basis of Respiration* by R. M. Peters, 1969, p. 49. Boston: Little, Brown.

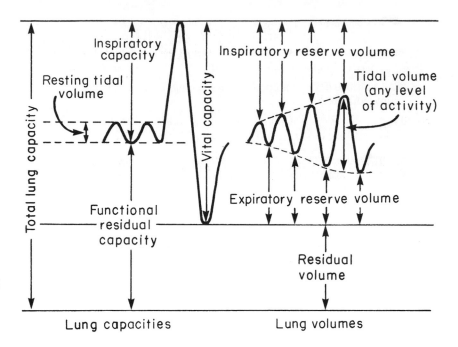

Figure 4-6. Lung volumes and capacities as displayed on a spirogram. (Modified from Pappenheimer et al., 1950.)

Volumes

Tidal Volume (TV)

The volume of air that we breathe in during a respiratory cycle is referred to as tidal volume (TV). The definition of tidal volume makes precise measurement difficult, because tidal volume varies as a function of physical exertion, body size, and age. **Quiet tidal volume** (tidal volume at rest) has an average for adult males of around 600 cc, and for adult females of approximately 450 cc. This works out to an average of 525 cc for adults, or approximately one-quarter of the volume of a 2-liter soda bottle every 5 seconds. You will fill up three of these bottles every minute. As shown in Table 4-1, tidal volume increases markedly as effort increases.

> **quiet tidal volume:** *the volume of air exchanged during one cycle of quiet respiration*

Inspiratory Reserve Volume (IRV)

The second volume of interest is **inspiratory reserve volume** (IRV). Inspiratory reserve volume is the volume that can be inhaled after a tidal inspiration. It is the volume of air that is in reserve for use *beyond* the volume you would breathe in tidally.

> **inspiratory reserve volume:** *the volume of air that can be inhaled after a tidal inspiration*

To help remember the inspiratory reserve volume, do the following exercise. Sit quietly and breathe in and out tidally until you become aware of your breath, and tag each breath mentally with the word "in" and "out." After a few "outs and ins," stop breathing at the end of one of your inspirations. This is the peak of the tidal inspiration. Instead of breathing out (which is what you want to do), breathe in as deeply as you can. The amount you inspired after you stopped is the inspiratory reserve volume, and if you are an average adult the volume is about 2,475 cc (2.475 liters).

Expiratory Reserve Volume (ERV)

The parallel volume for expiration is the **expiratory reserve volume** (ERV). Expiratory reserve volume is the amount of air that can be expired following passive, tidal expiration. To experience this, breathe as you did before, but this time stop before you breathe in following expiration. (This point is easier to reach, because you can just *relax* your muscles and air will flow out without muscular effort.) Expire as completely as you can and you will have experienced expiratory reserve volume: It is the amount of air you could expire after that tidal expiration, amounting to about 1,000 cc (1.0 liters). This volume is also referred to as **resting lung volume** (RLV), because it is the volume present in the resting lungs after a passive exhalation.

expiratory reserve volume: *the volume of air that can be expired after a tidal expiration*

Residual Volume (RV)

A third volume of interest is **residual volume** (RV), the volume remaining in the lungs after a maximum exhalation. No matter how forcefully or completely you exhale, there is a volume of air (about 1.1 liters) that cannot be eliminated. This volume exists because the lungs are stretched as a result of the relatively expanded thorax, so it should come as no shock to know that it is not present in the newborn. You might think of it as an acquired space. By the way, this does not mean we do not use that air, but rather simply that it is a *volume* that is not eliminated during expiration.

residual volume: *in respiration, the volume of air remaining after a maximum exhalation*

Dead Space Air

We have accommodated the major volumes, but we must deal with the volume that cannot be involved in gas exchange. The air in the conducting passageways cannot be involved in gas exchange because there are no alveoli there. You will recall that the conducting passageways of the lungs are constructed largely of cartilage, and the upper respiratory passageway (consisting of the mouth, pharynx, and nose) certainly does not have alveoli. The volume that cannot undergo gas exchange in the lungs is referred to as **dead space air** and in the adult has a volume of about 150 cc. This varies also with age and weight, but is approximately equal (in cubic centimeters) to your weight in pounds. The volume associated with dead air is included in residual volume, because both are volumes associated with air that cannot be expelled.

The concept of dead air (and its importance) may become more vivid if you consider a swimmer using a tube or snorkel to breathe from underwater. This person has additional dead air associated with the

dead space air: *the air within the conducting passageways that cannot be involved in gas exchange*

tube: the longer the tube is, the greater the volume he or she will have to inhale to pull air from the surface into the lungs. In pathological conditions, the term *dead space* takes on new meaning. In the healthy individual, **anatomical dead space** (that described previously) and **physiological dead space** (wasted ventilation) are the same. As you found in the clinical notes of Chapter 3, there are conditions that contribute to increased physiological dead space; that is, pathological conditions of the respiratory system often result in wastage of respiratory effort and air.

Capacities

The volumes may be combined in a number of ways to characterize physiological needs. The following four capacities are useful combinations of volumes.

Vital Capacity (VC)

vital capacity: *the total volume of air that can be inspired after a maximal expiration*

Of the capacities, **vital capacity** (VC) is the most often cited in speech and hearing literature, because it represents the capacity available for speech (see Figure 4-7). Vital capacity is the combination of inspiratory reserve volume, expiratory reserve volume, and tidal volume. That is, vital capacity represents the total volume of air that can be inspired after a maximal expiration. Because VC = IRV + ERV + TV, you can quickly see that it is approximately 4,000 cc in the average adult.

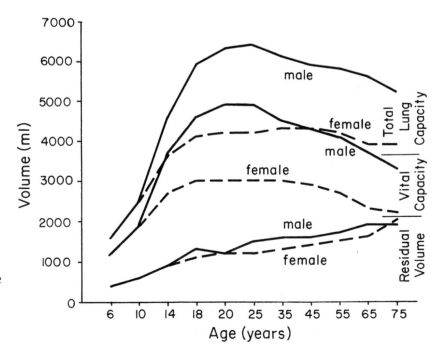

Figure 4-7. Vital capacity, total lung volume, and residual volume as a function of age. (Data from *Handbook of Biological Data* by W. S. Spector, 1956, p. 267. Philadelphia: W. B. Saunders.)

Functional Residual Capacity (FRC)

Functional residual capacity is the volume of air remaining in the body after a passive exhalation (FRC = ERV + RV). In the average adult this comes to approximately 2,100 ml.

Total Lung Capacity (TLC)

Total lung capacity is the sum of all the volumes (TLC = TV + IRV + ERV + RV), totaling approximately 5,100 cc. Note that this is different from vital capacity. Vital capacity represents the volume of air that is involved in a maximal respiratory cycle, whereas total lung capacity includes the residual volume. Residual volume serves as a buffer in respiration because it is not immediately involved in interaction with the environment. Oxygen-rich air is diluted by mixing with the air of the residual volume, so that during brief periods of fluctuating air quality relatively constant oxygenation will occur.

Inspiratory Capacity (IC)

Inspiratory capacity is the maximum inspiratory volume possible after tidal expiration (IC = TV + IRV). This refers to the capacity of the lungs for inspiration and represents a volume of approximately 3,000 cc in the adult.

▶ **functional residual capacity:** *the volume of air remaining in the body after a passive exhalation*

▶ **total lung capacity:** *sum of tidal volume, inspiratory reserve volume, expiratory reserve volume, and residual volume*

▶ **inspiratory capacity:** *the maximum inspiratory volume possible after tidal expiration*

Effect of Age on Volumes

As we age, tissue changes. What may surprise you is how rapidly your body reaches its peak function and how steady is the decline. Vital capacity is a function of body weight, age, and height, the relationship for which can be expressed mathematically, as seen in Table 4-4 and graphically in Figure 4-8.

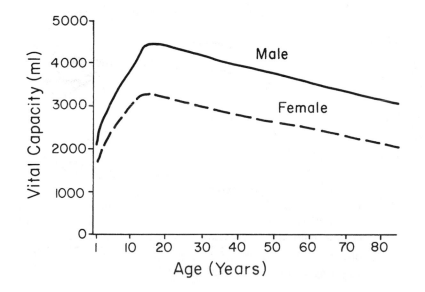

Figure 4-8. Mathematically predicted changes in vital capacity based on age and gender.

Muscle Weakness and Respiratory Function

Many disease processes reduce respiratory function, which can have a remarkable effect on other systems as well. Diseases that produce spasticity can result in paradoxical contraction of the muscles of expiration during inspiration, greatly reducing the vital capacity. Likewise, individuals may have flaccid or hypotonic (low muscle tone) conditions that reduce the degree and strength of muscular contraction. When you think about it, it makes perfect sense that diseases that cause muscular weakness could reduce respiratory capacity.

We have a warning about quickly blaming the muscles of respiration for apparent deficits in vital capacity, inspiratory reserve, and so on. When testing an individual with a compromised motor system, remember that you are testing the whole system. An individual being evaluated in our clinic had weak labial muscles that caused her to have difficulty getting an adequate seal around the mouthpiece of the spirometer. Readings from this instrument thus implied respiratory deficit when, in reality, the problem was with the articulatory system! Likewise, insufficiency of the soft palate, whether due to muscular weakness or inadequate tissue, can result in nasal leakage during respiratory tasks. Again, this can masquerade as an apparent respiratory deficit.

What you can see from the formula is that as age increases, vital capacity decreases by about 100 ml per year in adulthood. What the formula also shows is that vital capacity increases steadily with body growth up to about 20 years of age, holds constant through about age 25, and then begins a steady decline. Females have smaller vital capacity throughout the life span, as reflected in the height element (males tend to be taller).

To summarize:

- There are several volumes and capacities of importance to your study of respiration.
- The volumes, which indicate arbitrary partitioning of the respiratory system, include **tidal volume** (the volume inspired and expired in a cycle of respiration), **inspiratory reserve volume** (air inspired beyond tidal inspiration), **expiratory reserve volume** (air expired beyond tidal expiration), **residual volume** (air that remains in the lungs after maximal expiration), and **dead air**, which cannot undergo gas exchange.
- **Vital capacity** is the volume of air that can be inspired after a maximal expiration.
- **Functional residual capacity** is the air that remains in the body after passive exhalation. **Total lung capacity** represents the sum of all lung volumes.
- **Inspiratory capacity** is the volume that can be inspired from resting lung volume.

PRESSURES OF THE RESPIRATORY SYSTEM

There are five specific pressures for nonspeech and speech function: alveolar pressure, intrapleural pressure, subglottal pressure, intraoral pressure, and atmospheric pressure (see Figure 4-9).

The atmosphere surrounding the earth and within which we live exerts a sizable pressure on the surface of the earth (760 mm Hg; that is, sufficient pressure to elevate a column of mercury 760 mm against gravity). Atmospheric pressure (P_{atm}) is actually our reference in discussions of the respiratory system, and so we will treat it as a constant zero against which to compare respiratory pressures. **Intraoral** or **mouth pressure** (P_m) is the pressure that could be measured within the mouth,

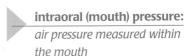

intraoral (mouth) pressure:
air pressure measured within the mouth

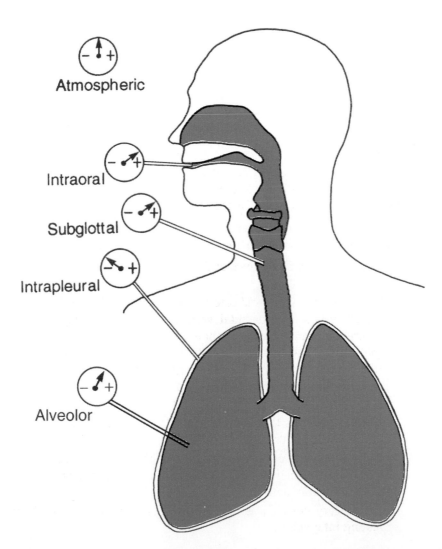

Figure 4-9. Pressures of respiration.

while **subglottal pressure** (P_s) is the pressure below the vocal folds. During normal respiration with open vocal folds, we may assume that subglottal and intraoral pressures are equal to alveolar pressure. As we progress more deeply into the lungs we can estimate alveolar or pulmonic pressure (P_{al}), the pressure that is present within the individual alveolus. If we were to measure the pressure in the space between parietal and visceral pleurae, we would refer to it as pleural or intrapleural pressure (P_{pl}). Intrapleural pressure will be negative throughout respiration. Recall that the lungs, inner thorax, and diaphragm are wrapped in a continuous sheet of pleural lining. When one attempts to separate the visceral from parietal pleurae, a negative pressure ensues.

These pressure measurements are all made relative to atmospheric pressure. When we refer to alveolar pressure as being, for instance, +3 cm H_2O, it means that, through muscular effort, we have generated +3 cm H_2O pressure above and beyond atmospheric pressure (if atmospheric pressure is 1,033 cm H_2O, then alveolar pressure would be 1,036 cm H_2O). Alveolar pressure may be indirectly estimated by having an individual swallow a balloon and breathe. Because the trachea and esophagus are adjacent structures sharing a common wall, the pressure changes within the trachea produce analogous changes in the esophagus, and a pressure sensor in the balloon will permit estimation of air pressure below the level of the vocal folds.

When the diaphragm is pulled down for tidal inspiration, Boyle's law predicts that alveolar pressure will drop (relative to atmospheric pressure). In quiet tidal inspiration, alveolar pressure drops to approximately –2 cm H_2O until equalized with atmospheric pressure by inspiratory flow. Likewise, during expiration the pressure at the alveolar level becomes positive with reference to the atmosphere, increasing to +2 cm H_2O during quiet tidal breathing.

alveolar (pulmonic) pressure: *air pressure measured at the level of the alveolus in the lung*

pleural (intrapleural) pressure: *pressure measured within the pleural linings of the lungs*

Pneumothorax

Pneumothorax (*pneumo* = air) is aggregation of air in the pleural space between the lungs and the chest wall, with subsequent loss of the negative intrapleural pressure. It can arise through one of several means, but the product is always a "collapsed" lung. In "open" pneumothorax, air is introduced into the space through a breach of the thoracic wall, typically by means of a puncture wound (knife wound, automobile accident, etc.). When air is introduced into the intrapleural space, the result is a loss of the constant negative intrapleural pressure. Recall that this pressure maintains the close bond between the visceral pleural lining of the lungs and that of the inner thorax. When that bond is broken by the open wound, the lungs will collapse. This collapse arises from the fact that the lungs are in a state of constant outward distension, arising from the difference between adult thorax size and adult lung size (see detail on lung development).

The work of expanding the lungs is one of overcoming resistance within the lungs. Surface active solution (surfactant) is released into the alveoli, and the result is greatly reduced surface tension. This decrease in surface tension reduces the pressure of the alveoli, keeps the alveolar walls from collapsing, and keeps fluid from the capillaries from being drawn into the lungs. Pressure in any network of tubes is greatest at the source of the pressure, which in this case is at the alveolus.

The surfactant protects the alveolus, promotes airflow, and facilitates effort-free respiration. During respiration, oxygen is perfused into the bloodstream across the alveolar-capillary membrane barrier, while carbon dioxide is perfused into the alveolus.

When the thorax is expanded by means of muscular contraction, the lungs will follow faithfully, with the result being expansion of the 300 million alveoli within the lungs. Secreting cells within the visceral pleurae release a lubricating fluid into the potential space between visceral and parietal pleurae, and presence of this fluid lets the lungs and thorax make a slippery, extremely low-friction contact. At the alveolus, oxygen and carbon dioxide diffuse across the alveolus-capillary boundary.

Figure 4-10 is a schematic of the alveolar pressures, intrapleural pressures, and change in lung volume during quiet tidal breathing. This figure shows the alveolar pressure associated with a cycle of respiration and illustrates what we have been talking about. We have placed markers on it so that we can discuss how this whole system of pressures and flows works together.

Look at the "volume" portion of the graph and notice the periodic function representing tidal respiration. Point "A" represents the peak of that inspiration, and the lungs have about 500 cc of air in them. Point "B" represents the end of the expiratory cycle, where our subject has relaxed the forces of inspiration and the lungs have passively evacuated down to resting lung volume. The point marked "C" represents the electromyographic activity recorded from the diaphragm as it contracts. Putting these two traces together, you can see that as the diaphragm contracts the volume increases to a maximum, ending at the point where the diaphragmatic contraction is complete.

Let us examine the "flow" component. As the diaphragm contracts, there is a fairly steady flow of air into the lungs (measured in ml/second), indicated by point "D." When the inspiratory effort is completed (represented by termination of the diaphragm activity and the volume peak at "A"), the flow of air into the lungs ends. That is, when the diaphragm stops contracting, air stops flowing. As air leaves the lungs, the airflow becomes negative at point "E" (which simply means that the air is flowing in a different direction). Alveolar pressure goes positive (+2 cm H_2O) during expiration, a change you would predict from what you know about the lungs. To summarize, when the diaphragm contracts, airflow begins and is fairly steady throughout the inspiratory cycle; when the diaphragm stops contracting, the air begins to flow out of the lungs.

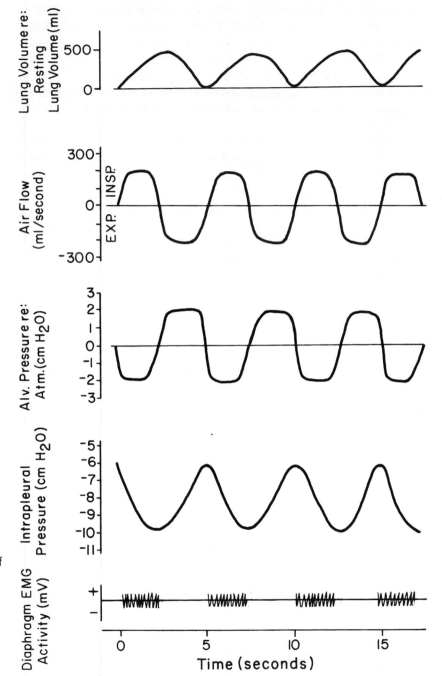

Figure 4-10. Relationships of pressures, flows, and volumes to diaphragm activity. Contraction of the diaphragm causes a drop in intrapleural pressure, which results in an increase in airflow and lung volume. (Data from *Physiology of Respiration* by J. H. Comroe, 1965. Chicago: Year Book Medical Publishers.)

This is a good point at which examine the pressures driving this process. Recall that contraction of the diaphragm causes the alveolar pressure to drop, and the point marked "F" will make sense: When the diaphragm is active ("C"), pressure deep within the lungs drops. Alveolar pressure reaches its maximum negativity during this tidal respiration (–2 cm H_2O relative to atmospheric pressure), because the negative pressure is responsible for airflow into the lungs. Looking at "G" will explain why that pressure drops. You will recall that intrapleural pressure is constantly negative relative to atmospheric pressure, arising from the fact that the lungs are in a state of continued expansion within the thoracic cavity. This is reflected in the fact that the highest pressure on the intrapleural plot is negative.

When the diaphragm contracts, the intrapleural pressure becomes even more negative as the diaphragm attempts to pull the diaphragmatic pleurae away from the visceral pleurae. During the entire period of contraction of the diaphragm, the pressure continues to drop: The diaphragm is pulling farther away from its resting point and the pressure between the pleurae increases proportionately. As the diaphragm reaches the end of its contraction, intrapleural pressure reaches a maximum negativity ("H") that reverses upon relaxation of the diaphragm. When the diaphragm contracts, the volume (space) between the two pleural linings increases; Boyle's law dictates that pressure will drop, and it does.

Depression of the diaphragm for quiet tidal inspiration results in an intrapleural pressure of approximately –10 cm H_2O, but relaxing the diaphragm during quiet expiration does not return the pressure to atmospheric, but rather returns it to a constant rest pressure of –6 cm H_2O. In the normal, healthy individual, intrapleural pressure remains negative at all times, becoming increasingly negative as muscles of inspiration act on the lungs.

The fact that this intrapleural pressure remains negative underscores two important notions. First, the lungs are in a state of continual expansion because the thorax is larger than the lungs that fill it. Second, the lungs are never completely deflated under normal circumstances, because of the residual volume discussed earlier.

During inspiration and expiration, two more pressures are of interest to us. Subglottal pressure is the pressure measured beneath the level of the vocal folds (*glottis* refers to the space between the vocal folds). Above the vocal folds, the respiratory pressure measured within the oral cavity is referred to as intraoral pressure. When the vocal folds are open, intraoral pressure, subglottal pressure, and alveolar pressure are the same.

The pressure beneath and above the vocal folds is directly related to what is happening in the lungs, as long as the vocal folds are open for air passage. If the lungs are drawing air in, there will be a negative pressure at both of these locations. If the lungs are in expiration, the pressure will be relatively positive. Things get more complicated when the vocal folds are closed.

When we close vocal folds for phonation (voicing), we place a significant blockage in the flow of air through the upper respiratory pathway. Closing the vocal folds causes an immediate increase in the subglottal air pressure as the lungs continue expiration. At the same time, closing the vocal folds causes the intraoral pressure to drop to near atmospheric, resulting in a large difference in pressure between the supraglottal (above vocal folds) and subglottal regions. If this increased pressure exceeds 3–5 cm H_2O, the vocal folds will be blown open and voicing will begin. This turns out to be a critical pressure in itself, because it marks the minimal requirement of respiration for speech.

You can now view these critical pressures as a system: We are continually playing the respiratory system against the relatively stable **atmospheric pressure**. Contraction of the diaphragm and muscles of inspiration causes the intrapleural pressure to decrease markedly, which in turn causes the lungs to be expanded. When the lungs expand, alveolar pressure drops relative to atmospheric pressure, causing air to enter the lungs. Relaxing the muscles of inspiration permits the natural recoil of the lungs and cartilage to draw the chest back to its original position, and the relaxed diaphragm again returns to its relatively elevated position in the thorax. When this happens, intrapleural pressure increases (but still stays negative) and alveolar pressure becomes positive relative to atmospheric pressure. Air leaves the lungs.

In summary:

- Volumes and pressures vary as a direct function of the forces acting on the respiratory system.
- With the vocal folds open, **oral pressure**, **subglottal pressure**, and **alveolar pressure** are roughly equivalent.
- **Intrapleural pressure** will remain constantly negative, increasing in negativity during inspiration.
- These pressures are all measured relative to **atmospheric pressure**.
- During inspiration, expansion of the thorax decreases the already negative intrapleural pressure, and the increased lung volume results in a **negative alveolar pressure**.
- Air from outside the body will flow into the lungs as a result of the pressure difference between the lungs and the atmosphere.
- During expiration, this pressure differential is reversed, with air escaping the lungs to equalize the **positive alveolar pressure** with the relatively negative atmospheric pressure.

Pressures Generated by the Tissue

At this point we should address the forces of expiration in earnest. The process of inspiration is one of exerting force to overcome **gravity**. Inspiration is generally active, requiring muscular action to complete it.

Expiration capitalizes on torque, elasticity, and gravity to reclaim some of the energy expended during inspiration. When muscles of inspiration contract, they stretch tissue, torque cartilage of the ribs, and distend the abdomen. When these muscles relax during expiration, the stretched tissues tend to return to their original dimension due to their elastic nature, the chondral portions of the ribs return to their original positions due to the elastic restoration following torquing, and gravity works to depress the rib cage. To breathe in, you have to move all of these muscles and bones, and as you relax they return to their original positions.

These restoring forces actually generate pressures themselves. Recoil of the chest during exhalation obeys the laws applying to any elastic material: The greater you distend or distort the material, the greater is the force required to hold it in that position, and the greater is the force with which it returns to rest.

You can get commonsense validation of this if you recall loading a stapler with staples. As you pull back the spring that holds the staples, you reach a point where the spring almost wins. The force required to hold the spring back is much greater as it gets farther from its point of rest. You know also the force with which your finger can get whacked if you do not get out of the way in time; the farther you have pushed the spring, the more it hurts when it is inadvertently released.

The same elastic forces govern how much effort is required to inhale. Close your eyes and breathe in as deeply as you can and hold it for a few seconds. Feel how much pressure you are fighting to hold your chest in that position. Next, take in a quiet breath and hold it: Do you feel the difference in pressure?

This relationship is described in the curve of Figure 4-11. What this figure shows is the result of pressure generated by all that force

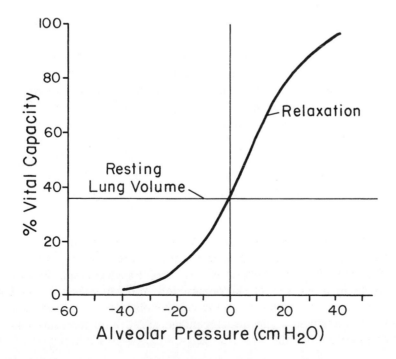

Figure 4-11. Relaxation pressure curve representing pressures generated by the passive forces of the respiratory system.

(remember that pressure is force exerted over an area). The farther the rib cage is expanded, the greater the force that is trying to return the rib cage to rest.

This curve is called the *relaxation pressure curve,* and it was generated by asking people to do what you just did with your eyes closed. Subjects were told to inhale to some percentage of their vital capacity and then to relax their musculature while their intraoral pressure (which approximates both subglottal and alveolar pressure) was measured using a manometer. Repeated measures of this sort at various percentages of vital capacity resulted in the upper positive portion of the curve. It is positive because the tissue is attempting to return to rest. This is a measure of the strength of those physical restoring forces. Note that you are capable of generating some reasonably large forces with this tissue recoil. Pressures on the order of 60 cm H_2O are fairly significant, considering that phonation requires only about 5 cm H_2O.

The bottom half of the curve is produced in much the same way, only this time people were asked to exhale down to a percentage of their vital capacity. The dashed line is the relaxation point, the point where no pressure is generated, because all parts of the system are at equilibrium. (Breathe out and then do not breathe in again: This "relaxation" point before you inhale a new breath is one of three times during a respiratory cycle when atmospheric pressure equals alveolar pressure.) The relaxation point of zero pressure represents about 38% of vital capacity. When you relax entirely with open airway, the lungs still have 38% of the total exchangeable volume left, and this could be forcefully exhaled. Said another way, from this point you can actively inhale 62% of your vital capacity.

Examine the bottom portion of the curve in Figure 4-11 and you will recognize that the pressures generated are not as great, and that they are negative. These negative pressures are predominantly the result of the recoil of the chest wall attempting to return to stasis, whereas the positive pressures are governed by the contribution of lung elasticity arising from the recoil of the muscles and cartilage in bronchi, bronchioles, and blood vessels, as well as elastic tissue throughout the lung. Agostoni and Mead (1964) demonstrated that above about 55% of vital capacity, the chest wall does not add anything to the pressure of the curve; below about 55%, the elasticity of the lungs contributes little to the curve. That is, the lungs compress the air nicely above resting lung volume (RLV), while the chest works very hard below RLV to pull air into the system. Likewise, below 55% you start to use the muscles of expiration to maintain constant subglottal pressure.

The relaxation pressures reveal the recoil forces of respiration without considering active muscular contraction. You can generate a similar set of responses by asking people to completely deflate their lungs and then inflate them to a specific percentage of VC, and then have them either exhale or inhale as forcefully as they can. This measures the result of forces that can be generated by actual work associated with muscular contraction.

Look at Figure 4-12 to see that the respiratory system works as you would expect. On the right side is the expiratory pressure. This is the result of trying to breathe out when you have achieved a specific lung volume. The greater your lung volume is, the more force you can generate for exhalation. On the left side, notice that your ability to draw air in is also intimately related to the amount of air in the lungs: The less air there is in your lungs, the greater is the force you can generate to bring air in. What is that curve in the middle? It is the same one we just looked at—the relaxation curve!

In summary:

- The process of contracting musculature deforms the cartilage and connective tissue, and **recoil forces** drive the respiratory system back to equilibrium after inspiration or expiration.

- **Relaxing** the musculature after inspiration results in a **positive alveolar pressure** that decreases as volume approaches resting lung volume.

- When the pressure is measured following forced expiration, a **negative relaxation pressure** is found, increasing to equity at resting lung volume.

- The negative pressures are a function of the chest wall recoil; the positive pressures arise from the expanded lungs and torqued cartilage.

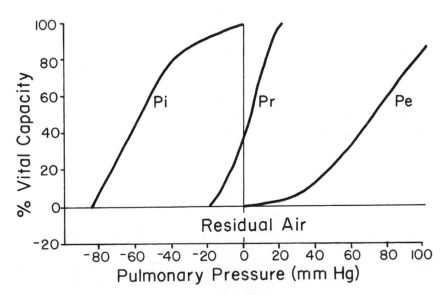

Figure 4-12. Pressure-volume relationship for muscular activity by percentage of vital capacity. Pi = Pressure from muscles of inspiration; Pe = Pressure from muscles of expiration; Pr = Pressure from relaxation of muscles of inspiration and expiration. (Based on data from "The Pressure-Volume Diagram of the Thorax" by H. Rahn, A. Otis, L. E. Chadwick, & W. Fenn, 1946, p. 164. *American Journal of Physiology, 146,* 161–178.)

EFFECTS OF POSTURE ON SPEECH

Body posture is a significant contributor to efficiency of respiration, and any condition that compromises posture also compromises respiration (see Figure 4-13). As the body is shifted from an erect, sitting posture to supine, the relationship between the physical structures of respiration and gravity changes. In the sitting posture, gravity is pulling the abdominal viscera down (supporting inspiration), as well as pulling the rib cage down (supporting expiration). When the body achieves the supine position, gravity is pulling the abdominal viscera toward the spine. The result of this is spread of the viscera toward the thorax and further distension of the diaphragm into the thoracic cavity. In supine position, gravity supports neither expiration nor inspiration: Muscles of inspiration must elevate both abdomen and rib cage against gravity.

Although vital capacity is not affected, the ability to completely inflate the lungs is. The resting lung volume is significantly reduced from approximately 38% of vital capacity in sitting position to 20% in supine, arising from the shift in viscera and effects of gravity on the rib cage. The elastic forces that would normally inflate the lungs to that 38% point only inflate them to 20%, leaving muscular effort to account for the additional 18%.

You can demonstrate the effects of posture easily for yourself. First, stand up, take a deep breath, and hold a sustained vowel as long as you

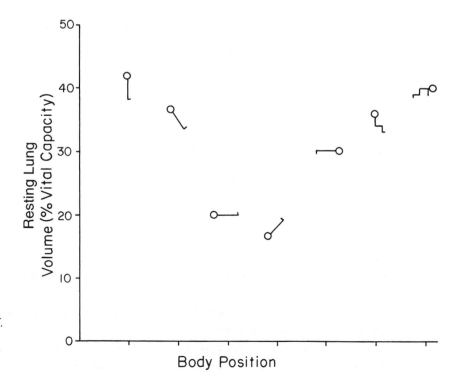

Figure 4-13. Vital capacity changes resulting from postural adjustment. (Data from "Kinematics of the Chest Wall During Speech Production: Volume Displacement of the Rib Cage, Abdomen, and Lung." By T. J. Hixon, M. D. Goldman, & J. Mead, 1973. *Journal of Speech & Hearing Research, 16,* 78–115.)

Muscular Weakness and Respiration

Individuals with diseases that weaken the muscles of inspiration are at significant respiratory risk for a number of reasons. Although gravity is the friend of respiration in a person with normal function, we must realize that inspiration requires muscular effort and that effort is aimed very specifically at overcoming gravity.

Individuals in the later stages of demyelinating diseases, such as amyotrophic lateral sclerosis (ALS), suffer from extreme muscular weakness as a result of the disease, but are still faced with the oxygenation demands typically met with respiratory work. If the patient is placed in the supine position (on the back), gravity will conspire against the respiratory effort, and this "resting" position will actually put him or her at risk for respiratory distress. Here's why: When lying in supine, gravity is pushing on the abdominal viscera, forcing them toward the patient's back. When the individual attempts to take a breath in, the abdomen should protrude, but with compromised muscular strength that will require more effort than the person is capable of. When in supine the abdominal viscera are one more thing to overcome, and it turns out to be one thing too many.

To overcome this, patients in the later stages of ALS often remain in a semi-reclined position to permit rest but capitalize on gravity to assist with respiration. By the way, this might also give you a clue as to why individuals with weakened musculature are more prone to pneumonia than healthy individuals: It takes a great deal of work to clear the lungs and to keep them clear.

can. You will want to keep track of the duration of the vowel. Next, lie on your back (in supine), take a deep breath, and perform the same task. What you will notice is that you were not able to sustain the vowel for as long. Finally, lie in prone (on your "stomach") and sustain the vowel again.

If you did all three of these activities, you found that the most efficient posture for respiration is erect. The reclining positions required more effort for the same gesture and were less efficient for sustained phonation.

You may have already realized the danger this poses to a person whose illness requires that he or she stay in bed for long periods of time. It should not surprise you that pneumonia is a major complication in conditions that immobilize a person.

To summarize:

- **Posture** and **body position** play an important role in volumes for respiration.
- When the body is placed in a reclining position, the abdominal contents shift rostrally as a result of the forces of gravity.
- Aside from reducing the resting lung volume, the force of **gravity** on the abdomen increases the effort required for inspiration.

PRESSURES OF SPEECH

The respiratory system operates at two levels of pressure virtually simultaneously. The first level is the relatively constant supply of subglottal pressure required to drive the vocal folds, a topic with which you will become familiar in the next chapter. To produce sustained voicing of a given intensity, this pressure is relatively constant. As we will see, the minimum driving pressure to make the vocal folds move would elevate a column of water between 3–5 cm (3–5 cm H_2O), with conversational speech requiring between 7 and 10 cm H_2O. Loud speech requires a concomitant increase in pressure.

The second level of pressure is one requiring micro-control. Even as we maintain the constant pressure needed for phonation, we can rapidly change the pressure for linguistic purposes such as syllable stress. With quick bursts of pressure (and laryngeal adjustments) we can create rapid increases in vocal intensity and vocal pitch. These bursts are small and fast: We will increase subglottal pressure by about 2 cm H_2O to add stress, but we will return to the previous subglottal pressure within one tenth of a second. We will see that these two modes of control use the same mechanical structures.

To maintain constant pressure for speech, we must first charge the system. During normal respiration, inhalation takes up approximately 40% of the cycle, while expiration takes up about 60%. When you realize that you speak only on expiration, you will realize also that it would not take many minutes of talking like this to drive you (and your communication partner) to distraction! Imagine every 6 seconds of speaking followed by 4 seconds of silence while you inhale, and you will see why we have modified this plan for speech (see Figure 4-14).

In fact, the respiratory cycle for speech is markedly different. You need a long, drawn-out expiration to produce long utterances, and you need a very short inspiration to maintain the smooth flow of communication. When you breathe in for speech, you actually spend only 10% of the respiratory cycle on inspiration, and about 90% breathing out.

This does not change the amount of air we breathe in and out. We will still breathe exactly the volume we need for our metabolic processes (too much and we take in too much oxygen, or hyperventilate; too little and we take in too little oxygen and become **hypoxic**). All we need to do is alter how long we spend in either stage of the process.

Earlier we said that we need to hold a reasonably constant subglottal pressure to maintain phonation, but we did not say *how* we achieve it. You already have all the pieces, so let us pose the puzzle to you. If you take in a deep breath as if you were about to speak, but just let the air flow out unimpeded, you run out of air within one or two quick words. That burst of air is not going to work for speech.

Instead of letting the air out through total relaxation, let the air out slowly. As you do this, pay attention to the fact that you are using mus-

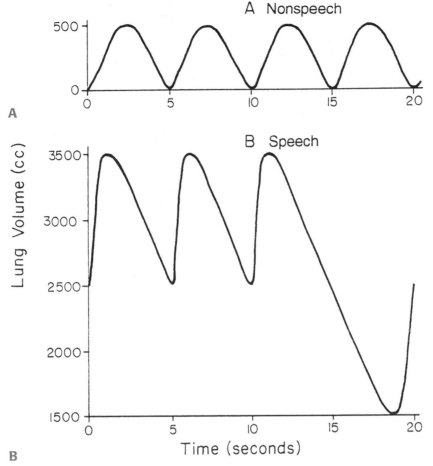

A Nonspeech

B Speech

Lung Volume (cc)

Time (seconds)

A

B

Figure 4-14. Modification of respiratory cycle during speech compared with nonspeech respiratory cycle. **A.** This trace represents quiet tidal respiration, with volume related to resting lung volume. **B.** This trace is related to total lung capacity. The speaker rapidly inhales a markedly larger volume than during quiet tidal inspiration and then slowly exhales the air during speech. Note that inspiration occurs with the same timing in both speech and nonspeech, but that the expiratory phase is proportionately longer during speech. In the final portion of the trace, the speaker is called on to speak on expiratory reserve volume.

cles to restrain the airflow. If you remember that the lungs are attempting to empty as a result of their being stretched for inspiration, then you might realize that if you were to *hold* that inspiration position you would impede the outflow of air. This process is called *checking action*. That is, you "check" (impede) the flow of air out of your inflated lungs by means of the muscles that got it there in the first place—the muscles of inspiration.

Checking action is extremely important for respiratory control of speech, because it directly addresses a person's ability to restrain the flow of air. When a person has a deficit associated with checking action (as in paralysis), the person is at a tremendous disadvantage, because he or she will be restricted to extremely short bursts of speech.

Checking action permits us to maintain the constant flow of air through the vocal tract, and that in turn lets us accurately control the pressure beneath vocal folds that have been closed for phonation. We will see that this is very important when it comes to maintaining constant vocal intensity and frequency of vibration.

There is an expiratory parallel to checking action, and that is the process of speaking on expiratory reserve. Take another look at Figure 4-11 and examine the relaxation pressure curve. Checking action lets us stay within the upper portion of the curve for quite a while, making maximum use of our respiratory charge for speech.

What happens when we get down to that resting lung volume point of 38% during speech? If we have more to say before we inhale, we simply keep talking. Instead of using the muscles of inspiration we used to keep the air from flowing out, we have to enlist the muscles of *expiration* to push beyond that resting lung volume. Using the muscles of expiration, we continue talking beyond the point where we would normally take another breath, letting us control when we break for inspiration so that our speech is fluid and nicely controlled.

A graphic demonstration of how well we perform this feat is fairly simple. Do the following steps and note the times:

Take a maximally deep breath, and time yourself as you hold a sustained vowel as long as you can only using your chest muscles (do not force using your abdominal muscles, but rather just let your inspiratory muscles do all the work).

Take another breath, but this time sustain the vowel just as long as you can by running all the way into the region of expiratory reserve. If you continue your vowel to the point where you are forcing with muscles of expiration, you will find that the duration has increased 40 to 50%. Of course, you do not normally speak as far down on your respiratory charge as that, but your teacher regularly gets into expiratory reserve while lecturing, we guarantee.

It is wise to say, one more time, that the speaker will always take care of business first: The body's needs will be met in a constant fashion in the face of using respiration for communication. The next time your instructor is lecturing, count the number of breaths she or he takes per minute and you will see that it is right around 15. Despite what you may have heard, teaching *is* work, so respiration may be a little faster than the 12 breaths per minute of quiet tidal respiration.

Remember, however, that this checking action and speaking on expiratory reserve do not come without a cost. We have to work to overcome the recoil forces in each case, and the deeper our inhalation or the farther we go below resting lung volume, the greater is the force we have to overcome. If you are a cheerleader you know exactly what we mean: Speaking loudly and with continuity requires effort. Look again at that relaxation pressure curve and realize that the effort you must exert in the upper part of the curve to keep the air from rapidly leaving the lungs is directly proportional to the pressure those forces generate. Likewise, it requires a great deal of effort to squeeze the last bit of expiratory reserve air out of the lungs.

If you look back on this discussion, you will find a common thread: Respiration is work. Generating pressure requires muscular activity, and restraining that pressure for speech requires even more effort. Respiration is truly the battery of the speech production mechanism, and it provides the energy source for our oral communication. Our next task is to see how respiration is used to produce a major component of this speech signal—voicing.

▶ CHAPTER SUMMARY

Respiration requires the balance of **pressures**. Decreased **alveolar pressure** is the product of expansion of the thorax. When the thorax expands, the pressure between the pleurae decreases as the thorax and diaphragm are pulled away from the lungs. The force of the distended lungs will increase the **negative intrapleural pressure**, and the expansion will cause a drop in alveolar pressure as well. The relatively lower alveolar pressure represents an imbalance between pressures of the lungs and the atmosphere, and air will enter the lungs to equalize the imbalance. **Expiration** requires reduction in thorax size that results in a **positive pressure** within the alveoli, with air escaping through the oral cavity. The **intrapleural pressure** becomes less negative during expiration, but never reaches atmospheric pressure.

Several **volumes** and **capacities** may be identified within the respiratory system. **Tidal volume** is the volume inspired and expired in a cycle of respiration, while **inspiratory reserve volume** is the air inspired beyond tidal inspiration. **Expiratory reserve volume** is air expired beyond tidal expiration, and **residual volume** is air that remains in the lungs after maximal expiration. **Dead space air** is air that cannot undergo gas exchange. **Vital capacity** is the volume of air that can be inspired after a maximal expiration, and **functional residual capacity** is the air that remains in the body after passive exhalation. Inspiratory capacity is the volume that can be inspired from resting lung volume. **Total lung capacity** is the sum of all lung volumes.

For speech we must work within the confines of pressures and volumes required for life function. We alter the respiratory cycle to capitalize on expiration time and restrain that expiration through **checking action**. We also generate pressure through contraction of the muscles of expiration when the lung volume is less than resting lung volume. With these manipulations we will maintain a respiratory rate to match our metabolic needs, and even use the accessory muscles of inspiration and expiration to generate small bursts of pressure for **syllabic stress**.

►STUDY QUESTIONS

1. Passive expiration involves the forces of _____, _____, and _____.

2. Identify the indicated volumes and capacities described below.

   a. _____ volume: The volume of air that we breathe in during a respiratory cycle.

   b. _____ volume: The volume that can be inhaled after a tidal inspiration.

   c. _____ volume: The volume that can be exhaled after a tidal expiration.

   d. _____ volume: The volume remaining in the lungs after a maximal exhalation.

   e. _____ capacity: The combination of inspiratory reserve volume, expiratory reserve volume, and tidal volume.

   f. _____ capacity: The volume of air remaining in the body after a passive exhalation.

   g. _____ capacity: The sum of all the volumes.

3. _____ is the volume of air that cannot undergo gas exchange.

4. _____ pressure is the air pressure measured within the oral cavity.

5. _____ pressure is the air pressure measured below the vocal folds.

6. _____ pressure is the pressure within the alveolus.

7. _____ pressure is the pressure between the visceral and parietal pleural membranes.

8. When the diaphragm contracts, pressure within the alveolus _____ (increases/decreases).

9. When air pressure within the lungs is lower than that of the atmosphere, air will _____ (enter/leave) the lungs.

10. When the body is placed in a reclining position, the resting lung volume _____ (increases/decreases).

11. Use of the muscles of inspiration to impede the outward flow of air during speech is termed _____.

12. Coordination of muscular activity is largely the responsibility of the cerebellum of the brain. An individual with neuropathology involving the cerebellum will have a deficit in coordination of motor function. What impact would this deficit have on speech function?

STUDY QUESTION ANSWERS

1. Passive expiration involves the forces of <u>TORQUE</u>, <u>ELASTICITY</u>, and <u>GRAVITY</u>.
2. Identify the indicated volumes and capacities described below.
   a. <u>TIDAL VOLUME</u>
   b. <u>INSPIRATORY RESERVE</u> volume
   c. <u>EXPIRATORY RESERVE</u> volume
   d. <u>RESIDUAL</u> volume
   e. <u>VITAL</u> capacity
   f. <u>FUNCTIONAL RESIDUAL</u> capacity
   g. <u>TOTAL LUNG</u> capacity
3. <u>DEAD SPACE AIR</u> is the volume of air that cannot undergo gas exchange.
4. <u>INTRAORAL</u> pressure is the air pressure measured within the oral cavity.
5. <u>SUBGLOTTAL</u> pressure is the air pressure measured below the vocal folds.
6. <u>ALVEOLAR</u> or <u>PULMONIC</u> pressure is the pressure within the alveolus.
7. <u>INTRAPLEURAL</u> or <u>PLEURAL</u> pressure is the pressure between the visceral and parietal pleural membranes.
8. When the diaphragm contracts, pressure within the alveolus <u>DECREASES</u>.
9. When air pressure within the lungs is lower than that of the atmosphere, air will <u>ENTER</u> the lungs.
10. When the body is placed in a reclining position, the resting lung volume <u>DECREASES</u>.
11. Use of the muscles of inspiration to impede the outward flow of air during speech is termed <u>CHECKING ACTION</u>.
12. Neuromuscular conditions that affect cerebellar function can result in loss of coordination of diaphragm contraction, difficulty maintaining constant subglottal pressure due to a deficit in checking action, and difficulty coordinating the respiratory effort with phonation, among other problems.

REFERENCES

Agostoni, E., & Mead, J. (1964). Statics of the respiratory system. In W. Fenn, & H. Rahn (Eds.), *Handbook of physiology, respiration* (Vol. 1, Sect. 3). Washington, DC: American Physiological Society. Baltimore: Williams & Wilkins.

Baken, R., & Cavallo, S. (1981). Prephonatory chest wall posturing. *Folia phoniatrica, 33,* 193–202.

Baken, R., Cavallo, S., & Weissman, K. (1979). Chest Wall movements prior to phonation. *Journal of Speech and Hearing Research, 22,* 862–872.

Baken, R. J., & Orlikoff, R. F. (1999). *Clinical measurement of speech and voice* (2nd ed.). San Diego, CA: Singular Publishing Group.

Basmajian, J. V. (1975). *Grant's method of anatomy.* Baltimore, MD: Williams & Wilkins.

Bateman, H. E., & Mason, R. M. (1984). *Applied anatomy and physiology of the speech and hearing mechanism.* Springfield, IL: Charles C. Thomas.

Beck, E. W. (1982). *Mosby's atlas of functional human anatomy.* St. Louis, MO: C. V. Mosby.

Bergman, R., Thompson, S., & Afifi, A. (1984). *A catalog of human variation.* Baltimore: Urban & Schwarzenberg.

Burrows, B., Knudson, R. J., & Kettel, L. J. (1975). *Respiratory insufficiency*. Chicago: Year Book Medical Publishers.

Campbell, E. (1958). An electromyographic examination of the role of the intercostal muscles in breathing in man. *Journal of Physiology, 129,* 12–26.

Campbell, E., Agostoni, E., & Davis, J. (1970). *The respiratory muscles, mechanics and neural control*. Philadelphia: W. B. Saunders.

Chusid, J. G. (1985). *Correlative neuroanatomy and functional neurology* (17th ed.). Los Altos, CA: Lange Medical Publications.

Comroe, J. H. (1974). *Physiology of respiration*. Chicago: Year Book Medical Publishers.

Creasy, R. K. (1997). *Management of labor and delivery*. Malden, MA: Blackwell Science.

Des Jardins, T., & Burton, G. G. (2001). *Clinical manifestation and assessment of respiratory disease*. Chicago: Mosby.

Draper, M., Ladefoged, P., & Whitteridge, D. (1959). Respiratory muscles in speech. *Journal of Speech and Hearing Research, 2,* 16–27.

Ganong, W. F. (2003). *Review of medical physiology* (21st ed.). New York: McGraw-Hill/Appleton & Lange.

Gordon, M. S. (1972). *Animal physiology: Principles and adaptations*. New York: Macmillan.

Gosling, J. A., Harris, P. F., Humpherson, J. R., Whitmore, I., & Willan, P. L. T. (1985). *Atlas of human anatomy*. Philadelphia: J. B. Lippincott.

Gray, H., Bannister, L. H., Berry, M. M., & Williams, P. L. (Eds.). (1995). *Gray's anatomy*. London: Churchill Livingstone.

Grobler, N. J. (1977). *Textbook of clinical anatomy* (Vol. 1). Amsterdam: Elsevier Scientific.

Hixon, T. J. (1973). Respiratory function in speech. In F. D. Minifie, T. J. Hixon, & F. Williams (Eds.), *Normal aspects of speech, hearing, and language* (pp. 73–126). Englewood Cliffs, NJ: Prentice-Hall.

Hixon, T. J., Goldman, M. D., & Mead, J. (1973). Kinematics of the chest wall during speech production: Volume displacement of the rib cage, abdomen, and lung. *Journal of Speech and Hearing Research, 16,* 78–115.

Kahane, J. (1982). Anatomy and physiology of the organs of the peripheral speech mechanism. In N. Lass, L. McReynolds, J. Northern, & D. Yoder (Eds.), *Speech, language, and hearing. Vol. 1: Normal processes* (pp. 109–155). Philadelphia: W. B. Saunders.

Kao, F. F. (1972). *An introduction to respiratory physiology*. Amsterdam: Exerpta Medica.

Kaplan, H. (1960). *Anatomy and physiology of speech*. New York: McGraw-Hill.

Kent, R. D. (1997). *The speech sciences*. San Diego, CA: Singular Publishing Group.

Konno, K., & Mead, J. (1968). Measurement of the separate volume changes of rib cage and abdomen during breathing. *Journal of Applied Physiology, 22,* 407–422.

Lass, N., McReynolds, L., Northern, J., & Yoder, D. (Eds.). (1982). *Speech, language, and hearing. Vol. I: Normal processes*. Philadelphia: W. B. Saunders.

Miller, A. D., Bianchi, A. L., & Bishop, B. P. (1997). *Neural control of the respiratory muscles*. Boca Raton, FL: CRC Press.

Moser, K. M., & Spragg, R. G. (1982). *Respiratory emergencies*. St. Louis, MO: C. V. Mosby.

Murray, J. F. (1976). *The normal lung. The basis for diagnosis and treatment of pulmonary disease*. Philadelphia: W. B. Saunders.

Netter, F. H. (1997). *Atlas of human anatomy*. Los Angeles, CA: Icon Learning Systems.

Pace, W. R. (1970). *Pulmonary physiology*. Philadelphia: F. A. Davis.

Pappenheimer, J. R., Comroe, J. H., Cournand, A., Ferguson, J. K. W., Filley, G. F., Fowler, W. S., Gray, J. S., Helmholtz, H. F., Otis, A. B., Rahn, H., & Riley, R. L. (1950). Standardization of definitions and symbols in respiratory physiology. *Federation proceedings, Federation of the American Society for Experimental Biology* (pp. 602–605).

Peters, R. M. (1969). *The mechanical basis of respiration.* Boston, MA: Little, Brown.

Rahn, H., Otis, A., Chadwick, L. E., & Fenn, W. (1946). The pressure-volume diagram of the thorax and lung. *American Journal of Physiology, 146,* 161–178.

Rohen, J. W., Yokochi, C., Lutjen-Drecoll, E., & Romrell, L. J. (2002). *Color atlas of anatomy* (5th ed.). Philadelphia: Williams & Wilkins.

Rosse, C., Gaddum-Rosse, P., & Rosse, G. (1997). *Hollinshead's textbook of anatomy.* Philadelphia: Lippincott-Raven.

Scott, J. R., Disaia, P. J., Hammond, C. B., & Spellacy, W. N. (1994). *Danforth's obstetrics and gynecology* (7th ed.). Philadelphia: J. B. Lippincott.

Snell, R. S. (1978). *Gross anatomy dissector.* Boston: Little, Brown.

Spector, W. S. (1956). *Handbook of biological data.* Philadelphia: W. B. Saunders.

Taylor, A. (1960). The contribution of the intercostal muscles to the effort of respiration in man. *Journal of Physiology, 151,* 390.

Tokizane, T., Kawamata, K., & Tokizane, H. (1952). Electromyographic studies on the human respiratory muscles. *Japan Journal of Physiology, 2,* 232.

Twietmeyer, A., & McCracken, T. D. (1992). *Coloring guide to regional human anatomy* (2nd ed.). Philadelphia: Lea & Febiger.

Zemlin, W. R. (1998). *Speech and hearing science: Anatomy and physiology* (4th ed.). Needham Heights, MA: Allyn & Bacon.

CHAPTER 5

Anatomy of Phonation

Spoken communication uses both voiceless and voiced sounds, and this chapter is concerned with that critical distinction. **Voiceless** phonemes or speech sounds are produced without use of the vocal folds; for example, the /s/ or /f/ sounds. **Voiced** sounds are produced by action of the vocal folds; for example, the /z/ and /v/ sound. **Phonation**, or voicing, is the product of vibrating vocal folds, and this occurs within the larynx. Just as we referred to respiration as the source of *energy* for speech, phonation is the source of voice for speech. Respiration is the energy source that permits phonation to occur; without respiration there would be no voicing.

The vocal folds are actually five layers of tissue, with the deepest layer being muscle. The space between the vocal folds is called the **glottis** (or **rima glottidis**), and the area below the vocal folds is the **subglottal** region. The vocal folds are located within the airstream at the superior end of the trachea. As the airstream passes between the vocal folds, they may be made to vibrate, much as a flag flaps in the wind. Try this: Place your hand on the side of your neck and hum. You will feel a tickling vibration. This is the mechanical correlate of the sound you hear. If you alternately produce /a/ and /h/, you will feel your vocal folds as they start vibrating and stop, because /a/ is a voiced sound and /h/ is voiceless.

rima glottidis: *L., "slit of the glottis"*

Biological Functions of the Larynx

Although we capitalize on the larynx for phonation, it has a much more important function in nature. The larynx is an exquisite sphincter, in that the vocal folds are capable of a very strong and rapid clamping of the airway in response to threat of intrusion by foreign objects. As evidence of this primary function, there are three pairs of laryngeal muscles directly responsible for either approximating or tensing the vocal folds, although there is only one pair of muscles responsible for opening them. The vocal folds are "wired" to close immediately on stimulation by outside agents, such as food or liquids, a response which is followed quickly by a rapid and forceful exhalation. This combination of gestures is designed to stop intrusion by foreign matter and to rapidly expel that matter away from the opening of the airway.

It has other important functions as well. Because the vocal folds provide an excellent seal to the respiratory system, they permit you to hold your breath, thus capturing a significant respiratory charge for such activities as swimming.

Holding your breath serves other functions as well. Lifting heavy objects requires you to "fix" your thorax by inspiring and clamping your laryngeal sphincter (vocal folds). This gives the muscles of the upper body a solid framework with which to work. You'll also note from the margin notes in Chapter 3 that tightly clamping the vocal folds plays an important part of childbirth and defecation.

When you felt the vibrations of the vocal folds, you also might have noted a very important aspect of phonation. You were able to turn your voice on and off to produce the alternating voiced and voiceless sounds. When you alternated those two sounds, you were actually moving the vocal folds into and out of the airstream to cause them to start or stop vibrating. The vocal folds are bands of tissue set into vibration. Now we are ready to look at the structure of the vocal mechanism (see Figure 5-1).

A TOUR OF THE PHONATORY MECHANISM

This is a good opportunity to walk you through the vocal mechanism. We will get into details soon enough, but for now let us look at the larger picture.

Framework of the Larynx

The larynx is a musculo-cartilaginous structure located at the superior (upper) end of the trachea. It is comprised of three unpaired and three paired cartilages bound by ligaments and lined with mucous membrane.

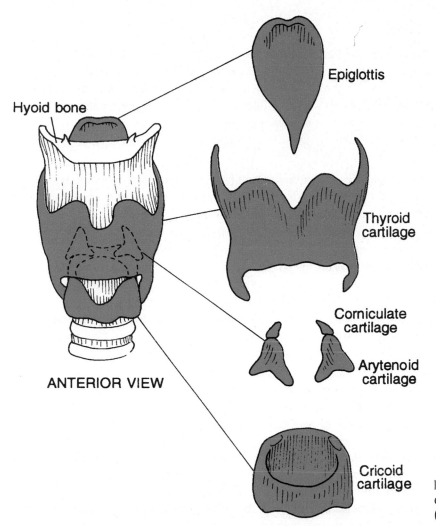

Figure 5-1. Larynx (*left*) and cartilages making up the larynx (*right*).

If you examine Figure 5-1, you can see the relation between the trachea and larynx. As you recall, the trachea is composed of a series of cartilage rings, connected and separated by fibroelastic membrane. As seen in Figure 5-1, the larynx sits as an oddly shaped box atop the last ring of the trachea. It is adjacent to cervical vertebrae 4 through 6 in the adult, but the larynx of an infant will be higher. The average length of the larynx in adult males is 44 mm; in females it is 36 mm.

The **cricoid cartilage** is a complete ring resting atop the trachea and is the most inferior of the laryngeal cartilages. From the side, the cricoid cartilage takes on the appearance of a signet ring, with its back arching up relative to the front. The **thyroid cartilage** is the largest of the laryngeal cartilages, articulating with the cricoid cartilage below by means of paired processes that let it rock forward and backward at that joint. With this configuration, the paired **arytenoid cartilages** ride on

▶ **cricoid:** *Gr., krikos, ring; "ring-form"*

▶ **arytenoid:** *Gr., arytaina, ladle; "ladle-form"*

Laryngectomy

Patients who undergo **laryngectomy** (surgical removal of the larynx) lose the voicing source for speech. The larynx is removed and the oral cavity is sealed off from the trachea and lower respiratory passageway as a safeguard, because the protective function of the larynx is also lost. **Laryngectomees** (individuals who have undergone laryngectomy) must alter their activities, because they now breathe through a **tracheostoma**, an opening placed in the trachea through a surgical procedure known as a **tracheostomy**.

Loss of the ability to phonate is but one of the difficulties facing the laryngectomee. This patient will have difficulty with **expectoration** (elimination of phlegm from respiratory passageway) and coughing, and will no longer able to enjoy swimming or other activities that would expose the **stoma** to water or pollutants. The air entering the patient's lungs is no longer humidified or filtered by the upper respiratory passageway, and a filter must be kept over the stoma to prevent introduction of foreign objects. The patient may be restricted from having house pets that shed hair, as the hair can work its way into the unprotected airway. The flavor of foods is greatly reduced, because the patient may no longer breathe through his or her nose, and our perception of food relies heavily on the sense of smell. Depending on pre- and postoperative treatment, patients may experience extreme dryness of oral tissues (xerostomia) arising from damage to salivary glands from radiation therapy. One result of this dryness may be swallowing dysfunction (dysphagia). Recognize that since the trachea has been completely separated from the esophagus, the risk of aspiration is reduced after healing occurs, although the stoma will always have to be protected from intrusion of foreign bodies or liquids.

corniculate: *L., cornu, horn;* *"little horn"*

epiglottis: *Gr., epi, over;* *"over glottis"*

An orifice is an opening.

the high-backed upper surface of the cricoid cartilage, forming the posterior point of attachment for the vocal folds (or plicae vocalis). The **corniculate cartilages** ride on the superior surface of each arytenoid and are prominent landmarks in the aryepiglottic folds. The inner surface of the thyroid cartilage provides the anterior point of attachment for the vocal folds.

The thyroid cartilage articulates with the **hyoid bone** by means of a pair of superior processes. Medial to the hyoid bone and thyroid cartilage is the **epiglottis**, a leaf-like cartilage. The epiglottis is potentially a protective structure, in that it will drop to cover the **orifice** of the larynx during swallowing. Although there is debate among physiologists and speech scientists as to whether the epiglottis protects the airway in humans, there is no doubt that it serves this function in animals that walk on four feet.

To summarize:
- The **larynx** is a musculo-cartilaginous structure located at the upper end of the trachea. It is comprised of the **cricoid**, **thyroid**, and **epiglottis cartilages**, as well as the paired **arytenoid**, **corniculate**, and **cuneiform cartilages**.

- The thyroid and cricoid cartilages articulate by means of the **cricothyroid joint** that lets the two cartilages come closer together in front.
- The **arytenoid** and **cricoid cartilages** also articulate with a joint that permits a wide range of arytenoid motion.
- The **corniculate cartilages** rest on the upper surface of the arytenoids, while the **cuneiform cartilages** reside within the **aryepiglottic folds**.

Inner Larynx

When these cartilages are combined with the trachea and the airway above the larynx, the result is a rough tube-like space with a constriction caused by the cartilages. This construction is unique, however, in that it is an *adjustable* constriction. The vocal folds are bands of mucous membrane, connective tissue, and muscle that are slung between the arytenoid cartilages and the thyroid cartilage so that they may be moved into and out of the airstream. (Alternately, some anatomists consider the vocal folds as the mucous membrane and connective tissue only, excluding the thyrovocalis muscle.) Muscles attached to the arytenoids provide both adductory and abductory functions, with which we control the degree of airflow by means of muscular contraction.

Laryngeal Membranes. The cavity of the larynx is a constricted tube with a smooth and reasonably aerodynamic surface (see Figure 5-2). This tube is created by developing a deep structure of cartilages, connecting those cartilages through sheets and cords of ligament and membrane, and lining the entire structure with a wet, smooth mucous membrane. Let us work from the inside out to identify these connective structures. The extrinsic ligaments provide attachment between the hyoid or trachea and the cartilage of the larynx. The **thyrohyoid membrane**

Valleculae and Swallow

The valleculae are "little valleys," formed by the membrane between the tongue and the epiglottis. During a normal swallow, the larynx elevates and the epiglottis folds down to protect the airway from food and liquid. The food and liquid pass over the back of the tongue, through the valleculae, into the pyriform sinuses, and finally into the esophagus (this will be discussed in detail in Chapter 9). When swallowing is compromised, as in the deficit arising from cerebrovascular accident (see Chapter 13), the larynx may not elevate properly, and food can accumulate in the valleculae. From this you can see that malodorous breath in an individual who is neurologically compromised may be a significant indicator of a dangerous swallowing dysfunction, because if the epiglottis is not covering the airway there is a good chance that the vocal folds are not doing their job in protecting the lungs and that the lungs are being penetrated by food and drink.

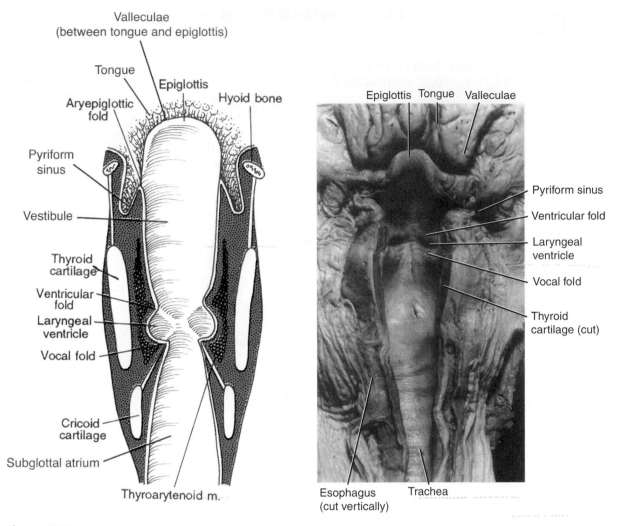

Figure 5-2. Cavity of the larynx with landmarks, as viewed from behind. Note that the laryngeal space has been revealed by a sagittal incision, and the post-laryngeal wall has been spread for access to the structure.

stretches across the space between the greater cornu of the hyoid and the lateral thyroid. Posterior to this is the **lateral thyrohyoid ligament**, which runs from the superior cornu of the thyroid to the posterior tip of the greater cornu hyoid. A small **triticial cartilage** may or may not be found here. In front, running from the corpus hyoid to the upper border of the anterior thyroid, is the **median thyrohyoid ligament**. Together, the median thyrohyoid ligament, thyrohyoid membrane, and lateral thyrohyoid ligament connect the larynx and the hyoid bone. There are other extrinsic ligaments. The **hyoepiglottic ligament** and **thyroepiglottic ligament** attach the epiglottis to the corpus hyoid and the inner thyroid cartilage, just below the notch, respectively. The epiglottic attachment to the tongue is made by means of the **lateral** and **median glossoepiglottic ligaments**, and the overlay of mucous membrane on these ligaments produces the "little valleys" or **valleculae** between the tongue and the epiglottis. The trachea must attach to the larynx as well, and this is performed through the **cricotracheal membrane**.

The **intrinsic ligaments** connect the cartilages of the larynx and form the support structure for the cavity of the larynx, as well as that of the vocal folds themselves. The **fibroelastic membrane** of the larynx is composed of the upper quadrangular **membranes** and **aryepiglottic folds**, the lower conus elasticus, and the **vocal ligament**, which is actually the upward free extension of the conus elasticus.

The quadrangular membranes are the undergirding layer of connective tissue running from the arytenoids to the epiglottis and thyroid cartilage and forming the false vocal folds. They originate at the inner thyroid angle and sides of the epiglottis, and form an upper cone that narrows as it approaches and terminates in a free margin at the arytenoid and corniculate cartilages. The **aryepiglottic muscles** course from the side of the epiglottis to the arytenoid apex, forming the upper margin of the quadrangular membrane and laterally, the aryepiglottic folds. These folds are simply the ridges marking the highest elevation of these membranes and muscles slung from epiglottis to arytenoids. The **pyriform sinus** is the space between the aryepiglottic fold and the thyroid cartilage, marking an important point of transit for food and liquid during a swallow, as will be discussed in Chapter 9.

To summarize:

- The **cavity** of the **larynx** is a constricted tube with a smooth surface.
- Sheets and cords of ligaments connect the cartilages, while smooth **mucous membrane** covers the medial-most surface of the larynx.
- The **thyrohyoid membrane**, **lateral thyrohyoid ligament**, and **median thyrohyoid ligament** cover the space between the hyoid bone and the thyroid.
- The **hyoepiglottic** and **thyroepiglottic ligaments** attach the epiglottis to the corpus hyoid and the inner thyroid cartilage, respectively.
- The **valleculae** are found between the tongue and the epiglottis, within folds arising from the lateral and median glossoepiglottic ligaments.
- The **cricotracheal ligament** attaches the trachea to the larynx.
- The **fibroelastic membrane** is composed of the upper **quadrangular membranes** and **aryepiglottic folds**, the lower **conus elasticus**, and the **vocal ligament**, which is actually the upward free extension of the conus elasticus. The **pyriform sinus** is the

[margin note, handwritten:] extrinsic

quadrangular: *L., quadri, four; angulus, right; "right-angled"*

conus elasticus: *L., elastic cone*

space between the fold of the aryepiglottic membrane and the thyroid cartilage laterally.

* The **aryepiglottic folds** course from the side of the epiglottis to the arytenoid apex.

Fine Structure of the Vocal Folds. The vocal folds are composed of five layers of tissue. Figure 5-3 shows the most superficial layer to be an extremely thin (less than 0.1 mm thick) sheet of squamous epithelium with an underlying layer of basement membrane to adhere it to the next layer. This epithelial layer gives the vocal folds the glistening white appearance seen during laryngoscopic examination (use of a **laryngo-scope**, a device typically used by **laryngologists** or speech-language pathologists to view the larynx). The superficial epithelial layer aids in hydration of the vocal folds by assisting in fluid retention.

Deep to this layer is the **lamina propria**, which is composed of three different tissues. Lamina propria is connective tissue that underlies mucosal epithelia throughout the body. The first (superficial) layer is made up of elastin fibers, so named because of their physical elastic qualities which permit them to be extensively stretched. The fibrous and elastic elements of the superficial lamina propria cushion the vocal folds. Moving medially, the intermediate lamina propria (1–2 mm thick) is composed of elastin fibers as well, but these fibers have an anterior-posterior orientation as compared with the more-or-less random orientation of the first layer of lamina propria. The deep lamina propria (also 1–2 mm thick) shares the anterior-posterior orientation of the second layer, but is

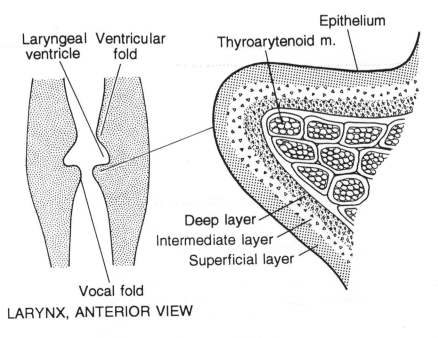

Figure 5-3. Microstructure of vocal folds. (From Titze, 1994.)

LARYNX, ANTERIOR VIEW

composed of collagen fibers which, in contrast to elastin, prohibit extension. The vocal ligament consists of the combination of the intermediate and deep lamina propria.

Deep to the lamina propria is the fifth layer of the vocal folds, the **thyrovocalis muscle**. This makes up the bulk of the vocal fold. Because the muscle course is anterior-posterior, the fibers are arranged in this orientation. This combination of tissues provides both active and passive elements. The thyrovocalis is the active element of the vocal folds, while the passive elements consist of the layers of lamina propria that provide strength, cushioning, and elasticity.

The **mucosal lining** of the vocal folds is actually a combination of the epithelial lining and the disorganized first lamina propria layer. The second and third layers (elastin and collagen) constitute the **vocal ligament**, a structure giving a degree of stiffness and support to the vocal folds. Some authors refer alternately to the **cover** of the vocal folds (superficial epithelium, primary and secondary layers of lamina propria) and the **body** (third layer of lamina propria and thyrovocalis) of the vocal folds.

Cavities of the Larynx

If you look at the profile of the larynx in Figure 5-4, you will appreciate some of the relationships among the structures. The aditus laryngis or **aditus** is the entry to the larynx from the pharynx above. (Some anatomists define the aditus as the first space of the larynx; others view it simply as the entryway to the first cavity—the vestibule—to be discussed.) You may think of the aditus as the door frame through which you would pass when entering a house. The anterior boundary of the "frame" of the aditus is the epiglottis, with the fold of membrane and muscle slung between the epiglottis and the arytenoids (the **aryepiglottic folds**) comprising the lateral margins of the aditus. In Figure 5-5 you can see two "bumps" under the aryepiglottic folds. These are caused by the cuneiform cartilages embedded within the folds. The second set of prominences posterior to the first two are from the corniculate cartilages on the arytenoids.

The first cavity of the larynx is the **vestibule**, or entryway. The vestibule is the space between the entryway or aditus and the **ventricular** (or **vestibular**) folds. The ventricular folds are known also as the **false vocal folds**, because they are not used for phonation except in rare (and clinically significant) cases. The vestibule is wide at the aditus but narrows at the ventricular folds. The lateral walls are comprised of the **aryepiglottic folds**, and the posterior walls are made up of the membrane covering the arytenoid cartilages, which project superiorly to the false folds. The false vocal folds are made up of mucous membrane and a fibrous **vestibular ligament**, but not muscular tissue. The space between the false vocal folds is termed the **rima vestibuli**.

aditus laryngis: *L., entrance; "laryngeal entrance"*

aryepiglottic: *ary(tenoid) + epiglottis*

rima vestibuli: *L., "slit of the vestibule"*

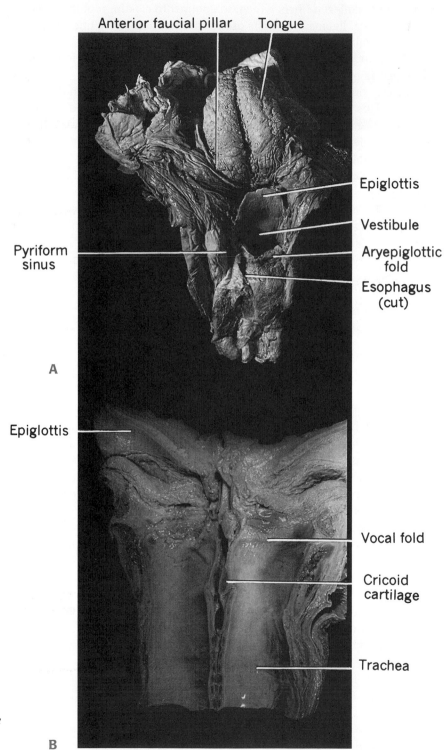

Anterior faucial pillar

Tongue

Epiglottis

Vestibule

Aryepiglottic fold

Esophagus (cut)

Pyriform sinus

A

Epiglottis

Vocal fold

Cricoid cartilage

Trachea

Figure 5-4. A. Larynx, as seen from behind and above. **B.** Larynx that has been cut sagittally and the sides reflected, revealing the two halves of the larynx. *(continues)*

B

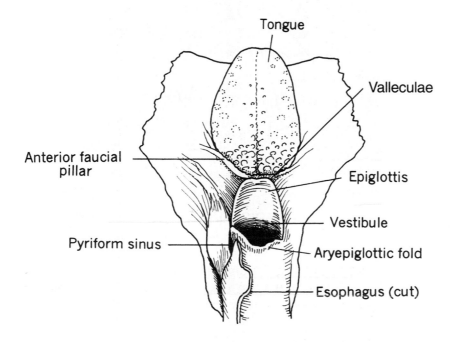

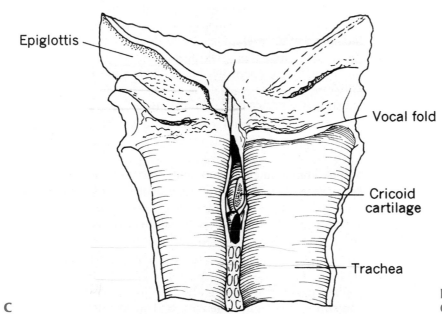

Figure 5-4. *(continued)*
C. Drawing showing landmarks.

C

171

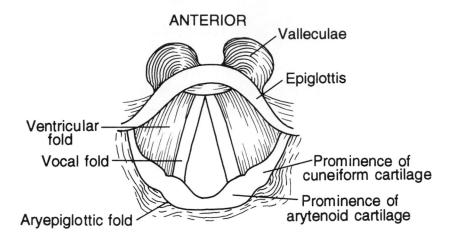

ANTERIOR

SUPERIOR VIEW

Figure 5-5. Vocal folds as seen from above.

In apes the laryngeal saccules are so well developed that they contribute to the resonance of the voice!

The middle space of the larynx lies between the margins of the false vocal folds and the true vocal folds below. This space is the **laryngeal ventricle** (or **laryngeal sinus**), and the anterior extension of this space is the **laryngeal saccule**. The saccule (or pouch) is endowed with more than 60 mucous glands that secrete lubricating mucus into the laryngeal cavity. These sacs are actually endowed with muscle to squeeze the mucus out for lubrication. The mucus also assists in eliminating errant food particles that enter the airway by encapsulating them, thereby enabling them to be eliminated through coughing.

The glottis is the space between the vocal folds, inferior to the ventricle and superior to the conus elasticus. This is the most important laryngeal space for speech, because it is defined by the *variable sphincter* that permits voicing. The length of the glottis is approximately 20 mm in adults at rest from the **anterior commissure** (anterior-most opening posterior to the angle of the thyroid cartilage) to the **posterior commissure** (between the arytenoid cartilages). The glottis area is variable, dependent upon the moment-by-moment configuration of the vocal folds. At rest the posterior glottis is approximately 8 mm wide, although that dimension will double during times of forced respiration.

The lateral margins of the glottis are the vocal folds and the arytenoid cartilage. The anterior three-fifths of the vocal margin is made up of the soft tissue of the vocal folds. (You will see this referred to as the **membranous glottis**, because some anatomists define the glottis as the entire vocal mechanism.) In adult males, the free margin of the vocal folds is approximately 15 mm in length, and in females it is approximately 12 mm. This free margin of the vocal folds is the vibrating element that provides voice. The posterior two-fifths of the vocal folds is comprised of the cartilage of the arytenoids. (This is often referred to as

Vocal Fold Hydration

The vocal folds are extremely sensitive to internal and external environment. Although the cigarette smoke and other pollutants are known to cause irritation to the tissues of the vocal folds, the internal environment appears to have an impact as well.

When the vocal folds are subject to abuse, several problems may arise, among them contact ulcers and vocal nodules. Hydration therapy is a frequent prescription to counteract the problems of irritated tissue. Dry tissue does not heal as well as moist tissue, so the client will be told to increase the environmental humidity, drink fluids, or even take medications to promote water retention. This type of therapy makes more than medical sense. Verdolini, Titze, and Fennell (1994) found that the *effort* of phonation increased as individuals became dehydrated, and decreased when they were hydrated beyond normal levels. Indeed, the airflow required to produce the same phonation is greatly increased by a poorly lubricated larynx. In addition, the vocal folds vibrate much more periodically (they have greatly reduced perturbation, or cycle-by-cycle variation) when lubricated (Fukida et al., 1988). When the relative periodicity of the vocal folds decreases, the voice sounds "hoarse," a perception that you will agree with if you think of the last time you had laryngitis.

the **cartilaginous glottis**, because "glottis" can refer also to the entire vocal mechanism.) This portion of the vocal folds is between 4 and 8 millimeters long, depending on gender and body size.

The conus elasticus begins at the margins of the true vocal folds and extends to the inferior border of the cricoid cartilage, widening from the vocal folds to the base of the cricoid.

In summary:

- The **vocal folds** are made up of five layers of tissue.
- Deep to the thin **epithelial layer** is the **lamina propria**, made up of two layers of elastin and one layer of collagen fibers. The thyrovocalis is the deepest of the layers.
- The **vocal ligament** is made of elastin. The **aditus** is the entryway of the larynx, marking the entry to the **vestibule**.
- The **ventricular** and **vocal folds** are separated by the **laryngeal ventricle**.
- The **glottis** is the variable space between the vocal folds.

Structure of the Larynx

Cricoid Cartilage

The unpaired cricoid cartilage can be viewed as an expanded tracheal cartilage (Figure 5-6). As the most inferior cartilage of the larynx, the cricoid cartilage is the approximate diameter of the trachea. It is higher in the back than in the front.

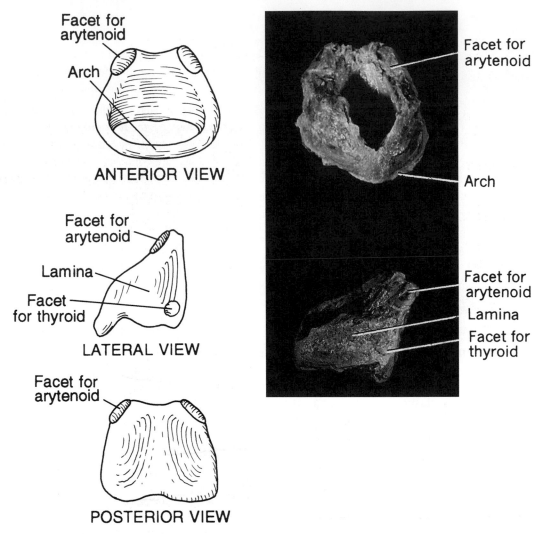

Facet for arytenoid

Arch

ANTERIOR VIEW

Facet for arytenoid

Lamina

Facet for thyroid

LATERAL VIEW

Facet for arytenoid

POSTERIOR VIEW

Facet for arytenoid

Arch

Facet for arytenoid

Lamina

Facet for thyroid

Figure 5-6. Cricoid cartilage and landmarks.

There are several important landmarks on the cricoid. The low, anterior cricoid arch provides clearance for the vocal folds that will pass over that point, while the posterior elevation, the superior surface of the **posterior quadrate lamina**, provides the point of articulation of the arytenoid cartilages. On the lateral surfaces of the cricoid are articular facets or "faces," marking the point of articulation of the inferior horns of the thyroid cartilage. This **cricothyroid joint** is a diarthrodial, pivoting joint that permits rotation of the two articulating structures. highly movable

One more note on the cricoid. The figures and photographs are quite misleading concerning the size of laryngeal structures. For perspective, your cricoid cartilage would fit loosely upon your little finger, which is about the diameter of your trachea. The laryngeal structures are *small*.

facets: *Fr., facette, small face*

Thyroid Cartilage

The unpaired thyroid cartilage is the largest of the laryngeal cartilages. As you can see in Figure 5-7, the thyroid has a prominent anterior surface made up of two plates called the thyroid laminae, joined at the midline

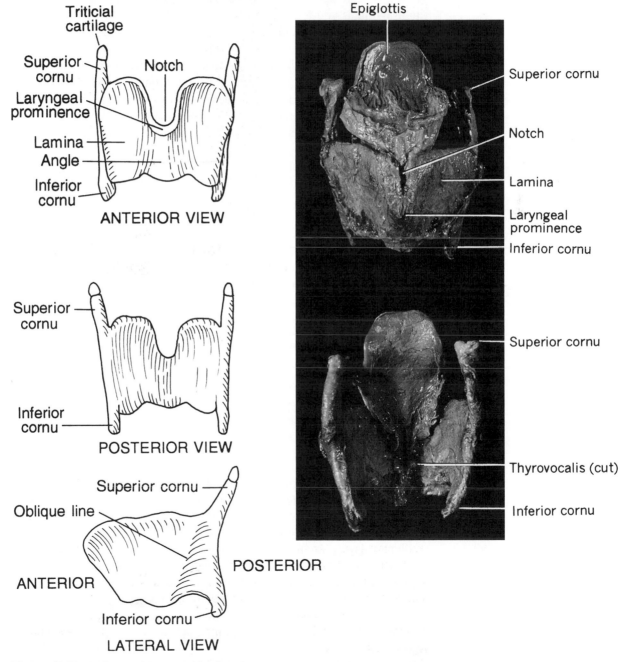

Figure 5-7. Thyroid cartilage and landmarks.

at the **thyroid angle**. At the superior-most point of that angle you will see the **thyroid notch**, which you can palpate if you do the following. Place your finger under your chin and on your throat, and bring it downward to the point you might refer to as your adam's apple (more prominent in males than females, for a good reason). When you have found the top of that structure you have identified the thyroid notch. Look at the drawing as you feel the indentation in your own thyroid. Now draw your finger down the midline a little until you feel the angle. If you put your index finger on the angle and your thumb and second finger on the sides, you will have digits on the angle and both laminae. Do take a moment to discover these regions on yourself, because they provide you with a reference that is near and dear to you. By the way, when you had your finger on the notch you were as close as you could be to touching your vocal folds, because they attach to the thyroid cartilage just behind that point.

Drawing your attention back to Figure 5-7, on the lateral superficial aspect of the thyroid laminae you will see the **oblique line**. This marks the point of attachment for two of the muscles we will talk about shortly.

The posterior aspect of the thyroid is open, and is characterized by two prominent sets of **cornu** or horns. The **inferior cornua** project downward to articulate with the cricoid cartilage, while the **superior cornua** project superiorly to articulate with the hyoid. In some individuals a small, **triticial cartilage** (*cartilago triticea*) may be found between the superior cornu of the thyroid cartilage and the hyoid bone.

cornu: *L., horn (as in cornucopia, the "horn of plenty")*

triticial: *L., triticeus, wheat; "wheat-like"*

Arytenoid and Corniculate Cartilages

The paired arytenoid cartilages are among the most important of the larynx. They reside on the superior posterolateral surface of the cricoid cartilage, and provide the mechanical structure that permits onset and offset of voicing. The form of the arytenoid may be likened to a pyramid to aid in visualization (see Figure 5-8). Each cartilage has two processes and four surfaces.

The apex is the truncated superior portion of the pyramidal arytenoid cartilage, and on the superior surfaces of each arytenoid is a **corniculate cartilage**, projecting posteriorly to form the peak of the distorted pyramid. The inferior surface of the cartilage is termed the **base**, and its concave surface is the point of articulation with the convex arytenoid facet of the cricoid cartilage.

The names of the two processes of the arytenoid give a hint as to their function. The **vocal processes** project anteriorly toward the thyroid notch, and it is these processes to which the posterior portion of the vocal folds themselves will attach. The **muscular process** forms the lateral outcropping of the arytenoid pyramid and, as its name implies, is the point of attachment for muscles that adduct and abduct the vocal folds.

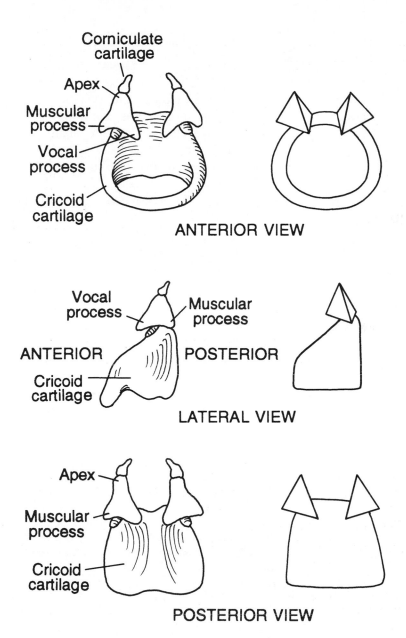

ANTERIOR VIEW

LATERAL VIEW

POSTERIOR VIEW

Figure 5-8. Arytenoid cartilages articulated with cricoid cartilage.

Epiglottis

The unpaired epiglottis is a leaflike structure that arises from the inner surface of the angle of the thyroid cartilage just below the notch, being attached there by the thyroepiglottic ligament. The sides of the epiglottis are joined with the arytenoid cartilages via the aryepiglottic folds, which are the product of the membranous lining draping over muscle and connective tissue.

The epiglottis projects upward beyond the larynx and above the hyoid bone and is attached to the root of the tongue by means of the median **glosso-epiglottic fold** and the paired **lateral glosso-epiglottic ligaments**. This juncture produces the valleculae, landmarks which will become important in your study of swallowing and swallowing deficit. During swallowing, food passes over the epiglottis, and from there laterally to the **pyriform** (also piriform) sinuses, which are small fossae or indentations between the aryepiglottic folds medially and the mucous lining of the thyroid cartilage. Together, the pyriform sinuses and valleculae are called the **pharyngeal recesses** (see Figure 5-5).

The epiglottis is attached to the hyoid bone via the **hyoepiglottic ligament**. The surface of the epiglottis is covered with mucous membrane lining, and beneath this lining on the posterior, concave surface may be found branches of the internal laryngeal nerve of the X vagus that conduct sensory information from the larynx.

See Chapter 12 for a discussion of the X vagus nerve.

vagus: *L., wandering*

cuneiform: *L., cuneus, wedge; "wedge-shaped"*

Cuneiform Cartilages

The cuneiform cartilages are small cartilages embedded within the aryepiglottic folds. They are situated above and anterior to the corniculate cartilages, and cause a small bulge on the surface of the membrane that looks white under illumination. These cartilages apparently provide support for the membranous laryngeal covering.

Hyoid Bone

Although not a bone of the larynx, the hyoid is the union between the tongue and the laryngeal structure. This unpaired small bone articulates loosely with the superior cornu of the thyroid cartilage, and has the distinction of being the only bone of the body that is not attached to other bone (see Figure 5-9).

As you can see from the view of the hyoid bone from above, this structure is U-shaped, being open in the posterior. There are three major elements of the hyoid bone. The corpus or body of the hyoid is the prominent shieldlike structure forming the front of the bone, and is a structure you can palpate. If you place your finger on your thyroid notch and push *lightly* back toward your vertebral column, you will feel the hard structure of the corpus near your fingernail. As you are doing this, take one more look at the figure showing the structures together (see Figure 5-1), to become acquainted with the relationship of these structures.

The front of the corpus is convex, and the inner surface is concave. The corpus is the point of attachment for six muscles, no small feat for such a small structure.

The **greater cornu** arises on the lateral surface of the corpus, projecting posteriorly. At the junction of the corpus and greater cornu you can see the **lesser cornu**. Three additional muscles attach to these two structures.

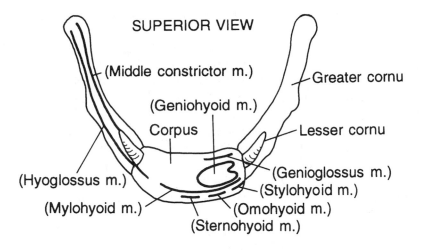

SUPERIOR VIEW

(Middle constrictor m.)

(Geniohyoid m.)

Corpus

Greater cornu

Lesser cornu

(Genioglossus m.)
(Stylohyoid m.)
(Omohyoid m.)

(Hyoglossus m.)

(Mylohyoid m.)

(Sternohyoid m.)

POSTERIOR VIEW

(Hyoepiglottic ligament)

Lesser cornu

(Thyrohyoid membrane)

(Thyrohyoid m.)

Figure 5-9. Hyoid bone as seen from above and behind. Points of attachment of muscles and membranes are indicated in parentheses.

Movement of the Cartilages

The cricothyroid and cricoarytenoid joints are the only functionally mobile points of the larynx, and both of these joints serve extremely important laryngeal functions.

The cricothyroid joint is the junction of the cricoid cartilage and inferior cornu of the thyroid cartilage, as mentioned earlier. These are synovial joints that permit the cricoid and thyroid to rotate and glide relative to each other. As seen in Figure 5-10, rotation at the cricothyroid joint permits the thyroid cartilage to rock down in front, and the joint also permits the thyroid to glide forward and backward slightly relative to the cricoid. This joint provides the major adjustment for change in vocal pitch.

The **cricoarytenoid joint** is the articulation formed between the cricoid and arytenoid cartilages. As you will recall, the base of the arytenoid cartilage is concave, mating with the smooth convex superior surface of the cricoid cartilage. These synovial joints permit rocking, gliding, and perhaps minimal rotation. The arytenoid facet of the cricoid is a convex, oblong surface, and the axis of motion is around a line projecting back along the superior surface of the arytenoid and converging

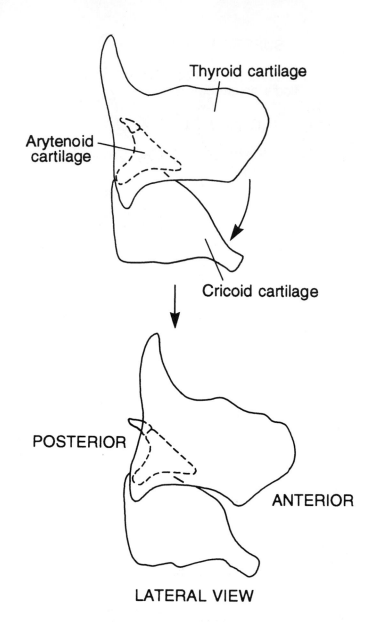

Figure 5-10. Movement of the cricoid and thyroid cartilages about the cricothyroid joint. When the cricoid and thyroid move toward each other in front, the arytenoid cartilage moves farther away from the thyroid cartilage, tensing the vocal folds.

above at a point above the arytenoid (see Figure 5-11). This rocking action rocks the two vocal processes toward each other, permitting the vocal folds to **approximate** (make contact). The arytenoids are capable also of gliding on the long axis of the facet, facilitating changes in vocal fold length. The arytenoids also may rotate upon a vertical axis drawn through the apex of the arytenoid, but this motion appears to be limited to extremes of abduction (Fink & Demarest, 1978). The combination of these gestures provides the mechanism for vocal fold approximation and abduction.

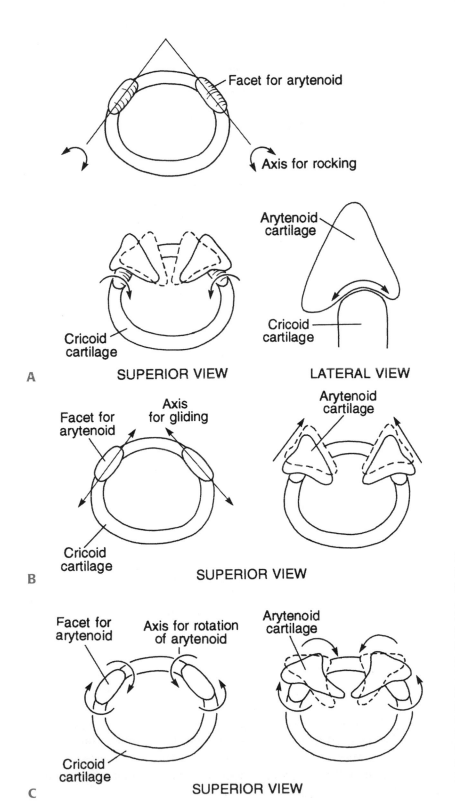

Figure 5-11. The articular facet for the arytenoid cartilage permits rocking, gliding, and rotation. **A.** The shape of the articular facet for the arytenoid cartilage promotes inward rocking of the arytenoid cartilage and vocal folds, as shown by the arrows. **B.** The long axis of the facet permits limited anterior-posterior gliding. **C.** The arytenoids may also rotate as shown, although this does not appear to be a functional gesture for adduction. (Based on data of Broad, 1973; Fink & Demarest, 1978; Netter, 1997; Zemlin, 1998.)

Palpation of the Larynx

To palpate the larynx, first identify the prominent thyroid notch or "adam's apple" (see Figure 5–7). Once you have found it, place your index finger on the notch itself, with your thumb and second finger on either side. Your thumb and second finger should feel a fairly flat surface, the thyroid lamina. Now bring your index finger straight down a little bit, and you will feel the prominent thyroid angle. Bring your finger back up to the top of the notch; when your finger is on top of the notch, the hard region contacting your fingernail is the corpus of the hyoid bone. In some people this is very hard to differentiate from the thyroid.

Palpate lateral to the notch on the superior surface and you will feel the superior cornu of thyroid. With a little discomfort you may feel the articulation of the hyoid and thyroid. If you draw your finger down the angle again you can find the lower margin of the thyroid, and feel the cricoid beneath. By carefully placing your thumb at the junction of the cricoid and thyroid, you can hum up and down the scale and feel the thyroid and cricoid moving closer together and farther apart as you do this. You will also feel the entire larynx elevate as you reach the upper end of your range. Finally, draw your finger to find the lower margin of the cricoid, marking the beginning of the trachea. Palpate the tracheal rings.

Your understanding of the movement of these cartilages in relation to each other will provide a valuable backdrop to understanding the laryngeal physiology presented in Chapter 6.

To summarize:
- The laryngeal cartilages have a number of important landmarks to which muscles are attached.
- The **cricoid** cartilage is shaped like a signet ring, higher in back.
- The **arytenoid** cartilages ride on the superior surface of the cricoid, with the cricoarytenoid joint permitting rotation, rocking, and gliding.
- The **muscular** and **vocal processes** provide attachment for the **thyromuscularis** and **thyrovocalis** muscles.
- The **corniculate** cartilages attach to the upper margin of the arytenoids.
- The **thyroid** cartilage has two prominent laminae, superior and inferior horns, and a prominent thyroid notch.
- The **hyoid bone** attaches to the superior cornu of the thyroid, while the **cricoid** cartilage attaches to the inferior horn via the cricothyroid joint.
- The **epiglottis** attaches to the tongue and thyroid cartilage, dropping down to cover the larynx during swallowing.
- The **cuneiform** cartilages are embedded within the aryepiglottic folds.

LARYNGEAL MUSCULATURE

As summarized in Table 5-1, muscles of the larynx may be conveniently divided into muscles that have both origin and insertion on laryngeal cartilages (**intrinsic laryngeal muscles**) and those with one attachment on a laryngeal cartilage and the other attachment on a nonlaryngeal

Table 5-1. Muscles associated with laryngeal function.

INTRINSIC MUSCLES OF LARYNX

Adductors
Lateral cricoarytenoid
Transverse arytenoid
Oblique arytenoid

Abductor
Posterior cricoarytenoid

Tensors
Thyrovocalis (medial thyroarytenoid)
Cricothyroid, pars recta, and pars oblique

Relaxers
Thyromuscularis (lateral thyroarytenoid)

Auxiliary Musculature
Thyroepiglotticus*
Superior thyroarytenoid
Thyroarytenoid
Aryepiglotticus

SUPRAHYOID AND INFRAHYOID MUSCLES

Hyoid and Laryngeal Elevators
Stylohyoid
Mylohyoid
Geniohyoid
Genioglossus
Hyoglossus
Inferior pharyngeal constrictor
Digastricus anterior and posterior

Hyoid and Laryngeal Depressors
Sternothyroid
Sternohyoid
Omohyoid
Thyrohyoid

*Note that the thyroepiglottic muscle is included here by virtue of its relevance to the swallowing function.

Referral in Voice Therapy

The phonatory mechanism is extremely sensitive, and vocal signs can be indicators for a broad range of problems. We must always refer an individual to a physician when we identify vocal dysfunction, even though we may be fairly certain that the problem is behavioral in nature. When a client comes to us with a hoarse voice, we may find out that the person is abusing his or her phonatory mechanism by spending too much time in loud, smoky settings that require raising the voice when speaking. What we don't know from this information is whether there is a vocal pathology, perhaps secondary to the same behavioral conditions, that is developing on the vocal folds. Although we suspect vocal nodules, the client could also be showing early signs of laryngeal cancer.

In a similar vein, a client who comes to us with a voice that is progressively weaker during the day, and for whom muscular effort of any sort is extremely difficult as the day wears on, will easily merit a referral, although it will be to a neurologist. Myasthenia gravis is a myoneural disease that results in a complex of speech disorders, including progressive weakening of phonation, progressive degeneration of articulatory function, and progressive hypernasality, all arising from use of the speech mechanism over the course of a day or briefer time. The condition is quite treatable, but often the speech-language pathologist is the individual to first recognize the signs because the client sees it primarily as a speech problem.

structure (**extrinsic laryngeal muscles**). The extrinsic muscles make major adjustments of the larynx, such as elevating or depressing it, while the intrinsic musculature makes fine adjustments of the vocal mechanism itself. Extrinsic muscles tend to work in concert with articulatory gestures of the tongue, and many are important in swallowing. Intrinsic muscles assume responsibility for opening, closing, tensing, and relaxing the vocal folds. We will begin with a discussion of the intrinsic muscles. The summary information of Appendix D may be helpful to your studies.

Intrinsic Laryngeal Muscles

Adductors

- **Lateral cricoarytenoid**
- **Transverse arytenoid**
- **Oblique arytenoid**

Lateral Cricoarytenoid Muscle. This extremely important muscle is one of the more difficult laryngeal muscles to visualize. The **lateral cricoarytenoid muscle** attaches to the cricoid and the muscular process of the arytenoid, causing the muscular process to move forward and medially (see Figure 5-12). The origin of the lateral cricoarytenoid muscle is the superior-lateral surface of the cricoid cartilage. The muscle courses up and back to insert into the muscular process of the arytenoid cartilage.

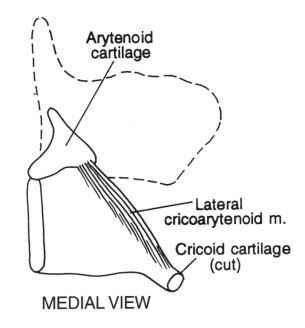

MEDIAL VIEW

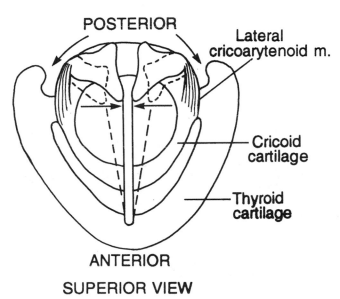

SUPERIOR VIEW

Figure 5-12. Course and effect of lateral cricoarytenoid muscle. Note that the cricoid cartilage in the upper figure has been cut so that you are viewing the left arytenoid from a medial perspective. The lower figure shows that contraction of the lateral cricoarytenoid muscle pulls the muscular process forward, adducting the vocal folds (seen from above).

As you can see from this figure, the course of the muscle dictates that the muscular process will be drawn forward, and that motion will rock the arytenoid inward and downward. This inward-and-downward rocking is the major adjustment associated with adduction of the vocal folds. In addition, this movement may lengthen the vocal folds (Hirano, Kiyokawa, & Kurita, 1988).

Innervation of all intrinsic muscles of the larynx is by means of the X vagus nerve. The vagus is a large, wandering nerve with multiple

Muscle:	Lateral cricoarytenoid
Origin:	Superior-lateral surface of the cricoid cartilage
Course:	Up and back
Insertion:	Muscular process of the arytenoid
Innervation:	X vagus, recurrent laryngeal nerve
Function:	Adducts vocal folds; increases medial compression

responsibilities for sensation and motor function in the thorax, neck, and abdomen. The vagus arises from the nucleus ambiguus of the medulla oblongata and divides into two major branches, the recurrent (inferior) laryngeal nerve (RLN) and the superior laryngeal nerve (SLN). The RLN is so named because of its course. The left RLN "re-courses" beneath the aorta, after which it ascends to innervate the larynx. The right RLN courses under the subclavian artery before ascending to the larynx. (This close association to the vascular supply results in voice problems arising from vascular disease, because **aneurysm** or enlargement of the aorta or subclavian artery may compress the left RLN and cause vocal dysfunction).

aneurysm: *Gr., anyeurysma, widening*

Transverse Arytenoid Muscle. The **transverse arytenoid muscle** also may be called the **transverse interarytenoid** muscle. This unpaired muscle is a band of fibers spanning the posterior surface of both arytenoid cartilages. As you can see from Figure 5-13, it is a band of fibers running from the lateral margin of the posterior surface of one arytenoid to the corresponding surface of the other arytenoid. Its function is to pull the two arytenoids closer together, and, by association, to approximate the vocal folds. It provides additional support for tight occlusion or closing of the vocal folds, and is an important element of medial compression. **Medial compression** refers to the degree of force that may be applied by the vocal folds at their point of contact. Increased medial compression is a function of increased force of adduction, and this is a vital element in vocal intensity change, as you shall see. Motor innervation of the transverse arytenoid muscles is by means of the inferior branch of the recurrent laryngeal nerve arising from the X vagus.

Muscle:	Transverse arytenoid
Origin:	Lateral margin of posterior arytenoid
Course:	Laterally
Insertion:	Lateral margin of posterior surface, opposite arytenoid
Innervation:	X vagus, recurrent laryngeal nerve
Function:	Adducts vocal folds

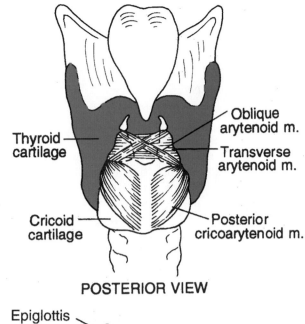

POSTERIOR VIEW

A

Thyroid cartilage

Cricoid cartilage

Oblique arytenoid m.

Transverse arytenoid m.

Posterior cricoarytenoid m.

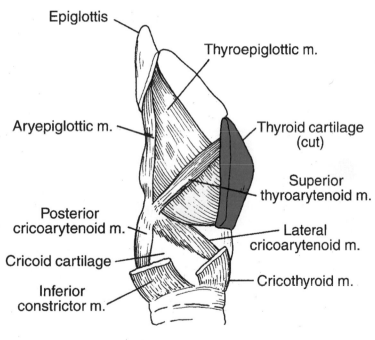

Epiglottis

Thyroepiglottic m.

Aryepiglottic m.

Posterior cricoarytenoid m.

Cricoid cartilage

Inferior constrictor m.

Thyroid cartilage (cut)

Superior thyroarytenoid m.

Lateral cricoarytenoid m.

Cricothyroid m.

B   **LATERAL VIEW**

Figure 5-13. A. Schematic of posterior cricoarytenoid muscle and transverse and oblique arytenoid muscles. Contraction of the transverse and oblique arytenoid muscles will pull the arytenoids closer together, thereby supporting adduction. Contraction of the posterior cricoarytenoid muscle pulls the muscular process back, abducting the vocal folds. **B.** Schematic illustrating relationship among posterior cricoarytenoid, lateral cricoarytenoid, superior thyroarytenoid, and aryepiglottic muscle.

Oblique Arytenoid Muscles.   The **oblique arytenoid muscles** also are known as the **oblique interarytenoid muscles**. The oblique arytenoid muscles are immediately superficial to the transverse arytenoid muscles, and perform a similar function. The paired oblique arytenoid muscles take

Muscle: Oblique arytenoid
Origin: Posterior base of the muscular processes
Course: Obliquely up
Insertion: Apex of the opposite arytenoid
Innervation: X vagus, recurrent laryngeal nerve
Function: Pulls the apex medially

their origins at the posterior base of the muscular processes to course obliquely up to the apex of the opposite arytenoid. This course results in a characteristic "X" arrangement of the muscles, as well as in the ability of these muscles to pull the apex medially. This action promotes adduction, enforces medial compression, and rocks the arytenoid (and vocal folds) down and in. Working in concert with the aryepiglottic muscle, the oblique arytenoid muscle aids in pulling the epiglottis to cover the opening to the larynx as it also serves tight adduction. Innervation of the oblique arytenoid muscles is the same as for the transverse arytenoid muscles.

Abductor

- **Posterior cricoarytenoid muscle**

Posterior Cricoarytenoid Muscle. The **posterior cricoarytenoid muscle** is the sole abductor of the vocal folds. It is a small but prominent muscle of the posterior larynx. As you can see from Figure 5-13, the posterior cricoarytenoid muscle originates on the posterior cricoid lamina. Fibers project up and out to insert into the posterior aspect of the muscular process of the arytenoid cartilage. By virtue of their attachments to the muscular processes, the posterior cricoarytenoid muscles are direct antagonists to the lateral cricoarytenoids (see Figures 5–13 and 5–14).

Contraction of this muscle pulls the muscular process posteriorly, rocking the arytenoid cartilage out on its axis and abducting the vocal folds. This muscle is quite active during physical exertion, broadly abducting the vocal folds to permit greater air movement into and out of the lungs. The posterior cricoarytenoid is innervated by the recurrent laryngeal nerve, a branch of the X vagus.

Muscle: Posterior cricoarytenoid
Origin: Posterior cricoid lamina
Course: Obliquely up
Insertion: Posterior aspect of the opposite arytenoid
Innervation: X vagus, recurrent laryngeal nerve
Function: Pulls the apex medially

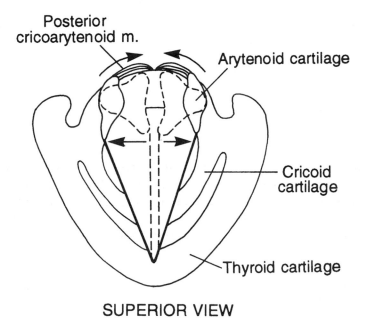

Figure 5-14. Superior view of action of the posterior cricoarytenoid muscle.

Glottal Tensors

- **Cricothyroid muscle**
- **Thyrovocalis muscle**

Cricothyroid Muscle. The primary tensor of the vocal folds achieves its function by rocking the thyroid cartilage forward relative to the cricoid cartilage. The **cricothyroid muscle** is composed of two heads, the pars recta and pars oblique, as seen in Figure 5-15.

The **pars recta** is the medial-most component of the cricothyroid muscle, originating on the anterior surface of the cricoid cartilage immediately beneath the arch. The pars recta courses up and out, to insert into the lower surface of the thyroid lamina. The **pars oblique** arises from the cricoid cartilage lateral to the pars recta, coursing obliquely up to insert into the point of juncture between the thyroid laminae and inferior horns.

The angle of incidence of these two segments speaks to their relative functions. Although both tense the vocal folds, individually these muscles have differing effects on the motion of the thyroid. Let us look at both of them.

By virtue of its more directly superior course, contraction of the pars recta rocks the thyroid cartilage downward, rotating upon the cricothyroid joint. Due to the flexibility of the loosely joined tracheal cartilages below, the cricoid will rise to meet the thyroid as well. This is a good time to remind you that the points of attachment of the vocal folds are the inner margin of the thyroid cartilage and arytenoid cartilages, and that the arytenoid cartilages are attached to the posterior

pars recta: *L., part + straight*

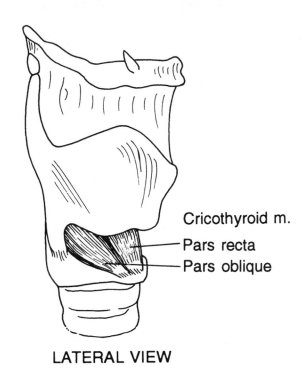

Cricothyroid m.
Pars recta
Pars oblique

LATERAL VIEW

Figure 5-15. Cricothyroid muscle, pars recta, and pars oblique.

cricoid cartilage. The effect of rocking the thyroid cartilage forward is that the vocal folds, slung between the posterior cricoid and anterior thyroid, are stretched. That is, rocking the thyroid and cricoid closer together in front makes the posterior cricoid more distant from the thyroid.

Vocal Hyperfunction

We have emphasized the notion that the larynx is a *small* structure, but we should add that even small muscles are capable of being misused. **Vocal hyperfunction** refers to using excessive adductory force, often resulting in **laryngitis**, which is inflammation of the vocal folds. Excessively forceful contraction of the lateral cricoarytenoid and the arytenoid muscles is undoubtedly the primary contributor to this problem, although it is also likely that laryngeal tension arising from contraction of the thyroarytenoid (thyromuscularis and thyrovocalis) and cricothyroid (with support by posterior cricoarytenoid) are contributors to this extraordinary force. In case you did not notice, that list included virtually all of the significant intrinsic laryngeal musculature, which should emphasize the notion that vocal hyperfunction is the result of general laryngeal tension. Vocal hyperfunction can result in laryngitis, vocal nodules, contact ulcers, vocal polyps, and vocal fatigue, and is usually behavioral in etiology.

Treatment typically requires a significant behavioral change in the client, but this is not without a cost. The voice is an extremely personal entity and is very tightly woven to an individual's self-concept. Approaching a client to change his or her voice is a delicate and challenging task for a clinician.

Muscle:	Cricothyroid
Origin:	Pars recta: anterior surface of the cricoid cartilage beneath the arch
	Pars oblique: cricoid cartilage lateral to the pars recta
Course:	Pars recta: up and out
	Pars oblique: obliquely up
Insertion:	Pars recta: lower surface of the thyroid lamina
	Pars oblique: thyroid cartilage between laminae and inferior horns
Innervation:	External branch of superior laryngeal nerve of X vagus
Function:	Depresses thyroid relative to cricoid; tenses vocal folds

The cricothyroid joint also permits the thyroid to slide forward and backward. The forward sliding motion is a function of the pars oblique, and the result is to tense the vocal folds as well. Together, the pars recta and oblique are responsible for the major laryngeal adjustment associated with pitch change. The cricothyroid is innervated by the external branch of the superior laryngeal nerve (SLN) of the X vagus. This branch courses lateral to the inferior pharyngeal constrictor to terminate on the cricothyroid muscle.

Thyrovocalis Muscle. The **thyrovocalis muscle** is actually the medial muscle of the vocal folds. Many anatomists define a singular muscle coursing from the posterior surface of the thyroid cartilage to the arytenoid cartilages, labeling it as the thyroarytenoid. There is ample *functional* evidence to support differentiating the thyroarytenoid into two separate muscles, the thyromuscularis and the thyrovocalis, although anatomical support for dividing it into two muscles is questionable. Although the thyromuscularis is discussed as a glottal relaxer, the contraction of the thyrovocalis distinctly tenses the vocal folds, especially when contracted in concert with the cricothyroid muscle.

The thyrovocalis (abbreviated as vocalis) originates from the inner surface of the thyroid cartilage near the thyroid notch. The muscle courses back to insert into the lateral surface of the arytenoid vocal process. Contraction of this muscle draws the thyroid and cricoid cartilages farther apart in front, making this muscle a functional antagonist of the cricothyroid muscle (which draws the anterior cricoid and anterior

Muscle:	Thyrovocalis (medial thyroarytenoid)
Origin:	Inner surface, thyroid cartilage near notch
Course:	Back
Insertion:	Lateral surface of the arytenoid vocal process
Innervation:	Recurrent laryngeal nerve, X vagus
Function:	Tenses vocal folds

thyroid closer together). This antagonistic function has earned the thyrovocalis classification as a glottal tensor, because contraction of the thyrovocalis (balanced by contraction of the cricothyroid muscle) tenses the vocal folds. The thyrovocalis is innervated by the recurrent laryngeal nerve, a branch of the X vagus.

Relaxers
- **Thyromuscularis**
- **Superior thyroarytenoid muscle**

Thyromuscularis Muscle.   The paired **thyromuscularis muscles** (or simply, muscularis) are considered to be the muscle masses immediately lateral to each thyrovocalis, and which, with the thyrovocalis, make up the thyroarytenoid muscle. The **thyromuscularis** or **external (lateral) thyroarytenoid** originates on the inner surface of the thyroid cartilage, near the notch and lateral to the origin of the thyrovocalis. It runs back to insert into the arytenoid cartilage at the muscular process and base.

Although there are questions about whether this muscle is truly differentiated from the vocalis, functional differences are clearly seen. As you can see from Figure 5-16, the forces exerted on the arytenoid from pulling differentially on the vocal or muscular process would produce markedly different effects. Contraction of the thyromuscularis has essentially the same effect on the vocal folds as contraction of the lateral cricoarytenoid. The vocal folds adduct and lengthen (Hirano, Kiyokawa, & Kurita, 1988).

Contraction of the medial fibers of the thyromuscularis may relax the vocal folds as well. By virtue of their attachment on the anterior surface

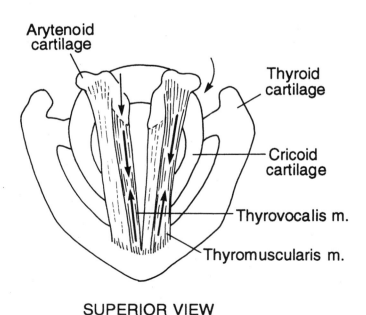

Figure 5-16. The thyromuscularis muscle is the lateral muscular component of the vocal folds; the thyrovocalis is the medial-most muscle of the vocal folds. Together they are often referred to as the thyroarytenoid muscle.

Muscle:	Thyromuscularis (lateral thyroarytenoid)
Origin:	Inner surface of thyroid cartilage near the notch
Course:	Back
Insertion:	Muscular process and base of arytenoid cartilage
Innervation:	Recurrent laryngeal nerve, X vagus
Function:	Relaxes vocal folds

of the arytenoid, these fibers pull the arytenoids toward the thyroid cartilage without influencing medial rocking. Thus, the thyromuscularis muscle is classically considered to be a laryngeal relaxer. The thyromuscularis is innervated by the recurrent laryngeal nerve, a branch of the X vagus.

Auxiliary Musculature

- **Thyroepiglottic (thyroepiglotticus) muscle**
- **Superior thyroarytenoid muscle**
- **Aryepiglottic muscle**

Thyroarytenoid, Thyroepiglotticus, and Aryepiglotticus. As discussed previously, the thyroarytenoid muscle (see Figure 5-16), which consists of the thyrovocalis and thyromuscularis muscles, arises from the lower thyroid angle. The thyroarytenoid courses back to insert into the anterolateral

Muscle:	Superior thyroarytenoid
Origin:	Inner angle of thyroid cartilage
Course:	Back
Insertion:	Muscular process of arytenoid
Innervation:	Recurrent laryngeal nerve, X vagus
Function:	Perhaps relaxes vocal fold

Muscle:	Thyroepiglottic muscle
Origin:	Inner surface of thyroid at angle
Course:	Back and up
Insertion:	Lateral epiglottis
Innervation:	Recurrent laryngeal nerve, X vagus
Function:	Dilates airway

Muscle:	Aryepiglottic muscle
Origin:	Continuation of oblique arytenoid muscle from arytenoid apex
Course:	Back and up as muscular component of aryepiglottic fold
Insertion:	Lateral epiglottis
Innervation:	Recurrent laryngeal nerve, X vagus
Function:	Constricts laryngeal opening

surface of the arytenoid cartilages. The medial fibers of the thyroarytenoid constitute the thyrovocalis muscle, while the superior fibers are continuous with the thyroepiglotticus superiorly. The superior thyroarytenoid is inconsistently present, arising from the inner angle of the thyroid cartilage and coursing to the muscular process of the arytenoid. The aryepiglottic muscle (see Figure 5-17) arises from the superior aspect of the oblique arytenoid muscle (i.e., the arytenoid apex), and continues as the muscular component of the aryepiglottic fold as it courses to insert into the lateral epiglottis. The thyroepiglotticus dilates the laryngeal opening,

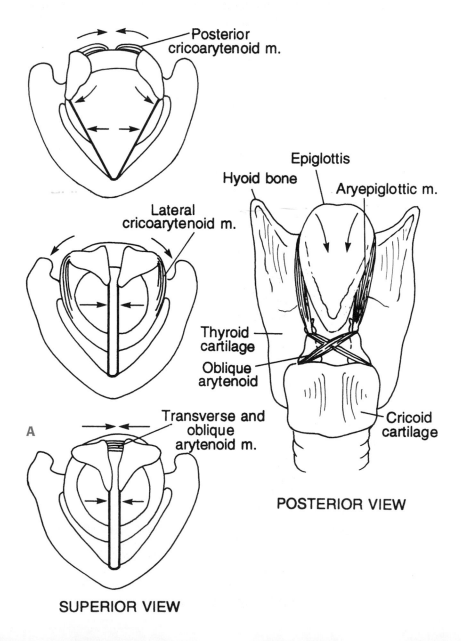

Figure 5-17. A. Thyrovocalis and thyromuscularis are tensed upon contraction of the cricothyroid muscle. *(continues)*

while the aryepiglotticus assists in protecting the airway during swallowing by deflecting the epiglottic cartilage over the laryngeal aditus (Gray et al., 1995). It is assumed that the superior thyroarytenoid serves as a relaxer of the vocal folds, like the thyromuscularis, although this has not been demonstrated.

Summary of Intrinsic Muscle Activity

Figure 5-17 will help us proceed with this discussion. Intrinsic muscles of the larynx include the thyrovocalis, thyromuscularis, cricothyroid, lateral and posterior cricoarytenoid, transverse arytenoid and oblique interarytenoid, superior thyroarytenoid muscles, and thyroepiglotticus. The

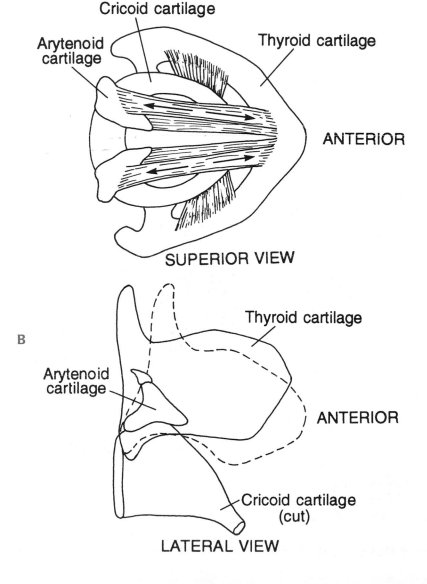

Figure 5-17. *(continued)* **B.** Contraction of muscle causes the thyroid to rock forward and down as the cricoid rocks up in front.

"Ain't Misbehavin' "

The range of phonatory "misbehavior" is broad and deep. The larynx is an exquisite structure made up of delicate tissues designed for use as a protective mechanism. When we use it as a phonatory source we capitalize on its flexibility. When we overuse the mechanism, we can get into trouble. Here are a few of the problems that can occur from laryngeal misuse.

Vocal nodules arise from excessively loud phonation or excessively forceful adduction. Contact ulcers apparently arise from excessive force on the posterior aspect of the vocal folds, applied by attempting to force the vocal folds into a lower vocal range and higher-than-appropriate vocal intensity.

The addition of toxins into your laryngeal environment can cause trouble as well. Alcohol consumption can irritate the vocal folds, as can cigarette and cigar smoke (primary or secondary smoke). Likewise, excessively dry air can irritate the vocal folds, leading to laryngitis. A diet that causes esophageal reflux can cause laryngeal irritation.

thyrovocalis and thyromuscularis muscles make up the muscular portion of the vocal folds. The cricothyroid pulls the anterior cricoid and anterior thyroid closer together, thereby stretching the vocal folds. The lateral cricoarytenoid adducts the vocal folds by rocking the arytenoids medially, while the posterior cricoarytenoid muscle abducts the vocal folds. The oblique and transverse arytenoid muscles pull the arytenoids closer together, assisting adduction. The superior thyroarytenoid muscle is variously present, serving to relax the vocal folds. The thyroepiglotticus has no apparent function in speech, but it is active during the pharyngeal stage of the swallow, as discussed in Chapter 9.

Movement of the vocal folds into and out of approximation (adduction and abduction) is achieved by coordinated effort of many of the intrinsic muscles of the larynx. The lateral cricoarytenoid muscle is responsible for rocking the arytenoid cartilage on its axis, causing the vocal folds to tip in and slightly down. This action is directly opposed by contraction of the posterior cricoarytenoid muscle, which rocks the arytenoid (and vocal folds) out on that same axis. Contraction of the transverse arytenoid muscle draws the posterior surfaces of the two arytenoids closer together, but it is most effective as an adductor if the lateral cricoarytenoid muscle is contracted as well. Contraction of the oblique arytenoid helps the vocal folds dip downward as they are adducted.

The thyroepiglotticus and aryepiglotticus are antagonists, in that the thyroepiglotticus increases the size of the laryngeal opening while the aryepiglotticus narrows it. These two functions are probably not components of communication, but rather assist in deep respiratory effort (thyroepiglotticus) and protection of the airway (aryepiglotticus).

The fact that the vocal folds rock in and down is not trivial. The force vector associated with this movement improves the ability of the vocal folds to impede outward flow of air, because more force is directed in an inferior direction than if the arytenoid rotated on a vertical axis.

The muscles of abduction and adduction work in concert to complete their task in one more way. Although you know that the vocal folds must be adducted and abducted, you should start becoming aware that a full range of laryngeal adjustments is possible, from completely abducted to tightly adducted. We use this full range during phonation, and the bulk of the voice clients on the caseload of a public school clinician will arise from inadequate control of this musculature (vocal nodules secondary to laryngeal hyperfunction).

Recalling the physical parameters that can be altered to change pitch will help you realize that either mass or tension is a likely candidate. Increasing the tension on the vocal folds will stretch them and thereby reduce the mass per unit length. Stretching the vocal folds does not decrease the mass of the muscle, but does decrease it relative to overall length. Both increased tension and reduced mass per unit length will increase frequency of vibration of the vocal folds, while relaxing the vocal folds will cause the frequency to drop.

Note that when the cricothyroid is contracted, the thyrovocalis will be stretched. If you also contract the thyrovocalis, the vocal folds will become tenser and the pitch raised.

Extrinsic Laryngeal Muscles

The extrinsic musculature consists of muscles with one attachment to a laryngeal cartilage. These include the sternothyroid, thyrohyoid, and thyropharyngeus muscles. A number of muscles attached to the hyoid also move the larynx, and these are described as infrahyoid muscles, which run from the hyoid to a structure below, and **suprahyoid muscles**, which attach to a structure above the hyoid. Infrahyoid muscles consist of the sternohyoid and omohyoid muscles, while the suprahyoid muscles are digastricus, stylohyoid, mylohyoid, geniohyoid, genioglossus, and hyoglossus muscles. They are often called the *strap muscles*.

A more functional categorization is based on function relative to the larynx. Muscles that elevate the hyoid and larynx are termed **laryngeal elevators** (digastricus, stylohyoid, mylohyoid, geniohyoid, genioglossus, hyoglossus, and thyropharyngeus muscles) and those that depress the larynx and hyoid are **laryngeal depressors** (sternohyoid, omohyoid, thyrohyoid, and sternothyroid muscles).

Hyoid and Laryngeal Elevators
- **Digastricus anterior and posterior**
- **Stylohyoid muscle**
- **Mylohyoid muscle**
- **Geniohyoid muscle**

- Genioglossus muscle
- Hyoglossus muscle
- Thyropharyngeus muscle

digastricus: *L., two + belly*

symphysis: *Gr., growing together*

Digastricus. As seen in Figure 5-18, the **digastricus muscle** is actually composed of two separate bellies. The anterior and posterior bellies of the digastricus muscle converge at the hyoid bone, and their paired contraction elevates the hyoid. The **digastricus anterior** originates on the inner surface of the mandible at the digastricus fossa, near the point of fusion of the two halves of the mandible, the **symphysis**. The muscle courses medially and down to the level of the hyoid, where it joins with the posterior digastricus by means of an **intermediate tendon**. The **posterior digastricus** originates on the mastoid process of the temporal bone, behind and beneath the ear. The intermediate tendon passes through and separates the fibers of another muscle, the stylohyoid, as it inserts into the hyoid at the juncture of the hyoid corpus and greater cornu.

The structure and attachment of the digastricus bellies define their function. Contraction of the anterior component results in the hyoid being drawn up and forward, whereas contraction of the posterior belly causes the hyoid to be drawn up and back. Simultaneous contraction

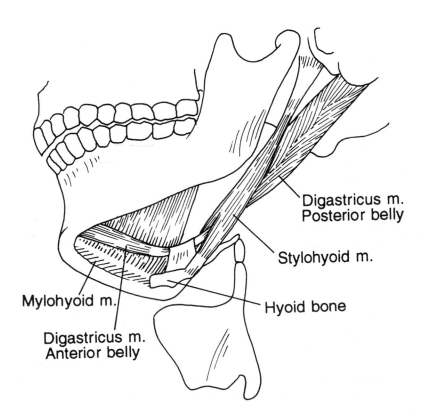

Figure 5-18. Schematic of digastricus, stylohyoid, and mylohyoid muscles. (After data and view of Netter, 1997.)

Muscle: Digastricus, anterior and posterior
Origin: Anterior: inner surface of the mandible, near symphysis
              Posterior: mastoid process of temporal bone
Course: Medial and down
Insertion: Hyoid, by means of intermediate tendon
Innervation: Anterior: V trigeminal nerve, mandibular branch, via the mylohyoid branch of the
              inferior alveolar nerve
              Posterior: VII, digastric branch
Function: Anterior belly: draws hyoid up and forward
              Posterior belly: draws hyoid up and back
              Together: elevate hyoid

results in hyoid elevation without anterior or posterior migration. You will see a great deal of activity in the digastricus during swallowing.

At this point, it is wise to point out that muscles attached to the mandible, such as the digastricus, also may be **depressors** of the mandible. That is, the digastricus could help to pull the mandible down if the musculature *below* the hyoid were to fix it in place. You will want to retain this notion for our discussion of the role of hyoid musculature in oral motor development and control. The anterior belly is innervated by the mandibular branch of V trigeminal nerve via the mylohyoid branch of the inferior alveolar nerve. This branch courses along the inner surface of the mandible in the mylohyoid groove, and exits to innervate the mylohyoid (to be discussed) and the anterior digastricus. The posterior belly is supplied by the digastric branch of the VII facial nerve.

trigeminal: *L., tres, three; gemina, twin*

Stylohyoid Muscle.   The **stylohyoid muscle** originates on the prominent styloid process of the temporal bone, a point medial to the mastoid process (see Figure 5-18). The course of this muscle is medially down, such that it crosses the path of the posterior digastricus (which actually passes through the stylohyoid) and inserts into the corpus of hyoid.

Contraction of the stylohyoid elevates and retracts the hyoid bone. The stylohyoid and posterior digastricus are closely allied in development, function, and innervation. Both the stylohyoid and posterior belly of the digastricus are innervated by the motor branch of the VII facial nerves.

Mylohyoid Muscle.   As with the digastricus anterior, the **mylohyoid muscle** originates on the underside of the mandible and courses to the corpus hyoid. Unlike the digastricus, the mylohyoid is fanlike, originating along the lateral aspects of the inner mandible on a prominence known as the mylohyoid line. The anterior fibers converge at the median fibrous raphe (ridge), a structure that runs from the **symphysis mente** (the juncture of the fused paired bones of the mandible) to the hyoid.

The posterior fibers course directly to the hyoid. Taken together, the fibers of the mylohyoid form the floor of the oral cavity. The relationship between the digastricus and the mylohyoid muscles may be seen in Figure 5-19. As may be derived from examination of its fiber course, the mylohyoid elevates the hyoid and projects it forward, or alternately depresses the mandible, in much the manner of the digastricus anterior. Unlike the digastricus, the mylohyoid muscle is responsible for elevation of the floor of the mouth during the first stage of deglutition.

The mylohyoid is allied with the anterior belly of the digastricus, through proximity, development, and innervation. As with the anterior digastricus, the mylohyoid is innervated by the alveolar nerve, arising

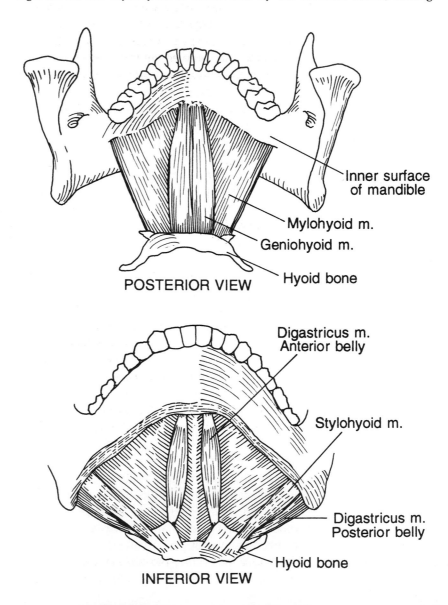

Figure 5-19. Schematic of the relationship among geniohyoid, mylohyoid, digastricus, and stylohyoid muscles.

Muscle:	Mylohyoid
Origin:	Mylohyoid line, inner surface of mandible
Course:	Fanlike to median fibrous raphe and hyoid
Insertion:	Corpus of hyoid
Innervation:	Alveolar nerve, V trigeminal, mandibular branch
Function:	Elevates hyoid or depresses mandible

from the V trigeminal nerve, mandibular branch. As stated for the digastricus anterior, this nerve courses within the mylohyoid groove of the inner surface of the mandible, branches, and innervates the mylohyoid.

Geniohyoid Muscle. The **geniohyoid muscle** is superior to the mylohyoid, originating at the mental spines projecting in a course parallel to the anterior belly of the digastricus from the inner mandibular surface (see Figure 5-19). Fibers of this narrow muscle course back and down to insert into the hyoid bone at the corpus. When contracted, the geniohyoid elevates the hyoid and draws it forward. It may depress the mandible also if the hyoid is fixed. The geniohyoid is innervated by the XII **hypoglossal** nerve. Although most of the hypoglossal originates in the hypoglossal nucleus of the medulla oblongata of the brainstem, those fibers innervating the geniohyoid arise from the first cervical spinal nerve.

hypoglossal: *L., glossa, tongue; under + tongue*

Hyoglossus Muscle. The **hyoglossus** and genioglossus provide another example of the interrelatedness of musculature. These muscles also are lingual (tongue) depressors (see Figure 7–38), because they have

Muscle:	Geniohyoid
Origin:	Mental spines, inner surface of mandible
Course:	Back and down
Insertion:	Corpus, hyoid bone
Innervation:	XII hypoglossal nerve
Function:	Elevates hyoid bone; depresses mandible

Muscle:	Hyoglossus
Origin:	Side of tongue
Course:	Down
Insertion:	Greater cornu hyoid
Innervation:	Motor branch of the XII hypoglossal
Function:	Elevates hyoid; depresses tongue

hyoglossus: *L., hyo, hyoid +
glossus, tongue*

*See the Clinical Note in
Chapter 3 for a discussion of
trunk stability and upper body
mobility.*

attachments on both of these structures. Speech-language pathologists concerned about oral motor control are painfully aware of these relationships, and studying them will benefit you as well. The **hyoglossus** is a laterally placed muscle. It arises from the entire superior surface of the greater cornu of the hyoid, and courses up to insert into the side of the tongue. The point of insertion in the tongue is near that of the styloglossus, a muscle we will discuss in the chapter covering the articulators. The muscle has a quadrilateral appearance and is a lingual depressor or hyoid elevator. The hyoglossus muscle is innervated by the motor branch of the XII hypoglossal.

Genioglossus Muscle.   Although the **genioglossus muscle** is more appropriately considered a muscle of the tongue (see Figure 7–38), it definitely is a hyoid elevator. The genioglossus originates on the inner surface of the mandible at the symphysis and courses up, back, and down to insert into the tongue and anterior surface of the hyoid corpus. We will discuss the lingual function of this muscle in Chapter 7, but the attachment at the hyoid guarantees that this muscle will elevate the hyoid. The genioglossus muscle is innervated by the motor branch of the XII hypoglossal.

Thyropharyngeus Muscle of Inferior Constrictor.   The **thyropharyngeus** and **cricopharyngeus muscles** constitute the **inferior pharyngeal constrictor**, to be discussed in detail later. The cricopharyngeus is the sphincter muscle at the orifice of the esophagus. The thyropharyngeus is involved in propelling food through the pharynx. Its attachment to the

Muscle:	Genioglossus
Origin:	Inner surface of mandible at symphysis
Course:	Up and back
Insertion:	Tongue and corpus hyoid
Innervation:	Motor branch of XII hypoglossal
Function:	Elevates hyoid

Muscle:	Thyropharyngeus of inferior pharyngeal constrictor
Origin:	Posterior pharyngeal raphe
Course:	Down, fanlike laterally
Insertion:	Thyroid lamina and inferior cornu
Innervation:	X vagus, recurrent laryngeal nerve (external laryngeal branch); X vagus, superior laryngeal nerve (pharyngeal branch)
Function:	Elevates larynx and constricts pharynx

cricoid and thyroid provides an opportunity for laryngeal elevation (see Figure 7–43).

The thyropharyngeus arises from the posterior pharyngeal raphe, coursing down fanlike and laterally to the thyroid lamina and inferior cornu. Contraction of this muscle promotes elevation of the larynx while constricting the pharynx. The inferior constrictors are innervated by branches from the X vagi, and by the recurrent laryngeal nerves off the vagi.

Hyoid and Laryngeal Depressors

- **Sternohyoid muscle**
- **Omohyoid muscle**
- **Sternothyroid muscle**
- **Thyrohyoid muscle**

Laryngeal depressors depress and stabilize the larynx via attachment to the hyoid, but also stabilize the tongue by serving as antagonists to the laryngeal elevators. The interconnectedness of the laryngeal and tongue musculature may at first be imposing, but take heart. Mastery of the components will greatly enhance your clinical competency, because oral motor control has its foundation in these interactions. We will discuss this in detail in Chapter 6.

Sternohyoid Muscle. As the name implies, the **sternohyoid** runs from sternum to hyoid. It originates from the posterior-superior region of the manubrium sterni, as well as from the medial end of the clavicle. It courses superiorly to insert into the inferior margin of the hyoid corpus.

Contraction of the sternohyoid depresses the hyoid or, if suprahyoid muscles are in contraction, fixes the hyoid and larynx. The lowering function is clearly evident following the pharyngeal stage in swallowing. The sternohyoid is innervated by the ansa cervicalis (ansa = loop; i.e., cervical loop), arising from C1 through C3 spinal nerves.

Omohyoid Muscle. As you can see in Figure 5-20, the **omohyoid** is a muscle with two bellies. The superior belly terminates on the side of the hyoid corpus, while the inferior belly has its origin on the upper

Muscle:	Sternohyoid
Origin:	Manubrium sterni and clavicle
Course:	Up
Insertion:	Inferior margin of hyoid corpus
Innervation:	Ansa cervicalis from spinal C1–C3
Function:	Depresses hyoid

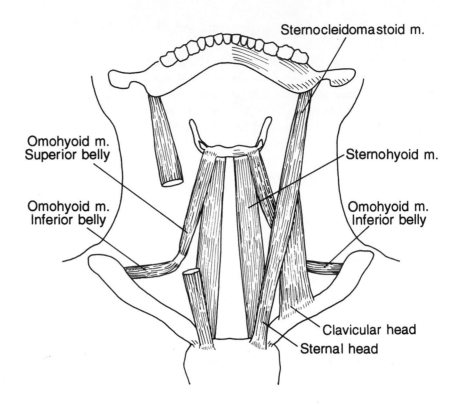

Sternocleidomastoid m.

Omohyoid m.
Superior belly

Sternohyoid m.

Omohyoid m.
Inferior belly

Omohyoid m.
Inferior belly

Clavicular head
Sternal head

Figure 5-20. Schematic of the relationship among omohyoid, sternocleidomastoid, and sternohyoid muscles.

See Chapters 3 and 8 for discussion of spinal nerves.

border of the scapula. The bellies are joined at an intermediate tendon. As you can see from this figure, the omohyoid passes deep to the sternocleidomastoid, which, along with the deep cervical fascia, restrains the omohyoid muscle to retain that characteristic "dogleg" angle. When contracted, the omohyoid depresses the hyoid bone and larynx. The superior belly is innervated by the superior ramus of the ansa cervicalis arising from C1 spinal nerve, whereas the inferior belly is innervated by the main ansa cervicalis, arising from C2 and C3 spinal nerves.

Muscle:	Omohyoid, superior and inferior heads
Origin:	Superior: corpus hyoid
	Inferior: upper border, scapula
Course:	Superior: down
	Inferior: down and laterally
Insertion:	Via intermediate tendon to hyoid
Innervation:	Superior belly: superior ramus of ansa cervicalis from C1
	Inferior belly: ansa cervicalis, spinal C2–C3
Function:	Depress hyoid

Laryngeal Stability

Laryngeal stability is the key to laryngeal control, and this stability is gained through development of the infra- and suprahyoid musculature. You can think of the larynx as a box connected to a flexible tube on one end (trachea) and loosely bound above. This "box" has liberal movement in the vertical dimension and some horizontal movement as well, but there must be a great deal of control in contraction of all of this musculature for this arrangement to work.

The larynx is intimately linked, via the hyoid bone, to the tongue, so that movement of the tongue is translated to the larynx. During development, an infant begins to gain control of neck musculature as early as four weeks, as seen in the ability to elevate the neck in prone. This ability to extend the previously flexed neck heralds the beginning of oral motor control, because the ability to balance neck extension with flexion permits the child to control the gross movement of the head. During this stage, the larynx is quite elevated, so much so that you can easily see the superior tip of the epiglottis behind the tongue of a two-year-old. In the early stages, the elevated larynx facilitates the anterior tongue protrusion required in infancy for nursing.

As the child develops, the larynx descends, starting a process of muscular differentiation between the tongue and the larynx. In the "nursing" position of the tongue, laryngeal stability is not as important, but the ability to move semi-hard and hard food around in the oral cavity is quite important as the child begins to eat solid foods. Now the child will develop the ability to move the tongue and larynx independently, permitting a much wider set of oral gestures. With this differentiation comes the control needed for accurate speech production. For information on head and neck control in children with motor dysfunction, you may wish to examine Jones-Owens (1991), and certainly you will want to read the work of Bly (1994) for insight into the development of muscle control.

Sternothyroid Muscle. As shown in Figure 5-21, contraction of the **sternothyroid muscle** depresses the thyroid cartilage. This muscle originates at the manubrium sterni and first costal cartilage, coursing up and out to insert into the oblique line of the thyroid cartilage. It is active during swallowing, drawing the larynx downward following elevation for the pharyngeal stage of deglutition. The sternothyroid is innervated by fibers from the spinal nerves C1 and C2 that pass in the hypoglossal nerve.

Muscle:	Sternothyroid
Origin:	Oblique line, thyroid cartilage
Course:	Down and in
Insertion:	Manubrium sterni
Innervation:	XII hypoglossal and spinal nerves C1, C2
Function:	Depresses thyroid cartilage

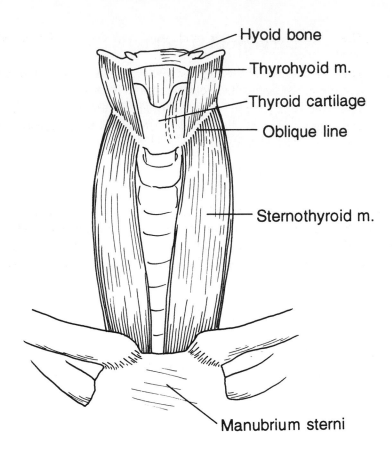

Hyoid bone

Thyrohyoid m.

Thyroid cartilage

Oblique line

Sternothyroid m.

Manubrium sterni

Figure 5-21. The sternothyroid and thyrohyoid muscles.

Thyrohyoid Muscle. This muscle is easily seen as the superior counterpart to the sternothyroid (see Figure 5-21). Coursing from the oblique line of the thyroid cartilage to the inferior margin of the greater cornu of the hyoid bone, the **thyrohyoid muscle** will either depress the hyoid or raise the larynx. The thyrohyoid is innervated by the fibers from spinal nerve C1 that course in the hypoglossal nerves.

In summary:

- The **extrinsic muscles** of the larynx include the **infrahyoid** and **suprahyoid** muscles.

Muscle: Thyrohyoid
Origin: Oblique line, thyroid cartilage
Course: Up
Insertion: Greater cornu, hyoid
Innervation: XII hypoglossal nerve and fibers from spinal C1
Function: Depresses hyoid or elevates thyroid

- The **digastricus** anterior and posterior elevate the hyoid, whereas the **stylohyoid** retracts it.
- The **mylohyoid** and **hyoglossus** elevate the hyoid, and the **geniohyoid** elevates the hyoid and draws it forward.
- The **thyropharyngeus** and **cricopharyngeus** muscles elevate the larynx, and the **sternohyoid**, **sternothyroid**, **thyrohyoid**, and **omohyoid** muscles depress the larynx.

Interaction of Musculature

The larynx is virtually suspended from a broad sling of muscles that must work in concert to achieve the complex motions required for speech and nonspeech function. Movement of the larynx and its cartilages requires both gross and fine adjustments. It appears that the gross

Vocal Fold Paralysis

Paralysis refers to loss of voluntary motor function, whereas **paresis** refers to weakness. Either can arise from damage to **upper motor neurons**, which are neurons that arise from the brain and end in the spinal column or brainstem; or damage to **lower motor neurons**, which are neurons that leave the spinal column or brainstem to innervate the muscles involved.

Vocal fold paralysis may take several forms, depending on the nerve damage. If only one side of the recurrent laryngeal nerve (lower motor neuron) is damaged, the result will be unilateral vocal fold paralysis. Bilateral vocal fold paralysis would result from bilateral lower motor neuron damage.

If the result of damage is **adductor paralysis**, the muscles of adduction are paralyzed and the vocal folds remain in the abducted position. If the damage results in **abductor paralysis**, the individual will not be able to abduct the vocal folds, and respiration will be compromised (you may want to read the note on "laryngeal stridor" in Chapter 6 to get a notion of what happens). If the superior laryngeal nerve is involved, the individual will suffer loss of the ability to alter vocal pitch, because the cricothyroid is innervated by this branch of the vagus.

In unilateral paralysis, one vocal fold is still capable of motion. Phonation can still occur, but production will be markedly breathy. Bilateral adductor paralysis will result in virtually complete loss of phonation.

There are several causes of vocal fold paralysis, but among the leaders are damage to the nerve during thyroid surgery and blunt trauma, often from the steering wheel of an automobile. **Cerebrovascular accidents** (CVA: hemorrhage or other condition causing loss of blood supply to the brain) may damage upper or lower motor neurons, resulting in paralysis, and a host of neurodegenerative diseases can weaken or paralyze the vocal folds. You should also be aware that paralysis may occur as a result of **aneurysm** of the aortic arch. An aneurysm is a focal "ballooning" of a blood vessel caused by a weakness in the wall. When the aneurysm balloons out, it compresses the recurrent laryngeal nerve, causing paresis or paralysis. A **phonatory sign** (objective evidence of phonatory deficit) is not to be taken lightly.

movements associated with laryngeal elevation and depression provide the background for the fine adjustments of phonatory control. The supra- and infrahyoid muscles raise and lower the larynx, changing the vocal tract length, but the intrinsic laryngeal muscles are responsible for the fine adjustments associated with phonation control.

To say that the musculature works as a unit is clearly an understatement. The simple gesture of laryngeal elevation must be countered with the controlled antagonistic tone of the laryngeal depressors. Elevation of the tongue will tend to elevate the larynx and increase the tension of the cricothyroid, and this must be countered through intrinsic muscle adjustment to keep the articulatory system from driving the phonatory mechanism. It is time to move to Chapter 6 to see how these components work together.

CHAPTER SUMMARY

The **larynx** is comprised of the **cricoid, thyroid,** and **epiglottis** cartilages, as well as the paired **arytenoid, corniculate,** and **cuneiform** cartilages. The thyroid and cricoid cartilages articulate by means of the **cricothyroid joint** that lets the two cartilages come closer together in front. The arytenoid and cricoid cartilages also articulate with a joint that permits a wide range of arytenoid motion. The epiglottis is attached to the thyroid cartilage and base of the **tongue**. The corniculate cartilages rest on the upper surface of the arytenoids, while the cuneiform cartilages reside within the **aryepiglottic folds**.

The **cavity** of the larynx is a constricted tube with a smooth surface. Sheets and cords of **ligaments** connect the cartilages, while smooth **mucous membrane** covers the medial-most surface of the larynx. The **valleculae** are found between the tongue and the epiglottis, within folds arising from the **lateral** and **median glossoepiglottic ligaments**. The **fibroelastic membrane** is composed of the upper **quadrangular membranes** and **aryepiglottic folds**, the lower **conus elasticus**, and the **vocal ligament**, which is actually the upward free extension of the conus elasticus.

The **vocal folds** are made up of five layers of tissue, the deepest being the muscle of the vocal folds. The **aditus** is the entryway of the larynx, marking the entry to the **vestibule**. The **ventricular** and vocal **folds** are separated by the laryngeal ventricle. The **glottis** is the variable space between the vocal folds.

Intrinsic muscles of the larynx include the **thyrovocalis, thyromuscularis, cricothyroid, lateral** and **posterior cricoarytenoid, transverse arytenoid** and **oblique interarytenoid, superior thyroarytenoid,**

and **thyroepiglotticus** muscles. **Extrinsic muscles** of the larynx include the **infrahyoid** and **suprahyoid** muscles. The **digastricus anterior** and **posterior** elevate the hyoid, while the **stylohyoid** retracts it. The **mylohyoid** and **hyoglossus** elevate the hyoid, and the **geniohyoid** elevates the hyoid and draws it forward. The **thyropharyngeus** and **cricopharyngeus** muscles elevate the larynx, and the **sternohyoid**, **sternothyroid**, and **omohyoid** muscles depress the larynx.

The thyroepiglotticus and **aryepiglotticus** both serve nonspeech functions. The thyroepiglotticus increases the size of the laryngeal opening for forced inspiration, while the aryepiglotticus protects the airway by narrowing the aditus and vestibule.

Movement of the vocal folds into and out of approximation requires coordinated effort of the intrinsic muscles of the larynx. The **lateral cricoarytenoid** muscle rocks the arytenoid cartilage on its axis, tipping the vocal folds in and slightly down. The **posterior cricoarytenoid** muscle rocks the arytenoid out. The **transverse arytenoid** muscle draws the posterior surfaces of the arytenoids closer together. The **oblique arytenoid** assists the vocal folds to dip downward when they are adducted. The thyroepiglotticus has no phonatory function but is involved in the swallowing function. Vocal fundamental frequency is increased by increasing tension, a function of the thyrovocalis and cricothyroid.

STUDY QUESTIONS

1. Identify the indicated structures on the figure below.

   a. _____ cartilage
   b. _____ cartilage
   c. _____ cartilage
   d. _____ cartilage
   e. _____ cartilage
   f. _____ bone

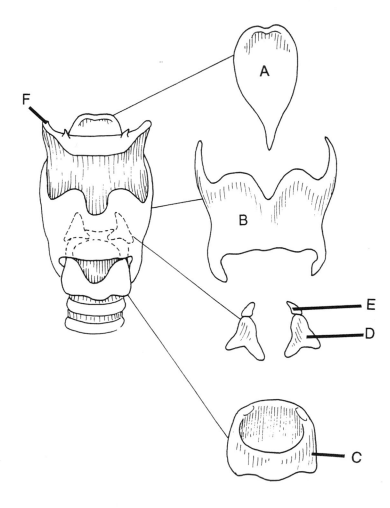

2. Identify the indicated landmarks on the figure below.

a. _____

b. _____

c. _____

d. _____

e. _____

f. _____

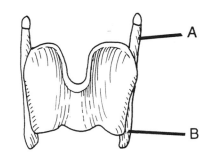

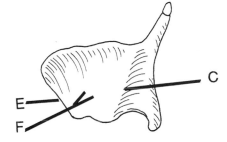

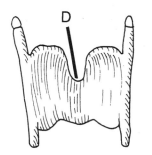

3. Identify the indicated landmarks on the figure below.

a. _____ process

b. _____ process

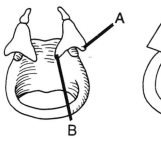
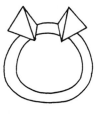
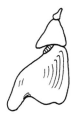
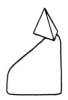
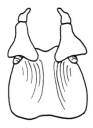

4. Identify the muscles indicated below.

    a. ———————————————

    b. ———————————————

    c. ———————————————

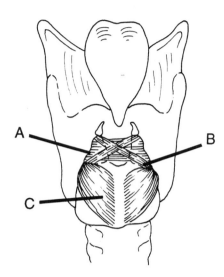

5. Identify the muscles indicated below.

a. _____

b. _____

c. _____

d. _____

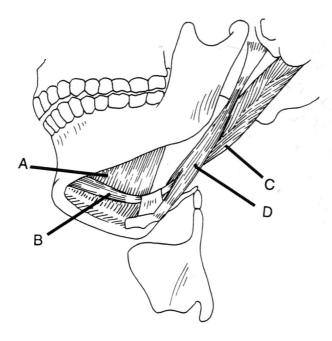

6. Identify the muscles indicated below.

a. _____

b. _____

c. _____

d. _____

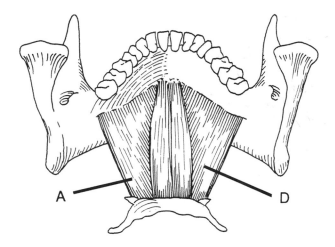

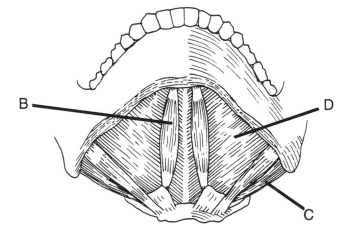

7. This is a view of the laryngeal opening from above. Identify the structures indicated below.

a. _____

b. _____

c. _____

d. _____

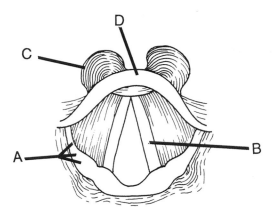

8. Identify the two muscles indicated below.

a. _____

b. _____

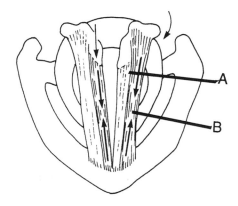

9. The _____ muscle is the primary muscle responsible for change of vocal fundamental frequency.

10. The space between the vocal folds is termed the _____.

11. Laryngeal cancer sometimes necessitates complete removal of the larynx. Because the respiratory and digestive systems share the pharynx, removal of this protective mechanism poses a problem for accounting for the needs of breathing and swallowing. What surgical changes would permit both processes?

STUDY QUESTION ANSWERS

1. Identify the indicated structures on the figure below.
   a. <u>EPIGLOTTIS</u> cartilage
   b. <u>THYROID</u> cartilage
   c. <u>CRICOID</u> cartilage
   d. <u>ARYTENOID</u> cartilage
   e. <u>CORNICULATE</u> cartilage
   f. <u>HYOID</u> bone
2. Identify the indicated landmarks on the figure below.
   a. <u>GREATER CORNU</u>
   b. <u>LESSER CORNU</u>
   c. <u>OBLIQUE LINE</u>
   d. <u>THYROID NOTCH</u>
   e. <u>ANGLE OF THYROID</u>
   f. <u>LAMINA</u>
3. Identify the indicated landmarks on the figure below.
   a. <u>MUSCULAR</u> process
   b. <u>VOCAL</u> process
4. Identify the muscles indicated below.
   a. <u>TRANSVERSE ARYTENOID</u>
   b. <u>OBLIQUE ARYTENOID</u>
   c. <u>POSTERIOR CRICOARYTENOID</u>
5. Identify the muscles indicated below.
   a. <u>MYLOHYOID</u>
   b. <u>DIGASTRICUS ANTERIOR</u>
   c. <u>DIGASTRICUS POSTERIOR</u>
   d. <u>STYLOHYOID</u>
6. Identify the muscles indicated below.
   a. <u>GENIOHYOID</u>
   b. <u>DIGASTRICUS ANTERIOR</u>
   c. <u>DIGASTRICUS POSTERIOR</u>
   d. <u>MYLOHYOID</u>
7. This is a view of the laryngeal opening from above. Identify the structures indicated below.
   a. <u>ARYEPIGLOTTIC FOLD</u>
   b. <u>TRUE VOCAL FOLDS</u>
   c. <u>VALLECULAE</u>
   d. <u>EPIGLOTTIS</u>
8. Identify the two muscles indicated below.
   a. <u>THYROVOCALIS</u>
   b. <u>THYROMUSCULARIS</u>
9. The <u>CRICOTHYROID</u> muscle is the primary muscle responsible for change of vocal fundamental frequency.
10. The space between the vocal folds is termed the <u>GLOTTIS</u>.

11. Removal of the larynx would leave the airway unprotected from intrusion of foreign matter during swallowing. To avoid this danger, the airway is sealed off surgically, and a stoma is surgically opened up through the trachea to permit unhampered respiration.

REFERENCES

Abrahams, P. H., McMinn, R. M. H., Hutchings, R. T., Sandy, C., & Mark, S. (2003). *McMinn's color atlas of human anatomy* (5th ed.). Philadelphia: Mosby.

Aronson, E. A. (1985). *Clinical voice disorders.* New York: Thieme.

Baer, T., Sasaki, C., & Harris, K. (1985). *Laryngeal function in phonation and respiration.* Boston: College-Hill Press.

Baken, R. J., & Orlikoff, R. F. (1999). *Clinical measurement of speech and voice* (2nd ed.). San Diego, CA: Singular Publishing Group.

Bateman, H. E. (1977). *A clinical approach to speech anatomy and physiology.* Springfield, IL: Charles C. Thomas.

Beck, E. W., Monson, H., & Groer, M. (1982). *Mosby's atlas of functional human anatomy.* St. Louis, MO: C. V. Mosby.

Berkovitz, B. K. B., & Moxham, B. J. (2002). *Head and neck anatomy: A clinical reference.* London: Martin Dunitz Ltd.

Bless, D. M., & Abbs, J. H. (1983). *Vocal fold physiology.* San Diego, CA: College-Hill Press.

Bly, L. (1994). *Motor skills acquisition in the first year.* Tucson, AZ: Therapy Skill Builders.

Boone, D. R. (1999). *The voice and voice therapy.* Englewood Cliffs, NJ: Prentice-Hall.

Broad, D. J. (1973). Phonation. In F. D. Minifie, T. J. Hixon, & F. Williams (Eds.), *Normal aspects of speech, hearing, and language.* Englewood Cliffs, NJ: Prentice-Hall.

Carrau, R. L., & Murry, T. (1999). *Comprehensive management of swallowing disorders.* San Diego, CA: Singular Publishing Group.

Childers, D. G., Hicks, D. M., Moore, G. P., Eskenazi, L., & Lalwani, A. L. (1990). Electroglottography and vocal fold physiology. *Journal of Speech and Hearing Research, 33,* 245–254.

Chusid, J. G. (1985). *Correlative neuroanatomy and functional neurology* (17th ed.). Los Altos, CA: Lange Medical Publications.

Daniloff, R. G. (1989). *Speech science.* San Diego, CA: College-Hill Press.

Doyle, P. C., Grantmyre, A., & Myers, C. (1989). Clinical modification of the tracheostoma breathing valve for voice restoration. *Journal of Speech and Hearing Disorders, 54,* 189–192.

Durrant, J. D., & Lovrinic, J. H. (1995). *Bases of hearing science.* Baltimore: Williams & Wilkins.

Eckel, F., & Boone, D. (1981). The s/z ratio as an indicator of laryngeal pathology. *Journal of Speech and Hearing Disorders, 46,* 147–149.

Fink, B. R. (1975). *The human larynx.* New York: Raven Press.

Fink, B. R., & Demarest, R. J. (1978). *Laryngeal biomechanics.* Cambridge, MA: Harvard University Press.

Frable, M. A. (1961). Computation of motion of the cricoarytenoid joint. *Archives of Otolaryngology, 73,* 551–556.

Fucci, D. J., & Lass, N. J. (1999). *Fundamentals of speech science.* Boston: Allyn & Bacon.

Fujimura, O. (1988). *Vocal fold physiology. Vol. 2. Vocal physiology.* New York: Raven Press.

Fukida, H., Kawaida, M., Tatehara, T., Ling, E., Kita, K., Ohki, K., Kawasaki, Y. & Saito, S. (1988). A new concept of lubricating mechanisms of the larynx. In O. Fujimura (Ed.), *Vocal physiology: Voice production, mechanisms and functions* (pp. 83–92). New York: Raven Press.

Ganong, W. F. (2003). *Review of medical physiology* (21st ed.). New York: McGraw-Hill/Appleton & Lange.

Gosling, J. A., Harris, P. F., Humpherson, J. R., Whitmore, I., & Willan, P. L. T. (1985). *Atlas of human anatomy.* Philadelphia: J. B. Lippincott.

Gray, H., Bannister, L. H., Berry, M. M., & Williams, P. L. (Eds.). (1995). *Gray's anatomy.* London: Churchill Livingstone.

Grobler, N. J. (1977). *Textbook of clinical anatomy* (Vol. 1). Amsterdam: Elsevier Scientific.

Hirano, M. (1974). Morphological structure of the vocal cord as a vibrator and its variations. *Folia Phoniatrica, 26,* 89–94.

Hirano, M., Kirchner, J. A., & Bless, D. M. (1987). *Neurolaryngology.* Boston: College-Hill Press.

Hirano, M., Kiyokawa, K., & Kurita, S. (1988). Laryngeal muscles and glottic shaping. In O. Fujimura (Ed.), *Vocal physiology: Voice production, mechanisms and functions* (pp. 49–65). New York: Raven Press.

Jones-Owens, J. L. (1991). Prespeech assessment and treatment strategies. In M. B. Langley, & L. J. Lombardino (Eds.), *Neurodevelopmental strategies for managing communication disorders in children with severe motor dysfunction.* Austin, TX: Pro-Ed.

Kaplan, H. M. (1971). *Anatomy and physiology of speech.* New York: McGraw-Hill.

Kent, R. D. (1997). *The speech sciences.* San Diego, CA: Singular Publishing Group.

Kirchner, J. A., & Suzuki, M. (1968). Laryngeal reflexes and voice production. In M. Krauss (Ed.), Sound Production in Man. *Annals of the New York Academy of Sciences, 155,* 98–109.

Kuehn, D. P., Lemme, M. L., & Baumgartner, J. M. (1989). *Neural bases of speech, hearing, and language.* Boston: Little, Brown.

Langley, M. B., & Lombardino, L. J. (1991). *Neurodevelopmental strategies for managing communication disorders in children with severe motor dysfunction.* Austin, TX: Pro-Ed.

Lieberman, P. (1968). *Intonation, perception, and language.* Research Monograph No. 38. Cambridge, MA: The M.I.T. Press.

Lieberman, P. (1977). *Speech physiology and acoustic phonetics: An introduction.* New York: Macmillan.

Liebgott, B. (2001). *The anatomical basis of dentistry.* St. Louis, MO: Mosby.

McMinn, R. M. H., Hutchings, R. T., & Logan, B. M. (1994). *Color atlas of head and neck anatomy.* London: Mosby-Wolfe.

Netter, F. H. (1983). *The CIBA collection of medical illustrations. Vol. 1. Nervous System. Part I. Anatomy and physiology.* West Caldwell, NJ: CIBA Pharmaceutical.

Netter, F. H. (1983). *The CIBA collection of medical illustrations. Vol. 1. Nervous system. Part II. Neurologic and neuromuscular disorders.* West Caldwell, NJ: CIBA Pharmaceutical.

Netter, F. H. (1997). *Atlas of human anatomy.* Los Angeles: Icon Learning Systems.

Proctor, D. F. (1968). The physiologic basis of voice training. In M. Krauss (Ed.), Sound Production in Man. *Annals of the New York Academy of Sciences, 155,* 208–228.

Rohen, J. W., Yokochi, C., Lutjen-Drecoll, E. L., & Romrell, L. J. (2002). *Color atlas of anatomy: A photographic study of the human body* (5th ed.). Philadelphia: Lippincott, Williams & Wilkins.

Rosse, C., Gaddum-Rosse, P., & Rosse, G. (1997). *Hollinshead's textbook of anatomy.* Philadelphia: Lippincott-Raven.

Shepard, T. H. (1998). *Catalog of teratogenic agents* (9th ed.). Baltimore: The Johns Hopkins University Press.

Sonninen, A. (1968). The external frame function in the control of pitch in the human voice. In M. Krauss (Ed.), Sound Production in Man. *Annals of the New York Academy of Sciences, 155,* 68–89.

Titze, I. R. (1994). *Principles of voice production*. Englewood Cliffs, NJ: Prentice-Hall.

Van den Berg, J. (1968). Sound production in isolated human larynges. In M. Krauss (Ed.), Sound Production in Man. *Annals of the New York Academy of Sciences, 155,* 18–27.

Verdolini, K., Titze, I. R., & Fennell, A. (1994). Dependence of phonatory effort on hydration level. *Journal of speech & hearing research, 37,* 1001–1007.

Whillis, J. (1946). Movements of the tongue in swallowing. *Journal of anatomy, 80,* 115–116.

Williams, P. & Warrick, R. (1980). *Gray's anatomy* (36th Brit. ed.). Philadelphia: W. B. Saunders.

Zemlin, W. R. (1998). *Speech and hearing science: Anatomy and physiology* (4th ed.). Needham Heights, MA: Allyn & Bacon.

CHAPTER 6

Physiology of Phonation

Discussion of the function of the larynx and vocal folds revolves around the movable components and the results of that movement. We will concentrate on the nonspeech functions initially, which will help as we talk about speech and vocal function. We use these nonspeech functions in our treatment of voice disorders, and this discussion may serve you well.

NONSPEECH LARYNGEAL FUNCTION

The protective function of the larynx is its most important role, because failure to prohibit entry of foreign objects into the lungs is life-threatening. This function is fulfilled through the cough and other associated reflexive gestures.

Coughing is a response by the tissue of the respiratory passageway to an irritant or foreign object, mediated by the visceral afferent (sensory) portion of the X vagus nerve innervating the bronchial mucosa. Coughing is a violent and broadly predictable behavior, which includes deep inhalation through widely abducted vocal folds, followed by tensing and tight adduction of the vocal folds and elevation of the larynx. The axis of movement of the arytenoids guarantees that as they are

cough: *forceful evacuation of the respiratory passageway, including deep inhalation through widely abducted vocal folds, tensing and tight adduction of the vocal folds, and elevation of the larynx, followed by forceful expiration*

221

rocked for adduction, they also are directed somewhat downward, providing more force in opposition to expiration. Significant positive subglottal pressure for the cough comes from tissue recoil and the muscles of expiration. The high pressure of forced expiration blows the vocal folds apart.

The aerodynamic benefit of this is that the person coughing generates a maximal flow of air through the passageway to expel the irritating object. The negative side of the cough is the force required for its production. Chronic irritation of the respiratory system leads to vocal abuse in the form of repeated coughing.

The "near cousin" of the cough is throat clearing. It is not as violent as the full cough, but is nonetheless stressful. If you spend a quiet moment clearing your throat and feeling its effects, you will sense increased respiratory effort that is countered by tightening of the laryngeal musculature. You build pressure in the subglottal region and clamp the vocal folds shut to restrain the pressure. Although this clamping serves a purpose, in that it permits you to clear your respiratory passageway of mucus, it also places the delicate tissues of the vocal folds under a great deal of strain, and the result can be catastrophic to a trained voice.

There is a positive clinical side to this gesture, as well. If a client cannot approximate the vocal folds because of muscular weakness, the clinician has a means of achieving this closure in the cough. If you can get a client to cough voluntarily, you can very likely get the client to phonate. Both of these gestures involve the muscles of adduction: lateral cricoarytenoid, arytenoids, and thyromuscularis. The medial compression generated in the cough is quite large, rivaled only by that required for abdominal fixation.

abdominal fixation:
process of impounding air in thorax to stabilize the torso

Abdominal fixation is the process of capturing air within the thorax to provide the muscles with a structure on which to push or pull. The laryngeal gesture of this effortful closure is one form of the Valsalva maneuver. The preparatory gesture for thorax/abdomen fixation is similar to that for the cough: Take in a large inspiratory charge, followed by tight adduction of the vocal folds. The effect is for the thorax to become a relatively rigid frame, so that the forces applied for lifting are translated to the legs. If the thorax is not fixed, those forces will act on the thorax instead, causing the rib cage to be depressed.

You may have wondered why you tend to grunt when lifting heavy objects or pushing your car. All of the components are there for phonation. You are using force that would cause expiration, and your vocal folds are adducted. With sufficient effort, some air escapes through the adducted vocal folds, and you hear the grunt.

Abdominal fixation plays an important role in childbirth, defecation, and vomiting. Review the Clinical Notes of Chapter 3 to refresh your memory.

So far we have dealt primarily with laryngeal functions focused only on tight adduction of the vocal folds, but abduction has its place as well. Abduction dilates the larynx, an important function for respiration during physical exertion. You will recall from Chapter 4 that physical requirements for oxygen increase significantly during work and exertion. During normal, quiet respiration, the vocal folds are abducted to provide a width of about 8 mm in the adult. During forced respiration, the needs for air cause you to **dilate** or open the respiratory tract as widely as possible, doubling that width (see Figure 6-1).

dilate: *to open or expand an orifice*

Reflexes are involuntary, although respiratory reflexes can come under some voluntary control (e.g., you can hold your breath or stifle a yawn). We eventually *must* breathe, which requires reflexively abducting the vocal folds. In cases of drowning and near-drowning, the victim may attempt to maintain adducted vocal folds, but must eventually attempt to breathe despite all logic that militates against it. In addition, individuals rapidly immersed in cold water will reflexively gasp for air, and the ability to inhibit this reflex is significantly reduced by alcohol consumption (a fact that explains one of the risks of combining drinking and boating).

We will discuss the swallowing reflex more fully in Chapter 9, but it should be mentioned here. During normal deglutition, a bolus of food will trigger a swallowing reflex as it passes into the region behind the

A bolus is a mass of chewed food formed into a ball in preparation for swallowing.

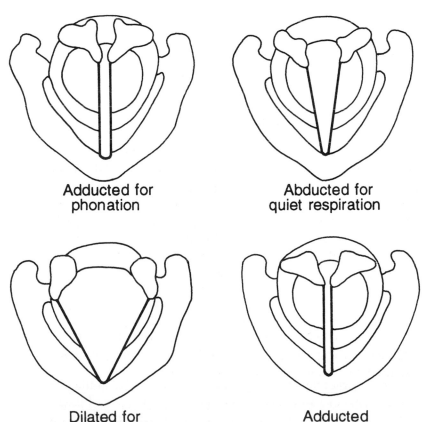

Adducted for phonation

Abducted for quiet respiration

Dilated for forced respiration

Adducted for whisper

Figure 6-1. Laryngeal postures for various functions. During adduction for phonation, the vocal folds are approximated. For quiet respiration, the folds are moderately abducted, but for forced respiration, they are widely separated. Adduction for whisper involves bringing the folds close together but retaining an open space between the arytenoid cartilages.

tongue and above the larynx. When the reflex is triggered, the larynx elevates, and the epiglottis (attached to the root of the tongue) drops down to cover the aditus. The aryepiglottic folds tense by action of the aryepiglottic muscle, and the vocal folds are adducted. Try this: Hold your finger lightly on your thyroid notch and swallow. You may feel your larynx elevate and tense up as you swallow. That finger on the thyroid, by the way, is one component of the clinical swallowing evaluation.

In summary:

- We use the larynx and associated structures for many **non-speech functions**, including coughing, throat-clearing, and abdominal fixation.
- These functions serve important biological needs, and provide us with the background for useful clinical intervention techniques.

LARYNGEAL FUNCTION FOR SPEECH

Before discussing phonation, we must look at the primary physical principle supporting phonation: the Bernoulli effect.

The Bernoulli Effect

Vocal folds are masses that may be set into vibration. The **larynx** is the cartilaginous structure housing the two bands of tissue we call the vocal folds. The paired vocal folds are situated on both sides of the larynx so that they actually intrude into the airstream, as you can see from the schematic in Figure 6-2. This figure is a view from above and a view from behind. From above, you can see that the vocal folds are bands of tissue that are actually visible from a point immediately behind your tongue, looking down toward the lungs. From behind, you can see that the vocal folds also are a constriction in the airway, a critical concept for phonation.

You will remember from our discussion of respiratory physiology that any constriction in the airway greatly increases airway turbulence. If you are the passenger in a car and put your hand out the window, you will feel the force of the wind dragging against your hand and you will hear the turbulence associated with it. You can rotate your hand so that the turbulence is reduced or increased, and as the force on your hand increases it becomes more difficult to keep your hand in the airstream.

The vocal folds also are a source of turbulence in the vocal tract. Without them, air would pass relatively unimpeded out of the lungs and into the oral cavity. The addition of the vocal folds results in air having

See Chapter 4 for a discussion of respiratory physiology.

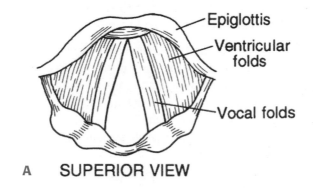

-Epiglottis
-Ventricular folds
-Vocal folds

A   SUPERIOR VIEW

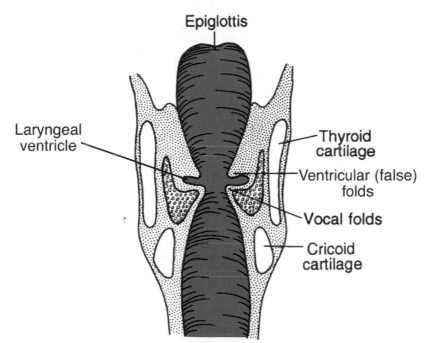

Epiglottis

Laryngeal ventricle

Thyroid cartilage
Ventricular (false) folds
Vocal folds
Cricoid cartilage

B   CORONAL SECTION, FROM BEHIND

Figure 6-2. A. Vocal folds from above. **B.** Anterior view of larynx, showing constriction in laryngeal space caused by the vocal folds.

to make a detour around the folds, and the result of that detour invokes a discussion of the Bernoulli effect.

Daniel Bernoulli, a seventeenth-century Swiss scientist, recognized the effects of constricting a tube during fluid flow. The **Bernoulli effect** states that, given a constant volume flow of air or fluid, *at a point of constriction there will be a decrease in air pressure perpendicular to the flow and an increase in velocity of the flow.* If you put a constriction in a tube, air flows faster as it detours around the constriction, and the pressure on the wall at the point of constriction will be lower than that of the surrounding area. Let us examine this statement.

Bernoulli Effect in Baseball

Examples of the Bernoulli effect are apparent throughout daily life. If you are a baseball fan, you will appreciate the amazing curve ball of your favorite pitcher more when you realize that the Bernoulli effect is the driving force behind it. In this case, the pitcher ensures that the ball *begins* its flight with the smooth surface toward the front and that the seam on the ball rotates to the side of the ball sometime during its brief flight. The seam acts as a constriction: The pressure on the seam side is lower than on the opposite smooth side, and the ball is "sucked" toward the seam.

For an excellent discussion of this effect, see Adair (2002).

Airflow Increase

Figure 6-3 shows a tube with a constriction in it representing the vocal folds. If you have placed your thumb over a garden hose, you know that the rate of water flow increases as a result of that constriction. Likewise, if you have ever been white-water rafting, you will immediately recognize that the white water comes from constriction in the flow of the river,

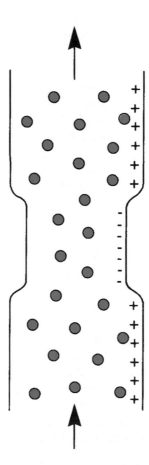

Figure 6-3. Rate of airflow through the tube will increase at the point of constriction, and air pressure will decrease at that point as well.

in the form of boulders. As the water flows through the constriction the rate of flow increases, giving you the thrill as you speed uncontrollably toward your fate.

Air Pressure Drop

To get an intuitive feel for the pressure drop, you must think about the flow in terms of molecules of air. Look again at Figure 6-3. We have drawn it so that you can count the number of molecules of air in the tube relative to the tube's length. In the unconstricted regions, you can count 10 molecules of air. Where the tube becomes narrower, there will be fewer air molecules because there is less space for them to occupy, and you only count five in that area. Where the constriction ends, you once again see 10 molecules.

When air is forced into a narrower tube, the same total volume of air has to squeeze through a smaller space. Because each unit mass of air becomes longer and narrower, it covers a longer stretch of the tube's walls. The pressure exerted by this mass, although the same in an over-all sense, is now distributed over more of the wall. The result is that each atom of the wall feels less force from the air molecules, and the narrow part of the tube is more likely to collapse. This effect only occurs when the air is forced to move; air without any forced movement will sooner or later equalize its pressure everywhere. If you remember that pressure is force exerted on an area ($F = P/A$), a drop in pressure makes perfect sense.

These two elements are the heart of the Bernoulli effect and help us to understand vocal fold vibration. Return to the notion of vocal folds being a constriction in a tube, as illustrated in Figure 6-4. You will want to refer to this figure as we discuss the Bernoulli principle applied to phonation.

See the Introduction *of Chapter 3 for a discussion of force, pressure, and area.*

The vocal folds are soft tissue, made up of muscle and epithelial tissue. Because of this, the folds are also capable of moving when sufficient force is exerted on them, as in the case of your hand extended out the moving car window.

By examining Panel A in Figure 6-4, you will see that the vocal folds are closed. In the next panel (B), the air pressure generated by the respiratory system is beginning to force the vocal folds open, but there is no transglottal flow because the folds are still making full contact. By Panel D the vocal folds have been blown open. Because the vocal folds are elastic, they will tend to return to the point of equilibrium, which is the point of rest. They cannot return to equilibrium, however, as long as the air pressure is so great that they are blown apart. When they are in that position, however, there is a drop in pressure at the point of constriction (the Bernoulli effect), and we already know that if there is a drop in pressure, something is going to move to equalize that pressure.

In the last three panels (E, F, and G) you can see the result of the negative pressure: The vocal folds are being sucked back toward midline

Figure 6-4. One cycle of vocal fold vibration as seen through a frontal section. **A.** Air pressure beneath the vocal folds arises from respiratory flow. **B.** Air pressure causes the vocal folds to separate in the inferior. **C.** The superior aspect of the vocal folds begins to open. **D.** The vocal folds are blown open, the flow between the folds increases, and pressure at the folds decreases. **E.** Decreased pressure and the elastic quality of vocal folds causes folds to move back toward midline. **F.** The vocal folds make contact inferiorly. **G.** The cycle of vibration is completed.

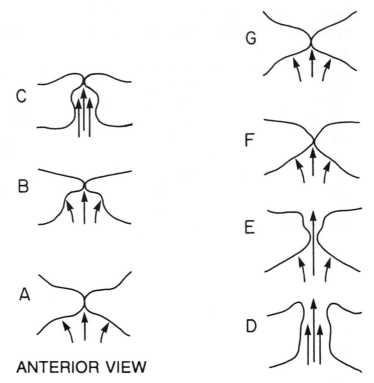

ANTERIOR VIEW

(E) as a result of the negative pressure and aided by tissue elasticity. The final panels (F and G) show the folds again making contact, with airflow completely halted. When the vocal folds are pulled back toward midline by their tissue-restoring forces, they completely block the flow of air for an instant as they make contact. At this point, the negative pressure related to flow is gone also. Instead, there is the force of respiratory charge beneath the folds ready to blow them apart once again. By the way, the minimum subglottal pressure that will blow the vocal folds apart to sustain phonation is approximately 3–5 cm H_2O, although much larger subglottal pressures are required for louder speech.

What you hear as voicing is the product of the repeated opening and closing of the vocal folds. The motion of the tissue and airflow disturb the molecules of air, causing the phenomenon we call sound.

The act of bringing the vocal folds together for phonation is referred to as **adduction**, and the process of drawing the vocal folds apart to terminate phonation is called **abduction**. As we shall see, both of these movements are achieved using specific muscles, but the actual vibration of the vocal folds is the product of airflow interacting with the tissue *in the absence of repetitive muscular contraction*.

If you have followed this introductory discussion of the principles governing vocal fold vibration, you are prepared to examine the structures of the larynx.

In summary:

- **Phonation**, or voicing, is the product of vibrating vocal folds within the larynx.
- The **vocal folds** vibrate as air flows past them; the Bernoulli phenomenon and tissue elasticity help maintain phonation.
- The **Bernoulli principle** states that, given a constant volume flow of air or fluid, at a point of **constriction** there will be a **decrease** in air **pressure** perpendicular to the flow and an **increase** in **velocity** of the flow.
- The interaction of **subglottal pressure**, **tissue elasticity**, and **constriction** within the airflow caused by the vocal folds produces sustained phonation as long as pressure, flow, and vocal fold approximation are maintained.

Attack

Phonation is an extremely important component of the speech signal. To accomplish phonation we must achieve three basic laryngeal adjustments. To *start* phonation, we must adduct the vocal folds, moving them into the airstream, referred to as **vocal attack**. We then hold the vocal folds in a fixed position in the airstream as the aerodynamics of phonation control the actual vibration associated with **sustained phonation**. Finally, we abduct the vocal folds to **terminate** phonation.

When we are *not* phonating, the vocal folds are sufficiently abducted to prohibit air turbulence in the airway to start audible vibration of the vocal folds. To initiate voicing, we bring the vocal folds close enough together that the forces of turbulence can cause vocal fold vibration. **Attack** is the process of bringing vocal folds together to *begin* phonation, and this requires muscular action. Vocal attack occurs quite frequently in running speech. If you were to say the sentence "Anatomy is not for the faint of heart," you would have brought the vocal folds together and drawn them apart at least six times in two seconds to accommodate voiced and voiceless phonemes.

There are three basic types of attack. When we initiate phonation using **simultaneous vocal attack**, we coordinate adduction and onset of respiration so that they occur simultaneously. The vocal folds reach the critical degree of adduction at the same time that the respiratory flow is adequate to support phonation. Chances are you are using simultaneous attack when you say the word "zany," because to start the flow of air before voicing would add the unvoiced /s/ to the beginning of the word, although adducting the vocal folds before producing the first sound would add a glottal stop to production.

Breathy vocal attack involves starting significant airflow before adducting the vocal folds. This occurs frequently during running speech, because we keep air flowing throughout production of long strings of

vocal attack: *movement of vocal folds into the airstream for the purpose of initiating phonation*

sustained phonation: *phonation which continues for long durations as a result of tonic contraction of vocal fold adductors*

simultaneous vocal attack: *vocal attack in which expiration and vocal fold adduction occur simultaneously*

breathy vocal attack: *vocal attack in which expiration occurs before the onset of vocal fold adduction*

words. Say the following sentence while attending to the airflow over your tongue and past your lips: "Harry is my friend." If you did this, you felt the constant airflow which indicates that some of the adductions involved had to be produced with air already flowing.

The third type of attack is glottal attack. In this attack, adduction of the vocal folds occurs prior to the airflow, much like a cough. Try this. Bring your vocal folds together (be gentle!) as if to cough, but instead of opening your vocal folds as you push air through the folds, keep them adducted and say /a/. That was a glottal attack. You might have felt a little tension or irritation from doing this exercise, a reminder of the delicacy of the vocal mechanism. We use glottal attack when a word begins with a stressed vowel. Say the following sentence and pay close attention to your vocal folds during production of the first phoneme of the words: "*Okay, I want the car.*" If you noticed a buildup of tension and pressure for those words, you were experiencing glottal attack.

All three of these attacks are quite functional in speech and are not at all pathological. Problems occur when an attack is misused. If a glottal attack becomes a **hard glottal attack**, the speaker may damage the delicate vocal mechanism tissues. If the speaker inadequately adducts the vocal folds, air may escape between them to produce a **breathy phonation**; a much more common phenomenon is breathy voice caused by a physical tissue change that obstructs adduction.

glottal attack: *the vocal attack in which expiration occurs after adduction of the vocal folds*

Termination

We bring the vocal folds together to begin phonation, and **termination** of phonation requires that we abduct them. We pull the vocal folds out of the airstream far enough to reduce the turbulence, using muscular action. When the turbulence is sufficiently reduced, the vocal folds stop vibrating. As with attack, we terminate phonation many times during running speech to accommodate voiced and voiceless speech sounds.

Both adduction and abduction occur very rapidly. Muscles controlling these functions can complete contraction within about 9 milliseconds (ms) (9/1,000 seconds). In running speech, you may see periods of

Ventricular Phonation

The false or ventricular vocal folds are technically unable to vibrate for voice, but in some instances clients may use them for this purpose. Boone (1999) cites instances in which clients used ventricular phonation as an adaptive response to severe vocal fold dysfunction, such as growths on the folds. Apparently the client forces the lateral superior walls close together during the adductory gesture, permitting the folds to make contact and vibrate.

The ventricular folds are thick, and the phonation heard is deep and often raspy. The false folds may **hypertrophy** (increase in size), facilitating ventricular phonation.

Vocal Fold Nodules

Vocal fold nodules are aggregates of tissue arising from abuse. This condition makes up a large share of the voice disorder cases seen by school clinicians. Common forms of vocal abuse are yelling, screaming, cheerleading, or "barking" commands (such as a drill sergeant). The result of this abuse is a sequence of events that can lead to permanent change in the vocal fold tissue. You are probably familiar with **laryngitis**, which is inflammation of the larynx. It causes hoarseness, often with loss of voice (**aphonia**). The laryngeal effect is swelling (**edema**) of the delicate vocal fold tissue, so that it is difficult to make the folds vibrate. In fact, they are often bowed so badly that expiratory flow will pass between them, even if you can produce phonation; we refer to this as a **breathy voice**. Laryngitis may easily be caused by **vocal hyperfunction**, which is over-adduction of the vocal folds. This is a form of **vocal abuse**, and you may have experienced it after a particularly thrilling football game.

The soreness is a message from your body to stop doing what made the vocal folds sore in the first place. Continued abuse results in formation of a protective layer of epithelium which is callous-like and is not a very effective oscillator. If the vocal hyperfunction continues, the hardened tissue will increase in size until a nodule forms on one (**unilateral**) or both (**bilateral**) vocal folds. The site of abuse is usually at the juncture of the anterior and middle thirds of the vocal folds, because this is the point of greatest impact during phonation. Although untreated vocal nodules may eventually have to be removed surgically, voice therapy to reverse the vocal behavior driving the phenomenon is always appropriate. If the vocal hyperfunction is not eliminated, the vocal nodules will return after surgery, and surgery may be avoided if therapy is sought in a timely manner.

vibration of the vocal folds as brief as three cycles of vibration (approximately 25 ms) for unstressed vowels, which would bring total adduction, phonation, and abduction time to only 53/1,000 of a second!

Adduction is a constant in all types of attack. The arytenoid cartilages are capable of moving in three dimensions, including **rotating**, **rocking**, and **gliding**. It appears that the primary arytenoid gesture for adduction is inward rocking. When the arytenoids are pulled medially on the convex arytenoid facet of the cricoid, the arytenoids rock down, with apices approaching each other. (You may wish to review Figure 5-11 in Chapter 5.) Some rotatory movement will occur during movement of the arytenoid, but it appears to be greatest at the extremes of lateral movement (i.e., nearly abducted; Fink, 1975). These motions are the product of the lateral cricoarytenoid muscle and the lateral portion of the thyromuscularis, facilitated by the oblique and transverse arytenoids. The arytenoid cartilages are also capable of limited gliding in the anterior-posterior dimension that could alter total vocal fold length. Adduction does not seem to affect the overall length of the glottis, although it tends to lengthen the membranous portion. The combined forces of the cricothyroid and posterior cricoarytenoid cause the entire glottis to lengthen (Hirano, Kiyokawa, & Kurita, 1988).

laryngitis: *inflammation of the larynx*

aphonia: *loss of ability to produce voicing for speech*

vocal hyperfunction: *excessive use of vocal mechanism, for speech or nonspeech function, which has the potential to produce organic pathology*

Sustained Phonation

Sustained phonation is the purpose of adduction and abduction for speech. Let us examine this closely.

Vocal attack requires muscular action, as does termination of phonation. In contrast, sustaining phonation simply requires *maintenance* of a laryngeal posture through **tonic** (sustained) contraction of musculature. This is a very important point. The vibration of the vocal folds is achieved by placing and holding the vocal folds in the airstream in a manner that permits their physical qualities to interact with the airflow, thereby causing vibration. The vocal folds are *held* in place during sustained phonation, and vibration of the vocal folds is *not the product of repeated adduction and abduction of the vocal folds.*

Phonation actually begins a few milliseconds prior to vocal fold approximation. As the vocal folds are brought together during attack, they begin vibrating as the turbulence increases, and this vibration is sustained as long as the folds are approximated and there is sufficient subglottal air pressure. By the way, vocal folds need not be touching to vibrate, as you can demonstrate for yourself. Begin the word "hairy" by stretching out the /h/ sound, and then let that breathiness carry forward into the vowel. The vocal folds very likely are not touching or are making only very light contact if you hear a breathy quality.

Vocal Register

Asking clients to practice adding /h/ to the beginning of words is a useful tool for reducing vocal hyperfunction.

Trained singers refer to combinations of thorax/oral/nasal cavity configurations, laryngeal gestures, and muscular "concentrations" to define registers that are perceptually differentiable but about which there are few acoustical or physiological data. See Titze (1994) for a lively discussion of register.

The "mode" is that which occurs most often in a distribution.

The **mode of vibration** of the vocal folds during sustained phonation refers to the pattern of activity that the vocal folds undergo during a cycle of vibration. Moving from one point in the vibratory pattern to the same point again defines one **cycle** of vibration, and within one cycle the vocal folds undergo some very significant changes. There are actually a number of modes or **vocal registers** that have been differentiated perceptually. Narrowly defined for purposes of phonatory discussion, **register** refers to differences in mode of vibration of the vocal folds.

The three registers most commonly referred to are modal register, glottal fry or pulse register, and falsetto. We will also be interested in the variant breathy and pressed phonatory modes, as well as whispered speech.

Modal Register

The first register, known as the **modal register** or modal phonation, refers to the pattern of phonation used in daily conversation. This pattern is the most important one for the speech-language pathologist, and it is the most efficient.

Figure 6-5 shows the vocal folds from the sides and from above, which will let us talk about the vertical and anterior-posterior modes of phonation. In the **vertical mode** of phonation, the vocal folds *open* from inferior to superior (bottom to top), and also *close* from inferior to superior.

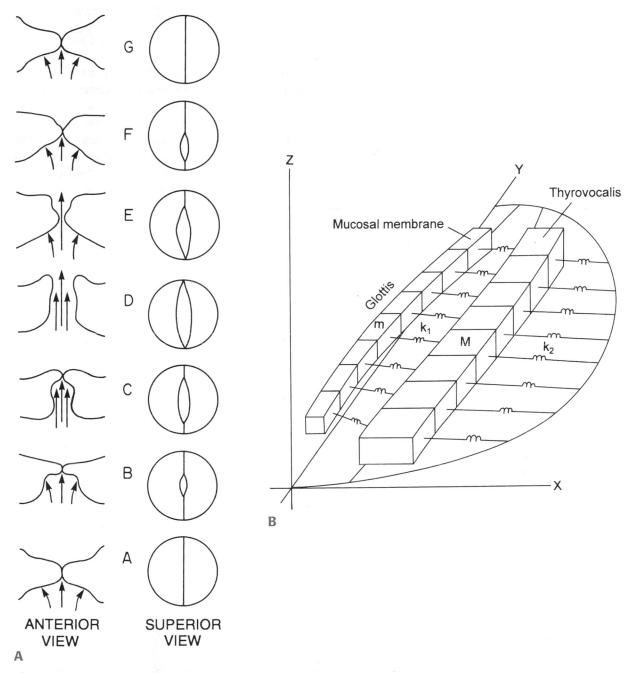

Figure 6-5. A. Graphic representation of vertical and transverse phase relationships during one glottal cycle. Notice that generally the vocal folds open from inferior to superior and also close from inferior to superior. Simultaneously, the glottis grows generally from posterior to anterior, but the vocal folds close from anterior to posterior. **B.** The mucoviscoaerodynamic theory of vocal fold vibration (Titze, 1973) holds that vocal fold vibration can best be explained if the mechanism is viewed as a series of masses (m) linked by spring elements (k). (Redrawn by permission, from Titze [1973] "The Human Vocal Cords: A Mathematical Model, Part I." *Phonetica, 28,* 129–170.)

You might suspect that they would open and close like a door swinging on a hinge, but that is not the case. The folds are an undulating wave of tissue, and it is more appropriate to think of air as "bubbling" through the adducted folds than of the folds opening and closing as if hinged.

You can see from the first panel of Figure 6-5 that the vocal folds are approximated at the beginning of a cycle of vibration. In the second panel, air pressure from beneath is forcing the folds apart in the inferior aspect. (This makes sense, because that is where the pressure is located.) In the third panel, the bubble of air has moved upward so that the superior portion of the folds is now open, and in Panel E you can see that they are closing again. Note that they begin closing at the bottom: They open at the bottom first, and they start closing first at the bottom as well. In the final panel the cycle is complete.

Sustained and Maximum Phonation

Physical systems, such as those encompassing the mechanisms of speech, are rarely employed at maximum output and stress. For instance, we generally do not breathe in maximally or speak using our entire vital capacity, although we are capable of doing this. When clinicians wish to examine whether there is a deficit in a system, one useful technique is to ask the client to perform a test of maximal output for a given parameter. In respiration, such tests would be examination of vital capacity, inspiratory reserve, and expiratory reserve.

This useful concept may be extended to voicing. If you ask a client to sustain a vowel for as long as he or she can, you are testing not only how well the vocal folds function, but also the vital capacity and checking action ability of the person under examination. If the respiratory system is intact, on average an adult female in the 17- to 41-year-old range will be able to sustain the /a/ vowel for approximately 15 seconds, and the male will be able to sustain that vowel for 23 seconds. This function changes with age, increasing through the second decade of life. Generally you may expect the phonation time of children to increase from about 10 seconds at 6 years, but you may be interested in looking at the norms by age as summarized by Kent, Kent, and Rosenbek (1987). By the way, did you wonder why males are able to phonate a little longer? If you attributed it to larger vital capacity, you were right.

Another phonation-related task involves maximum duration of the sustained sibilants, /s/ and /z/. Boone (1999) states that individuals are able to sustain these phonemes for approximately the same durations, but that the addition of physical change to the vocal folds (such as vocal nodules) will cause a significant reduction in the duration of the voiced /z/. Males again produce longer fricatives, and the duration increases with age. Clinicians calculate the ratio of s:z duration to aid their decisions. If the two durations are the same, the value is 1.0, whereas as the /z/ duration drops, the ratio will increase. The decline in /z/ duration arises from reduced phonatory efficiency caused by swelling (edema). Although the ratio undergoes continual examination for its clinical utility, many studies have substantiated the use of this clinical tool.

Titze (1994) has demonstrated that this phase difference in the mucosal wave from inferior to superior is a result of the mass and elasticity of the vocal folds, and that these conditions support continued oscillation by the vocal folds (i.e., the tissue continues to vibrate after the energy has been removed). You are able to change the tension and mass per unit length to arrive at a given, relatively constant laryngeal tone.

The vocal folds have one *primary* frequency of vibration, called the **vocal fundamental frequency**, but they produce an extremely rich set of harmonics as well, which are whole-number multiples of the fundamental. These harmonics provide important acoustical information for identification of voiced phonemes. If the vocal folds were simple tuning forks without these harmonics, we would not be able to tell one vowel from another. The complex vibrational mode of the vocal folds is extremely important.

The second mode of vibration of the vocal folds is in the **anterior-posterior** dimension. Whereas the vertical phase difference appears to be consistent in modal vibration, the anterior-posterior mode is less stereotypical. Zemlin (1998) reported that the vocal folds tend to open from posterior to anterior, but that closure at the end of a cycle is made by contact of the medial edge of the vocal fold, with the posterior closing last.

Because the vocal folds offer resistance to air flow, the **minimum driving pressure** of the vocal folds in modal phonation is approximately 3–5 cm H_2O subglottal pressure. If pressure is lower than this, the folds will not be blown apart. This is clinically important, because a client who cannot generate 3–5 cm H_2O and sustain it for 5 seconds will not be able to use the vocal folds for speech. (See the Clinical Note on measurement of subglottal pressure and Figure 6-6.)

> **vocal fundamental frequency:** *primary frequency of vibration of the vocal folds*

Glottal Fry

The second register is known as **glottal fry**, but is known also as **pulse register** and **Strohbass** ("straw bass"). What "fry," "pulse," and "straw bass" all allude to is the crackly, "popcorn" quality of this voice. Perceptually, this voice is extremely low in pitch and sounds rough, almost like eggs frying in a pan. Some voice scientists jokingly refer to it as the "I'm sick" voice, as it is the weak, low-pitched voice you might use to explain the reason you cannot come to work today.

Glottal fry is the product of a complex glottal configuration, and it occurs in frequencies ranging as low as 30 Hz, up to 80 or 90 Hz. This mode of vibration requires low subglottal pressure to sustain it (on the order of 2 cm H_2O), and tension of the vocalis is significantly reduced relative to modal vibration, so that the vibrating margin is flaccid and thick. The lateral portion of the vocal folds is tensed, so that there is strong medial compression with short, thick vocal folds and low subglottal

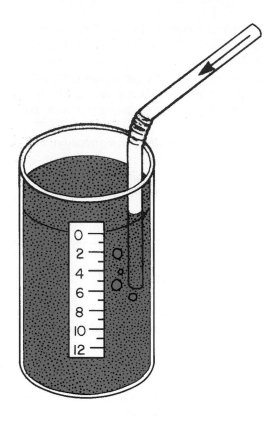

Figure 6-6. A useful clinical tool described by Hixon, Hawley, and Wilson (1982). This portable manometer gives the client feedback concerning respiratory ability and provides the clinician with a measure of function.

In music, syncopation *is the change in accent arising from stressing of a weak beat. In the case of glottal fry, this definition is stretched to accommodate the notion of including a weak beat in the rhythm. Glottal fry appears to include both weak and strong beats.*

pressure. If either vocalis tension or subglottal pressure is increased, the popcornlike perception of this mode of vibration is lost.

In glottal fry, the vocal folds take on a secondary, syncopated mode of vibration, such that there is a secondary beat for every cycle of the fundamental frequency. In addition to this syncopation, the vocal folds spend up to 90% of the cycle in approximation. Oscillographic waveforms of modal vibration and glottal fry are shown in Figure 6-7, and the presence of the extra beat may be clearly seen. This should re-emphasize the notion that the vocal folds are not simply vibrating at a slower rate than in modal phonation, but are vibrating *differently*.

Falsetto

The third and highest register of phonation, the **falsetto**, also is characterized by a vibratory pattern that varies from modal production. In falsetto, the vocal folds lengthen and become extremely thin and "reed-like." When set into vibration, they tend to vibrate along the tensed, bowed margins, in contrast to the complex pattern seen in other modes of phonation. The vocal folds make contact only briefly, as compared with modal phonation, and the degree of movement (amplitude of excursion) is reduced. The posterior portion of the vocal folds tends to be

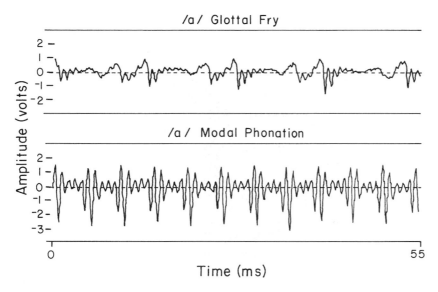

Figure 6-7. Oscillographic comparison of glottal fry (*top*) and modal phonation for the vowel /a/ (*bottom*).

damped, so that the length of the vibrating surface is decreased to a narrow opening. Contrast this to elevated pitch in modal phonation, which involves *lengthening* the vocal folds.

The perception of falsetto is one of an extremely "thin," high-pitched vocal production. The difference between falsetto and modal vibration is not simply one of the frequency of vibration (in the 300 to 600 Hz range). Although it is true that falsetto is the highest register, the modal and falsetto registers overlap.

Clinical Measurement of Subglottal Air Pressure

Hixon, Hawley, and Wilson (1982) have provided us with an excellent and simple tool to assess adequacy of subglottal pressure for speech. In their article, the authors recommend marking a cup of water in cm gradations (see Figure 6-6). Place a small pinhole in a flexible soda straw, and put a paper clip over the straw to hold it to the edge of the glass. Fill the glass up to the top centimeter mark.

As you push the straw deeper into the water, it becomes increasingly difficult to blow bubbles in the water through the straw. At the point where the straw is three centimeters below the water line, you must generate 3 cm H_2O of subglottal pressure to make bubbles.

When assessing a client for adequacy of subglottal pressure, you can have the individual begin blowing as you push the straw into the water. The point at which bubbles no longer flow is the limit of the individual's pressure ability. This is an excellent therapy tool as well, because it provides a practice device with visual feedback of progress toward improved respiratory support for speech. Realize that this is a measurement of respiratory ability, which is essential for phonation.

Whistle Register. There is actually a register above falsetto, known as the **whistle register**, but it is not apparently a mode of vibration as much as it is the product of turbulence on the edge of the vocal fold. It occurs at frequencies as high as 2,500 Hz, typically in females, and sounds very much like a whistle.

The shift from modal register to glottal fry or falsetto is clearly audible in the untrained voice. If you perform an up-glide of a sung note, reaching up to your highest production, you may hear an audible "break" in the voice as you enter that register. Trained singers learn to smooth that transition so that it is inaudible.

Pressed and Breathy Phonation

There are two variations on modal phonation that we should mention. In **pressed** phonation, medial compression is greatly increased. The product of pressed phonation is an increase in the strident or harsh quality, as well as an increase in abuse to the voice. Greater medial compression is translated as stronger, louder phonation, perhaps commanding greater attention. This forceful adduction often results in damage to the vocal fold tissue.

Breathy voice may be the product of the other end of this tension spectrum. If the vocal folds are inadequately approximated, so that the vibrating margins permit excessive airflow between them when in the closed phase, you will hear air escape as a **breathy** phonation. Breathiness is inefficient and causes air wastage, but is not a condition that will damage the phonatory mechanism.

Puberphonia

During normal development, children undergo a great deal of change during **puberty**, the time in a child's life when he or she becomes capable of reproduction. This occurs between 13 and 15 years of age for boys and between 9 and 16 years of age for girls. Puberty is characterized by rapid muscle development and height and weight gain. The thyroid cartilage and thyroarytenoid are not left out of development. They grow rapidly during this time, although the larynges of boys will grow considerably more than those of girls.

The result of this spurt of laryngeal growth is that the child (typically a boy) will have periods of voice change (**mutation**) in which his voice "breaks" down in pitch as he is speaking. This is, of course, a normal result of the changing tissue and the young man's attempt to control it for phonation, but it is nonetheless disturbing. **Puberphonia** refers to the maintenance of the childhood pitch despite having passed through the developmental stage of puberty. It surely represents an attempt to hold *something* constant during the roller-coaster ride of puberty, but the result is a significant mismatch between the large body of the developing teenaged boy and the high-pitched voice of the prepubescent child. Typically, the young man is speaking in falsetto but is aware of the "lower" voice. Therapy performed over the summer to help the individual alter habitual pitch, in the absence of peer pressures associated with the classroom regimen, is quite effective.

There is potential danger in the breathy voice, however. The under-lying factor keeping the vocal folds from approximating also could be any of a number of organic conditions, so that even when the speaker pushes the vocal folds tightly together, air escapes. In this case, breathy voice may signal the presence of vocal nodules, or even benign or malig-nant growths such as polyps or laryngeal cancer. In addition, if an indi-vidual attempts to overcome the breathy quality caused by nodules or other obstructing pathology, the vocal hyperfunction will be abuse.

Whispering

Whispering is not really a phonatory mode, because no voicing occurs. This does *not* mean that there are no laryngeal adjustments, but rather that they do not produce vibration in the vocal folds. Prove this to your-self. Exhale forcefully and attend to your larynx, and then on the next forceful exhalation *whisper* the word "Ha!" You probably felt the tension in your larynx increase during whispering. In respiration the vocal folds are abducted, but when whispering they must be partially adducted and tensed to develop turbulence in the airstream, and that turbulence is the noise you use to make speech. The arytenoid cartilages are rotated slightly in but are separated posteriorly, so that there is an enlarged "chink" in the cartilaginous larynx. It is *not* voiced, but it is strenuous and can cause vocal fatigue. Whispering is not economical, as you can prove to yourself by sustaining production of an /a/ in modal phonation and again in whispered production. You should see quite a difference in maximum duration.

In Chapter 5 we discussed the notion of frequency of vibration. As mentioned earlier in this chapter, the primary frequency of vibration of the vocal folds is called the *fundamental frequency*. This is the number of cycles the vocal folds go through per second, and it is audible. The movement of the vocal folds in air produces an audible disturbance in the medium of air known as **sound**. That sound is transmitted through

Electroglottography

The electroglottograph (EGG) is a useful and nonintrusive instrument for examination of vocal function. A pair of surface electrodes are placed on the thyroid lamina, typically held in place by an elastic band. An extremely small and imperceptible current is introduced through one electrode, and the impedance (resistance to current flow) is measured at the other electrode. When the vocal folds are approximated during phonation, there is less resistance to flow. The less contact the vocal folds make, the greater the impedance.

This nice arrangement permits researchers to examine at least some aspects of vocal fold function with ease. As you can see from the EGG trace of Figure 6-10, there are marked differences in the duration of vocal fold contact for quiet (A) versus loud (B) speech. For further reading, you may want to review Childers, Hicks, Moore, Eskenazi, and Lalwani (1990).

the air as a wave, with molecules being compressed by movement of the vocal folds.

intensity: *magnitude of sound, expressed as the relationship between two pressures or powers*

vocal intensity: *sound pressure level associated with a given speech production*

The interplay of the elasticity and mass of the vocal folds leads them to vibrate in a periodic fashion. However, we have not yet mentioned a final element of phonation, intensity. **Intensity** refers to the relative power or pressure of an acoustic signal, measured in decibels (abbreviated **dB**). In phonation, we may refer to the intensity of voice as **vocal intensity**. Intensity is a direct function of the amount of pressure exerted by the *sound wave* (as opposed to air pressure, as generated by the respiratory system). As molecules vibrate from movement of the vocal folds, the molecular movement exerts an extremely small but measurable force over an area, and that is defined as pressure. The larger the excursion of the vibrating body, the greater the intensity of the signal produced, because air will be displaced with greater force. The next two sections deal with frequency and intensity of vocal fold vibration.

To summarize:

- We must adduct the vocal folds to **initiate phonation**. This adduction may take several forms, including **breathy**, **simultaneous**, and **glottal attacks**.
- Conversational speech will naturally encompass all of these, although overuse of glottal attack in inappropriate contexts may be problematic.
- **Termination** of **phonation** requires abduction of the vocal folds, a process that must occur with the transition of voiced to voiceless speech sounds.
- **Sustained phonation** may take several forms, depending on the laryngeal configuration.
- **Modal phonation** will, by definition, characterize most speech.
- **Falsetto** occupies the upper range of laryngeal function, while **glottal fry** is found in the lower range.
- Vocal fold vibration varies for each of these phonatory modes, and the differences are governed by **laryngeal tension**, **medial compression**, and **subglottal pressure**.
- **Breathy phonation** occurs when there is inadequate medial compression to approximate the vocal folds. **Whispering** arises from tensing the vocal fold margins while holding the folds in a partially adducted position.

Frequency, Pitch, and Pitch Change

pitch: *the psychological (perceptual) correlate of frequency of vibration*

Pitch is the psychological correlate of frequency and is closely related to frequency: As frequency increases, pitch increases, and as frequency decreases, so does pitch. It is an important element in speech perception. Therefore, we should closely examine the mechanism of pitch change.

The vocal folds are made up of masses and elastic elements that tend to promote oscillation or repeated vibration at the same frequency. Because of these qualities, the vocal folds will tend to vibrate at the same frequency when mass and elastic elements remain constant. However, the frequency of vibration will change when these characteristics are altered.

There are several important terms with which we should become familiar. Unfortunately, most of these terms refer to perceived pitch when they really should refer to physical **frequency**! Let us take a look at optimal and habitual pitch, average fundamental frequency, and range of fundamental frequency.

Optimal Pitch

The term **optimal pitch** is used to refer to the pitch (actually, the *frequency*) of vocal fold vibration that is optimal or most appropriate for an individual. This frequency of vibration will be the most efficient for a given pair of vocal folds, and is a function of the mass and elasticity of the vocal folds. Some voice scientists and clinicians estimate optimal pitch directly from the individual's range of phonation, because it is considered to be approximately ¼ octave above the lowest frequency of vibration of an individual. Others will estimate it from a cough or throat-clearing, because the frequency of the vibrating vocal folds during throat-clearing will approximate conditions associated with conversational frequency, but without the psychological conditions associated with use of phonation for communication.

Optimal pitch varies as a function of gender and age. You can expect an adult female to have a fundamental frequency of approximately 212 Hz during a reading task, whereas the optimal fundamental frequency for adult males will be much lower, around 132 Hz, for the same task. Mean fundamental frequency will tend to be lower for spontaneous speech, and it tends to increase with each decade of life.

The reason for the difference in fundamental frequency between males and females has everything to do with tissue mass and length of vocal folds. During puberty, males undergo a significant growth of muscle and cartilage, resulting in greater muscle mass in males than in females. The laryngeal product of this growth is the prominent Adam's apple you can see in boys, as well as a significant drop in fundamental frequency arising from the increased mass of the folds (see Figure 6-8). Children will have fundamental frequency in the range of 300 Hz, but that rapidly changes in both boys and girls during puberty. Take a look at the Clinical Note on puberphonia to see what may occur when fundamental frequency *does not* change with puberty.

Habitual Pitch

We use the term **habitual pitch** to refer to the frequency of vibration of vocal folds that is habitually used during speech. In the ideal condition,

frequency: *number of cycles of vibration per second*

optimal pitch: *the perceptual characteristic representing the ideal or most efficient frequency of vibration of the vocal folds*

An octave is a doubling of frequency, so that the octave beginning at 120 Hz will end at 240 Hz, the octave beginning at 203 Hz will end at 406 Hz, and so forth.

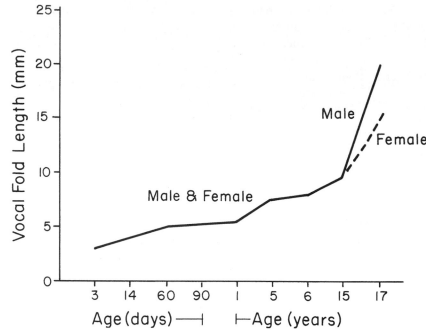

Figure 6-8. Changes in vocal fold length for males and females as a function of age. Note that males and females have essentially the same length of vocal folds until puberty, at which time both genders undergo marked physical development. (Data of Kaplan, 1971.)

this would be the same as optimal pitch. For some individuals, there are compelling reasons to alter their everyday pitch in speech beyond the range expected for their age, size, or gender. Although the choice to use an abnormally higher or lower fundamental frequency is often not a conscious decision, it will have an effect on phonatory efficiency and effort. When the vocal folds are forced into the extremes of their range of ability, greater effort is required to sustain phonation, and this will result in vocal and physical fatigue. Many different techniques are used to estimate this from a speech sample, including asking the individual to sustain a vowel or sustaining a vowel in a spoken word.

Habitual Use of Low Pitch

Habitual use of vocal pitch below optimum can result in **contact ulcers**, open sores on the delicate vocal fold epithelium. These lesions are most often found on the medial margins of the vocal processes and arise from repeated, forceful compression of the arytenoids at that point. Contact ulcers are frequently found in "driven" individuals under a great deal of stress who speak at a frequency habitually below optimum using hard glottal contact. They have also been associated with esophageal reflux, the regurgitation of small quantities of acidic esophageal contents into the pharynx.

Contact ulcers result in vocal fatigue but rarely aphonia. Treatment may include voice therapy to alter habitual pitch and vocal hyperfunction, or means to alleviate the reflux.

Average Fundamental Frequency

The **average fundamental frequency** of vibration of the vocal folds during phonation may reflect the frequency of vibration of *sustained phonation*, or some other condition, such as conversational speech. This actually reflects habitual pitch over a longer averaging period, and use of conversational speech or reading passages probably more accurately reflects an individual's true average rate of vocal fold vibration than a single vowel sample.

Pitch Range

Pitch range refers to the range of fundamental frequency for an individual and is calculated as the difference between the highest and lowest frequencies. The vocal mechanism is quite flexible and is capable of approximately two octaves of change in fundamental frequency from the lowest possible frequency to the highest. An individual with a low fundamental frequency of 90 Hz will be able to reach a high of about 360 Hz (octave 1 = 90 Hz to 180 Hz; octave 2 = 180 to 360 Hz). This range is often reduced by laryngeal pathology, for example, vocal nodules. It can be expanded through voice training as well. Let us examine how we make changes in vocal fundamental frequency, hence in perceived pitch.

Pitch-Changing Mechanism

Fundamental frequency increase comes from stretching and tensing the vocal folds using the cricothyroid and thyrovocalis muscles. Here is the mechanism of this change.

Tension, Length, and Mass. The changeable elements of the vocal folds are tension, length, and mass. We cannot actually change the mass of the vocal folds, but we can change the mass per unit length by spreading the muscle, mucosa, and ligament out over more distance. We also can change the tension of the vocal folds by stretching them tighter or relaxing them. Both of these changes arise from elongation.

↑ tension ↑ freq.

When the cricothyroid muscle is contracted, the thyroid tilts down, lengthening the vocal folds and increasing the fundamental frequency. *When the tension on the vocal folds is increased, the natural frequency of vibration will increase.*

The thyrovocalis is a tenser of the vocal folds as well, because contraction of this muscle will pull both cricoid and thyroid closer together, an action opposed by the simultaneously contracted cricothyroid. This tensing process must be opposed by contraction of the posterior cricoarytenoid, although it is not classified as a tenser of the vocal folds. The posterior cricoarytenoid is invested with **muscle spindles**, bodies responsible for monitoring and maintaining tonic muscle length. As the length of this muscle changes, its length may be reflexively controlled to compensate for the stretching force on the vocal folds.

The natural frequency of vibration refers to the frequency at which a body vibrates given the mass, tension, and elastic properties of the body.

See Chapter 13 for a discussion of the muscle spindle.

These tensers tend to operate together, but for slightly different function. It is currently believed that the cricothyroid contracts to approximate the degree of tension required for a given frequency of vibration. The thyrovocalis appears to fine-tune this adjustment. That is, the cricothyroid makes the gross adjustment, and the thyrovocalis causes the fine movement.

We still have not dealt with mass changes. *As the mass of a vibrating body decreases, frequency of vibration will increase.* The mass of the vocal folds is constant, because to actually increase or decrease mass would require growth of tissue or atrophy, and neither of these processes occurs quickly. Instead, the mass is rearranged by lengthening. When the vocal folds are stretched by contraction of the tensers, the mass of the folds will be distributed over a greater distance, thus reducing mass per unit length.

The effect of the lengthening and tensing gesture is to make vocal folds longer and thinner in appearance. Interestingly, there is evidence that the vocal folds do not lengthen continuously as fundamental frequency increases, but rather that, at some point near or in the falsetto range, the vocal folds again begin to shorten as frequency increases (Nishizawa, Sawashima, & Yonemoto, 1988). Others have found that increased medial compression may effectively shorten the vibrating surface, increasing frequency (Van den Berg & Tan, 1959).

Lowering fundamental frequency requires the opposite manipulation. *As mass per unit length increases and tension decreases, fundamental frequency will decrease.* We **relax** the vocal folds by shortening them, moving the cricoid and thyroid closer together in front. This process is achieved by contraction of the thyromuscularis. When it contracts, the vocal folds are relaxed and shortened so that they become more massive and less tense. It appears that there is help from some of the suprahyoid musculature that indirectly pulls up on the thyroid cartilage, shortening the vocal folds by distancing the thyroid from the cricoid.

Subglottal Pressure and Fundamental Frequency. There also are changes in subglottal pressure that must be reckoned with. *Increasing pitch requires increasing the tension of the system, thereby increasing the glottal resistance to airflow.* If airflow is to remain constant through the glottis, pressure must increase. It appears, however, that the increases in subglottal pressure are a *response* to the increased tension required for frequency change rather than a *cause.* Subglottal pressure does increase, but of itself has little effect on frequency change. It is a delicate balancing act that we perform.

To summarize:

- **Pitch** is the psychological correlate of frequency of vibration, although the term has come into common usage when referring to phenomena associated with the physical vibration of the vocal folds.

- **Optimal pitch** refers to the frequency of vibration that is most efficient for a given pair of vocal folds, and **habitual pitch** is the frequency of vibration habitually used by an individual.

- The **pitch range** of an individual will span approximately two octaves, although it will be reduced by pathology and may be increased through vocal training.

- Changes in **vocal fundamental frequency** are governed by the tension of the vocal folds and their mass per unit length.

- Increasing the length of the vocal folds will increase vocal fold tension as well as decrease the mass per unit area. This will increase the fundamental frequency.

- The **respiratory system** will respond to increased vocal fold tension with **increased subglottal pressure**, so that pitch and subglottal pressure tend to covary.

- Increased subglottal pressure is a response to increased vocal fold tension.

↑ subglottal pressure
↑ vocal fold tension

Intensity and Intensity Change

Just as pitch is the psychological correlate of frequency, **loudness** is the psychological correlate of intensity. **Intensity** (or its correlate, sound pressure level) is the physical measure of power (or pressure) ratios, but loudness is how we perceive power or pressure differences. As with pitch, there is a close relationship between loudness and intensity.

To increase vocal intensity of vibrating vocal folds, one must somehow increase the vigor with which the vocal folds open and close. In sustained phonation, the vocal folds move only as a result of the air pressure beneath them and the flow between them. Subglottal pressure and flow provide the energy for this vocal engine, so to increase the intensity or strength of the phonatory product we will have to increase the energy that drives it. *We increase subglottal pressure to increase vocal intensity.* To prove this to yourself, do the following. You need to feel what you do to produce loud speech. You may be in a quiet setting right now and you really may not want to yell, but that is fine. Pay attention to your lungs and larynx as you *prepare to yell as loudly as you can* to someone across the room. Without even yelling, you should have been able to feel your lungs take in a large charge of air, and you also should have felt your vocal folds tighten up. These are the two gestures of significance for increasing vocal intensity: increased subglottal pressure and medial compression.

Subglottal pressure and increased medial compression vary together, but the causal relationship is better established for vocal intensity than the tension-pressure relationship for pitch. For intensity to

↑ subglottal pressure
↑ vocal intensity
(loudness)

increase, the energy source also must increase, so subglottal pressure must rise. To explain the effect that medial compression has on vocal intensity requires a return to discussion of a cycle of vocal fold vibration.

We can break a cycle of vibration into stages, such as an **opening stage**, in which the vocal folds are opening up; a **closing stage**, in which the vocal folds are returning to the point of approximation; and a **closed stage**, in which there is no air escaping between the vocal folds (see Figures 6-9 and 6-10). In modal phonation at conversational intensities, it has been found that the vocal folds spend about 50% of their time in the

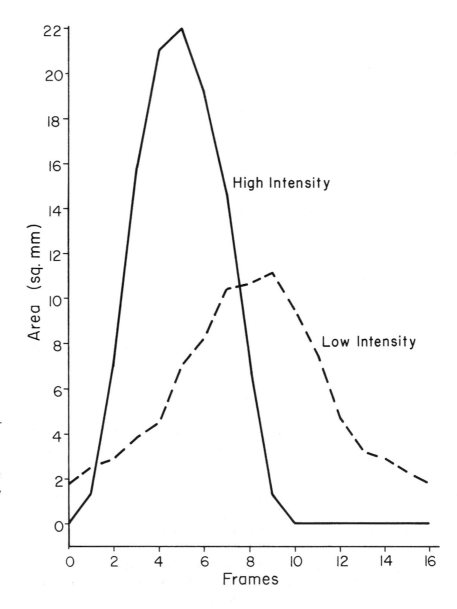

Figure 6-9. Effect of vocal intensity on vocal fold vibration. During low-intensity speech the opening and closing phases occupy most of the vibratory cycle, as revealed in the area of the glottis. During high-intensity speech the opening phase is greatly compressed, as is the closing phase, while the time spent in closed phase is greatly increased. (Data from Fletcher, 1950.)

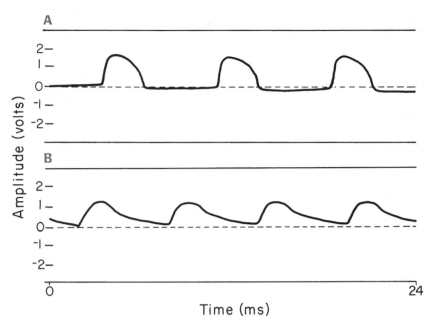

Figure 6-10. Effect of vocal intensity, as shown through electroglottographic trace. The electroglottograph measures impedance across the vocal folds, and the peak represents the closed phase of the glottal cycle. **A.** Conversational level sustained vowel. **B.** High level sustained vowel.

opening phase, 37% of the time in the closing phase, and 13% of the cycle completely closed. When the vocal folds are tightly adducted for increased vocal intensity, they tend to return to the closed position more quickly and to stay closed for a longer period of time. The opening phase reduces to approximately 33%, while the closed phase increases to more than 30%, depending on the intensity increase.

The concept you should retain is this: To increase vocal intensity, the vocal folds are tightly compressed, it takes more force to blow them open, they close more rapidly, and they tend to stay closed because they are tightly compressed. This is the *cause* side of the equation. The *effect* portion is that, because so much energy is required to hold the folds in compression, the release of the folds from this condition is markedly stronger. Each time the folds open, they do so with vigor, producing an explosive compression of the air medium. The harder that eruption of the vocal folds is, the greater is the amplitude of the cycle of vibration. Remembering that as the amplitude of the signal increases, so does the intensity, you will recognize the increase in intensity between the two panels of Figure 6-11.

The two waveforms in Figure 6-11 are different in intensity, but not in frequency. The time between the cycles is exactly the same, so the frequency must be the same. From this comes a very important point: *Intensity and frequency are controlled independently, and you can increase intensity without increasing frequency.* Here is the paradox. Increases in intensity and fundamental frequency depend upon the same

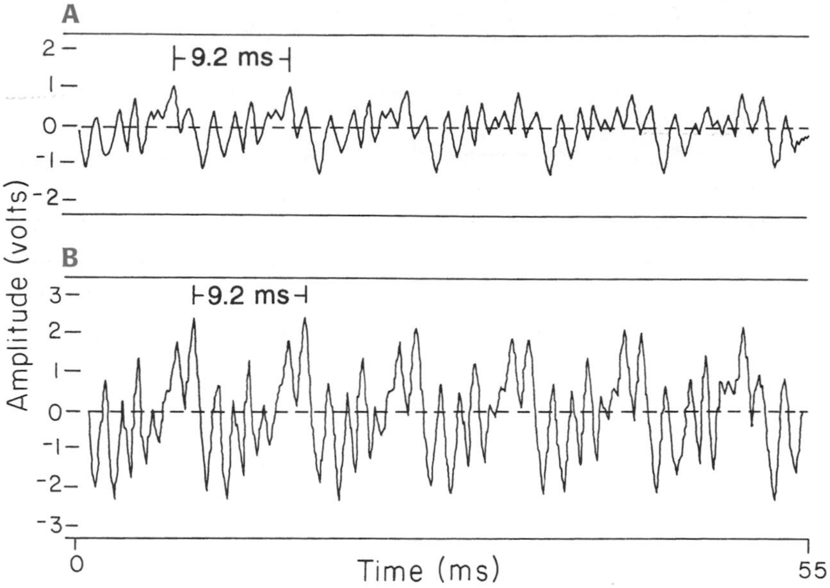

Figure 6-11. Oscillogram of sustained vowel at two vocal intensities. **A.** Sustained vowel at conversational level. **B.** Sustained vowel at increased vocal intensity. Although the vocal intensity increases, the period of each cycle of vibration remains constant at 9.2 milliseconds.

basic mechanism (tension/compression and subglottal pressure), so it is difficult to increase intensity without increasing pitch, but trained or well-controlled speakers can do this. The tendency is for frequency and intensity to increase together, which is a natural gesture that you can demonstrate to yourself. Find a place where you can shout, and then say a word before shouting it. Your pitch will most certainly go up, unless you try very hard to avoid it.

The relationship between subglottal pressure and the actual sound pressure level output of the vocal folds depends on the speaker. However, it appears that for every doubling of subglottal pressure, there is an increase of between 8 and 12 decibels in vocal intensity.

In summary:

- **Vocal intensity** refers to the increase in sound pressure of the speech signal.

- To increase vocal intensity of phonation, the speaker must increase **medial compression** through the muscles of adduction.

- This increased adductory force requires greater **subglottal pressure** to produce phonation and forces the vocal folds to remain in the closed portion of the phonatory cycle for a longer period of time.

- The increased **laryngeal tension** required for increasing intensity also will increase the vocal fundamental, although the trained voice is quite capable of controlling fundamental frequency and vocal intensity independently.

CLINICAL CONSIDERATIONS

The phonatory mechanism is extraordinarily sensitive to the physical well-being of the speaker. When individuals are ill, their voices often get weaker and, in the case of upper respiratory problems, "rough." Diseases that weaken individuals also tend to compromise phonatory effort, so that the voice weakens in intensity, and pitch range is reduced. Increasing muscle tension for pitch and intensity variation requires work, and illness tends to reduce the ability to exert such forces. A number of neuromuscular diseases have been shown to affect phonation, and many measures of phonatory stability and ability have gained clinical acceptance.

Frequency perturbation is a measure of cycle-by-cycle variability in phonation. Perturbation, or **vocal jitter**, provides an exquisite index of muscle tone and stability but requires instrumentation for measurement. The client is asked to sustain a vowel as steadily as possible while it is being recorded by computer. Following this, the computer program measures each cycle of vibration and calculates how closely each cycle corresponds to the next in duration. The computer measures the duration of the first cycle (e.g., 10.2 ms), and subtracts that of the next cycle (e.g., 10.4 ms) and stores that number. It performs this for all succeeding cycles of vibration and calculates the average of the (unsigned) differences as compared with the average period of vibration. The resulting **percent of perturbation** (or percent jitter) is an indication of how perfectly this imperfect system is oscillating. The broad rule of thumb is that variation in excess of 1–2% will be perceived as hoarse. This is a good measure of client change over time and a less effective means of comparing clients.

This measure has been shown to be sensitive to a number of characteristics. Individuals who are more physically fit will have lower perturbation values than those who are not. Individuals with **neuromotor dysfunction** (neurological conditions that affect motor function) will have higher perturbation than healthy individuals. Increased mass (such as vocal nodules) will increase perturbation, while therapy to reduce the mass will show a decrease in the jitter.

More prosaic measures do not require this degree of instrumentation, but nonetheless provide insight into phonatory function. The process of assessment often requires us to stress the system under examination so that its weakness can be seen with relation to normal abilities. (Kent, Kent, and Rosenbek [1987] provided an excellent overview of methods of stressing the phonatory system.) As mentioned earlier, **maximum phonation time** refers to the duration of phonation an individual is capable of sustaining. Sustained phonation provides an index of phonatory-plus-respiratory efficiency. You can examine the respiratory system by itself, to determine the ability of your client to sustain expiration in the absence of voicing, and have some confidence that length and steadiness of a sustained vowel are an indicator of laryngeal function.

vocal jitter: *cycle-by-cycle variation in fundamental frequency of vibration*

Another time-honored measure is diadochokinetic rate. Oral **diado-chokinesis** refers to the alternation of articulators (you may hear it referred to as *alternating motor rate* as well). Specifically, it is the number of productions of a single or multiple syllables an individual produces per second. This is an excellent tool for assessing the articulators (the topic of Chapters 7 and 8), but also helps assessment of the coordination of the phonatory and articulatory systems.

Pathological conditions often have an impact on vocal range and vocal intensity. For instance, the presence of vocal nodules may reduce an individual's vocal range from two octaves to one-half octave or less, and the breathy component will have a real impact on vocal intensity. Similarly, physical weakness may limit a client's ability to exert effort for either pitch or vocal intensity change.

The exquisitely sensitive vocal mechanism is an excellent window on the health and well-being of a client, as you will find in your advanced studies of voice.

suprasegmental: *parameters of speech that include prosody, pitch, and loudness changes for meaning*

prosody: *the system of stress used to vary the meaning of speech*

LINGUISTIC ASPECTS OF PITCH AND INTENSITY

Pitch and intensity play significant roles in the suprasegmental aspects of communication. **Suprasegmental** elements are the parameters of speech that are above the segment (phonetic) level. This term generally refers to elements of **prosody**, the system of stress used to vary meaning in speech. The prosodic elements include pitch, intonation, loudness, stress, duration, and rhythm; these elements not only convey a great

Prosody and Neuromuscular Disorder

The prosodic element of speech can be a window on speech physiology in neuropathology. *Prosody* is the combination of changes in fundamental frequency and vocal intensity that produce linguistically relevant intonation and stress characteristics. When the neuromuscular system is compromised, prosody may be affected. When muscle tone increases (hypertonus) due to spasticity, the individual may demonstrate prosody characterized by even and equal stress with inappropriately high vocal intensity on each syllable or word, in combination with a harsh phonatory quality.

When an individual has ataxic signs from cerebellar damage, she will have disrupted prosody from the discoordination of respiratory, phonatory, and articulatory systems. Speech syllable timing will be defective, and control of phonatory elements will be seriously deficient.

In many of the hyperkinetic dysarthrias, the element of speech control is overridden by movements of speech structures that are involuntary and uncontrollable. In these cases, prosody will be seriously affected, as the articulatory or phonatory gesture is interrupted by the spontaneous movements.

deal of information concerning emotion and intent, but also provide information that can disambiguate meaning. Even though it is not the purpose of an anatomy text to delve into these suprasegmental elements, pitch and intensity play such a heavy role that we should at least glance at them.

Intonation refers to the changes in pitch in speech, whereas **stress** refers to syllable or word emphasis relative to an entire utterance. For example, say the following sentence out loud: "That's a cat." You end it with a falling *intonation* and put more *stress* on "that's" than on "a" or "cat." To a large extent, these elements both arise out of variation in vocal intensity and fundamental frequency. Intonation may be considered the melodic envelope that contains the sentence, and may serve to mark sentence type. Generally, statements tend to have falling intonation at the end; questions tend to have rising intonation. Figure 6-12 shows traces of the fundamental frequency for the productions of "Bev bombed Bob." and "Bev bombed Bob?" If you say these two sentences, you can hear for yourself the changes that are so strong in the second sentence. Hirano, Ohala, and Vennard (1969) used this sentence contrast to show that the lateral cricoarytenoid, thyrovocalis, and cricothyroid were all quite active in making these rapid laryngeal adjustments.

Stress helps punctuate speech, providing emphasis to syllables or words through both intensity and frequency changes. To increase stress, we increase fundamental frequency and intensity by increasing subglottal pressure, medial compression, and laryngeal tension. As you will remember from our earlier discussion, both frequency and intensity involve adjustments of these variables. We capitalize on the fact that both intensity and fundamental frequency vary together, so stressed syllables

intonation: *the melody of speech, provided by variation of the fundamental frequency during speech*

stress: *the product of relative increase in fundamental frequency, vocal intensity, and duration*

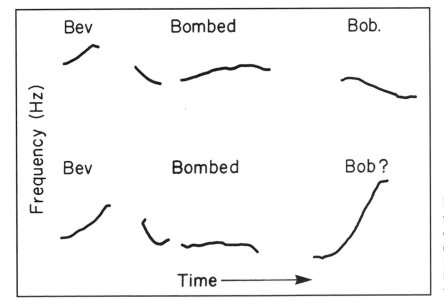

Figure 6-12. Fundamental frequency fluctuation for declarative statement and question form. Note the difference in falling and rising intonation between these two sentence forms.

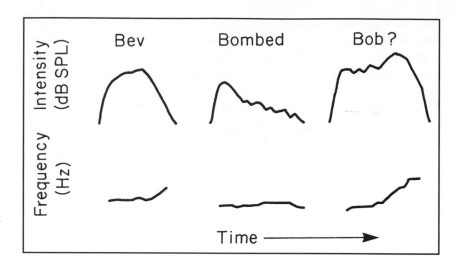

Figure 6-13. Fundamental frequency and intensity changes during production of a question form.

or words will show changes in both. If you look at the pitch and intensity traces of Figure 6-13, you can see how they vary together.

The musculature involved in stress is not unlike that of intonation, although we must factor in the increase in subglottal pressure. The changes in fundamental frequency will be on the order of 50 Hz (Netsell, 1973), governed by the lateral cricoarytenoid, thyrovocalis, and cricothyroid. The changes in subglottal pressure will be small but rapid, or pulsatile (Hixon, 1973). Because they require bursts of increased expiratory force, they are going to be driven by expiratory muscles.

Although stress and intonation are not *essential* for communication, they *are* essential for naturalness. Clearly you can speak in a **monopitch** (unvarying vocal pitch) or **monoloud** voice (unvarying vocal loudness), but the effect is so distracting that it certainly interferes with communication. You may find individuals with neurological impairments who show both of these characteristics. Treatment directed toward increased muscular effort at points requiring stress will greatly enhance the naturalness of speech, because increasing vocal effort at these points will inevitably increase both fundamental frequency and vocal intensity.

monopitch: *without variation in vocal pitch (the perception of frequency)*

monoloud: *without variation in vocal loudness (the perception of vocal intensity)*

THEORIES OF PHONATION

The history of theories of vocal fold vibration is long and colorful, leading certainly from Helmholtz of the 1800s to the present. Although it has long been known that the vocal folds are the source of voicing, only recently did we develop an understanding of the mechanism of phonation, and refinements continue. Certainly, the underlying principles discussed in this chapter are broadly accepted, although it has not always been so.

As discussed earlier, the myoelastic-aerodynamic theory of phonation states that vibration of the vocal folds depends on the elements embodied in the name of the theory. The myoelastic element is the elastic component of muscle (*myo* = muscle) and associated soft tissues of the larynx, and the aerodynamic component is that of the airflow and pressure through this constricted tube. Van den Berg (1958) recognized that the combination of tissue elasticity, which causes the vocal folds to return to their original position after being distended, and the Bernoulli effect, which helps promote this return by dropping the pressure at the constriction, could account for the sustained vibration shown in even a cadaverous specimen provided with an artificial source of expiratory charge.

Work by Titze (1994) has sought to explain how complex acoustic output can come from a simple oscillator such as the vocal folds. We have long recognized that the vocal folds are not simple oscillators, but rather undulate in the modes discussed earlier. Titze recognized that this complex vibration arises from the loosely bound masses associated with the membranous **cover** of the vocal folds (the epithelium and superficial layer of the lamina propria) and the **body** of the vocal folds (the intermediate and deep layers of lamina propria and thyrovocalis muscle). The loosely bound elastic tissue supports oscillation, and viewing the soft tissue as an infinite (or at least uncountable) number of masses reveals that a very large number of modes of vibration is possible. This discussion in no way gives justice to the elegance of this theory, and we recommend that you take time for the exceptionally readable work of Titze.

The phonatory mechanism is an important component of the speaking mechanism, providing the voiced source for speech. It is time for us to see what happens to the voice source after it leaves the larynx. See Chapter 7 for a continuation of this story.

Laryngeal Stridor

Laryngeal stridor refers to a harsh sound produced during respiration. The sound is associated with some obstruction in the respiratory passageway and is always a sign of dysfunction. Stridor may arise from a growth in the larynx or trachea causing turbulence during respiration, or it may arise from the vocal folds. If the vocal folds are paralyzed in the adducted position (**abductor paralysis**), they will not only obstruct the airway but also will vibrate as the air of inspiration passes by them. In this case, the harsh sound will be referred to as **inhalatory stridor**. You may want to imitate this in yourself so that you will come to recognize this sign of obstruction. Phonate while breathing out, and then, without abducting your vocal folds, force your inspiration through the closed vocal folds. You will notice not only a harsh sound but also the extreme difficulty of inhaling through an obstruction.

◤ CHAPTER SUMMARY

Phonation is the product of vibrating vocal folds within the **larynx**. The **vocal folds** vibrate as air flows past them, capitalizing upon the **Bernoulli phenomenon** and **tissue elasticity** to maintain phonation. The interaction of **subglottal pressure, tissue elasticity,** and **constriction** within the airflow caused by the vocal folds produces sustained phonation as long as **pressure,** flow, and **vocal fold approximation** are maintained.

The larynx is an important structure for a number of **nonspeech** functions as well, including **coughing, throat-clearing,** and **abdominal fixation**. The degree of muscle control during phonation is greatly increased, however, because the successful use of voice requires careful attention to vocal fold **tension** and **length**.

Adduction takes several forms, including **breathy, simultaneous,** and **glottal attacks,** and **termination** of phonation requires **abduction** of the vocal folds. **Sustained phonation** depends on the laryngeal configuration. The **modal pattern** of phonation is most efficient, capitalizing on the optimal combination of muscular tension and respiratory support for the vocal folds. **Falsetto** requires increased vocal fold tension, and **glottal fry** demands a unique glottal and respiratory configuration. Each of these modes of vocal fold vibration is different, and the variations are governed by laryngeal **tension, medial compression,** and **subglottal pressure**. **Breathy phonation** occurs when there is inadequate medial compression to approximate the vocal folds, and **whispering** results from tensing the vocal fold margins while holding the folds partially adducted.

Pitch is the psychological correlate of **frequency** of vibration, and **loudness** is the correlate of **intensity,** although both of the terms *pitch* and *intensity* have been used to represent physical phenomena. **Optimal pitch** is the most efficient frequency of vibration for a given pair of vocal folds, and **habitual pitch** is the frequency of vibration used by an individual habitually. The **pitch range** of an individual will span approximately two octaves, but can be reduced by pathology or increased through vocal training.

Vocal fundamental frequency changes are governed by vocal fold tension and mass per unit length. To increase fundamental frequency, we increase the **length** of the vocal folds, which will increase the **tension** of the vocal folds and decrease the **mass per unit length**. To compensate for increased tension, subglottal pressure will increase.

Medial compression is increased to produce an increase in vocal **intensity** of phonation, and this is performed largely through the muscles of adduction. Increased **adductory force** requires greater subglottal pressure to produce phonation, and this forces the vocal folds to remain in the closed portion of the phonatory cycle for a longer time. The **increased laryngeal tension** will increase the vocal fundamental frequency as well, although the fundamental frequency and vocal intensity may be controlled independently.

 ## END NOTE: MECHANICS OF VIBRATION

You are already familiar with the notion that things are capable of vibrating, because you have undoubtedly set a ruler into vibration on your desktop, or plucked a guitar string. When a physical body is set into vibration, it tends to continue vibrating (that is, oscillating), and that vibration tends to continue at the same rate.

Let us examine why a body tends to oscillate. If you have a guitar, pluck one of the strings. As you listen to the twang of the string, you will notice that it continues vibrating for quite a while before finally quieting down. The tone produced remains at about the same pitch throughout the audible portion of its vibration.

The actual process of vibration is determined by a lawful interplay among the elastic restoring forces of a material, the stiffness of the material, and inertia, a quality of its mass. **Elasticity** is that property of a material that causes it to return to its original shape after being displaced. **Stiffness** refers to the *strength* of the forces held within a given material that restore it to its original shape on being distended. **Inertia** is the property of mass dictating that a body in motion tends to stay in motion. If we discuss the vibration of the guitar string in detail, the interaction of these elements may become clearer. Look at Figure 6-14 as we discuss this.

In the first panel of Figure 6-14, the guitar string is at its resting point. At this point, all forces are balanced. Next, the string is being displaced by someone's finger. This displacing force is distending the string. In the next panel, the string has been released and is moving toward its starting point. This is a direct result of the restoring forces of the elastic material. The elastic qualities of the material from which the string is made and the stiffness of that material determine the efficiency with which the string returns. (If you were to try this with a highly inelastic material, such as a bar of lead or a slab of roast beef, would it return?)

In Panel D, when the string reaches the midpoint it is moving too fast to stop and sails on by that midpoint even though it is the point of equilibrium. Just as when you push someone in a swing, the swing does not simply return to the point of rest and stop, but rather overshoots that point. The reason the string travels past the point of rest is that it has mass. It takes energy to move mass and it takes energy to stop it once it

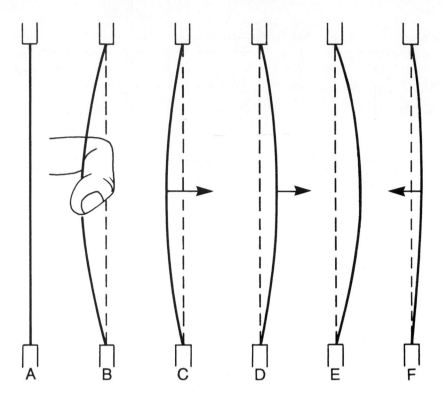

Figure 6-14. A guitar string illustrates oscillation. **A.** The string is at rest. **B.** A finger forces the string into displacement. **C.** The string is released and its elastic elements cause it to return toward the rest position. **D.** The string overshoots the rest position because of its inertia. **E.** The string reaches the extreme point of its excursion past the rest position. **F.** Elastic forces within the string cause the string to return toward the rest position.

has started moving. The string will not only return to its original resting position, due to elastic restoring forces, but will fly past that position due to the inertia associated with moving the mass of the object. In Panel E, the string eventually stops moving because it is now being distended in the opposite direction. The energy you expended in the first distension has now been translated into an opposite distortion as a result of inertia. In the final panel, the string may now begin its return trip toward the starting point, but it will once again overshoot that point because of inertia.

If you had set a pencil into vibration instead of a string and we had moved a sheet of paper in front of it as it vibrated, it might have drawn a picture something like shown in Figure 6-15, which depicts the periodic motion of a vibrating body. This picture is a graphic representation of the vibration of that object. The drawing represents a waveform, which is the representation of displacement of a body over time, and displays what the pencil or string was doing as it vibrated.

This waveform is **periodic**. When we say that vibration is periodic, we mean that it repeats itself in a predictable fashion. If it took the ruler 1/100 of a second to move from the first point of distension back to that point again, it will take 1/100 of a second to repeat that cycle if it is vibrating periodically.

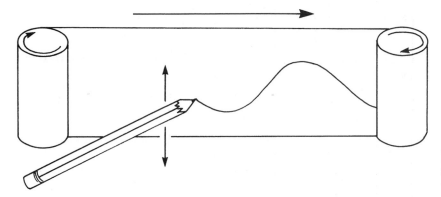

Figure 6-15. Periodic motion of a vibrating body graphically recorded.

Moving from one point in the vibratory pattern to the same point again defines one **cycle** of vibration, and the time it takes to pass through one cycle of vibration is referred to as the **period**. In our example, the period of vibration was 1/100 second, or 0.01 seconds. **Frequency** refers to how often something occurs, as in the frequency with which you shop for groceries (e.g., two times per month). The frequency of vibration is how often a cycle of vibration repeats itself, which, in our example, is 100 times per second. Frequency and period are the inverse of each other, and that relationship may be stated as $f = 1/T$ or $T = 1/f$. That is, frequency (f) equals 1 divided by period (T for "Time"). For our example, frequency = 1 / 0.01 seconds. If you will take a moment with your calculator, you will find that this calculation gives a result of 100.

Because frequency refers to the repetition rate of vibration, we speak of it in terms of number of **cycles per second**. The pencil vibrated with a frequency of 100 cycles per second, but shorthand notation for cycles per second is **Hertz (Hz)**, after Heinrich Hertz. When we set the pencil into vibration, it vibrated with a period of .01 seconds and a frequency of 100 Hz.

We said that frequency of vibration in a body was governed by the elasticity, stiffness, and mass. If you had added a large weight to the guitar string, it would have vibrated slower. As mass increases, frequency of vibration decreases.

If you were to make the string stiffer, it would vibrate more rapidly. Increased stiffness would drive the string to return to its point of equilibrium at a faster rate, increasing the frequency of vibration.

STUDY QUESTIONS

1. _____ is the process of capturing air within the thorax to provide the muscles with a structure upon which to push or pull.

2. In _____ attack, the vocal folds are adducted prior to initiation of expiratory flow.

3. In _____ attack, the vocal folds are adducted after the initiation of expiratory flow.

4. In _____ attack, the vocal folds are adducted simultaneous with initiation of expiratory flow.

5. During modal phonation, the vocal folds will open from _____ (inferior/superior) to _____ (inferior/superior). The folds will close from _____ (inferior/ superior) to _____ (inferior/superior).

6. The minimum subglottal driving pressure for speech is _____ cm H_2O.

7. In the mode of vibration known as _____, the vocal folds vibrate at a much lower rate than in modal phonation, and the folds exhibit a syncopated vibratory pattern.

8. In the mode of vibration known as _____, the vocal folds lengthen and become extremely thin and "reedlike."

9. Presence of vocal nodules or other space-occupying laryngeal pathology may result in _____ phonation.

10. To increase vocal intensity, one must _____ (increase/decrease) subglottal pressure and _____ (increase/decrease) medial compression.

11. To increase vocal fundamental frequency, one must _____ vocal fold tension by _____ (lengthening/shortening) the vocal folds.

12. _____ refers to the pitch of phonation that is most appropriate for an individual.

13. _____ refers to the vocal pitch that is habitually used during speech.

14. As vocal intensity increases, the closed phase of the vibratory cycle _____ (increases/decreases).

15. We had occasion to record the speech of an individual with a maxillary fistula secondary to squamous cell carcinoma. The cancerous condition had required removal of part of her maxilla, which meant that the oral cavity was continuous with the nasal cavity. While working with the physician who was

fitting her for an oral prosthesis, we recorded her speech, only to find that when speech was produced with the open fistula, the fundamental frequency was highly irregular, but became regular again when the oral prosthesis was in place. What could be the link between the vocal folds and the oral-nasal communication?

STUDY QUESTION ANSWERS

1. ABDOMINAL or THORACIC FIXATION is the process of capturing air within the thorax to provide the muscles with a structure upon which to push or pull.
2. In GLOTTAL attack, the vocal folds are adducted prior to initiation of expiratory flow.
3. In BREATHY attack, the vocal folds are adducted after the initiation of expiratory flow.
4. In SIMULTANEOUS attack, the vocal folds are adducted simultaneous with initiation of expiratory flow.
5. During modal phonation, the vocal folds will open from INFERIOR to SUPERIOR. The folds will close from INFERIOR to SUPERIOR.
6. The minimum subglottal driving pressure for speech is 3–5 cm H_2O.
7. In the mode of vibration known as GLOTTAL FRY, the vocal folds vibrate at a much lower rate than in modal phonation, and the folds exhibit a syncopated vibratory pattern.
8. In the mode of vibration known as FALSETTO, the vocal folds lengthen and become extremely thin and "reedlike."
9. Presence of vocal nodules or other space-occupying laryngeal pathology may result in BREATHY phonation.
10. To increase vocal intensity, one must INCREASE subglottal pressure and INCREASE medial compression.
11. To increase vocal fundamental frequency, one must INCREASE vocal fold tension by LENGTHENING the vocal folds.
12. OPTIMAL PITCH refers to the pitch of phonation that is most appropriate for an individual.
13. HABITUAL PITCH refers to the vocal pitch that is habitually used during speech.
14. As vocal intensity increases, the closed phase of the vibratory cycle INCREASES.
15. The vocal folds vibrate as a function of the transglottal pressure drop: The subglottal pressure is higher than the supraglottal (oral) pressure, so air flows through the glottis and the vocal folds vibrate. When the fistula was unoccluded, the transglottal pressure drop increased markedly, making control of the vocal folds difficult and causing the aperiodicity we saw. We have seen the same phenomenon in individuals with neurological diseases such as multiple sclerosis. In that case, we saw increased aperiodicity as a function of open vowel position, but the principle still holds.

REFERENCES

Adair, R. K. (1990). *The physics of baseball* (3rd ed.). New York: HarperCollins.

Adair, R. K. (1995). The physics of baseball. *Physics Today, 48*(5), 26–31.

Aronson, A. E. (1985). *Clinical voice disorders.* New York: Thieme.

Baer, T., Sasaki, C., & Harris, K. (1985). *Laryngeal function in phonation and respiration.* Boston: College-Hill Press.

Baken, R. J., & Orlikoff, R. F. (1999). *Clinical measurement of speech and voice* (2nd ed.). San Diego, CA: Singular Publishing Group.

Bateman, H. E., & Mason, R. M. (1984). *Applied anatomy and physiology of the speech and hearing mechanism.* Springfield, IL: Charles C. Thomas.

Bless, D. M., & Abbs, J. H. (1983). *Vocal fold physiology.* San Diego, CA: College-Hill Press.

Boone, D. R. (1999). *The voice and voice therapy.* Englewood Cliffs, NJ: Prentice-Hall.

Broad, D. J. (1973). Phonation. In F. D. Minifie, T. J. Hixon, & F. Williams (Eds.), *Normal aspects of speech, hearing, and language* (pp. 127–168). Englewood Cliffs, NJ: Prentice-Hall.

Childers, D. G., Hicks, D. M., Moore, G. P., Eskenazi, L., & Lalwani, A. L. (1990). Electroglottography and vocal fold physiology. *Journal of Speech and Hearing Research, 33*, 245–254.

Chusid, J. G. (1985). *Correlative neuroanatomy and functional neurology* (17th ed.). Los Altos, CA: Lange Medical Publications.

Daniloff, R. G. *Speech science.* San Diego, CA: College-Hill Press.

Doyle, P. C., Grantmyre, A., & Myers, C. (1989). Clinical modification of the tracheostoma breathing valve for voice restoration. *Journal of Speech and Hearing Disorders, 54*, 189–192.

Eckel, F., & Boone, D. (1981). The s/z ratio as an indicator of laryngeal pathology. *Journal of Speech and Hearing Disorders, 46*, 147–149.

Fink, B. R. (1975). *The human larynx.* New York: Raven Press.

Fink, B. R. & Demarest, R. J. (1978). *Laryngeal biomechanics.* Cambridge, MA: Harvard University Press.

Fletcher, W. W. (1950). *A study of internal laryngeal activity in relation to vocal intensity.* Doctoral dissertation, Northwestern University, Evanston, IL.

Fucci, D. J., & Lass, N. J. (1999). *Fundamentals of speech science.* Boston: Allyn & Bacon.

Fujimura, O. (1988). *Vocal fold physiology: Vol. 2. Vocal physiology.* New York: Raven Press.

Fukida, H., Kawaida, M., Tatehara, T., Ling, E., Kita, K., Ohki, K., Kawasaki, Y., & Saito, S. (1988). A new concept of lubricating mechanisms of the larynx. In O. Fujimura (Ed.), *Vocal physiology: Voice production, mechanisms and functions* (pp. 83–92). New York: Raven Press.

Ganong, W. F. (2003). *Review of medical physiology* (21st ed.). New York: McGraw-Hill/Appleton & Lange.

Gosling, J. A., Harris, P. F., Humpherson, J. R., Whitmore, I., & Willan, P. L. T. (1985). *Atlas of human anatomy.* Philadelphia: J. B. Lippincott.

Gray, H., Bannister, L. H., Berry, M. M., & Williams, P. L. (Eds.), (1995). *Gray's anatomy.* London: Churchill Livingstone.

Grobler, N. J. (1977). *Textbook of clinical anatomy* (Vol. 1). Amsterdam: Elsevier Scientific.

Hirano, M. (1974). Morphological structure of the vocal cord as a vibrator and its variations. *Folia Phoniatrica, 26*, 89–94.

Hirano, M., Kiyokawa, K., & Kurita, S. (1988). Laryngeal muscles and glottic shaping. In O. Fujimura (Ed.), *Vocal physiology: Voice production, mechanisms, and functions* (pp. 49–65). New York: Raven Press.

Hirano, M., Ohala, J., & Vennard, W. (1969). The function of laryngeal muscles in regulation of fundamental frequency and intensity of phonation. *Journal of Speech and Hearing Research, 12*, 616–628.

Hixon, T. J. (1973). Respiratory function in speech. In F. D. Minifie, T. J. Hixon, & F. Williams (Eds.), *Normal aspects of speech, hearing, and language* (pp. 73–126). Englewood Cliffs, NJ: Prentice-Hall.

Hixon, T. J. (1982). Speech breathing kinematics and mechanism inferences therefrom. In S. Grillner, A. Persson, B. Lindblom & J. Lubker (Eds.), *Speech motor control* (pp. 75–94). New York: Pergamon Press.

Hixon, T. J., Hawley, J. L., & Wilson, K. J. (1982). An around-the-house device for the clinical determination of respiratory driving pressure: A note on making simple even simpler. *Journal of Speech and Hearing Disorders, 47*, 413–415.

Hollien, H., & Moore, G. P. (1968). Stroboscopic laminography of the larynx during phonation. *Acta Otolaryngologica, 65*, 209–215.

Hufnagle, J., & Hufnagle, K. K. (1988). S/Z ratio in dysphonic children with and without vocal cord nodules. *Language, Speech, and Hearing Services in Schools, 19*, 418–422.

Husson, R. (1953). Sur la physiologie vocale. *Annals of Otolaryngology, 69*, 124–137.

Isshiki, N. (1964). Regulatory mechanisms of voice intensity variation. *Journal of Speech and Hearing Research, 7*, 17–29.

Kaplan, H. M. (1971). *Anatomy and physiology of speech.* New York: McGraw-Hill.

Kent, R. D. (1997). *The speech sciences.* San Diego, CA: Singular Publishing Group.

Kent, R. D., Kent, J. F., & Rosenbek, J. C. (1987). Maximum performance tests of speech production. *Journal of Speech and Hearing Disorders, 52*, 367–387.

Kirchner, J. A., & Suzuki, M. (1968). Laryngeal reflexes and voice production. In M. Krauss (Ed.), Sound production in man. *Annals of the New York Academy of Sciences, 155*, 98–109.

Kuehn, D. P., Lemme, M. L., Baumgartner, J. M. (1989). *Neural bases of speech, hearing, and language.* Boston: Little, Brown.

Langley, M. B., & Lombardino, L. J. (1991). *Neurodevelopmental strategies for managing communication disorders in children with severe motor dysfunction.* Austin, TX: Pro-Ed.

Lieberman, P. (1968a). *Intonation, perception, and language.* Research monograph No. 38. Cambridge, MA: The M.I.T. Press.

Lieberman, P. (1968b). Vocal cord motion in man. *Annals of the New York Academy of Sciences, 155*, 28–38.

Lieberman, P. (1977). *Speech science and acoustic phonetics: An introduction.* New York: Macmillan Publishing Co.

Logemann, J. (1983). *Evaluation and treatment of swallowing disorders.* Boston: College-Hill Press.

Netsell, R. (1973). Speech physiology. In F. D. Minifie, T. J. Hixon, & F. Williams (Eds.), *Normal aspects of speech, hearing, and language* (pp. 134–211). Englewood Cliffs, NJ: Prentice-Hall.

Netsell, R., & Hixon, T. J. (1978). A noninvasive method for clinically estimating subglottal air pressure. *Journal of Speech and Hearing Disorders, 43*, 326–330.

Nishizawa, N., Sawashima, M., & Yonemoto, K. (1988). Vocal fold length in vocal pitch change. In O. Fujimua (Ed.), *Vocal physiology: Voice production, mechanisms and functions* (pp. 49–65). New York: Raven Press.

Proctor, D. F. (1968). The physiologic basis of voice training. In M. Krauss (Ed.), Sound production in man. *Annals of the New York Academy of Sciences, 155*, 208–228.

Ptacek, P. H., & Sander, E. K. (1963). Maximum duration of phonation. *Journal of Speech and Hearing Disorders, 28*(2), 171–182.

Ramig, L. A., & Ringel, R. L. (1983). Effects of physiological aging on selected acoustic characteristics of voice. *Journal of Speech and Hearing Research, 26*, 22–30.

Rastatter, M. P., & Hyman, M. (1982). Maximum phoneme duration of /s/ and /z/ by children with vocal nodules. *Language, Speech, and Hearing Services in Schools, 13*, 197–199.

Rosse, C., Gaddum-Rosse, P., & Rosse, G. (1997). *Hollinshead's textbook of anatomy.* Philadelphia: Lippincott-Raven.

Sapienza, C. M., & Stathopoulos, E. T. (1994). Respiratory and laryngeal measures of children and women with bilateral vocal fold nodules. *Journal of Speech and Hearing Research, 37*, 1229–1243.

Sonninen, A. (1968). The external frame function in the control of pitch in the human voice. In M. Krauss (Ed.), Sound production in man. *Annals of the New York Academy of Sciences, 155*, 68–89.

Sorensen, D. N., & Parker, P. A. (1992). The voiced/voiceless phonation time in children with and without laryngeal pathology. *Language, Speech, and Hearing Services in Schools, 23*, 163–168.

Tait, N. A., Michel, J. F., & Carpenter, M. A. (1980). Maximum duration of sustained /s/ and /z/ in children. *Journal of Speech and Hearing Disorders, 15*, 239–246.

Timcke, R., Von Leden, H., & Moore, G. P. (1958). Laryngeal vibrations: Measurements of the glottic wave I: The normal vibratory cycle. *Archives of Otolaryngology, 68*, 1–19.

Titze, I. (1973). The human vocal cords: A mathematical model, Part I. *Phonetica, 28*, 129–170.

Titze, I. R. (1988). The physics of small amplitude oscillation of the vocal folds. *Journal of the Acoustical Society of America, 83*(4), 1536–1552.

Titze, I. R. (1994). *Principles of voice production*. Englewood Cliffs, NJ: Prentice-Hall.

Van den Berg, J. W. (1958). Myoelastic-aerodynamic theory of voice production. *Journal of Speech and Hearing Research, 1*, 227–244.

Van den Berg, J. W. (1968). Sound production in isolated human larynges. In M. Krauss (Ed.), Sound production in man. *Annals of the New York Academy of Sciences, 155*, 18–27.

Van den Berg, J. W., & Tan, T. S. (1959). Results of experiments with human larynxes. *Practica Oto-Rhino-Laryngologica, 21*, 425–450.

Verdolini, K., Titze, I. R., & Fennell, A. (1994). Dependence of phonatory effort on hydration level. *Journal of Speech and Hearing Research, 37*, 1001–1007.

Whillis, J. (1946). Movements of the tongue in swallowing. *Journal of Anatomy, 80*, 115–116.

Zemlin, W. R. (1998). *Speech and hearing science. Anatomy and physiology* (4th ed.). Needham Heights, MA: Allyn & Bacon.

CHAPTER 7

Anatomy of Articulation and Resonation

When the lay person thinks of the process of speaking, it is more than likely that he or she is actually thinking about articulation. You, of course, now know that there is much more to speech than moving the lips, tongue, mandible, and so forth. Nonetheless, the articulatory system is an extremely important element in our communication system.

Articulation is the process of joining two elements together, and the **articulatory system** is the system of mobile and immobile articulators brought into contact for the purpose of shaping the sounds of speech. As you will remember from Chapters 5 and 6, laryngeal vibration produces the sound required for voicing in speech. We are capable of rapidly starting and stopping phonation, depending on whether we want voiced or voiceless production. This chapter focuses on what happens after that sound reaches the oral cavity. In this cavity, the undifferentiated buzz produced by the vocal folds is shaped into the sounds we call *phonemes*. Let us present an overview of how the oral cavity is capable of such a creation.

articulation for speech:
the process of bringing two or more moveable speech structures together to form the sounds of speech

SOURCE-FILTER THEORY OF VOWEL PRODUCTION

A widely accepted description of how the oral cavity is capable of creating speech sounds is the **source-filter theory** of vowel production. In general terms, the theory states that a voicing source is generated by the vocal folds and routed through the vocal tract where it is shaped into the sounds of speech. Changes in the shape and configuration of the tongue, mandible, soft palate, and other articulators govern the resonance characteristics of the vocal tract, and the resonances of the tract determine the sound of a given vowel. Here is how that works.

The **vocal tract**, consisting of the mouth (oral cavity), the region behind the mouth (pharynx), and the nasal cavity, may be thought of as a series of linked tubes (see Figure 7-1). From your experience you know that if you blow carefully across the top of a soda bottle, you will hear a tone. If you decrease the volume of the air in the bottle by adding fluid to it, the frequency of vibration of the tone increases. Likewise, if you blow across the top of a bottle with larger volume, the tone decreases in frequency. As the volume of the air in the bottle increases, the frequency of the tone decreases. As the volume decreases, the frequency increases. You are experimenting with the **resonant frequency** of a cavity, which is the frequency of sound to which the cavity most effectively responds. You might think of the bottle as a filter that lets only one frequency of sound through and rejects the other frequencies, much as a coffee filter lets the liquid through but traps the grounds. The airstream blowing across the top of the bottle is actually producing a very broad-spectrum

resonant frequency:
frequency of stimulation to which a resonant system responds most vigorously

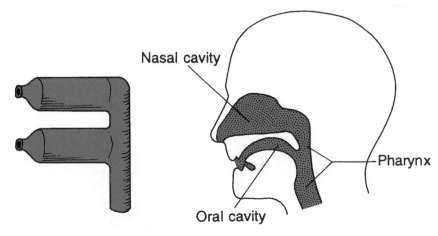

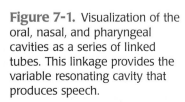

Figure 7-1. Visualization of the oral, nasal, and pharyngeal cavities as a series of linked tubes. This linkage provides the variable resonating cavity that produces speech.

signal, but the bottle selects the frequency components that are at its resonant frequency. The resonant frequency of a cavity is largely governed by its volume and length. Now, if you were somehow able to blow across two bottles (one low-resonant frequency, one high-frequency), the two tones would combine.

When you move your tongue around in your mouth, you are changing the shape of your oral cavity, making it smaller or larger, lengthening or shortening it. It is as if you had a series of bottles that you could manipulate in your mouth, changing their shape at will. When you change the shape of the oral cavity, you are changing the resonant frequencies, and therefore you are changing the sound that comes out of the mouth.

This, then, is the source-filter theory view of speech production. The vocal folds produce a quasi-periodic tone (see Chapters 5 and 6), and that tone is passed through the filter of your vocal tract. The vocal tract filter is manipulable, so that you are able to change its shape and therefore change the sound.

The resonant frequencies govern our perception of vowels. To prove that it is *not* your vocal folds that govern the nature of a vowel, whisper the words *he* and *who*. Could you tell the difference? The vocal folds were not vibrating, but you excited the oral cavity filter through the turbulence of your whispered production, and the vowels were quite intelligible.

The source-filter theory can be easily expanded to other phonemes as well. The source of the sound may vary. With vowels, the source will always be phonation in normal speech. With consonants, other sources will include the turbulence of frication or combinations of voicing and turbulence. In all cases, you produce a noise source and pass it through the filter of the oral cavity that has been configured to meet your acoustic needs. One example will prove this to you.

Look at Figure 7-2, and notice the difference between production of the /s/ and /ʃ/ phonemes. Sustain an /s/ and realize that when you produce it, your tongue is high, forward, and tense. You pass a compact stream of air over the surface of the tongue, and then between the tongue tip and the upper front teeth. Now produce the /ʃ/ and recognize that the tongue is farther back in your mouth, much as in the figure. The source in both cases is the turbulence associated with the airstream escaping from its course between your tongue and an immobile structure of your mouth (front teeth or roof of your mouth). The turbulence excites the cavity in front of the constriction and you have a recognizable sound. Which of the two phonemes has the larger cavity distal to the constriction? The /ʃ/ has a larger resonant cavity than the /s/, so its resonant frequency will be lower, following our discussion of bottles. Now make the /s/ again, but without stopping, slide your tongue back in your mouth until you reach the /ʃ/ position. As you do this you will hear the

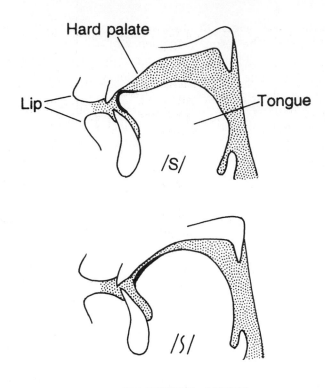

Figure 7-2. Comparison of the articulatory posture used for production of /s/ and /ʃ/. (After data and view of Shriberg and Kent, 2002.)

noise drop in frequency because the cavity is increasing in size. The source-filter theory dictates this change.

To summarize:

- The source-filter theory states that speech is the product of sending an acoustic source, such as the sound produced by the vibrating vocal folds, through the filter of the vocal tract that shapes the output.
- The ever-changing speech signal is the product of moving articulators.
- Sources may be voicing, as in the case of vowels, or the product of turbulence, as in fricatives. Articulators may be moveable (such as the tongue, lips, pharynx, mandible, and velum) or immobile (such as the teeth, hard palate, and alveolar ridge).

Let us now examine the structures of the articulatory system. As with the phonatory system, we must examine the support structure (the skull and bones of the face) and the muscles that move the articulators. Before we begin, we will define the articulators used in speech production.

THE ARTICULATORS

As noted, articulators may be either mobile or immobile. In speech we will often move one articulator to make contact with another, thus positioning a mobile articulator in relation to an immobile articulator.

The largest mobile articulator is the *tongue*, with the lower jaw (*mandible*) a close second (see Figure 7-3). The *velum* or *soft palate* is another mobile articulator, used to differentiate nasal sounds such as /m/ or /n/ from non-nasal sounds. The *lips* are moved to produce different speech sounds, and the *cheeks* play a role in changes of resonance of the cavity. The region behind the oral cavity (the *fauces* and the *pharynx*) may be moved through muscular action, and the *larynx* and *hyoid bone* both change to accommodate different articulatory postures.

There are three immobile articulators. The *alveolar ridge* of the upper jaw (*maxillae*) and the *hard palate* are both significant articulatory surfaces. The *teeth* are used in production of a variety of speech sounds.

The process of articulation for speech is quite automatic. To get a feel for changes in speech that occur when you alter the function of an articulator, try this. Place a small stack of tongue depressors between your molars on one side of your mouth and bite lightly (this is a *bite block*). Now say "You wish to know all about my grandfather." Now say the same sentence after placing your tongue between your front teeth, and biting lightly. Finally, say the sentence while pulling your cheeks out with your fingers. There are two important points to this demonstration. First, your speech changed when you altered the articulatory and resonatory characteristics of the tract. You restrained articulators and had to work harder to make yourself understood. Second, you were able to overcome these difficulties. Despite having a bite block or clamped tongue tip, you were able to make yourself understood. In fact, you automatically adjusted your articulation to match the new physical constraints. As a student in speech-language pathology, you should be quite heartened by the extraordinary flexibility of motor planning exhibited in this demonstration, because you can use this to your advantage in treatment.

Of these mobile and immobile articulators, the tongue, mandible, teeth, hard palate, and velum are the major players, although all surfaces and cavities within the articulatory/resonatory system are contributors to the production of speech.

You may wish to refer to Figures 7–4 through 7–9 as we begin our discussion of the bones of the facial and cranial skeleton. In addition, Table 7-1 may help you to organize this body of material.

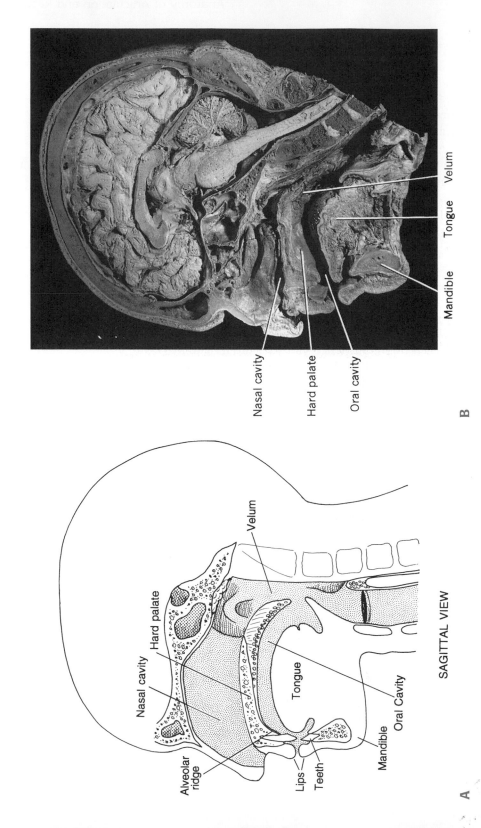

Nasal cavity

Hard palate

Oral cavity

Velum

Tongue

Mandible

B

Velum

Hard palate

Nasal cavity

Tongue

Alveolar ridge

Lips

Teeth

Mandible

Oral Cavity

SAGITTAL VIEW

A

Figure 7-3. A. Relationships among the articulators. **B.** Photograph of articulators seen through sagittal section.

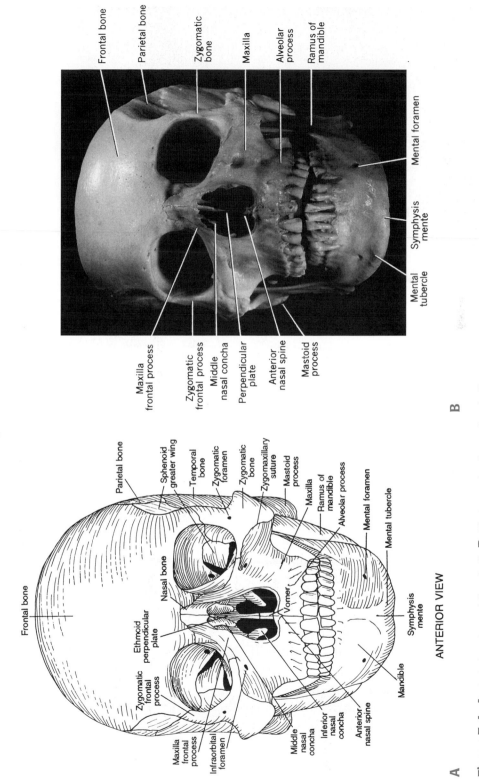

ANTERIOR VIEW

A

B

Figure 7-4. A. Anterior view of the skull. B. Photograph of anterior skull.

269

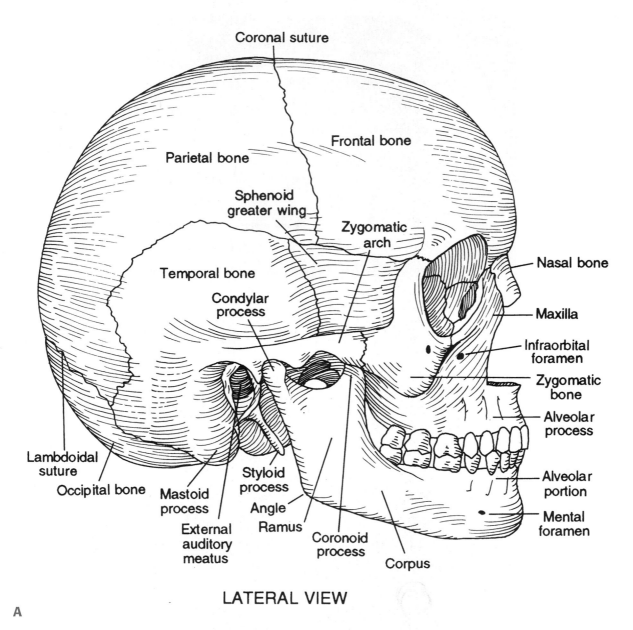

Coronal suture

Parietal bone

Frontal bone

Sphenoid
greater wing

Zygomatic
arch

Temporal bone

Condylar
process

Nasal bone

Maxilla

Infraorbital
foramen

Zygomatic
bone

Alveolar
process

Lambdoidal
suture

Occipital bone

Mastoid
process

Styloid
process

Angle

Ramus

Alveolar
portion

Mental
foramen

External
auditory
meatus

Coronoid
process

Corpus

LATERAL VIEW

A

Figure 7-5. A. Lateral view of the skull. *(continues)*

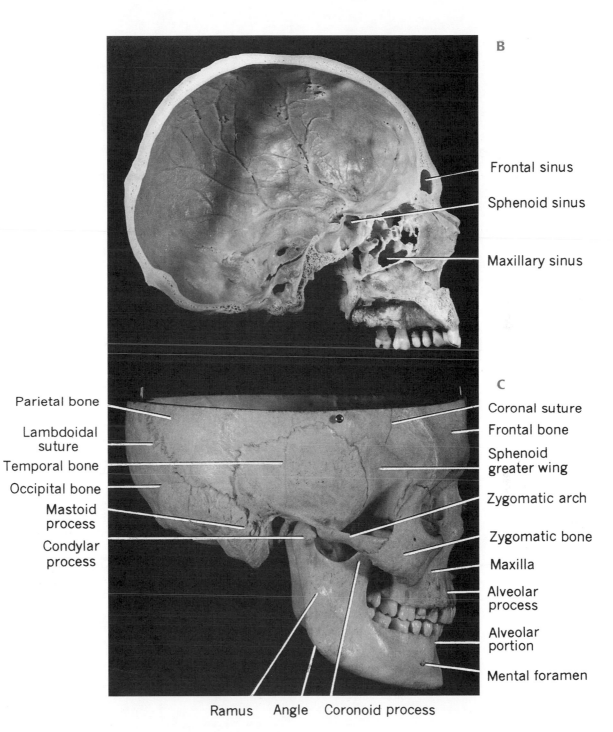

B

Frontal sinus

Sphenoid sinus

Maxillary sinus

C

Parietal bone

Lambdoidal suture

Temporal bone

Occipital bone

Mastoid process

Condylar process

Coronal suture

Frontal bone

Sphenoid greater wing

Zygomatic arch

Zygomatic bone

Maxilla

Alveolar process

Alveolar portion

Mental foramen

Ramus   Angle   Coronoid process

Figure 7-5. *(continued)* **B.** Medial surface of the skull. **C.** Photo of lateral skull.

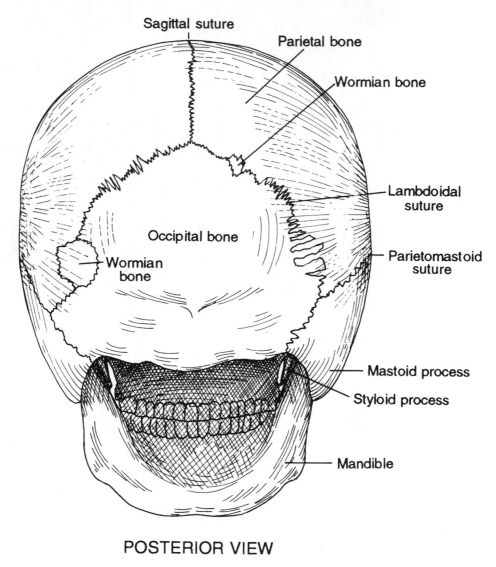

Sagittal suture

Parietal bone

Wormian bone

Lambdoidal
suture

Parietomastoid
suture

Occipital bone

Wormian
bone

Mastoid process

Styloid process

Mandible

POSTERIOR VIEW

Figure 7-6. Posterior view of skull.

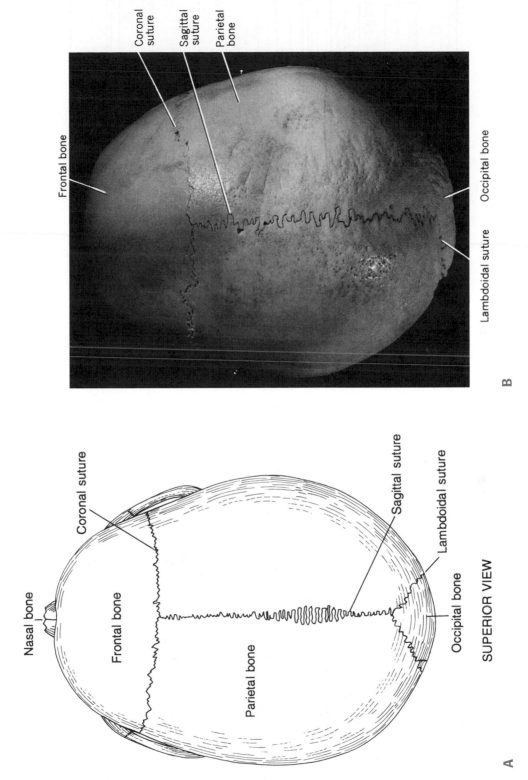

Figure 7-7. A. Superior view of skull. **B.** Superior view photo of skull.

Coronal suture
Sagittal suture
Parietal bone
Frontal bone
Occipital bone
Lambdoidal suture

B

Nasal bone
Coronal suture
Frontal bone
Parietal bone
Sagittal suture
Lambdoidal suture
Occipital bone

SUPERIOR VIEW

A

273

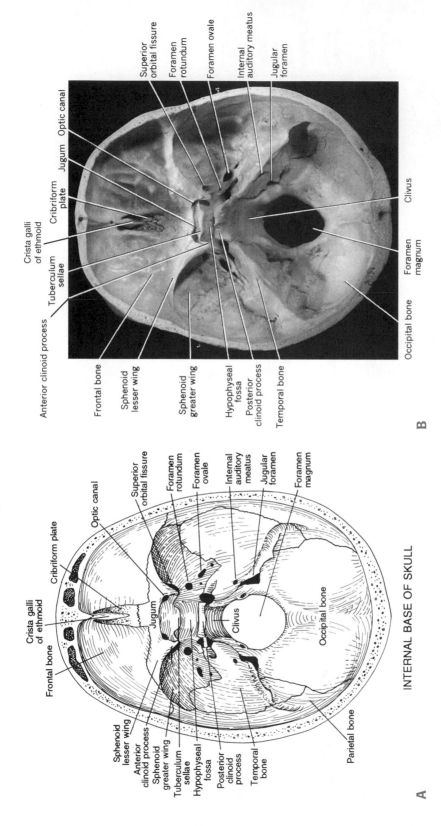

Figure 7-8. A. Internal view of base of skull. **B.** Photo of internal skull.

INTERNAL BASE OF SKULL

Labels for A:

Crista galli of ethmoid
Frontal bone
Sphenoid lesser wing
Anterior clinoid process
Sphenoid greater wing
Tuberculum sellae
Hypophyseal fossa
Posterior clinoid process
Temporal bone
Parietal bone
Cribriform plate
Optic canal
Jugum
Superior orbital fissure
Foramen rotundum
Foramen ovale
Internal auditory meatus
Jugular foramen
Foramen magnum
Clivus
Occipital bone

Labels for B:

Crista galli of ethmoid
Cribriform plate
Jugum
Optic canal
Superior orbital fissure
Foramen rotundum
Foramen ovale
Internal auditory meatus
Jugular foramen
Tuberculum sellae
Anterior clinoid process
Frontal bone
Sphenoid lesser wing
Sphenoid greater wing
Hypophyseal fossa
Posterior clinoid process
Temporal bone
Clivus
Foramen magnum
Occipital bone

274

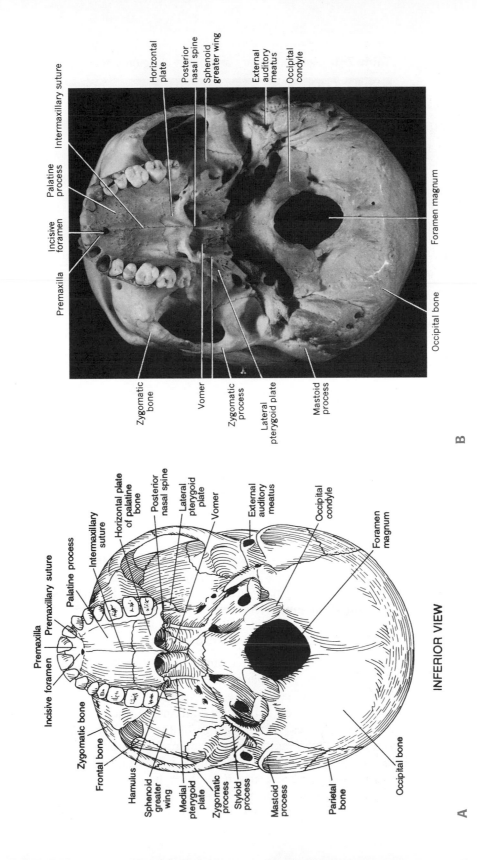

INFERIOR VIEW

Figure 7-9. **A.** Inferior view of skull. **B.** Photo of inferior view of skull.

275

Table 7-1. Bones of the face and cranial skeleton.

BONES OF THE FACE	BONES OF THE CRANIAL SKELETON
Mandible	Ethmoid bone
Maxillae	Sphenoid bone
Nasal bone	Frontal bone
Palatine bone and nasal conchae	Parietal bone
Vomer	Occipital bone
Zygomatic bone	Temporal bone
Lacrimal bone	
Hyoid bone	

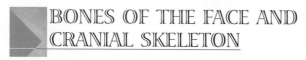

BONES OF THE FACE AND CRANIAL SKELETON

Bones of the Face

- **Mandible**
- **Maxillae**
- **Nasal bone**
- **Palatine bone and nasal conchae**
- **Vomer**
- **Zygomatic bone**
- **Lacrimal bone**
- **Hyoid bone**

There are numerous bones of the face with which you should become familiar. As with the respiratory and phonatory systems, learning the landmarks will serve you well as you identify the course and function of the muscles of articulation.

Mandible

The mandible is the massive unpaired bone making up the lower jaw of the face. It begins as a paired bone but fuses at the midline by the child's first birthday. As you can see from Figure 7-10, there are several landmarks of interest on both outer and inner surfaces. The point of fusion of the two halves of the mandible is the **symphysis mente** or **mental symphysis**, marking the midline **mental protuberance** and separating the paired **mental tubercles**. Lateral to the tubercles on either side is the **mental foramen**, the hole through which the mental nerve of V trigeminal passes in life. The lateral mass of bone is the **corpus** or body, and the point at which the mandible angles upward is the **angle**.

mental: *L., mentum, chin*

symphsis: *Gr., growing together*

protuberance: *Gr., pro, before + tuber, bulge*

tubercle: *L., tuberculum, little swelling*

foramen: *L., a passage, opening, orifice*

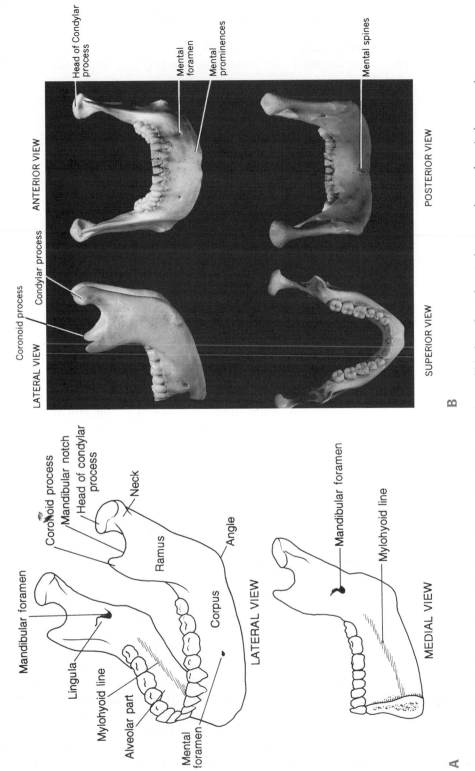

Figure 7-10. A. Lateral and medial views of mandible. **B.** Photo of mandible from lateral, anterior, superior, and posterior aspects.

On Use of the Bite Block

A *bite block* is a device used to stabilize the mandible so that other articulators can be evaluated or exercised. Bite blocks come in many shapes, sizes, and textures, ranging from acrylic blocks about 1 cm square to bite blocks that are created from dental impression material. The softer, more pliable dental impression bite block provides a better surface for sustained use, and is particularly good for clients who have limited motor control.

A bite block is used when you cannot differentiate the contribution of the mandible from that of the lips or tongue during articulation. For instance, if you say /ta ta ta ta/ repeatedly while lightly holding your mandible you will feel the mandible move, even though the dominant articulator is the tongue. If you wanted to strengthen the tongue, such as having it push toward the roof of the mouth against a resistance, you could place a bite block between the molars and have your client push up against a tongue depressor.

Needless to say, having your client perform oral motor activities such as the one mentioned here requires that you have a firm understanding of the anatomy and physiology of articulation, as well as a deep knowledge of motor development. Oral motor therapy focuses on remediating muscle imbalance, and inappropriate application of oral motor activities can create even greater problems! For an excellent discussion, see Langley and Lombardino, 1991.

ramus: *L., branch*

fovea: *L., a pit*

The rhomboidal plate rising up from the mandible is the **ramus**. The **condylar** and **coronoid** processes are important landmarks and are separated by the **mandibular notch**. The prominent **head** of the condylar process articulates with the skull, permitting rotation of the mandible. The **pterygoid fovea** on the anterior surface of the condylar process marks the point of attachment of the lateral pterygoid muscle, to be discussed. In the healthy mandible, teeth will be found within small **dental alveoli** (sacs) on the upper surface of the **alveolar arch** of the mandible.

On the inner surface of the mandible are prominent midline **superior** and **inferior mental spines** and the laterally placed **mylohyoid line**, landmarks that will figure prominently as we attach muscles to this structure. The **mandibular foramen** is the conduit for the inferior alveolar nerve of V trigeminal, providing sensory innervation for the teeth and gums.

Maxillae

Maxilla is the singular of maxillae.

The paired maxillae (singular, **maxilla**) are the bones making up the upper jaw. These bones deserve careful study, for they make up most of the roof of the mouth (**hard palate**), nose, and upper dental ridge and are involved in clefting of the lip and hard palate. As you study the landmarks of this complex bone, it might help you to realize that the various processes are logically named. That is, the *frontal* process of maxilla articulates with the *frontal* bone. Thus, learning the names of the larger structures will facilitate learning the processes and attachments.

In Figure 7-11 you can see the significant landmarks of the maxillae. As you can see, the **frontal process** is the superior-most point of this bone.

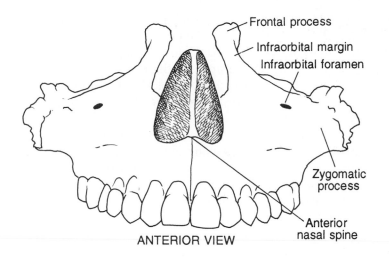

Frontal process

Infraorbital margin

Infraorbital foramen

Zygomatic process

Anterior nasal spine

ANTERIOR VIEW

Maxillary sinus

Frontal process

Palatine process

Nasal crest

Anterior nasal spine

Alveolar process

MEDIAL VIEW

A

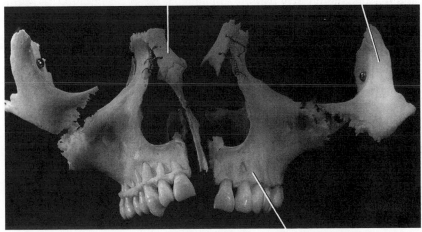

Nasal bone

Zygomatic bone

Alveolar process

B   ANTERIOR VIEW

Figure 7-11. **A.** Anterior and medial views of maxilla. **B.** Anterior view of maxillae, showing relationship with nasal and zygomatic bones.

You can palpate this process on yourself by placing your finger on your nose at the nasal side of your eye. You could run your finger down the **infraorbital margin** from there to the lower midpoint of your eye. Supporting your eye is the **orbital process**, the lower portion of the orbital surface. Just below your finger is the **infraorbital foramen**, the conduit for the infraorbital nerve arising from the maxillary nerve of the V trigeminal, providing sensory innervation of the lower eyelid, upper lip, and nasal alae. Lateral to your finger is the **zygomatic process** of the maxilla bone, which articulates with the zygomatic bone.

At the midline you can see the **anterior nasal spine** and **nasal crest**, and lateral to this is the **nasal notch**. The lower tooth-bearing ridge, the **alveolar process**, contains alveoli that hold teeth in the intact adult maxilla. The region between the **canine** eminence and the **incisive fossa** will become important as we discuss cleft lip.

A medial view requires disarticulation of left and right maxillae. This view reveals the **maxillary sinus**, the **palatine process**, and the important inner margin of the alveolar process.

Figure 7-12 shows an inferior view of the maxillae. As you can see from this, the two palatine processes of the maxilla articulate at the **intermaxillary suture** (also known as the **median palatine suture**). This suture marks the point of a cleft of the hard palate. The palatine process makes up three-fourths of the hard palate, with the other one-fourth being the horizontal plate of the palatine bone, to be discussed.

The **incisive foramen** in the anterior aspect of the hard palate serves as a conduit for the nasopalatine nerve serving the nasal mucosa. Trace the **premaxillary suture** forward from the incisive foramen to the alveolar process and you have identified the borders of the **premaxilla**. The premaxilla is difficult to see on the adult skull, but is nonetheless an important topic of discussion. Note that the premaxillary suture neatly separates the lateral incisors from the cuspids. A cleft of the lip will occur at this location and may include lip, alveolar bone, and the region of the premaxillary suture. Cleft lip may be either unilateral or bilateral, but in virtually all cases it will occur at this suture (there is very rarely a midline cleft lip).

canine: *L., caninus, related to dog*

fossa: *L., furrow or depression*

sinus: *L., curve or hollow*

suture: *L., sutura, seam; the fibrous union of skull bones*

Mandibular Hypoplasia and Micrognathia

Congenital mandibular hypoplasia is a condition in which there is inadequate development of the mandible. Although some specific genetic syndromes have this as a trait (e.g., Pierre Robin syndrome), **micrognathia** (small jaw) may occur without known mediating condition. The misalignment of the mandibular and maxillary arches may be corrected through surgery to extend the mandible. It is hypothesized that, during development, micrognathia may lead to cleft palate: The mandible may not develop adequately to accommodate the tongue, which in turn blocks the extension of the palatine processes of the maxillae.

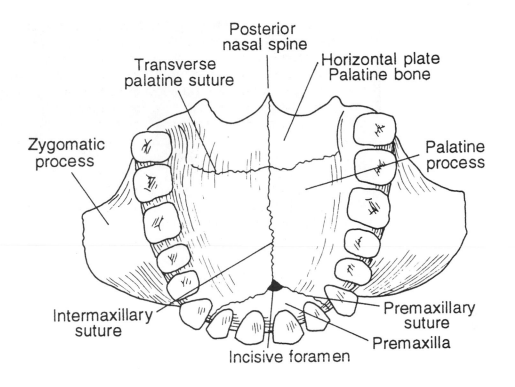

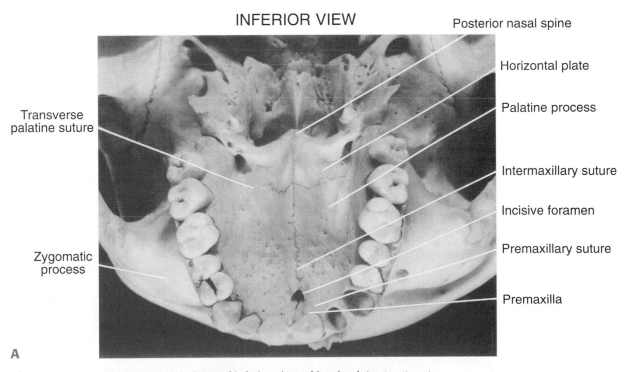

INFERIOR VIEW

A

Figure 7-12. A. Schematic and photo of inferior view of hard palate. *(continues)*

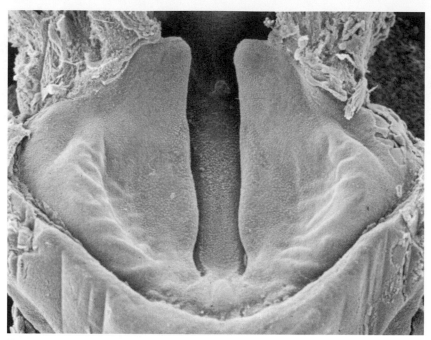

Figure 7-12. *(continued)*
B. Experimentally induced cleft palate in mouse. (Courtesy of Marilyn Russell, Ph.D.)

B

Nasal Bones

The nasal bones are small, making up the superior nasal surface. As you can see from Figure 7-4, the nasal bones articulate with the frontal bones superiorly, the maxillae laterally, and the perpendicular plate of the ethmoid bone and the nasal septal cartilage, all to be discussed.

Palatine Bones and Nasal Conchae

You will recall that the posterior one-fourth of the hard palate is made up of the horizontal plate of the palatine bone. Let us now examine this small but complex bone (see Figure 7-13).

When viewed from the front, you can see that the articulated palatine bones echo the nasal cavity defined by the maxillae. The **posterior nasal spine** and **nasal crest** provide midline correlates to the anterior nasal spine and nasal crest of the maxillae, while the **horizontal plate** parallels the palatine process of the maxilla. When viewing from the side, you can note the **perpendicular plate** that will make up the posterior wall of the nasal cavity. The **orbital process** makes up a small portion of the orbit cavity.

The **inferior nasal conchae** (**inferior turbinates**) are small, scroll-like bones located on the lateral surface of the nasal cavity (see Figure 7-4). These small but significant bones articulate with the maxilla, pala-

turbinate: *L., turbo, whirl*

RIGHT PALATINE BONE

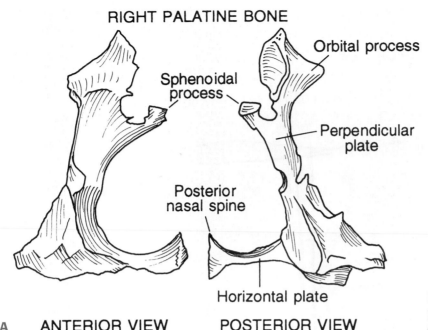

Orbital process

Sphenoidal
process

Perpendicular
plate

Posterior
nasal spine

Horizontal plate

A   **ANTERIOR VIEW**   **POSTERIOR VIEW**

Figure 7-13. A. Anterior and posterior views of palatine bones. *(continues)*

tine, and ethmoid bones. The **middle** and **superior nasal conchae**, processes of the ethmoid bone (to be discussed), are superiorly placed correlates of the inferior conchae, all of which have important function in mammals. The mucosal lining covering the nasal conchae is the thickest of the nose and is richly endowed with vascular supply. Air passing over the nasal conchae will be warmed and humidified before reaching the delicate tissues of the lower respiratory system. The shape of the conchae greatly increases the surface area available, promoting rapid heat exchange.

Vomer

The vomer (see Figure 7-14) is an unpaired, midline bone making up the inferior and posterior **nasal septum**, the dividing plate between the two nasal cavities (see Figure 7-15). The vomer has the appearance of a knife blade or a plowshare, with its point aimed toward the front. It articulates with the sphenoid **rostrum** and perpendicular plate of the ethmoid bone in the posterior-superior, and with the maxillae and palatine bones on the inferior margin. The posterior **ala** of the vomer marks the midline terminus of the nasal cavities. As you examine Figure 7-15, attend to the fact that the bony nasal septum is made up of two elements: the vomer, and the perpendicular plate of the ethmoid bone. With the addition of the midline **septal cartilage**, the nasal septum is complete.

septum: *L., partition*

rostrum: *L., beak or beaklike*

ala: *L., wing*

ANTERIOR VIEW

Orbital process Perpendicular plate Posterior nasal spine

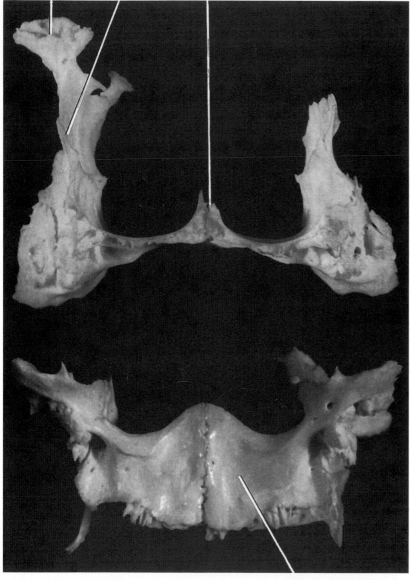

Horizontal plate

B   INFERIOR VIEW

Figure 7-13. *(continued)*
B. Articulated palatine bones from front and beneath. Note that the left perpendicular plate is incomplete.

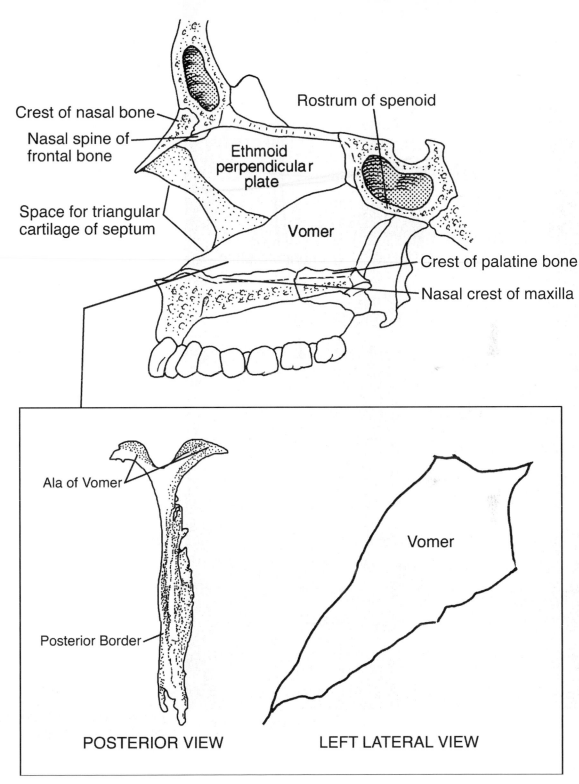

Crest of nasal bone

Nasal spine of frontal bone

Space for triangular cartilage of septum

Rostrum of spenoid

Ethmoid perpendicular plate

Vomer

Crest of palatine bone

Nasal crest of maxilla

Ala of Vomer

Posterior Border

POSTERIOR VIEW

Vomer

LEFT LATERAL VIEW

Figure 7-14. Lateral view of vomer.

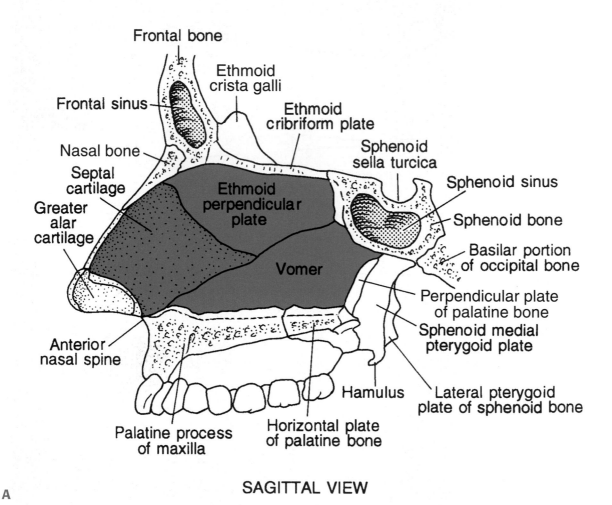

SAGITTAL VIEW

A

Figure 7-15. A. Medial view of nasal septum. Notice that the septum is composed of the perpendicular plate of the ethmoid, the vomer, and the septal cartilage. *(continues)*

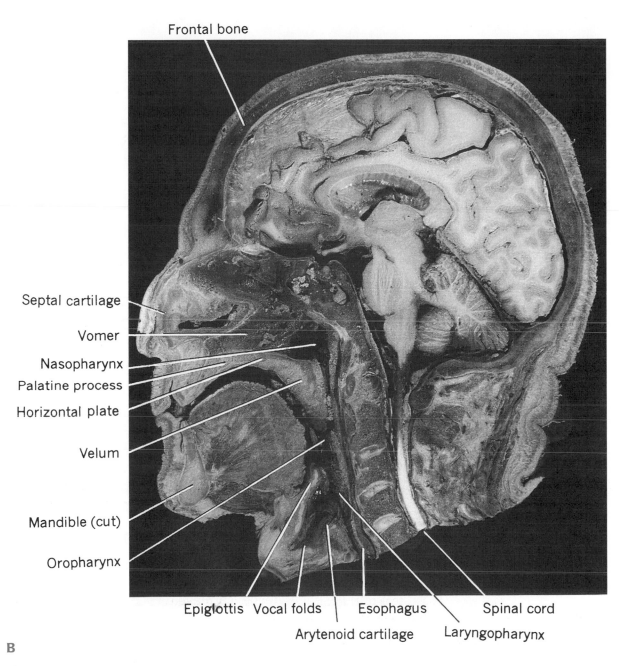

Frontal bone

Septal cartilage

Vomer

Nasopharynx

Palatine process

Horizontal plate

Velum

Mandible (cut)

Oropharynx

Epiglottis   Vocal folds   Esophagus   Spinal cord

Arytenoid cartilage   Laryngopharynx

B

Figure 7-15. *(continued)* **B.** Sagittal section through the nasal septum. *(continues)*

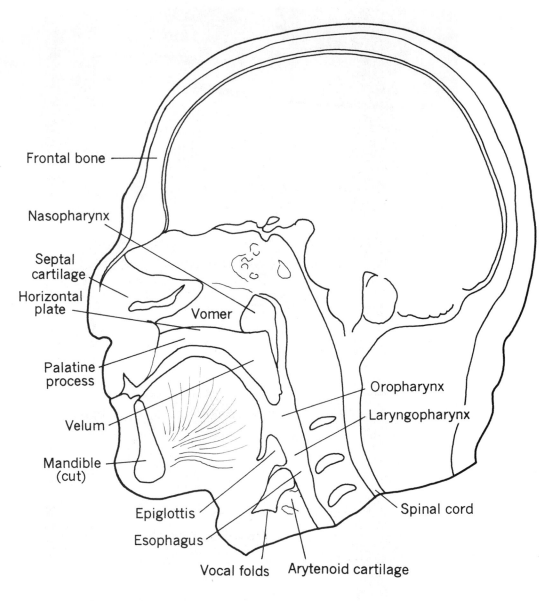

C

Figure 7-15. *(continued)* **C.** Drawing of sagittal section through the nasal septum. *(continues)*

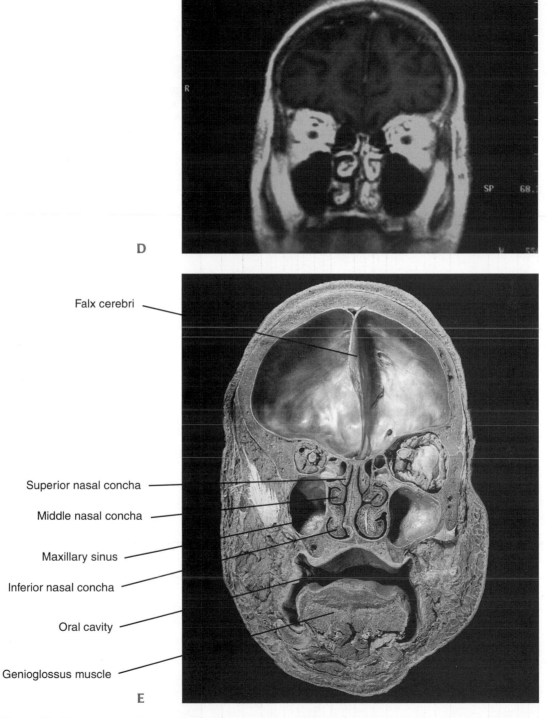

D

Falx cerebri

Superior nasal concha

Middle nasal concha

Maxillary sinus

Inferior nasal concha

Oral cavity

Genioglossus muscle

E

Figure 7-15. *(continued)* **D.** Frontal magnetic resonance image showing deviated nasal septum and hypertrophied nasal mucosa and turbinate. **E.** Frontal section revealing maxillary sinuses, nasal cavities, and relationship of oral articulators.

289

Zygomatic Bone

The zygomatic bone makes up the prominent structure we identify as cheekbones. As you can see from Figure 7-16, the zygomatic bone articulates with the maxillae, frontal bone, and temporal bone (you cannot see the articulation with the sphenoid bone), and makes up the lateral orbit. Fortunately, the landmarks of the zygomatic bone make intuitive sense.

orbital: *L., orbita, orbit*

At the base of the **orbital** margin is the **maxillary process**, the point of articulation of the zygomatic bone and maxilla. The **temporal process** seen in the lateral aspect projects back, forming half of the **zygomatic arch**. (The zygomatic arch consists of the temporal process of the zygomatic bone and the zygomatic process of the temporal bone.) The **frontal process** forms the articulation with the frontal and sphenoid bones.

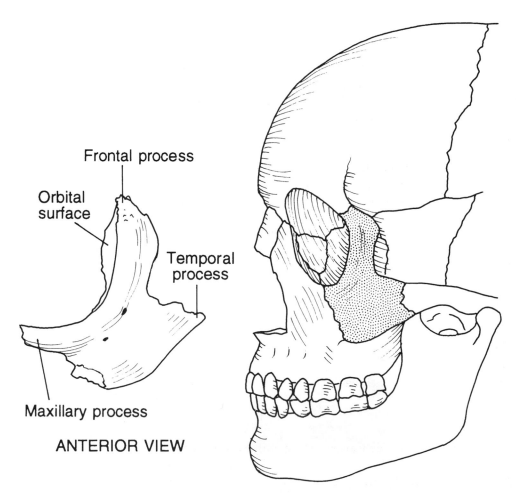

Frontal process

Orbital surface

Temporal process

Maxillary process

ANTERIOR VIEW

Figure 7-16. Anterior view of zygomatic bone.

Cleft Lip and Cleft Palate

Cleft lip and cleft palate arise during early development. Cleft lip may be either unilateral or bilateral, occurring along the premaxillary suture. Cleft lip will almost never be midline, but may involve soft tissue alone, or include a cleft of the maxilla up to the incisive foramen. Cleft palate may involve both hard and soft palates.

Cleft lip appears to result from a failure of embryonic facial and labial tissue to fuse during development. It looks as though tissues migrate and develop normally, but for some reason either fail to fuse or the fusion of the migrating medial nasal, maxillary, and lateral nasal processes breaks down. Cleft palate apparently arises from some mechanical intervention in development. Prior to the seventh embryonic week the palatine processes of the maxillae have been resting alongside the tongue so that the tongue separates the processes. As the oral cavity and mandible grow, the tongue drops away from the processes, and the processes can extend, make midline contact, and fuse. If something blocks the movement of the tongue (such as micrognathia), the palatine processes will not move in time to make contact. The head grows rapidly, and the plates will have missed their chance to become an intact palate.

Lacrimal Bones

The small **lacrimal** bones are almost completely hidden in the intact skull. They articulate with the maxillae, frontal bone, nasal bone, and inferior conchae. They constitute a small portion of the lateral nasal wall and form a small portion of the medial orbit as well.

lacrimal: *L., lacrima, tear*

Hyoid Bone

The hyoid bone was discussed in Chapters 5 and 6, but rightfully belongs in this chapter as well. Its presence in this listing should remind you of the interconnectedness of the phonatory and articulatory systems.

Bones of the Cranial Skeleton

- Ethmoid
- Sphenoid
- Frontal
- Parietal
- Occipital
- Temporal

The bones of the cranium include those involved in creation of the cranial cavity.

Ethmoid Bone

The **ethmoid** bone is a complex, delicate structure with a presence in the cranial, nasal, and orbital spaces. If the cranium and facial skeleton were an apple, the ethmoid would be the core. You may want to refer to Figure 7-17 for this discussion.

ethmoid: *Gr., ethmos, sieve + eidos, like*

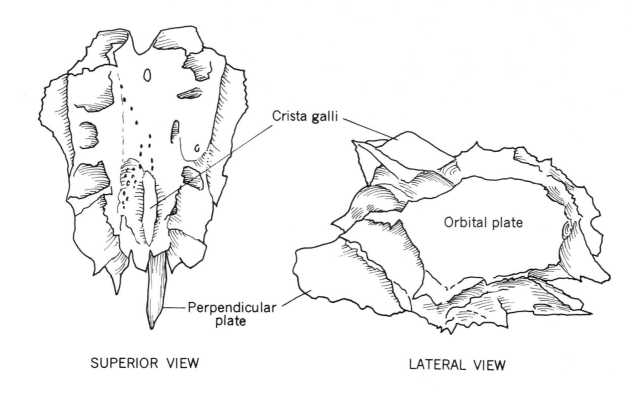

Crista galli

Perpendicular
plate

Orbital plate

SUPERIOR VIEW

LATERAL VIEW

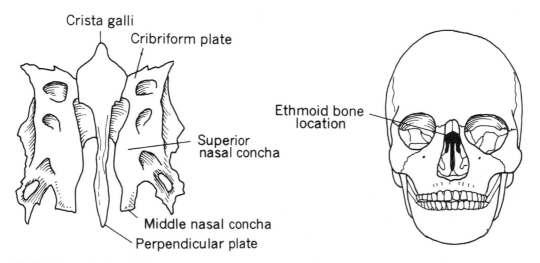

ANTERIOR VIEW

Crista galli

Cribriform plate

Superior
nasal concha

Middle nasal concha

Perpendicular plate

Ethmoid bone
location

Figure 7-17. Views of ethmoid bone.

When viewed from the front, the superior surface is dominated by the **crista galli**, which protrudes into the cranial space. Projecting down is the **perpendicular plate**, making up the superior nasal septum, and lateral to this plate are the **middle** and **superior nasal conchae**. On both sides of the perpendicular plate and perpendicular to it are the **cribriform plates**. The cribriform plates separate the nasal and cranial cavities, and provide the conduit for the olfactory nerves as they enter the cranial space. The lateral **orbital plates** articulate with the frontal bone, lacrimal bone, and maxilla to form the medial orbit.

crista: *L., crest*

conchae: *Gr., konche, shell*

cribriform: *L., cribum, sieve + forma, form*

Sphenoid Bone

The **sphenoid** bone exceeds the ethmoid bone in complexity. A glance at Figure 7-18 will show that the sphenoid is a significant contributor to the cranial structure. The sphenoid consists of a corpus and three pairs of processes, the greater wings of the sphenoid, lesser wings of the sphenoid, and pterygoid processes. The sphenoid also contains numerous foramina through which nerves and blood vessels pass.

sphenoid: *Gr., spheno, wedge + eidos, like*

When viewed from above, you can see that the medially placed **corpus** is dominated by the **hypophyseal fossa** (also known as the **sella turcica** or **pituitary fossa**), the indentation holding the pituitary gland (hypophysis) in life. This gland projects down from the hypothalamus and is placed at the point where the optic nerve decussates, the **chiasma**. The anterior portion of the fossa is the **tuberculum sellae** and the posterior aspect is the **dorsum sellae**. The **anterior clinoid processes** project from the lesser wing of the sphenoid, lateral to the tuberculum sellae. The optic nerve passes under these processes, having passed through the optic foramen anteriorly. The **clivus** forms the union with the foramen magnum of the occipital bone. Within the corpus are the air-filled **sphenoid sinuses**.

sella turcica: *L., Turkish saddle*

chiasma: *Gr., khiasma, cross; an X-shaped crossing*

tuberculum: *L., little swelling*

clivus: *L., slope*

The **lesser** and **greater wings** of the sphenoid are striking landmarks, likened to the wings of a bat. The lesser wings arise from the corpus and clinoid process, and partially cover the optic canal. The greater wings arise from the posterior corpus, making up a portion of the orbit. The greater wing comprises a portion of the anterolateral skull, and articulates with the frontal and temporal bones.

Projecting downward from the greater wing and corpus are the **lateral** and **medial pterygoid plates**. The fossa between the medial and lateral plates will be the point of attachment for one of the muscles of mastication (medial pterygoid muscle), and the tensor veli palatini will attach to the **scaphoid fossa**. A hamulus projects from each medial lamina, and the tendon of the tensor veli palatini passes around this on its course to the velum, as will be discussed.

The openings of the superior sphenoid are particularly significant. For example, the **optic canal** carries the II optic nerve, and the **foramen ovale** provides the conduit for the mandibular nerve of V trigeminal.

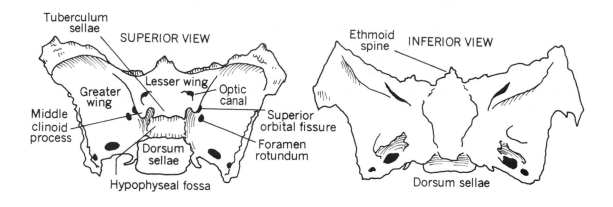

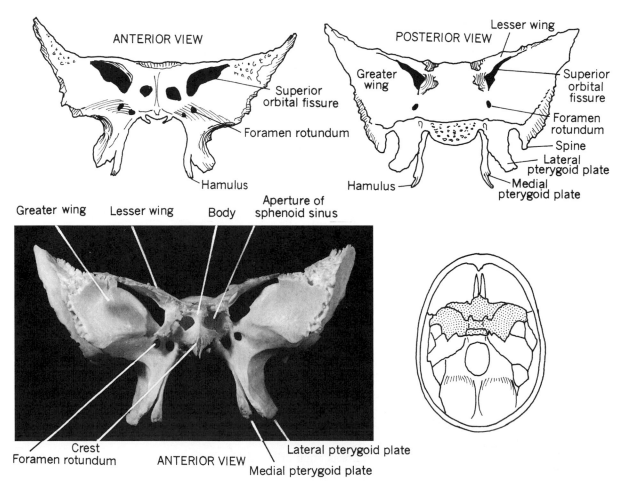

Figure 7-18. Photograph of anterior view of sphenoid bone and schematic drawings of sphenoid from four views.

The maxillary nerve arising from the V trigeminal passes through the **foramen rotundum**, and the **superior orbital fissure** conveys the III oculomotor, IV trochlear, several branches of the ophthalmic nerve of V trigeminal, and VI abducens nerves. The **body** of the sphenoid includes the anteriorly placed jugum and the **chiasmatic groove**, which accommodates the optic chiasm.

jugum: *L., a yoke*

Frontal Bone

The unpaired frontal bone shown in Figure 7-19 makes up the bony forehead, anterior cranial case, and supraorbital region. Near the middle of the intact skull, the coronal suture marks the point of articulation of the frontal and parietal bones. The frontal bone articulates with the zygomatic bones via the **zygomatic processes** and with the nasal bones by means of the **nasal portion**. From beneath, the **orbital portion** provides the superior surface of the eye socket.

Parietal Bones

The paired parietal bones overlie the parietal lobes of the cerebrum and form the middle portion of the braincase (see Figure 7-20). These bones are united at the midline by the sagittal suture, running from the frontal bone in front to the occipital bone in back, separated by the **lambdoidal suture**. Small, irregular **wormian** bones may be formed by the bifurcations of the lambdoidal suture. The lateral margin of the parietal bone is marked by the **squamosal** suture, forming the union between parietal and temporal bones.

lambdoidal: *Gr., "L"-like*

wormian: *after Olaus Worm, anatomist*

squamosal: *L., scale*

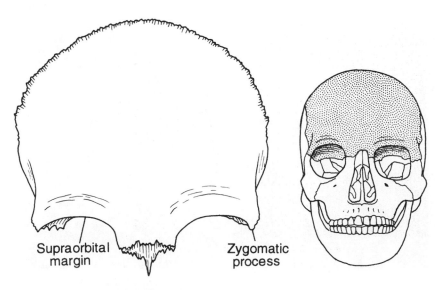

Supraorbital margin   Zygomatic process

ANTERIOR VIEW

Figure 7-19. Anterior view of frontal bone.

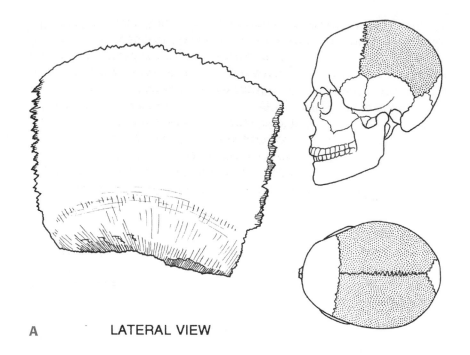

A   **LATERAL VIEW**

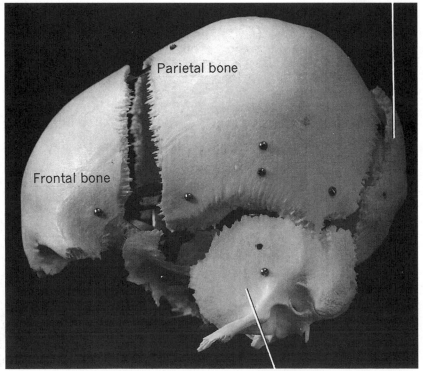

Occipital bone

Parietal bone

Frontal bone

Temporal bone

Figure 7-20. A. Lateral view of parietal bone. **B.** Photo of disarticulated parietal, frontal, temporal, and occipital bones.

B

Occipital Bone

The unpaired occipital bone is deceptively simple in appearance (see Figure 7-21). It overlies the occipital lobe of the brain and makes up the posterior braincase. It articulates with the temporal, parietal, and sphenoid bones. The **external occipital protuberance** is a midline prominence visible from behind. The **cerebral** and **cerebellar fossa** of the inner superior surface mark the locations of the occipital lobe and cerebellum, respectively in the intact braincase.

The most significant landmarks are those visible from beneath. From this vantage point, you can see that the occipital bone forms the base of the skull, wrapping beneath the brain. The **foramen magnum** provides the conduit for the spinal cord and beginning of the medulla oblongata, and the **condyles** mark the resting point for the first cervical vertebra. The **basilar part** articulates with the corpus of the sphenoid.

Temporal Bone

The temporal bone is an important structure for students of speech pathology and audiology. On gross examination of the lateral skull, you can see that the temporal bone is separated from the parietal bone by the **squamosal suture** (also known as the *parietomastoid suture*) and from the occipital bone by the **occipitomastoid suture** (see Figure 7-22).

The temporal bone seen from the side is extremely dense and is remarkably rich in important landmarks. This complex bone is divided into four segments: the squamous, tympanic, mastoid, and petrous portions.

The **squamous portion**, which abuts the squamosal suture, is fan-shaped and thin. The lower margin includes the roof of the **external auditory meatus**, the conduit for sound energy to the middle ear. The anteriorly directed **zygomatic process** also arises from the squamous portion, articulating with the temporal process of the zygomatic bone to form the **zygomatic arch** (see Figure 7-5A). Beneath the base of the zygomatic process is the **mandibular fossa** of the temporal bone with which the condyloid process of the mandible articulates to form the temporomandibular joint.

meatus: *L., opening*

The **mastoid portion** makes up the posterior part of the temporal bone. Air cells in the mastoid portion communicate with the **tympanic antrum**. Above the antrum is the **tegmen tympani**, a thin plate of bone, and medial to it is the lateral semicircular canal. The **mastoid process**, a structure you can easily palpate by feeling behind your ear, arises from this portion. The **tympanic portion** includes the anterior and inferior walls of the external auditory meatus. The prominent **styloid process** protrudes beneath the external auditory meatus and medial to the mastoid process. The **petrous portion** includes the cochlea and semicircular canals in life.

tympanic antrum: *L., drum cavity*

tegmen tympani: *L., drum covering*

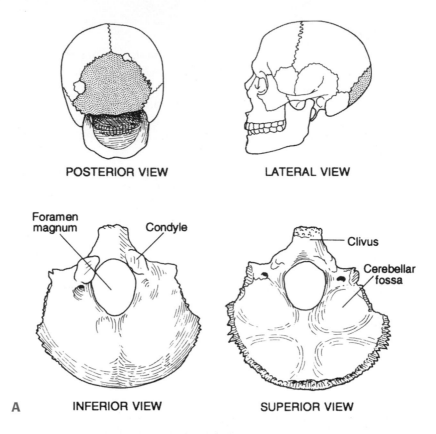

POSTERIOR VIEW   LATERAL VIEW

Foramen magnum   Condyle   Clivus

                                  Cerebellar fossa

A   INFERIOR VIEW   SUPERIOR VIEW

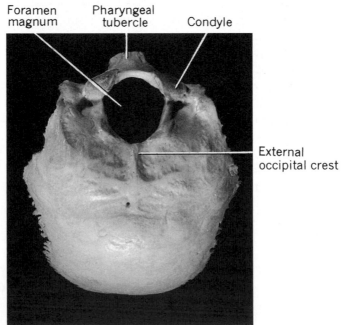

Foramen magnum   Pharyngeal tubercle   Condyle

External occipital crest

B   INFERIOR VIEW

Figure 7-21. A. Occipital bone seen from inferior and superior aspects. **B.** Photo of occipital bone, inferior view.

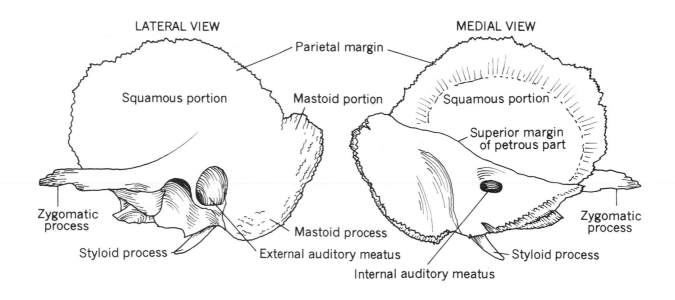

LATERAL VIEW

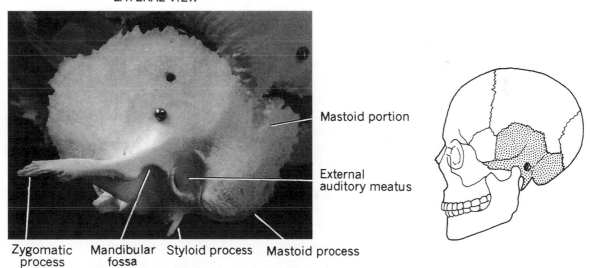

Figure 7-22. Schematic and photo of lateral and medial view of temporal bone.

The **temporal fossa** is a region including a portion of the temporal, parietal, and occipital bones. The temporal portion is the large region near the parietal and occipital bones. A band including the squamosal suture on the parietal bone and the superior portion of the occipitotemporal suture are included in the temporal fossa as well, with the entire region marking the point of origin of the fan-shaped temporalis muscle (to be discussed). The medial surface of the temporal bone reveals the **internal auditory meatus** through which the VIII cranial nerve will pass on its way to the brainstem.

To summarize, the bones of the **face** and **skull** work together in a complex fashion to produce the structures of **articulation**.

- The **mandible** provides the lower **dental arch**, **alveolar region**, and the resting location for the tongue.
- The **maxillae** provide the **hard palate**, point of attachment for the **soft palate**, **alveolar ridge**, upper **dental arch**, and dominant structures of the **nasal cavities**.
- The midline **vomer** articulates with the perpendicular plate of the **ethmoid** and the **cartilaginous septum** to form the **nasal septum**.
- The **zygomatic bone** articulates with the **frontal bone** and **maxillae** to form the cheekbone. The small **nasal bones** provide the upper margin of the nasal cavity.
- The **ethmoid bone** serves as the core of the skull and face, with the prominent **crista galli** protruding into the **cranium** and the **perpendicular plate** dividing the nasal cavities.
- The **frontal**, **parietal**, **temporal**, and **occipital** bones of the skull overlie the lobes of the brain of the same names.
- The **sphenoid bone** has a marked presence within the braincase, with the prominent **greater** and **lesser wings** of the sphenoid being found lateral to the **corpus**. The **hypophyseal fossa** houses the pituitary gland. The **clivus** joins the **occipital** bone near the **foramen magnum**.

DENTITION

The teeth are vital components of the speech mechanism. Housed within the alveoli of the maxillae and mandible, teeth provide the mechanism for mastication, as well as articulatory surfaces for several speech sounds.

Before we discuss the specific teeth, let us begin with an orientation to the dental arch itself. The upper and lower dental arches contain equal numbers of teeth of four types: incisors, cuspids, bicuspids, and molars. It is convenient to think of half-arches, knowing that left and right sides will have equal distribution of teeth (see Figure 7-23).

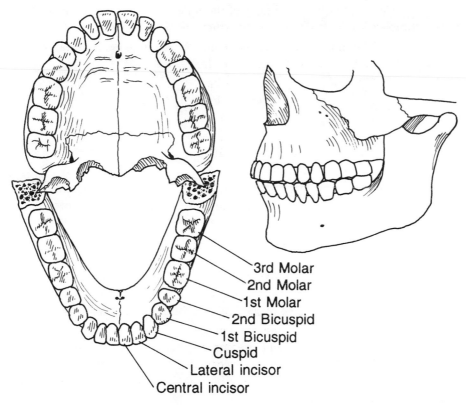

3rd Molar
2nd Molar
1st Molar
2nd Bicuspid
1st Bicuspid
Cuspid
Lateral incisor
Central incisor

MANDIBULAR DENTAL ARCH

A

Figure 7-23. A. Permanent dental arches. *(continues)*

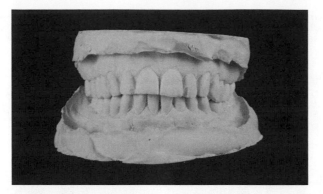

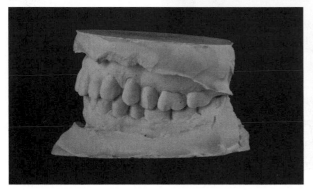
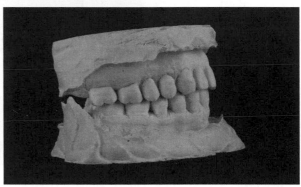

B

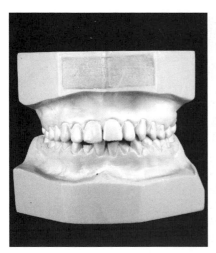
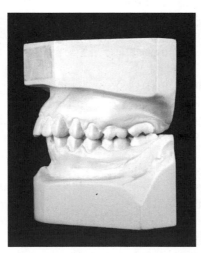
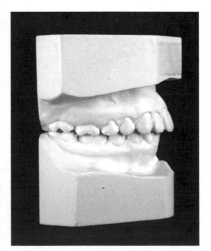

C

Figure 7-23. *(continued)* **B.** Anterior and lateral views of normal adult dental arch. **C.** Anterior and lateral views of deciduous dental arch. *(continues)*

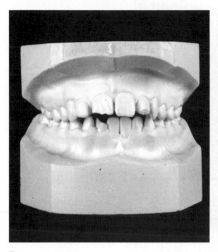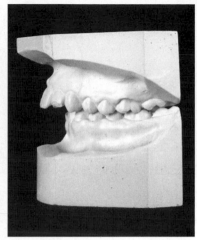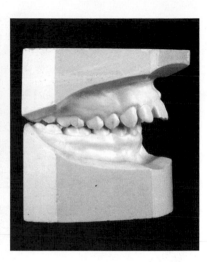

D

Figure 7-23. *(continued)* **D.** Deciduous dental arch of child with significant oromyofunctional disorder. Note the marked labioversion of the incisors, but presence of normal Class I occlusal relationship of molars.

Generally, teeth in the upper arch are larger than those in the lower arch, and the upper arch typically overlaps the lower arch in front. Each tooth has a **root**, hidden beneath the protective **gingival** or gum line (see Figure 7-24). The **crown** is the visible one-third of the tooth, and the juncture of the crown and root is termed the **neck**. The surface of the crown is composed of the dental **enamel**, an extremely hard surface that overlies the **dentin**, or ivory, of the tooth. At the heart of the tooth is the **pulp**, in which the nerve supplying the tooth resides. The tooth is held in its socket by **cementum**, which is a thin layer of bone. As teeth shift from pressures (such as the forces accompanying tongue thrust), the cementum will develop to ensure that the tooth remains firmly in its socket.

> **gingival:** *L., gingiva, gum*

> **dentin:** *L., dens, tooth*

Five surfaces are important when discussing teeth. To understand the terminology, you need to alter your thinking about the dental arch a bit. Examine Figure 7-25 and you will see that the center of the dental arch is considered to be the point between the two central incisors, in front. Follow the arch around toward the molars in back and you have traced a path distal to those incisors. That is, *medial* refers to movement along the arch toward the midline between the central incisors, whereas *distal* refers to movement along the arch away from that midpoint. From this you can see that the **medial surface** (or **mesial**) of any tooth is the surface "looking" along the arch toward the midpoint between the central incisors. The **distal surface** is the surface of any tooth that is farthest from that midline point. Every tooth has a medial and a distal surface. Table 7-2 provides descriptions of terms related to dentition.

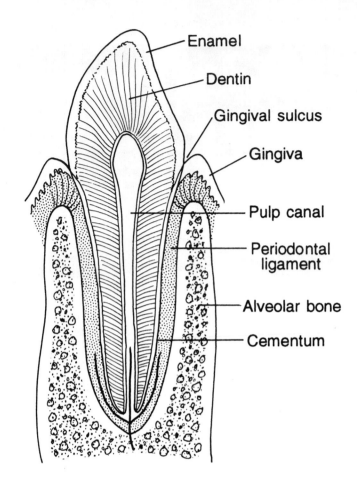

Figure 7-24. Components of a tooth.

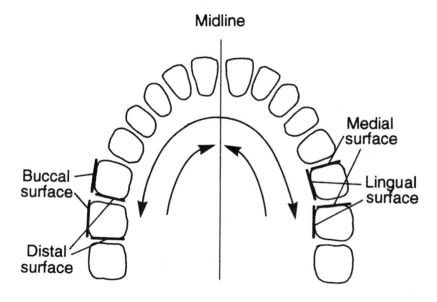

Figure 7-25. Surface referents of teeth and the dental arch.

Table 7-2. Terms related to dentition.

Surfaces:	
Medial/mesial	Surface of individual tooth closest to midline point on arch between central incisors.
Distal	Surface of individual tooth most distant from midline point on arch between central incisors.
Buccal	Surface of a tooth that could come in contact with the buccal wall.
Lingual	Surface of a tooth that could come in contact with the tongue.
Occlusal	The contact surface between teeth of the upper and lower arches.
Development:	
Intraosseous eruption	Eruption of teeth through the alveolar process.
Clinical eruption	Eruption of teeth into the oral cavity.
Successional teeth	Teeth that replace deciduous teeth.
Superadded teeth	Teeth in the adult arch not present within the deciduous arch.
Supernumerary	Teeth in excess of the normal number for an arch.
Dental Occlusion:	
Overjet	Normal projection of upper incisors beyond lower incisors in transverse plane.
Overbite	Normal overlap of upper incisors relative to lower incisors.
Class I occlusal relationship	Relationship between your upper and lower teeth in which the first molar of the mandibular arch is one-half tooth advanced of the maxillary molar.
Class I malocclusion	Occlusal relationship in which there is normal orientation of the molars, but an abnormal orientation of the incisors.
Class II malocclusion	Relationship of upper and lower arches in which the first mandibular molars are retracted at least one tooth from the first maxillary molars.
Class III malocclusion	Relationship of upper and lower arches in which the first mandibular molar is advanced more than one tooth beyond the first maxillary molar.
Relative micrognathia	Condition in which mandible is small in relation to the maxillae.
Axial Orientation:	
Torsiversion	Condition in which individual tooth is rotated or twisted on its long axis.
Labioverted	Condition in which individual tooth tilts toward the lips.
Linguaverted	Condition in which individual tooth tilts toward the tongue.
Buccoversion	Condition in which individual tooth tilts toward cheek.
Distoverted	Condition in which individual tooth tilts away from midline of dental arch.
Mesioverted	Condition in which individual tooth tilts toward the midline of the dental arch.
Infraverted	Condition in which tooth is inadequately erupted.
Supraverted	Condition in which a tooth protrudes excessively into the oral cavity, causing inadequate occlusion of other dentition.
Persistent open bite	Condition in which the front teeth do not occlude because of excessive eruption of posterior teeth.
Persistent closed bite	Condition in which the posterior teeth do not occlude because of excessive eruption of anterior dentition.

buccal: *L., bucca, cheek*

incisor: *L., cutter*

cingulum: *L., girdle*

cuspid: *L., cuspis, point*

The **buccal surface** of a tooth is that which could come in contact with the buccal wall (cheek), and the **lingual surface** is the surface facing the tongue. The **occlusal surface** is the contact surface between teeth of the upper and lower arches. Not surprisingly, the thickest enamel overlies the occlusal surface, because it receives the most abrasion. A habit of chewing ice can undo this plan of nature, however, causing premature **attrition** or wearing away of the dental enamel.

Incisors clearly are designed for cutting, as their name implies (see Figure 7-26). The **central incisors** of the upper dental arch present a large, spadelike surface with a thin cutting surface. The **lateral incisors** present a smaller but similar surface. If you feel your superior incisors with your tongue you will feel a prominent ridge or **cingulum**. The lower incisors are markedly smaller than the upper incisors, resting within the upper arch, and you must slightly open and protrude your mandible to make contact between the occlusal surfaces of the incisors.

The **cuspid** (also **canine; eye tooth**) is well named. It has a single cusp or point that is used for tearing. In carnivores this tooth is particularly well suited for separating the fibers of muscle to promote meat eating. Lateral to the cuspids are the **first** and **second bicuspids** or **premolars**. These teeth have two cusps on the occlusal surface, and are absent in the deciduous dental arch.

UPPER ARCH

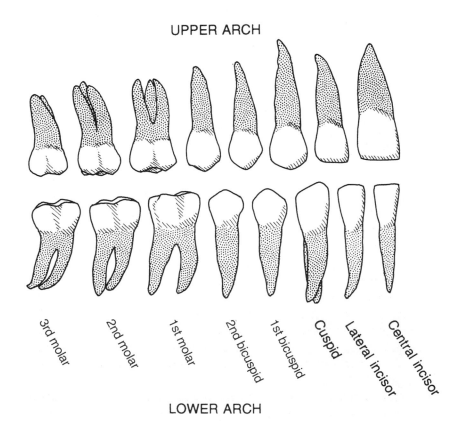

3rd molar   2nd molar   1st molar   2nd bicuspid   1st bicuspid   Cuspid   Lateral incisor   Central incisor

Figure 7-26. Types of teeth.

LOWER ARCH

Molars are large teeth with great occlusal surfaces designed to grind material, and their placement in the posterior arch capitalizes on the significant force available in the muscles of mastication. This mix of cutting teeth (incisors, cuspids, bicuspids) and grinding teeth (molars) is just right for omnivorous humans: We will eat virtually anything!

molar: *L., molaris, grinding*

There are three molars in each half of the adult dental arch. The medial-most **first molar** is the largest of the group, with the **second** and **third molars** descending in size. The first molar will have four cusps, the second molar may have three or four, and the third molar will have three. The third molar is sometimes known as the **wisdom tooth**, often erupting well into adulthood. The third molar is very likely a safeguard against losing teeth. In days before dental hygiene it was not uncommon to lose many teeth to **caries**. A late-emerging set of molars, useful for grinding grain and pulverizing fibers, would be just the item to extend the life of our ancestors. Now those wisdom teeth seem less "wise," as they tend to crowd the other teeth and often develop with an orientation that makes them not only useless, but a threat to the healthy teeth.

The roots of the teeth reflect the forces applied to the teeth. The incisors and cuspids have a single long root, with the cuspid, which has a great deal of force on it from tearing, having the longest root. The bicuspids have variously one or two roots, and the molars will have two or three roots to help anchor them against the massive forces of grinding.

Dental Development

Dental development clearly parallels that of the individual. Infants develop **deciduous** or **shedding teeth** (also known as **milk teeth**) that give way to the **permanent teeth** that must last a lifetime. Deciduous teeth actually begin development quite early in prenatal development, but start **erupting** through the bone (**intraosseous eruption**) and the gum (**clinical eruption**) when the child is between six and nine months of age. Tooth buds form when the developing mandible and maxillae are only 1 mm long, but by birth the buds have spread out to match the jaw that is 40 times longer. These teeth are not only much smaller than the adult teeth, matching the size of the arch, but are fewer in number. Generally, central incisors emerge first (lower, then upper), followed by lateral incisors (upper, then lower). The first molars emerge at approximately the same time as the cuspids (between 15 and 20 months), and the second molars will have erupted by the child's second birthday. You will notice that there is no third molar, and the first and second bicuspids are conspicuously absent. These teeth are reserved for the adult arch. Each deciduous arch has 10 teeth, whereas the adult arch has 16 (see Figure 7-27 and Table 7-3).

deciduous: *L., deciduus, falling off*

Your first-grade school photograph will remind you of the period during which shedding begins. That gap-toothed grin of the 6-year-old

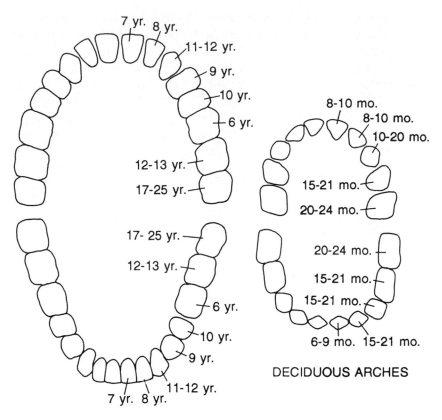

Figure 7-27. A. Age of eruption of teeth in the permanent and deciduous arches. *(continues)*

A   **PERMANENT ARCHES**

child comes from shedding of the deciduous arch, beginning with the incisors (6 through 9 years), followed by first molars and cuspids (9 to 12 years), and finally second molars (beginning around 10 years of age).

Shedding is not a passive process. If you have occasion to view a tooth shed by a child, you will see very little of the root. The deciduous

Dental Anomalies

There are numerous developmental dental anomalies. Children may be born with **supernumerary teeth** (teeth in addition to the normal number), or teeth may be smaller than appropriate for the dental arch (**microdontia**). Teeth may **fuse** together at the root or crown. In addition to this, enamel may be extremely thin or even missing from the surface of the tooth (**amelogenesis imperfecta**), or the enamel may be stained by use of the antibiotic tetracycline or fluoride.

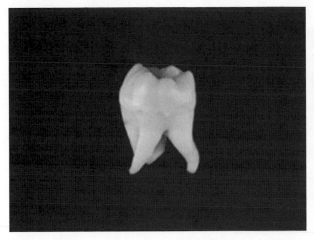
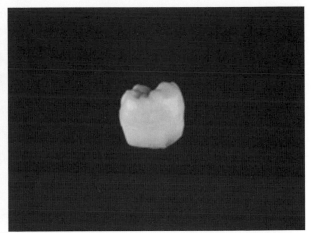

B

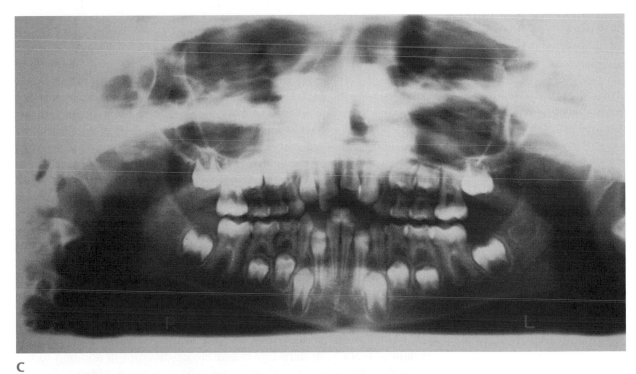

C

Figure 7-27. *(continued)* **B.** Individual deciduous and permanent teeth, with adult third molar (wisdom tooth) on left and deciduous molar on right. **C.** Pantomagraph of mixed dentition. Note presence of unerupted permanent teeth within the maxilla and mandible.

Table 7-3. Timeline for eruption of mandibular and maxillary dentition.

EARLIEST AGE OF EXPECTED ERUPTION	TYPE OF DENTITION	MANDIBULAR DENTITION	MAXILLARY DENTITION
5 mo.	Deciduous	Central incisors	
6 mo.	Deciduous		Central incisors
7 mo.	Deciduous	Lateral incisors	
8 mo.	Deciduous		Lateral incisors
10 mo.	Deciduous	First molars	
16 mo.	Deciduous	Cuspids	Cuspids
20 mo.	Deciduous	Second molars	
36 mo.			Second molars
6 years	Permanent	Central incisors First molars	First molars
7 years	Permanent	Lateral incisors	Central incisors
8 years	Permanent		Lateral incisors
9 years	Permanent	Cuspids	
10 years	Permanent	First bicuspids	First bicuspids Second bicuspids
11 years	Permanent	Second bicuspids	Cuspids
12 years	Permanent	Second molars	Second molars
17 years	Permanent	Third molars	Third molars

Source: Based on data of Behrman, Vaughan, & Nelson, 1987.

periodontal: *Gr., peri, around + odous, tooth*

tooth is suspended in the socket by means of a **periodontal ligament** that serves as a pressure sensor. As the permanent tooth migrates toward the surface, its proximity stimulates conversion of the deciduous periodontal ligament into osteoclasts that promote resorption of the root and enamel. Thus, by the time the permanent tooth is ready to erupt, the deciduous tooth has lost its anchor in the alveolus and comes out easily.

The permanent teeth that replace deciduous teeth are called **successional teeth**. The third molar and bicuspids erupt in addition to the original constellation, and thus are referred to as **superadded**.

Dental Occlusion

The primary purpose of dentition is mastication, and this fact makes the orientation of teeth of the utmost importance. **Occlusion** is the process of bringing the upper and lower teeth into contact, and proper occlusion is essential for successful mastication. Clearly, if the upper molars do not make contact with the lower molars, no grinding will occur. We will discuss orientation of the upper and lower dental arches, as well as orientation that the individual teeth can take within the arches. These terms of orientation will serve you well as you prepare for your clinical work, because they are central to the oral-peripheral examination of teeth.

To discuss this orientation, first examine your own dental arch relationship. Lightly tap your molars, and then bite down lightly and leave them occluded. This sets the orientation of the arches. With your teeth making contact in this manner, open your lips so that you can see the front teeth while looking in a mirror. If you have a **Class I occlusal relationship** between your upper and lower teeth, the first molar of the mandibular arch is one-half tooth advanced of the maxillary molar. Your upper incisors project beyond the lower incisors vertically by a few millimeters (termed **overjet**), and the upper incisors naturally hide the lower incisors (termed **overbite**) so that only a little of the lower teeth will show. This Class I occlusion (also known as **neutroclusion**) (see Figure 7-28) is considered the normal relationship between the molars of the dental arches.

In **Class II malocclusion**, the first mandibular molars are retracted at least one tooth from the first maxillary molars. This is sometimes the product of **relative micrognathia**, a condition in which the mandible is small in relation to the maxillae (see Figure 7-29).

A **Class III malocclusion** is identified if the first mandibular molar is advanced farther than one tooth beyond the first maxillary molar. Thus, in Class II malocclusion the mandible is retracted, whereas in Class III the mandible is protruded. There is a **Class I malocclusion**, as

micrognathia: *Gr., micro, small + gnathos, jaw*

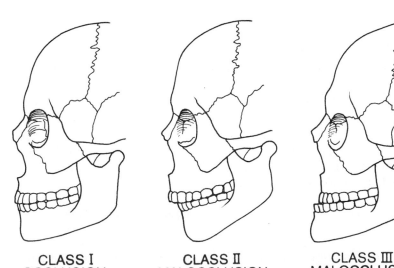

CLASS I
OCCLUSION

CLASS II
MALOCCLUSION

CLASS III
MALOCCLUSION

Figure 7-28. Types of malocclusion.

well. This is defined as an occlusion in which there is normal orientation of the molars, but an abnormal orientation of the incisors.

Individual teeth may be misaligned as well. If a tooth is rotated or twisted on its long axis, it has undergone **torsiversion**. If it tilts toward the lips, it is referred to as **labioverted**, whereas tilting toward the tongue is **linguaverted** (see Figure 7-29A). When molars tilt toward the cheeks, it is called *buccoversion*. A tooth that tilts away from the midline along the arch is said to be **distoverted**, whereas one tilting toward that midline between the two central incisors is **mesioverted**. When a tooth does not erupt sufficiently to make occlusal contact with its pair in the opposite arch, it is said to be **infraverted**; the tooth that erupts too far is said to be **supraverted**. In some cases the front teeth may not demonstrate the proper occlusion because teeth in the posterior arch prohibit anterior contact, a condition that is termed **persistent open bite**. If supraversion

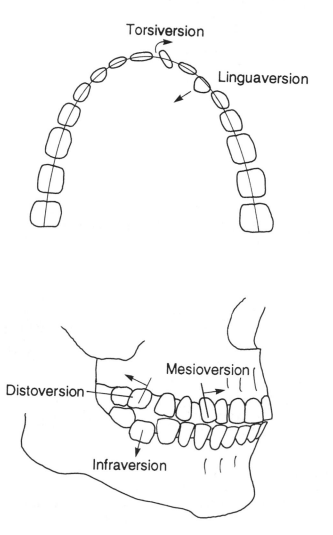

Figure 7-29. A. Graphic representation of torsiversion, linguaversion, infraversion, distoversion, and mesioversion.
(continues)

A

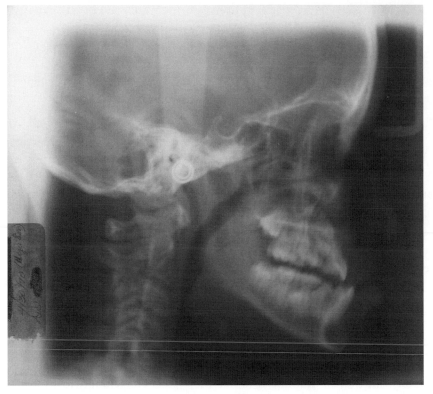

B

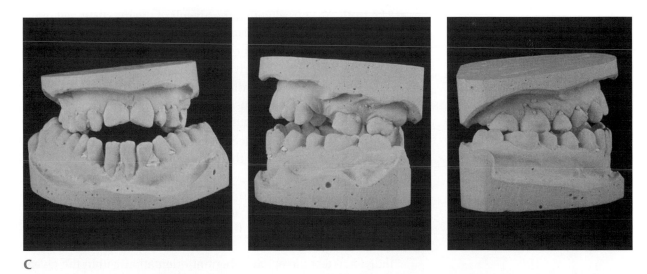

C

Figure 7-29. *(continued)* **B.** Radiograph of prognathic mandible that was later surgically corrected. **C.** Dental impression of young adult with significant oromyofunctional disorder, revealing extreme palatal arch, distoversion, torsiversion, linguaversion, and labioversion secondary to tongue thrust. Note evidence of gingival lesion (gum recession) secondary to retained tongue thrust.

Supernumerary Teeth

Supernumerary teeth arise from a developmental anomaly in which the embryonic dental lamina produces excessive numbers of tooth buds. When this occurs, the individual will be born with more teeth than predicted, often resulting in "twinning" of incisors. Below is a report from J. M. Harris, D.D.S., of a child he saw in his dental practice in Idaho Falls, Idaho.

An eight-year-old girl was brought to Dr. Harris's clinic with the complaint that one of her deciduous teeth needed to be extracted due to the patient's age. Dr. Harris performed panelipse radiography to verify that the permanent teeth were present prior to the extraction, but the radiograph revealed supernumerary teeth in the left mandibular arch in the bicuspid region.

Extraction of the decayed deciduous tooth revealed a pocket of 15 supernumerary teeth: Some were simply tooth buds, but some had developed small roots and looked like fully formed molars. In an arch built ultimately for 16 teeth, that would be a significant addition!

The cluster was removed, Gelfoam was placed in the cavity, and sutures closed the space. There were no further complications.

prohibits the posterior teeth from occlusion, it is called **persistent closed bite**. As you examine the dental orientation of the photographs in Figure 7-29B and 7-29C, attend closely to the variety of misalignments in this dentition. The cast in Figure 7-29C was made from the teeth of a young man with Down syndrome who had the typical congenitally low muscle tone as well as marked and uncorrected tongue thrust.

In summary:

- The **teeth** are housed within the **alveoli** of the **maxillae** and **mandible**, and consist of **incisors, cuspids, bicuspids,** and **molars.**
- Each tooth has a **root** and **crown**, with the surface of the crown composed of **enamel** overlying **dentin.**
- Each tooth has a **medial, distal, lingual, buccal** (or labial), and **occlusal** surface; the occlusal surface reflects the function of the teeth in the omnivorous human dental arch.
- **Clinical eruption** of the **deciduous** arch begins between six and nine months of age, while the **permanent arch** emerges between six and nine years.
- **Class I occlusion** refers to normal orientation of mandible and maxillae, while **Class II malocclusion** refers to a relatively retracted mandible. **Class III malocclusion** refers to a relatively protruded mandible.
- Individual teeth may have aberrant orientation within the alveolus, including **torsiversion, labioversion, linguaversion, distoversion,** and **mesioversion.**
- Inadequately erupted or hypererupted teeth are referred to as **infraverted** and **supraverted.**

CAVITIES OF THE VOCAL TRACT

We mentioned that the source-filter theory depends upon cavities to shape the acoustic output. Before we show you the muscles associated with articulation, let us discuss the cavities that will be shaped by moving those muscles. These are the oral, buccal, nasal, and pharyngeal cavities (see Figure 7-30).

The **oral cavity** is the most significant cavity of the speech mechanism, as it undergoes the most change during the speech act. Its shape can be altered by movement of the tongue or mandible.

The oral cavity extends from the oral opening, or mouth, in front to the faucial pillars in back. The oral opening is strongly involved in articulation, being the point of exit of sound for all orally emitted phonemes (i.e., all sounds except those emitted nasally). The lips of the mouth are quite important for articulation of a number of consonants and vowels.

This is a good opportunity to take a guided tour of your own mouth (see Figure 7-31). Palpate the roof of your mouth (you can use your tongue to feel this if you wish). The hard roof of your mouth is the **hard**

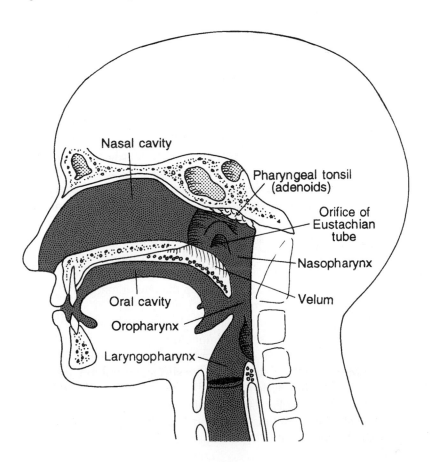

Figure 7-30. Oral, nasal, and pharyngeal cavities.

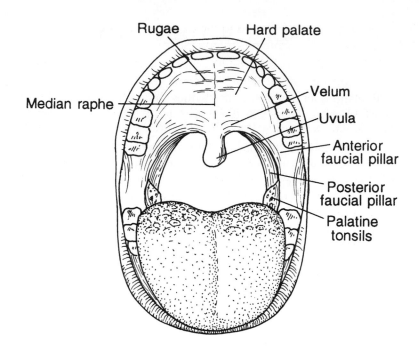

Figure 7-31. Anterior view of oral cavity.

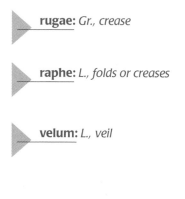

rugae: *Gr., crease*

raphe: *L., folds or creases*

velum: *L., veil*

fauces: *L., throat*

palate. The prominent ridges running laterally are the rugae, potentially useful structures in formation of the bolus of food during deglutition and serving as a landmark in articulation. The **median** raphe divides the hard palate into equal halves.

As you run your tongue or finger back along the roof of your mouth, you can feel the point at which the hard palate suddenly becomes soft. This is the juncture of the hard and soft palates, and the soft portion is the **soft palate** or velum, with the **uvula** marking the terminus of the velum. The velum is the movable muscle mass separating the oral and nasal cavities (or more technically, the oropharynx and nasopharynx, as you shall see). The velum is attached in front to the palatine bone and is thus a muscular extension of the hard palate.

On either side of the soft palate and continuous with it are two prominent bands of tissue. These are the **anterior** and **posterior** faucial **pillars**, and they mark the posterior margin of the oral cavity. The teeth and alveolar ridge of the maxillae make up the lateral margins of the oral cavity. The tongue occupies most of the lower mouth.

Between the anterior and posterior faucial pillars you may see the **palatine tonsils**. These masses of lymphoid tissue are situated between the pillars on either side, and even invade the lateral undersurface of the soft palate. Medial to these tonsils, on the surface of the tongue, are the lingual tonsils (to be discussed).

The **buccal cavity** lies lateral to the oral cavity, composed of the space between the posterior teeth and the cheeks of the face. It is bounded by the cheeks laterally, the lips in front, and the teeth medially.

The posterior margin is at the third molar. This space plays a role in oral resonance when the mandible is depressed to expose it, is involved in high-pressure consonant production, and is the source of the distortion heard in the misarticulation known as the lateral /s/.

The **pharyngeal cavity**, or **pharynx**, is broken into three logically named regions. You can envision the pharynx as a tube approximately 12 cm in length, extending from the vocal folds, below, to the region behind the nasal cavities, above. This tube is lined with muscle capable of constricting the size of the tube to facilitate deglutition, and this musculature plays an important role in effecting closure of the **velopharyngeal port**, the opening between the oropharynx and nasopharynx.

The **oropharynx** is the portion of the pharynx immediately posterior to the fauces, bounded above by the velum. The lower boundary of the oropharynx is the hyoid bone, which marks the upper boundary of the laryngopharynx. The **laryngopharynx** (or **hypopharynx**) is bounded anteriorly by the epiglottis and inferiorly by the esophagus.

The third pharyngeal space is the **nasopharynx**, the space above the soft palate, bounded posteriorly by the pharyngeal protuberance of the occipital bone and by the nasal choanae in front. The lateral nasopharyngeal wall contains the **orifice** of the **Eustachian tube** (also known as the **auditory tube**; see Figure 7-30).

Although minute, the Eustachian tube serves an extremely important function in that it provides a means of aerating the middle ear cavity. Recognize that the nasopharynx is on a level with the ears, so that the tube connecting the nasopharynx with the middle ear space must course slightly up, back, and out to reach that cavity. The Eustachian tube is actively opened through contraction of the tensor veli palatini muscle, as discussed later in this chapter. The bulge of tissue partially encircling the orifice of the Eustachian tube is the **torus tubarius**, and the ridge of tissue coursing down from the orifice is the **salpingopharyngeal fold**—actually the salpingopharyngeus muscle covered with mucous membrane.

salpingopharyngeal: *Gr., salpinx, tube + pharynx*

Also within the nasopharynx is the **pharyngeal tonsil** (also known as **adenoids**). This mass of lymphoid tissue typically is found to arise from the base of the posterior nasopharynx. By virtue of its proximity to the velopharyngeal port, the tissue of the pharyngeal tonsil may provide support for velar function. Removal of the adenoids from children with short or hypotrophied soft palates may result in persistent hypernasality.

The final cavities of concern to articulation are the nasal cavities (see Figure 7-32). The nasal cavities are produced by the paired maxillae, palatine, and nasal bones, and are divided by the nasal septum, made up of the singular vomer bone, perpendicular plate of the ethmoid, and the cartilaginous septum (as discussed in the previous section). The nasal cavities and turbinates are covered with mucous membrane endowed with beating and secreting epithelia, as well as a rich vascular supply. Air entering the nasal cavities is quickly warmed and humidified

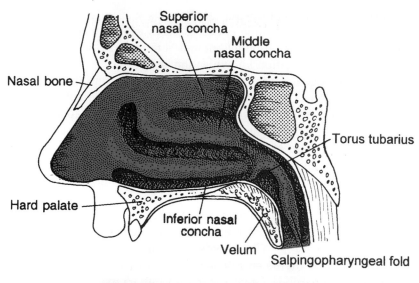

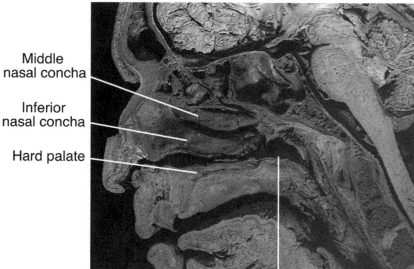

Figure 7-32. Nasal cavity and nasopharynx.

to protect the lungs, and fine nasal hairs help prevent particulate matter from entering the lower respiratory passageway. Beating epithelia propel encapsulated pollutants toward the nasopharynx, from whence they slowly work their way toward the esophagus, to be swallowed (a much better fate than being deposited in the lungs).

The **nares** or nostrils mark the anterior boundaries of the nasal cavities, while the **nasal choanae** are the posterior portals connecting the nasopharynx and nasal cavities. The floor of the nasal cavity is the hard palate of the oral cavity, specifically the palatine processes of the maxillae and horizontal plates of the palatine bones.

choaeae: *Gr., funnel*

Palpation of the Oral Cavity

This palpation exercise is best performed with one of your friends, and requires aseptic procedures. You will want to perform it under the guidance of your instructor, as this will be a procedure that will carry into the oral peripheral examination in your clinical practice. A flashlight will help you identify structures.

Have your friend open her mouth as you look inside. Ensure that your nondominant hand (e.g., left hand if you are right-handed) is the only hand that holds the flashlight, as the other hand is gloved and must not touch anything but your friend. Ask your friend to say "ah" and watch the velum in back elevate. Look for presence or absence of the palatine tonsils between the faucial pillars. Shine the light on the hard palate and note the median raphe and rugae. Now palpate both of these structures, running your finger back along both sides of the median raphe of the hard palate. Palpate the margin of the hard and soft palate, being sensitive to the fact that this may elicit a gag reflex in some people. As you palpate the hard palate, be sensitive to the potential presence of occult (hidden; submucous) clefts of the hard palate.

Have your friend bite lightly on her molars and hold her teeth closed but lips open for an /i/ vowel. With the gloved finger, palpate the lateral margins of the teeth and gums. With a tongue depressor, move the cheeks away from the teeth and examine the relationship between the upper and lower teeth for occlusion.

Pull the lower lip down gently and examine the labial frenulum. Ask your friend to open her mouth and elevate her tongue, and examine the lingual frenulum.

To summarize, the **cavities** of the articulatory system can be likened to a series of linked tubes.

- The most posterior of the tubes is the vertically directed **pharynx**, made up of the **laryngopharynx**, **oropharynx**, and **nasopharynx**.
- The horizontally coursing tube representing the nasal cavities arises from the nasopharynx, with the nasal and nasopharyngeal regions entirely separated from the oral cavity by elevation of the **soft palate**.
- The large tube representing the **oral cavity** is flanked by the small **buccal cavities**.
- The shape and size of the oral cavity is altered through movement of the tongue and mandible, and the nasal cavity may be coupled with the oral/pharyngeal cavities by means of the **velum**.
- The shape of the pharyngeal cavity is altered primarily by use of the **pharyngeal constrictor muscles** and by elevation or depression of the larynx.

Let us examine the muscles involved in the articulatory system. The summary table in Appendix E may assist you in your study of these muscles.

Eustachian Tube Development

The Eustachian tube is the communicative port between the nasopharynx and middle ear cavity. It is opened during deglutition and yawning and provides a means of aeration of the middle ear cavity. In the adult, the Eustachian tube courses down at an angle of about 45°. In the infant, the tube is more horizontal, with the shift in angle of descent brought about by head growth. It is felt that this horizontal course in the infant contributes to middle ear disease, with the assumption being that liquids and bacteria have a low-resistance path to the middle ear from the nasopharynx of an infant being bottle-fed in the supine position.

MUSCLES OF THE FACE AND MOUTH

The articulatory system is dominated by three significant structures, the lips, the tongue, and the velum. Movement of the lips for speech is a product of the muscles of the face, while the tongue capitalizes on its own musculature and that of the mandible and hyoid for its movement. The muscles of the velum elevate that structure to completely separate the oral and nasal regions. Table 7-4 may assist you in organizing the muscles of the face and mouth, while Figure 7-33 will help you recognize their functions.

Muscles of the Face

- **Orbicularis oris**
- **Risorius**
- **Buccinator**
- **Levator labii superioris**
- **Zygomatic minor**
- **Levator labii superioris alaeque nasi**
- **Levator anguli oris**
- **Zygomatic major**
- **Depressor labii inferioris**
- **Depressor anguli oris**
- **Mentalis**
- **Platysma**

Orbicularis Oris. The lips form the focus of the facial muscles, as their movement largely determines their function in both facial expression and speech (see Figure 7-33). The lips are comprised of muscle and mucous membrane that is richly invested with vascular supply, a trait made apparent by the translucent superficial epithelia. Although the lips

Table 7-4. Muscles of articulation.

MUSCLES OF THE FACE

Orbicularis oris	Levator anguli oris
Risorius	Zygomatic major
Buccinator	Depressor labii inferioris
Levator labii superioris	Depressor anguli oris
Zygomatic minor	Mentalis
Levator labii superioris alaeque nasi	Platysma

INTRINSIC TONGUE MUSCLES

Superior longitudinal
Inferior longitudinal
Transverse
Vertical

EXTRINSIC TONGUE MUSCLES

Genioglossus
Hyoglossus
Styloglossus
Chondroglossus
Palatoglossus

MANDIBULAR ELEVATORS AND DEPRESSORS

Masseter	Digastricus muscle
Temporalis muscle	Mylohyoid muscle
Medial pterygoid muscle	Geniohyoid muscle
Lateral pterygoid muscle	Platysma

MUSCLES OF THE VELUM

Levator veli palatini
Musculus uvulae
Tensor veli palatini
Palatoglossus
Palatopharyngeus

PHARYNGEAL MUSCULATURE

Superior pharyngeal constrictor	Thyropharyngeus muscle
Middle pharyngeal constrictor	Salpingopharyngeus muscle
Inferior pharyngeal constrictor	Stylopharyngeus muscle
Cricopharyngeal muscle	

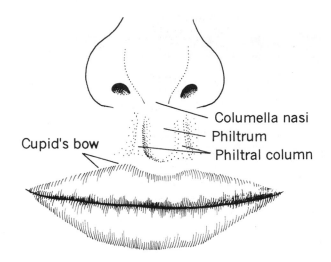

Columella nasi
Philtrum
Philtral column
Cupid's bow

Figure 7-33. Landmarks of the lips.

serve a significant articulatory function, their social, cultural, and aesthetic value as a central feature of the face is quite important. In cases where symmetry and morphology of the lips are compromised, as in clefting of the lip, the plastic surgeon will perform precise examination and measurement of the structure prior to performing exacting procedures to restore aesthetic balance.

To the plastic surgeon, the fine points of the **cupid's bow** are extremely important. The symmetry of this region is judged by the grace of its curve and its relationship to the columella and **philtrum**.

The **orbicularis oris** has been characterized as both a single muscle encircling the mouth opening (see Figure 7-34) and paired upper and lower muscles (**orbicularis oris superior** and **orbicularis oris inferior**). As we shall see in Chapter 8, there is ample evidence for *functional* differentiation of the upper and lower orbicularis oris. The upper and lower orbicularis oris act much like a drawstring to pull the lips closer together and effect a labial seal. The orbicularis oris is innervated by the mandibular marginal and lower buccal branches of the VII facial nerve.

The orbicularis oris serves as the point of insertion for many other muscles and interacts with the muscles of the face to produce the wide variety of facial gestures of which we are capable. The muscles inserting

columella: *L., small column*

Muscle:	Orbicularis oris inferior and superior
Origin:	Corner of lips
Course:	Laterally within lips
Insertion:	Opposite corner of lips
Innervation:	VII facial nerve
Function:	Constrict oral opening

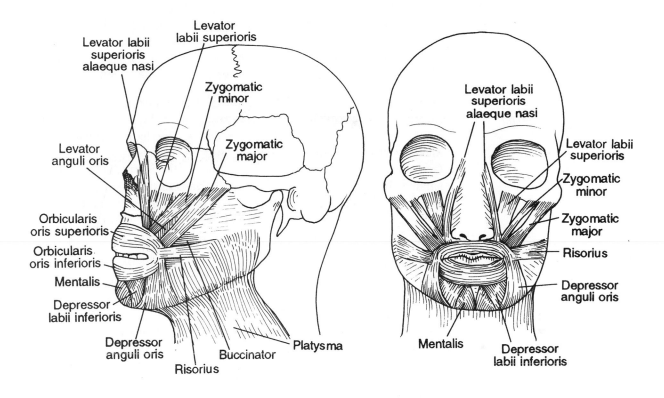

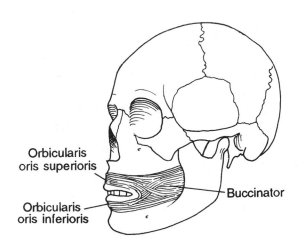

Figure 7-34. Muscles of the face.

into the orbicularis oris have different effects, based on their course and point of insertion into the lips. The risorius and buccinator muscles insert into the corners of the mouth and retract the lips. The depressor labii inferioris depresses the lower lip, and the levator labii superioris, zygomatic minor, and levator labii superioris alaeque nasi muscles elevate the upper lip. The zygomatic major muscle elevates and retracts the lips, whereas the depressor anguli oris depresses the corner of the mouth. The levator anguli oris pulls the corner of the mouth up and medially.

Risorius Muscle. It is evident from the course of the buccinator and risorius that they retract the corners of the mouth (see Figure 7-34). The buccinator is the dominant muscle of the cheeks. The **risorius muscle** is the most superficial of the pair, originating from the posterior region of the face along the fascia of the masseter muscle. The risorius is considerably smaller than the buccinator, coursing forward to insert into the corners of the mouth. The function of the risorius muscles is to retract the lips at the corners, facilitating smiling and grinning. Innervation of the risorius is by means of the buccal branch of the VII facial nerve.

Buccinator Muscle. The **buccinator muscle** ("bugler's muscle") lies deep to the risorius, following a parallel course. It originates on the pterygomandibular ligament, a tendinous slip running from the hamulus of the internal pterygoid plate of the sphenoid to the posterior mylohyoid line of the inner mandible. Fibers of the buccinator also arise from the posterior alveolar portion of the mandible and maxillae, while the posterior fibers appear to be continuous with those of the superior pharyngeal constrictor. The buccinator courses forward to insert into the upper and lower orbicularis oris.

The buccinator, like the risorius, is primarily involved in mastication. The buccinator is used to move food onto the grinding surfaces of the molars, and contraction of this muscle tends to constrict the oropharynx. The buccinator is innervated by the buccal branch of the VII facial nerve.

risorius: *L., laughing*

Muscle:	Risorius
Origin:	Posterior region of the face along the fascia of the masseter
Course:	Forward
Insertion:	Orbicularis oris at corners of mouth
Innervation:	Buccal branch of the VII facial nerve
Function:	Retracts lips at the corners

Muscle:	Buccinator
Origin:	Pterygomandibular ligament
Course:	Forward
Insertion:	Orbicularis oris at corners of mouth
Innervation:	Buccal branch of the VII facial nerve
Function:	Movement of food onto the grinding surfaces of the molars; oropharynx constriction

Levator Labii Superioris, Zygomatic Minor, and Levator Labii Superioris Alaeque Nasi Muscles. The levator labii superioris, zygomatic minor, and levator labii superioris alaeque nasi share a common insertion into the mid-lateral region of the upper lip, such that some anatomists refer to them as heads of the same muscle. The three hold the major responsibility for elevation of the upper lip.

The medial-most **levator labii superioris alaeque nasi** courses nearly vertically along the lateral margin of the nose, arising from the frontal process of the maxilla. The intermediate **levator labii superioris** originates from the infraorbital margin of the maxilla, coursing down and in to the upper lip. The **zygomatic minor** begins its downward course from the facial surface of the zygomatic bone.

Together, these three muscles are the dominant forces in lip elevation. Working in conjunction, these muscles readily dilate the oral opening, and fibers from the levator labii superioris alaeque nasi that insert into the wing of the nostril will flare the nasal opening. The levator labii superioris, zygomatic minor, and levator labii superioris alaeque nasi are innervated by the buccal branches of the VII facial nerve.

zygomatic: *Gr., zygoma, cheekbone*

Levator Anguli Oris. The **levator anguli oris** arises from the canine fossa of the maxilla, coursing to insert into the upper and lower lips. This muscle is obscured by the levator labii superioris. The levator

Muscle:	Levator labii superioris
Origin:	Infraorbital margin of the maxilla
Course:	Down and in to the upper lip
Insertion:	Mid-lateral region of the upper lip
Innervation:	Buccal branches of the VII facial nerve
Function:	Elevation of the upper lip

Muscle:	Zygomatic minor
Origin:	Facial surface of the zygomatic bone
Course:	Downward
Insertion:	Mid-lateral region of upper lip
Innervation:	Buccal branches of the VII facial nerve
Function:	Elevation of the upper lip

Muscle:	Levator labii alaeque nasi superioris
Origin:	Frontal process of maxilla
Course:	Vertically along the lateral margin of the nose
Insertion:	Mid-lateral region of the upper lip
Innervation:	Buccal branches of the VII facial nerve
Function:	Elevation of the upper lip

Muscle: Levator anguli oris
Origin: Canine fossa of maxilla
Course: Down
Insertion: Corners of upper and lower lips
Innervation: Superior buccal branches of VII facial nerve
Function: Draws corner of mouth up and medially

anguli oris draws the corner of the mouth up and medial-ward. The levator anguli oris is innervated by the superior buccal branches of the VII facial nerve.

Zygomatic Major.   The **zygomatic major muscle** (zygomaticus) arises lateral to the zygomatic minor on the zygomatic bone. It takes a more oblique course than the minor, inserting into the corner of the orbicularis oris. The zygomatic major elevates and retracts the angle of the mouth, as in the gesture of smiling. The zygomatic major muscle is innervated by the buccal branches of the VII facial nerve.

Depressor Labii Inferioris.   The **depressor labii inferioris** is the counterpart to the levator triad listed previously. It originates from the mandible at the oblique line, coursing up and in to insert into the lower lip. Contraction of the depressor labii inferioris dilates the orifice of the mouth by pulling the lips down and out. The depressor labii inferioris is innervated by the mandibular marginal branches of the VII facial nerve.

Muscle: Zygomatic major (zygomaticus)
Origin: Lateral to the zygomatic minor on zygomatic bone
Course: Obliquely down
Insertion: Corner of the orbicularis oris
Innervation: Elevates and retracts angle of mouth
Function: Buccal branches of the VII facial nerve

Muscle: Depressor labii inferioris
Origin: Mandible at the oblique line
Course: Up and in
Insertion: Lower lip
Innervation: Mandibular marginal branch of the VII facial nerve
Function: Dilates orifice by pulling lip down and out

Depressor Anguli Oris. The **depressor anguli oris** (triangularis) originates along the lateral margins of the mandible on the oblique line. Its
fanlike fibers converge on the orbicularis oris and upper lip at the corner. Contraction of the depressor anguli oris will depress the corners of
the mouth and, by virtue of attachment to upper lip, help compress the
upper lip against the lower lip, as well as help produce a frown. The
depressor anguli oris is innervated by the mandibular marginal branch
of the VII facial nerve.

Mentalis Muscle. The **mentalis muscle** arises from the region of the
incisive fossa of the mandible, inserting into the skin of the chin below.
Contraction of the mentalis elevates and wrinkles the chin and pulls the
lower lip out, as in pouting. The mentalis receives its innervation via the
mandibular marginal branch of the facial nerve.

Platysma. The **platysma** is more typically considered a muscle of the
neck, but it is discussed here because of its function as a mandibular
depressor. The platysma arises from the fascia overlying the pectoralis

platysma: *Gr., plate*

Muscle:	Depressor anguli oris
Origin:	Lateral margins of mandible on oblique line
Course:	Fanlike upward
Insertion:	Orbicularis oris and upper lip corner
Innervation:	Mandibular branch of the VII facial nerve
Function:	Depresses corners of mouth and helps to compress upper lip against lower lip

Muscle:	Mentalis
Origin:	Region of the incisive fossa of mandible
Course:	Down
Insertion:	Skin of the chin below
Innervation:	Mandibular marginal branch of the VII facial nerve
Function:	Elevates and wrinkles chin and pulls lower lip out

Muscle:	Platysma
Origin:	Fascia overlaying pectoralis major and deltoid
Course:	Up
Insertion:	Corner of the mouth, region below symphysis mente, lower margin of mandible, and skin near masseter
Innervation:	Cervical branch of the VII facial nerve
Function:	Depression of the mandible

major and deltoid, coursing up to insert into the corner of the mouth, the region below the symphysis mente, and the lower margin of the mandible, fanning as well to insert into the skin near the masseter. The platysma is highly variable, but appears to assist in depression of the mandible. Its proximity to the external jugular vein has led to speculation that it promotes venous drainage. The platysma is innervated by the cervical branch of the VII facial nerve.

In summary, the muscles of **facial expression** are important for articulation involving the lips.

- Numerous muscles insert into the **orbicularis oris** inferior and superior muscles, providing a flexible system for lip **protrusion**, **closure**, **retraction**, **elevation**, and **depression**.
- The **risorius** and **buccinator** muscles assist in retraction of the lips, as well as supporting entrapment of air within the oral cavity.
- Contraction of the **levator labii superioris**, **zygomatic minor**, and **levator labii superioris alaeque nasi** elevate the upper lip, and contraction of the **depressor labii inferioris** depresses the lower lip.
- Contraction of the **zygomatic major** muscle elevates and retracts the corners of the mouth, while the **depressor labii inferioris** pulls the lips down and out.
- The **depressor anguli oris** muscle depresses the corner of the mouth, the **mentalis** muscle pulls the lower lip out, and the **platysma** depresses the mandible.

Muscles of the Mouth

Musculature of the mouth is dominated by intrinsic and extrinsic muscles of the tongue, as well as those responsible for elevation of the soft palate. Movement of the tongue is an interesting engineering feat, as you shall see.

The Tongue

The tongue is a massive structure occupying the floor of the mouth. If you take a moment to examine Figure 7-35, you can get some notion of the magnitude of this organ. When a child uses the tongue as an expressive instrument, she or he protrudes only a small portion of it, leaving the bulk of the tongue within the mouth. We divide the muscles of the tongue into intrinsic and extrinsic musculature, a division that proves to be both anatomical and functional. The extrinsic muscles tend to move the tongue into the general region desired, while the intrinsic muscles tend to provide the fine, graded control of the articulatory gesture. The tongue is involved primarily in mastication and deglutition, being responsible for movement of food within the oral cavity to position it for chewing and to propel it backward for swallowing.

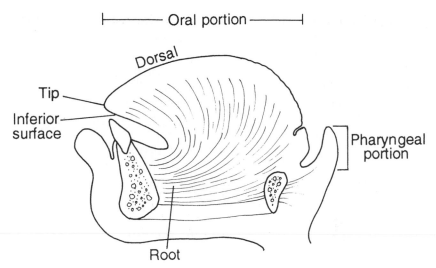

Figure 7-35. Demarcation of regions of the tongue.

The tongue is divided longitudinally by the **median fibrous septum**, a dividing wall between right and left halves that serves as the point of origin for the transverse muscle of the tongue. The septum originates on the body of the hyoid bone via the hyoglossal membrane, forming the tongue attachment with the hyoid. The septum courses the length of the tongue.

It is useful to divide the tongue into regions as we discuss its characteristics (see Figure 7-35). The superior surface is referred to as the **dorsum**, and the anterior-most portion is the **tip** or **apex**. The **base** of the tongue is the portion of the tongue that resides in the oropharynx. The portion of the tongue surface within the oral cavity, referred to as the **oral** or **palatine surface**, makes up about two-thirds of the surface of the tongue. The other third of the tongue surface lies within the oropharynx and is referred to as the **pharyngeal surface**.

The mucous membrane covering the tongue dorsum has numerous landmarks (see Figure 7-36). The prominent central or **median sulcus** divides the tongue into left and right sides. The posterior of the tongue is invested with **lingual papillae**, small, irregular prominences on the surface of the tongue. The **terminal sulcus** marks the posterior palatine surface, and the center of this groove is the **foramen cecum**, a deep recess in the tongue.

Beneath the membranous lining of the pharyngeal surface of the tongue are **lingual tonsils**, groups of lymphoid tissue. Taken in conjunction with the pharyngeal and palatine tonsils, the lingual tonsils form the final portion of the ring of lymph tissue in the oral and pharyngeal cavities. Tonsils tend to atrophy over time. Although the pharyngeal and palatine tonsils may be quite prominent during childhood, they are markedly diminished in size by puberty.

papillae: *L., nipple*

cecum: *L., caecum, blindness*

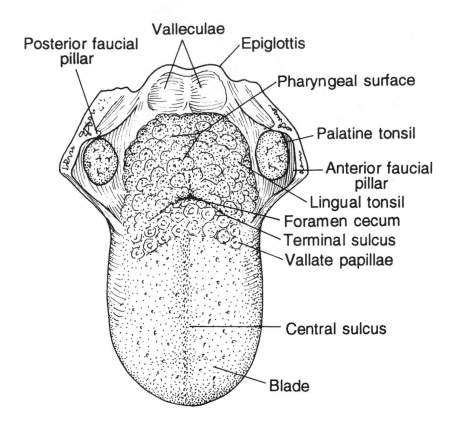

Figure 7-36. Landmarks of the tongue.

The tongue is invested with taste buds to convey the gustatory sense. The anterior tongue has receptors that are primarily sensitive to both sweet and sour tastes, and the sides of the tongue are sensitive primarily to sour tastes. Bitter tastes are sensed near the terminal sulcus. The sensors, or "taste buds," are located in the various papillae found on the tongue, as will be discussed in detail in Chapter 9.

If you examine the inferior surface of your tongue in a mirror, you will see three important landmarks (see Figure 7-37). Notice the rich vascular supply on that undersurface: Medications administered under the tongue will be very quickly absorbed into the bloodstream. You will see a prominent band of tissue running from the inner mandibular mucosa to the underside of the tongue. The **lingual frenulum** (or **lingual frenum**) joins the inferior tongue and the mandible, perhaps stabilizing the tongue during movement. Notice also the transverse band of tissue on either side of the tongue (the **sublingual fold**). At this point are the ducts for the sublingual salivary glands. Lateral to the lingual frenulum are the ducts for the submandibular salivary glands that are hidden under the mucosa on the inner surface of the mandible. These salivary glands and their function are discussed in detail in Chapter 9.

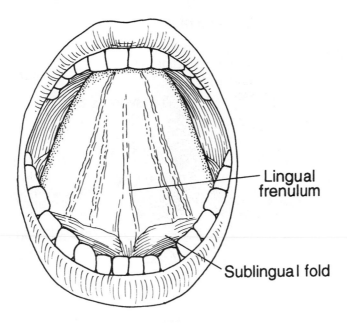

Lingual
frenulum

Sublingual fold

Figure 7-37. Inferior surface of tongue.

Intrinsic Tongue Muscles

The intrinsic muscles of the tongue include two pairs of muscles running longitudinally, as well as muscles coursing transversely and vertically. At the outset we should note that the intrinsic muscles of the tongue interact in a complex fashion to produce the rapid, delicate articulations needed for speech and nonspeech activities. As we discuss each muscle, we will provide you with the basic function, but will deal more fully with the integration of these muscles in Chapter 8. Examination of Figure 7-38 will assist you in our discussion of these very important lingual muscles.

- **Superior longitudinal**
- **Inferior longitudinal**
- **Transverse**
- **Vertical**

Tongue Tie

The *lingual frenulum* is a band of tissue connecting the tongue to the floor of the mouth. It appears to assist in stabilizing the tongue during movement, but occasionally may be too short for proper lingual function. This condition, colloquially referred to as **tongue tie**, will result in difficulty elevating the tongue for phonemes requiring palatal or alveolar contact. The tongue may appear heart-shaped when protruded, resulting from the excessive tension on the midline by the short frenulum. A surgical procedure to correct the condition may be useful, although such surgery is not minor.

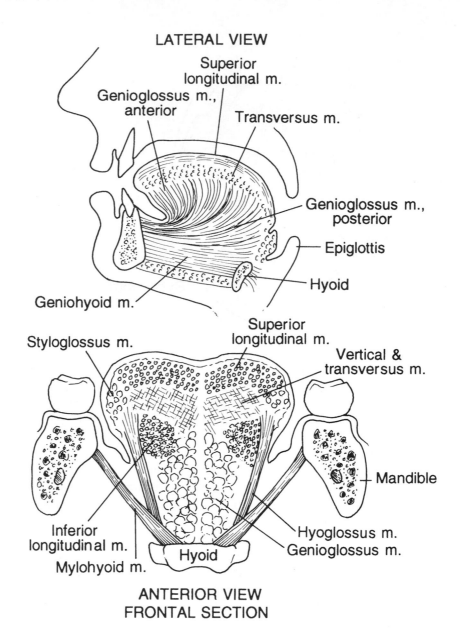

LATERAL VIEW

Figure 7-38. Intrinsic muscles of the tongue. (From data of Netter, 1997.)

ANTERIOR VIEW
FRONTAL SECTION

Superior Longitudinal Muscle of Tongue.   The **superior longitudinal muscle** courses along the length of the tongue, comprising the upper layer of the tongue. This muscle originates from the fibrous submucous layer near the epiglottis, the hyoid, and from the median fibrous septum. Its fibers fan forward and outward to insert into the lateral margins of the tongue and region of the apex. By virtue of their course and insertions, fibers of the superior longitudinal muscle tend to elevate the tip of

Muscle:	Superior longitudinal
Origin:	Fibrous submucous layer near the epiglottis, the hyoid, and from the median fibrous septum
Course:	Fans forward and outward
Insertion:	Lateral margins of the tongue and region of apex
Innervation:	XII hypoglossal nerve
Function:	Elevates, assists in retraction, or deviates tip of tongue

the tongue. If one superior longitudinal muscle is contracted without the other, it will tend to pull the tongue toward the side of contraction. Innervation of all intrinsic muscles of the tongue is by means of the XII hypoglossal nerve.

Inferior Longitudinal Muscle.   The **inferior longitudinal muscle** originates at the root of the tongue and corpus hyoid, with fibers coursing to the apex of the tongue. This muscle occupies the lower sides of the tongue, but is absent in the medial tongue base, which is occupied by the extrinsic genioglossus muscle (to be described in a later section). The inferior longitudinal muscle pulls the tip of the tongue downward and assists in retraction of the tongue if co-contracted with the superior longitudinal. As with the superior longitudinal, unilateral contraction of the inferior longitudinal will cause the tongue to turn toward the contracted side and downward. Innervation of all intrinsic muscles of the tongue is by means of the contralateral XII hypoglossal nerve.

Transverse Muscles of the Tongue.   The **transverse muscles of the tongue** provide a mechanism for narrowing the tongue. Fibers of these muscles originate at the median fibrous septum and course laterally to insert into the side of the tongue in the submucous tissue. Some fibers of the transverse muscle continue as the palatopharyngeus muscle, to be described in a later section. The transverse muscle of the tongue pulls the edges of the tongue toward the midline, effectively narrowing the tongue. Innervation of all intrinsic muscles of the tongue is by means of the XII hypoglossal nerve.

Muscle:	Inferior longitudinal
Origin:	Root of the tongue and corpus hyoid
Course:	Forward
Insertion:	Apex of the tongue
Innervation:	XII hypoglossal nerve
Function:	Pulls tip of tongue downward, assists in retraction, deviates tongue

Muscle: Transverse muscles of the tongue
Origin: Median fibrous septum
Course: Laterally
Insertion: Side of the tongue in the submucous tissue
Innervation: XII hypoglossal nerve
Function: Provide a mechanism for narrowing the tongue

Vertical Muscles of the Tongue. The **vertical muscles of the tongue** run at right angles to the transverse muscles and flatten the tongue. Fibers of the vertical muscle course from the base of the tongue and insert into the membranous cover. The fibers of the transverse and vertical muscles interweave. Contraction of the vertical muscles of the tongue will pull the tongue down into the floor of the mouth. Innervation of all intrinsic muscles of the tongue is by means of the XII hypoglossal nerve.

Extrinsic Tongue Muscles

- **Genioglossus**
- **Hyoglossus**
- **Styloglossus**
- **Chondroglossus**
- **Palatoglossus**

The intrinsic muscles of the tongue are responsible for precise articulatory performance and the extrinsic muscles of the tongue tend to move the tongue as a unit. It appears that they set the general posture for articulation, with the intrinsic muscles performing the refined perfection of that gesture.

Genioglossus Muscle. The **genioglossus** is the prime mover of the tongue, making up most of its deeper bulk. As you can see from Figure 7-39, the genioglossus arises from the inner mandibular surface at the symphysis and fans to insert into the tip and dorsum of the tongue, as well as to the corpus of the hyoid bone.

Muscle: Vertical muscles of the tongue
Origin: Base of the tongue
Course: Vertically
Insertion: Membranous cover
Innervation: XII hypoglossal nerve
Function: Pull tongue down into the floor of the mouth

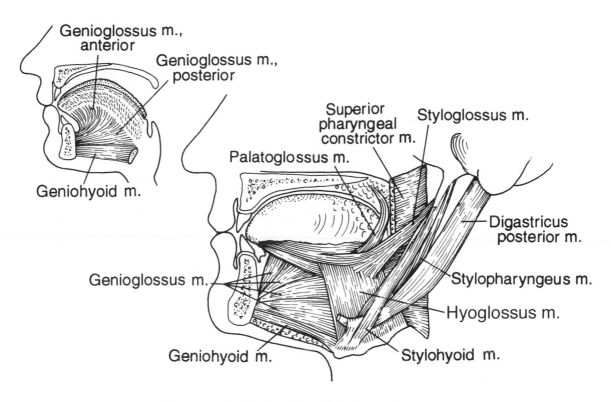

Genioglossus m.,
anterior

Genioglossus m.,
posterior

Superior
pharyngeal
constrictor m.

Styloglossus m.

Palatoglossus m.

Geniohyoid m.

Digastricus
posterior m.

Genioglossus m.

Stylopharyngeus m.

Hyoglossus m.

Geniohyoid m.

Stylohyoid m.

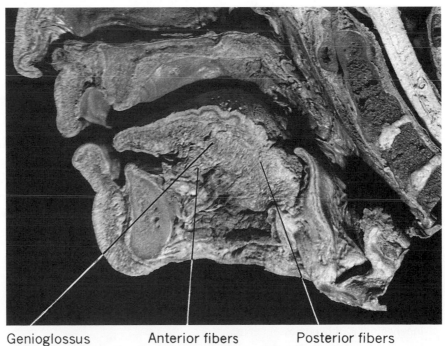

Genioglossus   Anterior fibers   Posterior fibers

A

Figure 7-39. A. Genioglossus and related muscles. *(continues)*

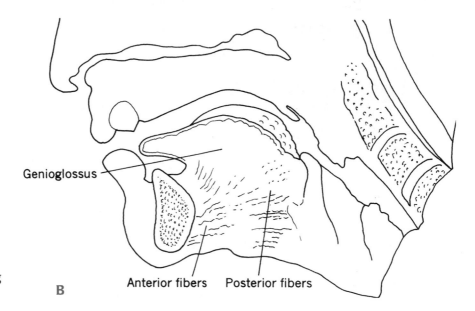

Figure 7-39. *(continued)*
B. Drawing of photo showing landmarks.

The genioglossus muscle occupies a medial position in the tongue, with the inferior longitudinal muscle, hyoglossus, and styloglossus being lateral to it. Fibers of the genioglossus insert into the entire surface of the tongue, but are sparse to absent in the tip. Contraction of the anterior fibers of the genioglossus muscle results in retraction of the tongue, whereas contraction of the posterior fibers draws the tongue forward to aid protrusion of the apex. If both anterior and posterior portions are contracted, the middle portion of the tongue will be drawn down into the floor of the mouth, functionally cupping the tongue along its length. Needless to say, we will return to the interaction of the genioglossus and intrinsic muscles when we discuss deglutition. The genioglossus is innervated by the XII hypoglossal nerve.

Hyoglossus Muscle.   As the name implies, the **hyoglossus** arises from the length of the greater cornu and lateral body of the hyoid bone, coursing upward to insert into the sides of the tongue between the styloglossus (to be discussed) and the inferior longitudinal muscles. The hyoglossus pulls the sides of the tongue down, in direct antagonism to

Muscle:	Genioglossus
Origin:	Inner mandibular surface at symphysis
Course:	Fans up, back, and forward
Insertion:	Tip and dorsum of tongue and corpus hyoid
Innervation:	XII hypoglossal nerve
Function:	Anterior fibers retract tongue; posterior fibers protrude tongue; together, anterior and posterior fibers depress tongue

Muscle:	Hyoglossus
Origin:	Length of greater cornu and lateral body of hyoid
Course:	Upward
Insertion:	Sides of tongue between styloglossus and inferior longitudinal muscles
Innervation:	XII hypoglossal nerve
Function:	Pulls sides of tongue down

the palatoglossus (to be discussed). The hyoglossus is innervated by the XII hypoglossal nerve.

Styloglossus.   If you examine Figure 7-39 again, you will see that the **styloglossus** originates from the anterolateral margin of the styloid process of the temporal bone, coursing forward and down to insert into the inferior sides of the tongue. It divides into two portions: one interdigitates with the inferior longitudinal muscle, and the other with the fibers of the hyoglossus. As you can guess from examination of the course and insertion of this muscle, contraction of the paired styloglossi will draw the tongue back and up. The styloglossus is innervated by the XII hypoglossal nerve.

Chondroglossus.   The **chondroglossus** muscle is often considered to be part of the hyoglossus muscle. As with the hyoglossus, the chondroglossus arises from the hyoid (lesser cornu), coursing up to interdigitate with the intrinsic muscles of the tongue medial to the point of insertion of the hyoglossus. The chondroglossus is a depressor of the tongue. The chondroglossus is innervated by the XII hypoglossal nerve.

chondroglossus: *Gr., chondros, cartilage + glossus, tongue*

Muscle:	Styloglossus
Origin:	Anterolateral margin of styloid process
Course:	Forward and down
Insertion:	Inferior sides of the tongue
Innervation:	XII hypoglossal nerve
Function:	Draws the tongue back and up

Muscle:	Chondroglossus
Origin:	Lesser cornu hyoid
Course:	Up
Insertion:	Interdigitates with intrinsic muscles of the tongue medial to hyoglossus
Innervation:	XII hypoglossal nerve
Function:	Depresses the tongue

Muscle:	Palatoglossus
Origin:	Anterolateral palatal aponeurosis
Course:	Down
Insertion:	Sides of posterior tongue
Innervation:	Pharyngeal plexus from the XI accessory and X vagus nerves
Function:	Elevates tongue or depresses soft palate

Palatoglossus. The **palatoglossus** may be functionally defined as a muscle of the tongue or of the velum, although it is more closely allied with palatal architecture and origin (see Figures 7-43 and 7-45). It will be described in a later section, but you should realize that it serves the dual purpose of depressing the soft palate or elevating the back of the tongue. The palatoglossus makes up the anterior faucial pillar.

To summarize:

- The **tongue** is a massive structure occupying the floor of the mouth. It is divided by a **median fibrous septum** that provides the origination for the transverse intrinsic muscle of the tongue.
- The tongue is divided into **dorsum**, **apex** (tip), and **base**.
- Fine movements are produced by contraction of the intrinsic musculature (**transverse**, **vertical**, **inferior longitudinal**, and **superior longitudinal** muscles of the tongue).
- Larger adjustments of lingual movement are completed through use of **extrinsic muscles**. The **genioglossus** retracts, protrudes, or depresses the tongue. The **hyoglossus** and **chondroglossus** depress the tongue, while the **styloglossus** and **palatoglossus** elevate the posterior tongue.

Muscles of Mastication: Mandibular Elevators and Depressors

mastication: *L., masticare, chewing*

The process of chewing food, or **mastication**, requires movement of the mandible so that the molars can make a solid, grinding contact. The muscles of mastication are among the strongest of the body, and the coordinated contraction of these muscles is required for proper food preparation. The muscles of mastication include the mandibular elevators (masseter, temporalis, medial pterygoid), muscles of protrusion (lateral pterygoid), and depressors (digastricus, mylohyoid, geniohyoid, platysma).

- **Masseter**
- **Temporalis**
- **Medial pterygoid**
- **Lateral pterygoid**
- **Digastricus**

- Mylohyoid
- Geniohyoid
- Platysma

Masseter.   As you may see from Figure 7-40, the **masseter** is the most superficial of the muscles of mastication. This massive quadrilateral muscle originates on the lateral, inferior, and medial surfaces of the zygomatic arch, coursing down to insert primarily into the ramus of the mandible, but with some of the deeper fibers terminating on the coronoid process. The course and attachments of the masseter make it ideally suited for placing maximum force on the molars. Contraction of this muscle elevates the mandible, and when the teeth are clenched, the prominent muscular belly is clearly visible. The masseter is innervated by the anterior trunk of the mandibular nerve arising from the V trigeminal.

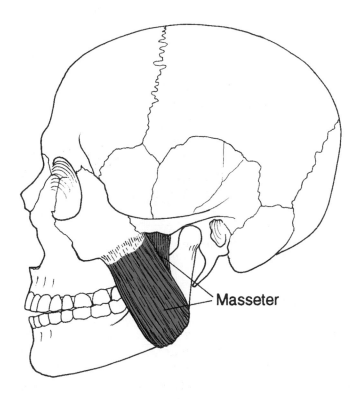

Masseter

Figure 7-40. Graphic representation of masseter.

Muscle:	Masseter
Origin:	Zygomatic arch
Course:	Down
Insertion:	Ramus of the mandible and coronoid process
Innervation:	Anterior trunk of mandibular nerve arising from the V trigeminal
Function:	Elevates mandible

Temporalis Muscle. The **temporalis muscle** is deep to the masseter, arising from a region of the temporal and parietal bones known as the **temporal fossa**. As you can see in Figure 7-41, it arises from a broad region of the lateral skull, converging as it courses down and forward. The terminal tendon of the temporalis passes through the zygomatic arch and inserts in the coronoid process and ramus. The temporalis elevates the mandible and draws it back if protruded. It appears to be capable of more rapid contraction than the masseter. The temporalis is innervated by the temporal branches arising from the mandibular nerve of V trigeminal.

pterygoid: *Gr., pterygodes, wing*

Medial Pterygoid Muscle. The **medial pterygoid muscle** (also known as the **internal pterygoid muscle**) originates from the medial pterygoid plate and fossa lateral to it (see Figure 7-42). Fibers from the muscle

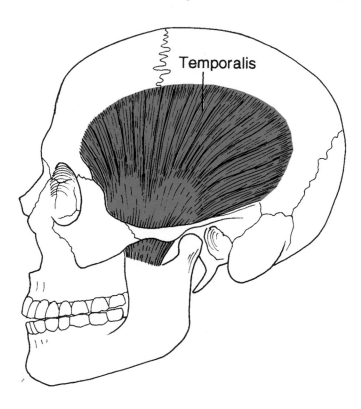

Temporalis

Figure 7-41. Graphic representation of temporalis.

Muscle:	Temporalis
Origin:	Temporal fossa of temporal and parietal bones
Course:	Converging downward and forward, through the zygomatic arch
Insertion:	Coronoid process and ramus
Innervation:	Temporal branches arising from the mandibular nerve of V trigeminal
Function:	Elevates the mandible and draws it back if protruded

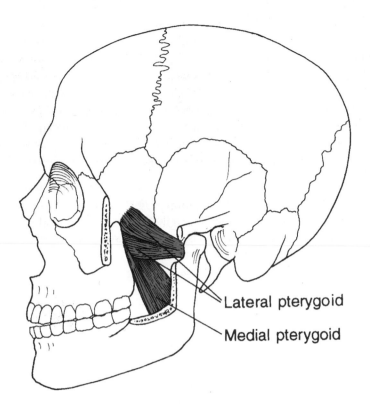

Figure 7-42. Lateral and medial pterygoid muscles.

course down and back to insert into the mandibular ramus. The medial pterygoid muscle elevates the mandible, acting in conjunction with the masseter. The medial pterygoid muscle is innervated by the mandibular division of the V trigeminal nerve.

Lateral Pterygoid Muscle.   The **lateral** (or external) **pterygoid muscle** arises from the sphenoid bone. One head of the lateral pterygoid arises from the lateral pterygoid plate (hence the name of the muscle); another head attaches to the greater wing of the sphenoid. Fibers course back to insert into the pterygoid fovea of the mandible, the lower inner margin of the condyloid process of the mandible (see Figure 7-42). Contraction of the lateral pterygoid muscle protrudes the mandible, and it works in contrast with the mandibular elevators for grinding action at the molars.

Muscle:	Medial pterygoid
Origin:	Medial pterygoid plate and fossa
Course:	Down and back
Insertion:	Mandibular ramus
Innervation:	Mandibular division of the V trigeminal nerve
Function:	Elevates the mandible

Tongue Thrust

As with other motor functions, swallowing develops from immature to mature forms. The immature swallow capitalizes on the needs of the moment: An infant needs to compress his or her mother's nipple to stimulate release of milk, so the tongue moves forward naturally during this process. As the infant develops teeth, anterior movement of the tongue is blocked even as the need for it diminishes. The child begins eating semisolid and solid food, and chewing becomes more important than sucking. The mature swallow propels a bolus back toward the oropharynx, a maneuver requiring posterior direction of the tongue.

If the child fails to develop the mature swallow, he or she has a condition known as **tongue thrust**. The anterior direction of the tongue will cause labioversion of the incisors. This child may have flaccid oral musculature, weak masseter action during swallow, and a disorganized approach to generation of the bolus. Considering that we swallow between 400 and 600 times per day, the immature swallow is difficult (but far from impossible) to reorganize into a mature swallow. Many speech-language pathologists specialize in **oral myofunctional therapy** directed toward remediation of such problems, a rich and rewarding practice that results in (literally) smiling clients (see Zickefoose, 1989). Chapter 9 discusses issues related to tongue thrust.

The lateral pterygoid muscle is innervated by the mandibular branch of the V trigeminal nerve.

digastric: *L., two + belly*

Digastricus.   The dual-bellied digastricus was described in Chapter 5, so it is only briefly discussed here. The **digastricus anterior** originates on the inner surface of the mandible at the digastricus fossa, near the symphysis, while the **digastricus posterior** originates on the mastoid process of the temporal bone. The anterior fibers course medially and down to the hyoid, where they join with the posterior digastricus by means of an intermediate tendon that inserts into the hyoid at the juncture of the hyoid corpus and greater cornu. If the hyoid bone is fixed by infrahyoid musculature, contraction of the anterior component will result in depression of the mandible. The anterior belly is innervated by the mandibular branch of the V trigeminal nerve via the mylohyoid branch of the inferior alveolar nerve. The posterior belly is supplied by the digastric branch of the VII facial nerve.

Muscle:	Lateral pterygoid (external pterygoid)
Origin:	Lateral pterygoid plate and greater wing of sphenoid
Course:	Back
Insertion:	Pterygoid fovea of the mandible
Innervation:	Mandibular branch of the V trigeminal nerve
Function:	Protrudes the mandible

Muscle: Digastricus anterior

Origin: Inner surface of mandible at digastricus fossa, near the symphysis

Course: Medially and down

Insertion: Intermediate tendon to juncture of hyoid corpus and greater cornu

Innervation: Mandibular branch of V trigeminal nerve via the mylohyoid branch of the inferior alveolar nerve

Function: Pulls hyoid forward; depresses mandible if in conjunction with digastricus posterior

Muscle: Digastricus posterior

Origin: Mastoid process of temporal bone

Course: Medially and down

Insertion: Intermediate tendon to juncture of hyoid corpus and greater cornu

Innervation: Digastric branch of the VII facial nerve

Function: Pulls hyoid back; depresses mandible if in conjunction with anterior digastricus

Mylohyoid Muscle. This muscle was described in Chapter 5. The **mylohyoid** originates on the underside of the mandible and courses to the corpus hyoid. This fanlike muscle courses from the **mylohyoid line** of the mandible to the median fibrous raphe and inferiorly to the hyoid, forming the floor of the mouth. With the hyoid fixed in position, the mylohyoid will depress the mandible. The mylohyoid is innervated by the alveolar nerve, arising from the V trigeminal nerve, mandibular branch.

Geniohyoid Muscle. Also described in Chapter 5, the **geniohyoid muscle** originates at the mental spines of the mandible, and projects parallel

Muscle: Mylohyoid

Origin: Mylohyoid line, inner mandible

Course: Back and down

Insertion: Median fibrous raphe and inferiorly to hyoid

Innervation: Alveolar nerve, arising from the V trigeminal nerve, mandibular branch

Function: Depresses the mandible

Muscle: Geniohyoid

Origin: Mental spines of the mandible

Course: Medially

Insertion: Corpus hyoid

Innervation: XII hypoglossal nerve

Function: Depresses the mandible

to the anterior digastricus from the inner mandibular surface to insert into the corpus hyoid. Contraction of the geniohyoid depresses the mandible if the hyoid is fixed. Innervation of the geniohyoid is by means of the XII hypoglossal nerve.

Platysma. The platysma was discussed in the "Muscles of the Face" section.

To summarize, the muscles of **mastication** include mandibular **elevators** and **depressors**, as well as muscles to **protrude** the mandible.

- Mandibular elevators include the **masseter, temporalis**, and **medial pterygoid** muscles, while the **lateral pterygoid** protrudes the mandible.
- Depression of the mandible is performed by the **mylohyoid, geniohyoid**, and **platysma** muscles. The grinding action of the molars requires coordinated and synchronized contraction of the muscles of mastication.

Muscles of the Velum

Only three speech sounds in English require that the soft palate be depressed (/m/, /ŋ/ and /n/). During most speaking time and during swallowing, the soft palate is actively elevated. We will discuss the general configuration of the soft palate and then discuss how we go about elevating and depressing this important structure.

The **soft palate** or **velum** is actually a combination of muscle, aponeurosis, nerves, and blood supply covered by mucous membrane lining. The **palatal aponeurosis** makes up the mid-front portion of the soft palate, being an extension of an aponeurosis arising from the tensor veli palatini (to be described). The palatal aponeurosis divides around the musculus uvulae, but serves as the point of insertion for other muscles of the soft palate. The mucous membrane lining is invested with lymph and mucous glands, and the oral side of the lining also has taste buds.

- **Levator veli palatini**
- **Musculus uvulae**
- **Tensor veli palatini**
- **Palatoglossus**
- **Palatopharyngeus**

Muscles of the soft palate include elevators (levator veli palatini, musculus uvulae), a tensor (tensor veli palatini), and depressors (palatoglossus and palatopharyngeus). Although the superior constrictor muscle is a pharyngeal muscle, it should be noted that it is an important muscle for function of the soft palate. We will discuss the muscles of the pharynx following discussion of the muscles of the soft palate. Figure 7-43 will assist you in the following discussion.

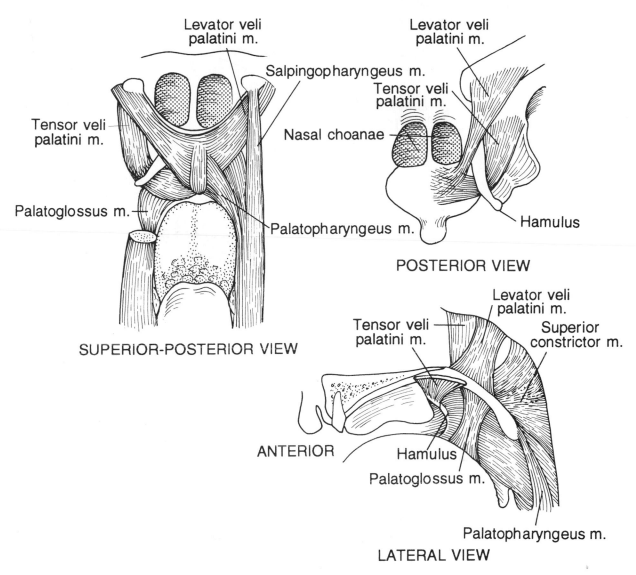

Figure 7-43. Muscles of the soft palate from superior-posterior (*left*), posterior (*right*), and the side (*lower figure*). (From data of Schprintzen & Bardach, 1995; Langley, Telford, & Christensen, 1969; and Williams & Warrick, 1980.)

Levator Veli Palatini Muscle. The **levator veli palatini** (or **levator palati**) is the palatal elevator, making up the bulk of the soft palate (see Figure 7-44). This muscle arises from the apex of the petrous portion of the temporal bone, as well as from the medial wall of the Eustachian tube cartilage. The levator veli palatini courses down and forward to insert into the palatal aponeurosis of the soft palate, lateral to the musculus uvulae. The levator veli palatini is the primary elevator of the soft palate. Contraction elevates and retracts the posterior velum.

levator: *L., lifter*

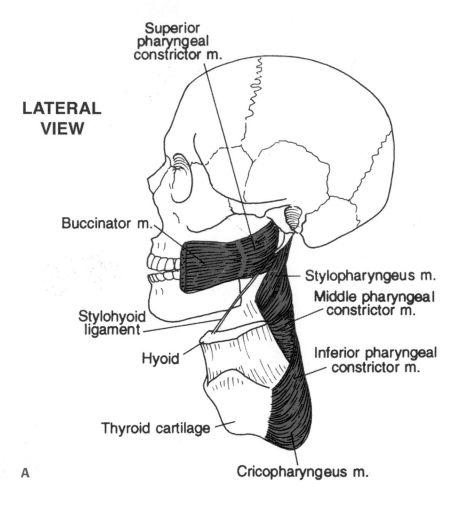

LATERAL
VIEW

Superior
pharyngeal
constrictor m.

Buccinator m.

Stylopharyngeus m.
Middle pharyngeal
constrictor m.

Stylohyoid
ligament

Hyoid

Inferior pharyngeal
constrictor m.

Thyroid cartilage

Cricopharyngeus m.

A

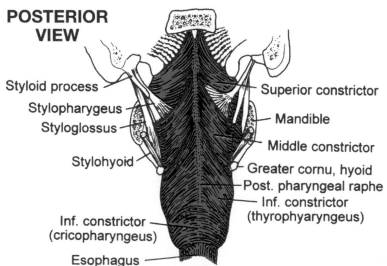

POSTERIOR
VIEW

Styloid process

Stylopharygeus

Styloglossus

Stylohyoid

Superior constrictor

Mandible

Middle constrictor

Greater cornu, hyoid

Post. pharyngeal raphe

Inf. constrictor
(thyrophyaryngeus)

Inf. constrictor
(cricopharyngeus)

Esophagus

B

Figure 7-44. A. Lateral view of
pharyngeal constrictor muscles.
B. Posterior view of pharyngeal
constrictor musculature.

Muscle:	Levator veli palatini (levator palati)
Origin:	Apex of petrous portion of temporal bone and medial wall of Eustachian tube cartilage
Course:	Down and forward
Insertion:	Palatal aponeurosis of soft palate, lateral to musculus uvulae
Innervation:	Pharyngeal plexus from the XI accessory and X vagus nerves
Function:	Elevates and retracts the posterior velum

The levator veli palatini is innervated by the pharyngeal plexus, arising from the XI accessory and X vagus nerves.

Musculus Uvulae.   Casual examination of the inner workings of your own mouth reveal the structure of the **musculus uvulae**. The **uvula** makes up the medial and posterior portions of the soft palate, and the musculus uvulae is the muscle embodied within this structure. This paired muscle arises from the posterior nasal spines of the palatine bones and from the palatal aponeurosis. Fibers run the length of the soft palate on either side of the midline, inserting into the mucous membrane cover of the velum. Contraction of the uvula shortens the soft palate, effectively bunching it up. The musculus uvulae is innervated by the pharyngeal plexus, arising from the XI accessory and X vagus nerves.

▶ **uvulae:** *L., little grapes*

Tensor Veli Palatini Muscle.   The **tensor veli palatini** (tensor veli palati) has long been viewed as a tensor of the soft palate, as well as the dilator of the Eustachian tube. In reality, the tensor veli palatini appears

Muscle:	Musculus uvulae
Origin:	Posterior nasal spines of the palatine bones and palatal aponeurosis
Course:	Runs the length of the soft palate
Insertion:	Mucous membrane cover of the velum
Innervation:	Pharyngeal plexus of XI accessory and X vagus nerves
Function:	Shortens the soft palate

Muscle:	Tensor veli palatini (tensor veli palati)
Origin:	Scaphoid fossa of sphenoid, sphenoid spine, and lateral Eustachian tube wall
Course:	Courses down, terminates in tendon that passes around pterygoid hamulus, then is directed medially
Insertion:	Palatal aponeurosis
Innervation:	Mandibular nerve of V trigeminal
Function:	Dilates Eustachian tube

only to function as a dilator of the Eustachian tube. This muscle arises from the sphenoid bone (scaphoid fossa between lateral and medial pterygoid plates, and sphenoid spine) as well as from the lateral Eustachian tube wall. The fibers converge to course down to terminate in a tendon. The tendon, in turn, passes around the pterygoid hamulus and then is directed medially. This tendon expands to become the palatal aponeurosis in conjunction with the tendon of the opposite side. Contraction of the tensor veli palatini dilates or opens the Eustachian tube, thereby permitting **aeration** (exchange of air) of the middle ear cavity. The tensor veli palatini muscle is the only muscle of the soft palate not innervated by the XI accessory nerve. This muscle receives its innervation by means of the mandibular nerve of the V trigeminal.

Palatoglossus Muscle. If you again look in your mouth using a mirror, you will be able to see the structure of the **palatoglossus** (see Figure 7-43). At the posterior of the oral cavity you will see two prominent arches that mark the entry to the pharynx. The arch closest to you is the anterior **faucial pillar**, and the muscle of which it is comprised is the palatoglossus. (While you are in there, take a look at the posterior faucial pillar, just behind it. That is the palatopharyngeus, to be discussed shortly.)

The palatoglossus muscle was discussed briefly as a muscle of the tongue, because it serves a dual purpose. This muscle originates at the anterolateral palatal aponeurosis, coursing down to insert into the sides of the posterior tongue. This muscle will either help to elevate the tongue, as mentioned earlier, or depress the soft palate. The fact that the soft palate, in its relaxed state, is depressed does not mean that we do not actively depress it, especially during speech. The palatoglossus is innervated by the pharyngeal plexus, arising from the XI accessory and X vagus nerves.

Palatopharyngeus Muscle. Although classically considered a pharyngeal muscle, the **palatopharyngeus** is included in this discussion because of its role in velar function (see Figure 7-43). Anterior fibers of the palatopharyngeus originate from the anterior hard palate, and posterior fibers arise from the midline of the soft palate posterior to the fibers of the levator veli palatini, attached to the palatal aponeurosis. Fibers of each muscle course laterally and down, forming the posterior faucial pil-

Muscle:	Palatoglossus
Origin:	Anterolateral palatal aponeurosis
Course:	Down
Insertion:	Sides of posterior tongue
Innervation:	Pharyngeal plexus from the XI accessory and X vagus nerves
Function:	Elevates tongue or depresses soft palate

Muscle:	Palatopharyngeus
Origin:	Anterior hard palate and midline of soft palate
Course:	Laterally and down
Insertion:	Posterior margin of the thyroid cartilage
Innervation:	Pharyngeal plexus from XI accessory and pharyngeal branch of X vagus nerve
Function:	Narrows pharynx; lowers soft palate

lar and inserting into the posterior thyroid cartilage. This muscle has wide variability, mingling with fibers of the stylopharyngeus and salpingopharyngeus muscles prior to its ultimate insertion into the posterior margin of the thyroid cartilage. This muscle will assist in narrowing the pharyngeal cavity, as well as lowering the soft palate. It may also help to elevate the larynx. The palatopharyngeus is innervated by the pharyngeal plexus, arising from the XI accessory and pharyngeal branch of the X vagus nerve.

Pharyngeal Musculature

- **Superior pharyngeal constrictor**
- **Middle pharyngeal constrictor**
- **Inferior pharyngeal constrictor**
- **Cricopharyngeal muscle**
- **Thyropharyngeus muscle**
- **Salpingopharyngeus**
- **Stylopharyngeus muscle**

Muscles of the pharynx are closely allied with the tongue, muscles of the face, and laryngeal musculature. It will help if you imagine the pharynx as a vertical tube. This tube is made of muscles wrapping more-or-less horizontally from the front to a midline point in the back, as well as by muscles and connective tissue running from skull structures. Thus, the pharynx is composed of a complex of muscles that, when contracted, will constrict the pharynx to assist in deglutition.

Pharyngeal Constrictor Muscles.   The superior, middle, and inferior **constrictor muscles** are the means by which the pharyngeal space is reduced in diameter. Of these, the superior constrictor is an important muscle of velopharyngeal function (see Figure 7-44).

Superior Pharyngeal Constrictor.   Conceptually, the **superior pharyngeal constrictor** forms a tube beginning at the pterygomandibular raphe (the point of attachment of the buccinator). It projects back from this structure on both sides to the **median pharyngeal raphe**, the midline tendinous component of the pharyngeal aponeurosis. This aponeurosis

Muscle:	Superior pharyngeal constrictor
Origin:	Pterygomandibular raphe
Course:	Posteriorly
Insertion:	Median raphe of pharyngeal aponeurosis
Innervation:	XI accessory nerve and X vagus via pharyngeal plexus
Function:	Pulls pharyngeal wall forward and constricts pharyngeal diameter

arises from the pharyngeal tubercle of the occipital bone (immediately anterior to the foramen magnum) and forms the superior sleeve of the pharyngeal wall by attaching to the temporal bone (petrous portion), medial pterygoid plate, and Eustachian tube. The median pharyngeal raphe is the midline portion of this structure, descending along the back wall of the pharynx and providing the points of insertion for pharyngeal muscles. The superior constrictor muscle forms the sides and back wall of the nasopharynx and part of the back wall of the oropharynx, a function requiring a variety of points of attachment.

The median pterygoid plate gives rise to the uppermost fibers of the muscle, and these fibers are the "landing pad" for the soft palate, known as **Passavant's pad**. When present, this pad of muscle at the posterior pharyngeal wall appears as a ridge at the point of articulation of the soft palate with the wall. Clearly, the addition of tissue at this point can only assist in effecting a seal with the soft palate, and in fact, this pad appears to develop most markedly in individuals with palatal insufficiency, perhaps from compensatory activity.

The fibers from the pterygomandibular raphe are parallel to those of the buccinator, coursing back to insert into the median raphe of the posterior pharynx. Beneath these fibers, another portion of the superior constrictor arises from the mylohyoid line on the inner mandibular surface, while some other fibers arise from the sides of the tongue. Contraction of the superior pharyngeal constrictor muscle pulls the pharyngeal wall forward and constricts the pharyngeal diameter, an especially prominent movement during swallowing. It assists in effecting the velopharyngeal seal and thereby prevents the bolus from entering the nasopharynx. The superior pharyngeal constrictor is innervated by the XI accessory nerve in conjunction with the X vagus, via the pharyngeal plexus.

Middle Pharyngeal Constrictor.　The **middle pharyngeal constrictor** arises from the horns of the hyoid bone, as well as from the **stylohyoid ligament** that runs from the styloid process to the lesser horn of the hyoid. The middle constrictor courses up and back, inserting into the median pharyngeal raphe. The middle constrictor narrows the diameter of the pharynx. The middle pharyngeal constrictor is innervated by the XI accessory nerve in conjunction with the X vagus, via the pharyngeal plexus.

Muscle:	Middle pharyngeal constrictor
Origin:	Horns of the hyoid and stylohyoid ligament
Course:	Up and back
Insertion:	Median pharyngeal raphe
Innervation:	XI accessory nerve and X vagus via pharyngeal plexus
Function:	Narrows diameter of pharynx

Inferior Pharyngeal Constrictor. The **inferior pharyngeal constrictor** makes up the inferior pharynx. The portion arising from the sides of the cricoid cartilage forms the cricopharyngeal portion, frequently referred to as a separate muscle, the **cricopharyngeal muscle** (or **cricopharyngeus**). This portion, which courses back to form the muscular orifice of the esophagus, is an important muscle for swallowing and is the structure set into vibration during esophageal speech. The upper thyropharyngeal portion (or **thyropharyngeus muscle**) arises from the oblique line of the thyroid lamina, coursing up and back to insert into the median pharyngeal raphe. Contraction of the inferior constrictor reduces the diameter of the lower pharynx. The inferior pharyngeal constrictor is innervated by the XI accessory nerve in conjunction with the X vagus, via the pharyngeal plexus.

Salpingopharyngeus. The **salpingopharyngeus muscle** arises from the lower margin of the Eustachian tube, descending the lateral pharynx to join the palatopharyngeus muscle (see Figure 7-45). The **salpingopharyngeal fold** is a crease in the lateral nasopharynx formed by the mucosa covering this muscle. The salpingopharyngeus assists in elevation of the

Muscle:	Inferior pharyngeal constrictor; cricopharyngeus
Origin:	Cricoid cartilage
Course:	Back
Insertion:	Orifice of esophagus
Innervation:	XI accessory nerve and X vagus via pharyngeal plexus
Function:	Constricts superior orifice of esophagus

Muscle:	Inferior pharyngeal constrictor; thyropharyngeus
Origin:	Oblique line of thyroid lamina
Course:	Up and back
Insertion:	Median pharyngeal raphe
Innervation:	XI accessory nerve and X vagus via pharyngeal plexus
Function:	Reduces diameter of lower pharynx

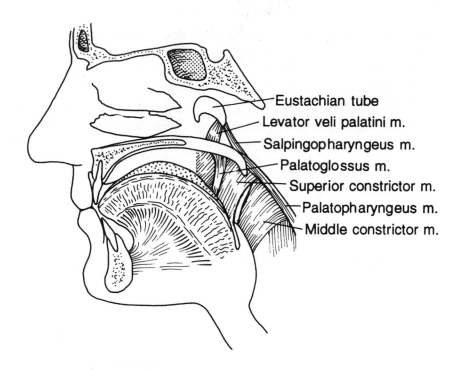

- Eustachian tube
- Levator veli palatini m.
- Salpingopharyngeus m.
- Palatoglossus m.
- Superior constrictor m.
- Palatopharyngeus m.
- Middle constrictor m.

Figure 7-45.
Salpingopharyngeus muscle.

lateral pharyngeal wall. The salpingopharyngeus is innervated by the X vagus and XI spinal accessory nerve via the pharyngeal plexus.

Stylopharyngeus Muscle.   As the name implies, the **stylopharyngeus** arises from the styloid process of the temporal bone, coursing down between the superior and middle pharyngeal constrictors (see Figure 7-44).

Muscle:	Salpingopharyngeus
Origin:	Lower margin of Eustachian tube
Course:	Down
Insertion:	Converges with palatopharyngeus muscle
Innervation:	X vagus and XI spinal accessory nerve via the pharyngeal plexus
Function:	Elevates lateral pharyngeal wall

Muscle:	Stylopharyngeus
Origin:	Styloid process
Course:	Down
Insertion:	Into pharyngeal constrictors and posterior thyroid cartilage
Innervation:	Muscular branch of IX glossopharyngeal nerve
Function:	Elevates and opens pharynx

Some fibers insert into the constrictors; others insert into the posterior thyroid cartilage in concert with the palatopharyngeus muscle. The stylopharyngeus elevates and opens the pharynx, particularly during deglutition. The stylopharyngeus muscle is innervated by the muscular branch of the IX glossopharyngeal nerve.

To summarize, the **soft palate** is a structure attached to the posterior hard palate and comprised of muscle and aponeuroses.

- The **levator veli palatini** muscle elevates the soft palate, and the **musculus uvulae** bunches the soft palate. The **tensor veli palatini** dilates the Eustachian tube.
- The soft palate is depressed by means of the **palatoglossus** and **palatopharyngeus**.
- The **superior pharyngeal constrictor** assists in gaining velopharyngeal closure, while peristaltic movement of food is facilitated by the **middle** and **inferior pharyngeal constrictors**.
- The **cricopharyngeal muscle**, a component of the inferior constrictor, forms the muscular orifice of the **esophagus**.
- Fibers of the **salpingopharyngeus** intermingle with those of the superior constrictor, providing assistance in elevation of the pharyngeal wall.
- The **stylopharyngeus** assists in elevation of the larynx.

As you can tell from this chapter, the structures of the articulatory system are extremely complex and mobile. We are capable of myriad movements that are incorporated into nonspeech and speech function. Let us move on to Chapter 8 and articulatory physiology.

CHAPTER SUMMARY

The **source-filter theory** states that speech is the product of sending an **acoustic source**, such as the sound produced by the vibrating vocal folds, through the **filter of the vocal tract** that shapes the output. Sources may be **voicing**, as in the case of vowels, or the product of **turbulence**, as in fricatives. Articulators may be **movable** (such as the tongue, lips, pharynx, mandible, and velum) or **immobile** (such as the teeth, hard palate, and alveolar ridge).

Facial bones and those of the skull work together in a complex fashion to produce the structures of articulation. The **mandible** provides the lower dental arch, alveolar regions, and the resting location for the tongue. The **maxillae** provide the bulk of the hard palate, alveolar ridge, upper dental arch, and dominant structures of the nasal cavities, and the **palatine bones** provide the rest of the hard palate and the point of attachment for the velum. The midline **vomer** articulates with the perpendicular plate of the **ethmoid** and the cartilaginous septum to form the **nasal septum**. The **zygomatic bone** articulates with the **frontal bone** and **maxillae** to form the cheekbone. The small **nasal bones** form the upper margin of the nasal cavity. The **ethmoid bone** serves as the core of the skull and face, with the prominent crista galli protruding into the **cranium** and the **perpendicular plate** dividing the nasal cavities. The **frontal**, **parietal**, **temporal**, and **occipital** bones of the skull overlie the lobes of the brain of the same name. The **sphenoid bone** has a marked presence within the braincase, with the prominent greater and lesser wings of the sphenoid located lateral to the corpus. The **hypophyseal fossa** houses the pituitary gland. The clivus joins the occipital bone near the foramen magnum.

Incisors, **cuspids**, **bicuspids**, and **molars** are housed within the alveoli of the maxillae and mandible. **Teeth** have roots and crowns, and the exposed tooth surface is covered with enamel. Each tooth has a **medial**, **lateral**, **lingual**, **buccal** (or labial), and **occlusal** surface. **Clinical eruption** of the deciduous arch begins between six and nine months, and eruption of the permanent arch begins at six years. **Class I occlusion** refers to normal orientation of mandible and maxillae. **Class II malocclusion** refers to a relatively retracted mandible, and **Class III malocclusion** refers to a relatively protruded mandible. Individual teeth may have aberrant orientations within the alveolus, including **torsiversion**, **labioversion**, **linguaversion**, **distoversion**, and **mesioversion**. Inadequately erupted or hypererupted teeth are referred to as **infraverted** and **supraverted**, respectively.

The cavities of the articulatory and resonatory system can be envisioned as a series of linked tubes. The vertically directed **pharynx** is comprised of the **laryngopharynx**, **oropharynx**, and **nasopharynx**. The nasal cavities arise from the nasopharynx, with the nasal and nasopharyngeal regions entirely separated from the oral cavity by the **soft palate** or **velum**. The oral cavity is flanked by the small **buccal cavities**. The shape and size of the oral cavity are altered through movement of the **tongue** and **mandible**, and the nasal cavity may be coupled with the oral and pharyngeal cavities by means of the soft palate. The shape of the pharyngeal cavity is altered by the **pharyngeal constrictor muscles**, but is secondarily changed by elevation or depression of the **larynx**.

Facial muscles are important for articulations involving the lips. Numerous muscles insert into the **orbicularis oris** inferior and superior muscles, permitting lip protrusion, closure, retraction, elevation, and depression. The **risorius** and **buccinator** muscles retract the lips and support entrapment of air within the oral cavity. The **levator labii superioris**, **zygomatic minor**, **levator labii superioris alaeque nasi**, and **levator anguli oris** elevate the upper lip, and the **depressor labii inferioris** depresses the lower lip. The **zygomatic major** muscle elevates and retracts the corner of the mouth. The **depressor labii inferioris** pulls the lips down and out. The **depressor anguli oris** muscle depresses the corner of the mouth, and the **mentalis** muscle pulls the lower lip out. The **platysma** depresses the mandible.

The **tongue**, which occupies the floor of the mouth, is divided into **dorsum**, **apex** (tip), and **base**. Fine movements are the product of the **intrinsic musculature** (**transverse, vertical, inferior longitudinal** and **superior longitudinal** muscles of the tongue). Larger adjustments of lingual movement require extrinsic muscles. The **genioglossus** retracts, protrudes, or depresses the tongue, and the **hyoglossus** and **chondroglossus** depress the tongue. The **styloglossus** and **palatoglossus** elevate the posterior tongue.

Muscles of **mastication** include mandibular elevators and depressors, as well as muscles to protrude the mandible. The **masseter, temporalis**, and **medial pterygoid** muscles elevate the mandible, and the **lateral pterygoids** protrude it. **Mandibular depression** is achieved by the **mylohyoid, geniohyoid**, and **platysma** muscles.

The **velum** or **soft palate** is attached to the posterior hard palate. The **levator veli palatini** muscle elevates the soft palate and the **musculus uvulae** bunches it. The **tensor veli palatini** dilates the Eustachian tube. The velum is depressed by the **palatoglossus** and **palatopharyngeus**. The **superior pharyngeal constrictor** assists in gaining velopharyngeal closure, while peristaltic movement of food is facilitated by the **middle** and **inferior pharyngeal constrictors**. The **cricopharyngeus** forms the muscular orifice of the esophagus. The **salpingopharyngeus** elevates the pharyngeal wall, and the **stylopharyngeus** assists in elevation of the larynx.

STUDY QUESTIONS

1. The _____ theory of vowel production states that the voicing source is routed through the vocal tract, where it is shaped into the sounds of speech by the articulators.

2. On the figure below, identify the bones and landmarks indicated.

   a. _____ (bone)

   b. _____ (bone)

   c. _____ bone

   d. _____ bone

   e. _____ bone

   f. _____ process

   g. _____ process

   h. _____

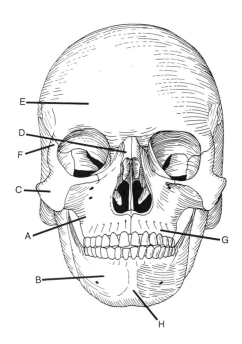

3. On the figure below, identify the bones and landmarks indicated.

a. _____ (bone)

b. _____ bone

c. _____ bone

d. _____

e. _____

f. _____

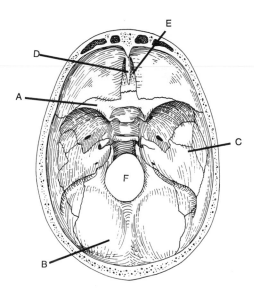

4. On the figure below, identify the bones and landmarks indicated.

a. _____ bone

b. _____ bone

c. _____ (bone)

d. _____ (bone)

e. _____ bone

f. _____ bone

g. _____ bone

h. _____ bone

i. _____

j. _____

k. _____ process

l. _____ process

m. _____ process

n. _____

o. _____ process

p. _____ process

q. _____

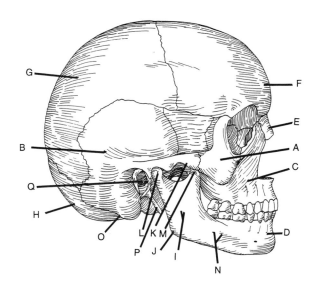

5. On the figure below, identify the structures indicated.

a. _____ process

b. _____ (bone)

c. _____ bone

d. _____

e. _____ foramen

f. _____ suture

g. _____ process

h. _____ plate

i. _____ plate

j. _____ process

k. _____

l. _____

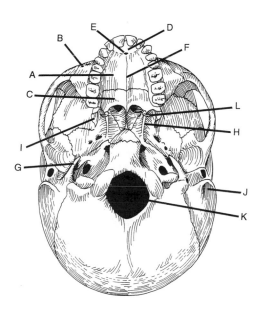

6. On the figure below, identify the muscles indicated.

a. _____

b. _____

c. _____

d. _____

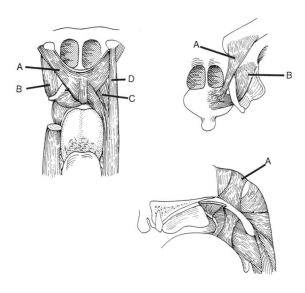

7. On the figure below, identify the muscles indicated.

a. _____

b. _____

c. _____

d. _____

e. _____

f. _____

g. _____

h. _____

i. _____

j. _____

k. _____

l. _____

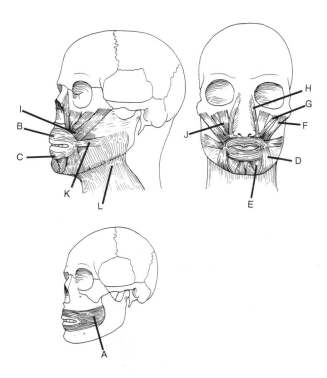

8. On the figure below, identify the muscles indicated.

a. _____

b. _____

c. _____

d. _____

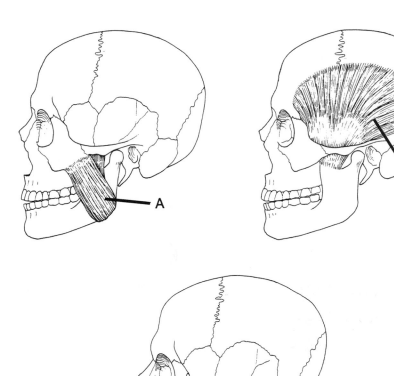

9. On the figure below, identify the muscles indicated.

a. _____

b. _____

c. _____

d. _____

e. _____

f. _____

g. _____

h. _____

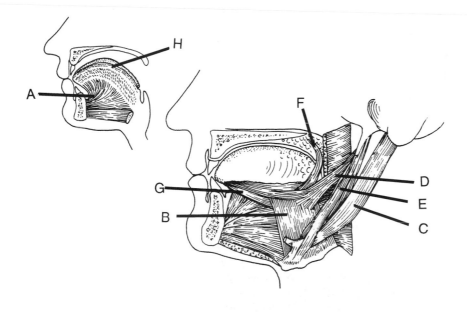

10. On the figure below, identify the structures indicated.
    a. _____ (bone)
    b. _____ process
    c. _____ plate
    d. _____ plate
    e. _____
    f. _____ bone

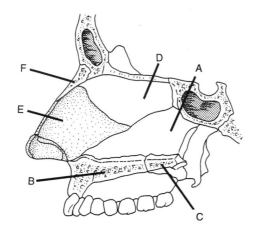

11. The soft palate is a diverse structure that typically serves us well, in that it separates the oropharynx and nasopharynx to protect against nasal regurgitation, not to mention keeping non-nasal phonemes from becoming nasalized. In our clinical practice, we have seen that low-back vowels tend to become nasalized more frequently in neurologically compromised clients than other vowels. What could be the source of this?

 STUDY QUESTION ANSWERS

1. The SOURCE-FILTER theory of vowel production states that the voicing source is routed through the vocal tract, where it is shaped into the sounds of speech by the articulators.

2. On the figure below, identify the bones and landmarks indicated.
    a. MAXILLA (bone)
    b. MANDIBLE (bone)
    c. ZYGOMATIC bone
    d. NASAL bone
    e. FRONTAL bone
    f. FRONTAL process
    g. ALVEOLAR process

h. SYMPHYSIS MENTE

3. On the figure below, identify the bones and landmarks indicated.

a. SPHENOID bone

b. OCCIPITAL bone

c. TEMPORAL bone

d. CRISTA GALLI

e. CRIBRIFORM PLATE

f. FORAMEN MAGNUM

4. On the figure below, identify the bones and landmarks indicated.

a. ZYGOMATIC bone

b. TEMPORAL bone

c. MAXILLAE (bone)

d. MANDIBLE (bone)

e. NASAL bone

f. FRONTAL bone

g. PARIETAL bone

h. OCCIPITAL bone

i. RAMUS

j. ANGLE

k. ZYGOMATIC process

l. CONDYLAR process

m. CORONOID process

n. CORPUS

o. MASTOID process

p. STYLOID process

q. EXTERNAL AUDITORY MEATUS

5. On the figure below, identify the structures indicated.

a. PALATINE process

b. MAXILLAE (bone)

c. PALATINE bone

d. PREMAXILLA

e. INCISIVE foramen

f. INTERMAXILLARY suture

g. STYLOID process

h. MEDIAL PTERYGOID plate

i. LATERAL PTERYGOID plate

j. MASTOID process

k. FORAMEN MAGNUM

l. PTERYGOID HAMULUS

6. On the figure below, identify the muscles indicated.

a. LEVATOR VELI PALATINI

b. TENSOR VELI PALATINI

c. PALATOGLOSSUS

d. PALATOPHARYNGEUS

7. On the figure below, identify the muscles indicated.
   a. <u>BUCCINATOR</u>
   b. <u>ORBICULARIS ORIS SUPERIORIS</u>
   c. <u>ORBICULARIS ORIS INFERIORIS</u>
   d. <u>DEPRESSOR ANGULI ORIS</u>
   e. <u>DEPRESSOR LABII INFERIORIS</u>
   f. <u>ZYGOMATIC MAJOR</u>
   g. <u>ZYGOMATIC MINOR</u>
   h. <u>LEVATOR LABII SUPERIORIS ALAEQUE NASI</u>
   i. <u>LEVATOR ANGULI ORIS</u>
   j. <u>LEVATOR LABII SUPERIORIS</u>
   k. <u>RISORIUS</u>
   l. <u>PLATYSMA</u>

8. On the figure below, identify the muscles indicated.
   a. <u>MASSETER</u>
   b. <u>TEMPORALIS</u>
   c. <u>LATERAL PTERYGOID</u>
   d. <u>MEDIAL PTERYGOID</u>

9. On the figure below, identify the muscles indicated.
   a. <u>GENIOGLOSSUS</u>
   b. <u>HYOGLOSSUS</u>
   c. <u>DIGASTRICUS POSTERIOR</u>
   d. <u>STYLOGLOSSUS</u>
   e. <u>STYLOHYOID</u>
   f. <u>PALATOGLOSSUS</u>
   g. <u>INFERIOR LONGITUDINAL</u>
   h. <u>SUPERIOR LONGITUDINAL</u>

10. On the figure below, identify the structures indicated.
    a. <u>VOMER</u> (bone)
    b. <u>PALATINE</u> process
    c. <u>HORIZONTAL</u> plate
    d. <u>PERPENDICULAR</u> plate
    e. <u>CARTILAGINOUS SEPTUM</u>
    f. <u>NASAL</u> bone

11. You remember that the palatoglossus (glossopalatine) is a shared muscle of the tongue and of the soft palate. When it contracts, either the soft palate is depressed or the back and sides of the tongue are elevated, depending on whether the tongue is anchored or the soft palate is anchored. In the case of neurological deficit resulting in muscular weakness, when the tongue is depressed for the low-back vowels, the soft palate may be pulled down due to inadequate resistance by the levator veli palatini and tensor veli palatini.

REFERENCES

Abrahams, P. H., McMinn, R. M. H., Hutchings, R. T., Sandy, C., & Mark, S. (2003). *McMinn's color atlas of human anatomy* (5th ed.). Philadelphia: Mosby.

Baken, R. J., & Orlikoff, R. F. (1999). *Clinical measurement of speech and voice* (2nd ed.). San Diego, CA: Singular Publishing Group.

Basmajian, J. V. (1975). *Grant's method of anatomy.* Baltimore: Williams & Wilkins.

Bateman, H. E. (1977). *A clinical approach to speech anatomy and physiology.* Springfield, IL: Charles C. Thomas.

Bateman, H. E., & Mason, R. M. (1984). *Applied anatomy and physiology of the speech and hearing mechanism.* Springfield, IL: Charles C. Thomas.

Beck, E. W., Monson, H., & Groer, M. (1982). *Mosby's atlas of functional human anatomy.* St. Louis, MO: C. V. Mosby.

Bly, L. (1983). *The components of normal movement during the first year of life and abnormal motor movement.* Chicago, IL: Neuro-Developmental Treatment Association.

Bly, L. (1994). *Motor skills acquisition in the first year.* Tucson, AZ: Therapy Skill Builders.

Chusid, J. G. (1985). *Correlative neuroanatomy and functional neurology* (17th ed.). Los Altos, CA: Lange Medical Publications.

Ettema, S. L., & Kuehn, D. P. (1994). A quantitative histologic study of the normal human adult soft palate. *Journal of Speech and Hearing Research, 37,* 303–313.

Gelb, H. (1985). *Clinical management of head, neck and TMJ pain and dysfunction.* Philadelphia: W. B. Saunders.

Gosling, J. A., Harris, P. F., Humpherson, J. R., Whitmore, I., & Willan, P. L. T. (1985). *Atlas of human anatomy.* Philadelphia: J. B. Lippincott.

Gray, H., Bannister, L. H., Berry, M. M., & Williams, P. L. (Eds.). (1995). *Gray's anatomy.* London: Churchill Livingstone.

Grobler, N. J. (1977). *Textbook of clinical anatomy* (Vol. 1). Amsterdam: Elsevier Scientific.

Hauser, G., Daponte, A., & Roberts, M. J. (1989). Palatal rugae. *Journal of Anatomy, 124,* 237–249.

Kahane, J. C., & Folkins, J. F. (1984). *Atlas of speech and hearing anatomy.* Columbus, OH: Charles E. Merrill.

Kapetansky, D. I. (1987). *Cleft lip, nose, and palate reconstruction.* Philadelphia: J. B. Lippincott.

Kaplan, H. (1960). *Anatomy and physiology of speech.* New York: McGraw-Hill.

Kent, R. D. (1997). *The speech sciences.* San Diego, CA: Singular Publishing Group.

Kuehn, D. P., Lemme, M. L., & Baumgartner, J. M. (1989). *Neural bases of speech, hearing, and language.* Boston: Little, Brown.

Kuehn, D. P., Templeton, P. J., & Maynard, J. A. (1990). Muscle spindles in the velopharyngeal musculature of humans. *Journal of Speech and Hearing Research, 33,* 488–493.

Langley, L. L., Telford, I. R., & Christensen, J. B. (1969). *Dynamic anatomy and physiology.* New York: McGraw-Hill.

Langley, M. B., & Lombardino, L. J. (1991). *Neurodevelopmental strategies for managing communication disorders in children with severe motor dysfunction.* Austin, TX: Pro-Ed.

Lieberman, P. (1977). *Speech physiology and acoustic phonetics: An introduction.* New York: Macmillan.

Liss, J. M. (1990). Muscle spindles in the human levator veli palatini and palatoglossus muscles. *Journal of Speech and Hearing Research, 33,* 736–746.

McMinn, R. M. H., Hutchings, R. T., & Logan, B. M. (1994). *Color atlas of head and neck anatomy.* London: Mosby-Wolfe.

Minifie, F. (1973). Speech acoustics. In F. D. Minifie, T. J. Hixon, & F. Williams (Eds.), *Normal aspects of speech, hearing, and language* (pp. 11–72). Englewood Cliffs, NJ: Prentice-Hall.

Moore, K. L. (1988). *The developing human.* Philadelphia: W. B. Saunders.

Netter, F. H. (1983). *The CIBA collection of medical illustrations. Vol. 1. Nervous system. Part I. Anatomy and physiology.* West Caldwell, NJ: CIBA Pharmaceutical Company.

Netter, F. H. (1997). *Atlas of human anatomy.* Los Angeles: Icon Learning Systems.

Pickett, J. M. (1980). *The sounds of speech communication.* Baltimore: University Park Press.

Rohen, J. W., Yokochi, C., Lutjen-Drecoll, E., & Romrell, L. J. (2002). *Color atlas of anatomy* (5th ed.). Philadelphia: Williams & Wilkins.

Rosse, C., Gaddum-Rosse, P., & Rosse, G. (1997). *Hollinshead's textbook of anatomy.* Philadelphia: Lippincott-Raven.

Sawashima, M., & Cooper, F. S. (1977). *Dynamic aspects of speech production.* Tokyo: University of Tokyo Press.

Shprintzen, R. J., & Bardach, J. (1995). *Cleft palate speech management.* St. Louis, MO: C. V. Mosby.

Shriberg, L. D., & Kent, R. D. (2002). *Clinical phonetics* (3rd ed.). New York: Allyn & Bacon.

Small, A. M. (1973). Acoustics. In F. D. Minifie, T. J. Hixon, & F. Williams (Eds.), *Normal aspects of speech, hearing, and language.* Englewood Cliffs, NJ: Prentice-Hall.

Snell, R. S. (1978). *Gross anatomy dissector.* Boston: Little, Brown.

Williams, P., & Warrick, R. (1980). *Gray's anatomy* (36th British ed.). Philadelphia: W. B. Saunders.

Zemlin, W. R. (1998). *Speech and hearing science: Anatomy and physiology* (4th ed.). Needham Heights, MA: Allyn & Bacon.

Zickefoose, W. (1989). *Techniques of oral myofunctional therapy.* Sacramento, CA: O.M.T. Materials, Inc.

CHAPTER 8

Physiology of Articulation and Resonation

INTRODUCTION

Clearly, the function of the articulatory system is of paramount importance in speech production. Although a review of acoustic phonetics is beyond the scope of an anatomy text, the source-filter theory of speech production discussed in Chapter 7 nonetheless provides the framework for our discussion. Intrinsic to that explanation of speech production is the notion that the movement of articulators shapes the resonant cavities of the vocal tract, and altered resonances give the acoustic output we call speech. We begin our discussion of the physiology of articulation and resonation by discussing speech function, and follow in Chapter 9 with our investigation of the biological function associated with swallowing.

SPEECH FUNCTION

Speech production requires execution of an extremely well-organized and integrated sequence of neuromotor events. Say the word "tube" and pay attention to the sequence of articulations. Ignoring respiratory preparation for the moment, your tongue must elevate to the alveolar ridge simultaneously with elevation and tensing of the velum. Air pressure builds behind your tongue, and then your tongue actively drops to release the pressure and produce the /t/. Even as it releases, your tongue must quickly draw back to produce the /u/, assisted by the rounding of your lips. Your lips must then clamp together to permit buildup of air pressure for the final /b/. This all happens in less than $3/10$ of a second, and quite easily for most of us.

As you can see, thinking about the interaction of articulators and the articulatory plan can get complex in a hurry. Let us begin with function of the individual movable articulators.

Lips

The lips are deceptively simple articulators. As discussed in Chapter 7, the orbicularis is primarily responsible for ensuring a labial seal, but numerous facial muscles insert into it. Those muscles are capable of exerting a distinct force on the lips, often in combination with other muscles. Contraction of these muscles becomes an exercise in physics and force vectors: The direction of lip movement is the result of adding the directional forces of these muscles.

The lips are deceptive in another sense as well. At first glance, one might assume that the upper and lower lips have very similar qualities. In reality, however, the lower lip achieves a greater velocity and force than the upper lip, and it seems to do most of the work in lip closure. The extra force is a function of the mentalis muscle, for which there is no parallel in the upper lip, and the doubled velocity is necessitated by the variable movement and placement of the mandible. The lower lip is attached to a movable articulator (the mandible), and it must quickly adapt to being closer or farther from the maxillary upper lip. That is, for sound to be accurately perceived as the chosen phoneme, the lips must make contact within closely timed tolerances. The lower lip is capable of rapidly altering its rate of closure to accommodate a variety of jaw positions, unflinchingly.

The notion of variable mandible position reinforces another fine point of labial function. The lips (as with the other articulators) are amazingly resistant to interference. We can easily adjust to perturbations of our articulators, or even to gross malformation. As an example, you could ask a friend to recite a poem with her eyes closed. At an unpredictable point you could briefly pull down on her lip, and she would quickly adjust to the distorted articulatory position and continue talking with the new configuration (within limits, of course).

Similarly, you are able to adapt to other restrictions on supportive articulators. Try this. Repeat the syllable "puh" as rapidly as you can, counting the number of syllables you can produce in five seconds. Notice that your mandible was helping, and it moved when you closed your lips. Now bite lightly on a pencil using your incisors and do the same task. Your rate of repetition was probably very similar, despite the fact that your mandible was no longer able to help your lips close.

We are amazingly resistant to interference with the articulatory mechanism. This resistance, by the way, is evidence that the plan for an articulatory gesture is not "micro-managed" by central cortical control, but rather that the details of motor execution are left to be worked out by some type of "coordinative structures," as will be discussed. If the neural command, for instance, said simply to elevate the lower lip 1.3 cm, either of the distortions mentioned previously would have resulted in a faulty articulation.

This does not mean that we do not use the proprioceptive information provided by sensors in our facial muscles to help us note muscle tone and position. Although we do not have spindles in facial muscles to assist in this process, we do have other sensors (such as those for pressure and touch) that provide feedback on the condition of facial muscles. Reflexive contraction of the orbicularis oris occurs with increased intraoral pressure, such as that produced during production of a bilabial stop plosive. The oral mucosa and lips have sensors for light mechanical stimulation such as would occur during lingua-dental articulation. Although there is little evidence of stretch receptors of the lips, a stretch reflex can be elicited through retraction of the angles of the mouth.

Evidence that you *do* use this type of information to control muscles may be found in remembering your last trip to the dentist. If the dentist's anesthetic deadened your lip, you may remember accidentally biting it while chewing or talking. Your unconscious perception of its position generally keeps that from happening. Mechanical stimulation of the lips affects other articulators as well. When the lower lip is stimulated, reflexive excitation in both the masseter and genioglossus can be recorded. The *degree* to which this information is *required* for speech accuracy is still a lively topic of debate.

Mandible

The mandible is something of an unsung hero among articulators. It quietly and unceremoniously goes about its business, assisting the lips, changing its position for tongue movement, and tightly closing when necessary. It *does* move, however, and you can remind yourself of that by placing one finger of your right hand on your upper lip, and another finger on your chin. Close your eyes and count to 20 quickly, paying attention to the degree of movement you feel. You probably felt very little movement, but the mandible *did* move. Now clamp your mandible and count to 20. Were you still intelligible? (Yes.) Now do the opposite: Let your mouth hang absolutely slack-jaw open, and count to 20.

If you really relaxed your jaw and refused to elevate it for your speech, you probably noticed that you were largely unintelligible. The mandible is an extremely important articulator in its supportive role of carrying the lips, tongue, and teeth to their targets in the maxilla (lips, teeth, alveolar ridge, hard palate), but its adjustments are rather minute in normal speech. For this reason, paralysis of the muscles of mastication can be devastating to speech intelligibility.

The muscles of mandibular elevation (temporalis, masseter, medial pterygoid) are endowed with muscle spindles, although those of mandibular depression (digastricus, mylohyoid, geniohyoid, lateral pterygoid) are not. You can easily see the effects of muscle spindles on yourself. Relax your jaw while looking into a mirror. Now apply a firm rubbing pressure to the masseter in a downward-pulling direction. You will see your mandible elevate slightly as you trigger the mandibular reflex. There are also sensors of joint position within the temporomandibular joint that permit extremely accurate positioning of the jaw (within one mm). If these sensors are anesthetized, the speaker's accuracy diminishes markedly.

The mandible is, of course, quite important for mastication, and the function of the muscles of mastication is distinctly different for speech than for chewing. It appears that there is a central pattern generator within the brainstem that produces the rhythmic muscular contraction needed for chewing. The mandible must elevate, grind laterally, and depress, requiring coordinated activation of the elevators and depressors in a synergistic, rhythmic fashion. We will discuss this pattern further in Chapter 9.

For speech, in contrast, the mandibular elevators and depressors stay in dynamic balance, so that slight modification in muscle activation (and inhibition of antagonists) permits a quick adjustment of the mandible (Moore, 1993). Indeed, depression of the mandible seems to be not only a function of the classically defined mandibular depressors (digastricus, mylohyoid, geniohyoid, lateral pterygoid) but also, to a significant extent, of the infrahyoid musculature (Westbury, 1988). The hyoid undergoes a great deal of movement during depression of the mandible.

Tongue

Arguably, the tongue is the most important of the articulators. It is involved in production of the majority of phonemes in English. Let us look at how we achieve the individual movements of the tongue.

As a first approximation, you can think of the tongue as a group of highly organized (intrinsic) muscles being carried on the "shoulders" of the extrinsic muscles. Much as the muscles of the legs and trunk move your upper body to a position where your arms and head can interact with the environment, the extrinsic muscles set the basic posture of the tongue, whereas the intrinsic muscles have a great deal of responsibility for the microstructure of articulation. The two groups of muscles work together closely to achieve the target articulatory gesture. Let us examine each of the basic gestures required for speech (see Table 8-1).

Tongue Tip Elevation

Elevation of the tongue is primarily the responsibility of the superior longitudinal muscle of the tongue. When these fibers are shortened, the tip and lateral margins of the tongue are pulled up.

Tongue Tip Depression

Depression of the tongue is the primary responsibility of the inferior longitudinal muscles. Their course along the lateral margins of the lower tongue make them perfectly suited to pull the tip and sides of the tongue down.

Table 8-1. Muscles of tongue movement.

MOVEMENT	MUSCLE
Elevate tongue tip	Superior longitudinal muscles
Depress tongue tip	Inferior longitudinal muscles
Deviate tongue tip	Simultaneous contraction of either left or right superior and inferior longitudinal muscles for left or right deviation
Relax lateral margin	Posterior genioglossus for protrusion; superior longitudinal for tip elevation; transverse intrinsic pulls sides medially
Narrow tongue	Transverse intrinsic
Deep central groove	Genioglossus depresses tongue body; vertical intrinsic depresses central dorsum
Broad central groove	Moderate genioglossus to depress tongue body; vertical intrinsic depresses dorsum; superior longitudinal elevates margins
Protrude tongue	Posterior genioglossus advances body; vertical muscles narrow tongue; superior and inferior longitudinal balance and point tongue
Retract tongue	Anterior genioglossus retracts into oral cavity; superior and inferior longitudinal shorten tongue; styloglossus retracts into pharyngeal cavity
Elevate posterior tongue	Palatoglossus elevates sides; transverse intrinsic bunches tongue
Depress tongue body	Genioglossus contraction depresses medial tongue; hyoglossus and chondroglossus depress sides if hyoid is fixed by infrahyoid muscles

Unilateral Tongue Weakness

One element of the **oral-peripheral examination** is examination for relative tongue strength. When you ask a client to push forcefully with his or her tongue sideways against a resistance, you are interested in identifying whether the client has adequate strength and symmetrical strength. If there appears to be greater strength in one direction than the other, you will consider activities to strengthen the musculature. Improving muscle strength will improve tone and muscle control.

Tongue Tip Deviation, Left and Right

Deviation of the tongue tip to the left requires simultaneous contraction of the left superior and inferior longitudinal muscles. This asymmetrical contraction will have the desired result, which is asymmetrical movement of the tongue tip.

Relaxation of Lateral Margins

The lateral margins of the tongue must be relaxed for the /l/ phoneme even as the tongue is protruded to the anterior alveolar ridge and slightly elevated. This complex gesture is accomplished by slight contraction of the posterior genioglossus (which helps to move the tongue forward) and the superior longitudinal (which elevates the tip). Contraction of the transverse intrinsic muscles of the tongue will pull the sides medially away from the lateral gum ridge, opening the lateral sulcus for resonation.

Tongue Narrowing

The transverse fibers coursing from the median fibrous septum to the lateral margins of the tongue are required for this gesture.

Central Tongue Grooving

The degree of tongue grooving determines the magnitude of muscle involvement in this gesture. Wholesale depression of the medial tongue is accomplished by contraction of the entire genioglossus in conjunction with the vertical fibers. A more moderate groove will involve the genioglossus to a lesser degree, but will still use the vertical muscles. A broadened groove could be accomplished by co-contraction of the superior longitudinal muscle, elevating the sides of the tongue as well.

Tongue Protrusion

Tongue protrusion requires use of the posterior genioglossus, and at least two of the intrinsic muscles. Contraction of the posterior genioglossus will draw the tongue forward, but will not let you point your tongue. To make a proper "statement" with your tongue, however, you will need assistance from vertical and transverse intrinsic muscles, and deviation (up, down, or to the sides) will require the use of superior and inferior

Tongue Deviation on Protrusion

Tongue musculature is paired, and unilateral weakness will produce asymmetry on protrusion. When the tongue is protruded, the bilateral musculature of the genioglossus must contract with equal force. If the left genioglossus is weak, it will not contribute equally to the protrusion, and the right genioglossus will overcome the left's effort. As a result, left genioglossus weakness will result in deviation toward the left side. Put another way, with lower motor neuron damage the tongue "points toward the lesion."

longitudinal intrinsics. The genioglossus posterior by itself would leave the tongue hanging down from your opened mouth.

Tongue Retraction

Retraction of the body of the tongue involves both intrinsic and extrinsic muscles. The anterior genioglossus will draw the protruded tongue into the oral cavity, and co-contraction of the superior and inferior longitudinal muscles will shorten the tongue. To retract the tongue into the pharyngeal space, as in the swallowing gesture, the styloglossus must be engaged.

Posterior Tongue Elevation

The palatoglossi insert into the sides of the tongue, and their contraction elevates the sides. Contraction of the transverse muscles in the posterior tongue would assist in bunching the tongue up in that region.

Tongue Body Depression

Contraction of the genioglossus as a unit depresses the medial tongue. The addition of the hyoglossus and chondroglossus will depress the sides of the tongue, assuming that the hyoid is fixed by the infrahyoid muscles.

Although the tongue is capable of generating a great deal of force through contraction, we typically only use about 20% of its potential force for speech activities. The tongue is endowed with muscle spindles, golgi tendon organs, and tactile sensors. Muscle spindles have been found in the tongue muscles, and golgi tendon organs have been found in the transverse intrinsic muscles. Passive movement of the tongue (pulling outward) will result in a reflexive retraction of the tongue, and mechanical stimulation of the tongue dorsum will cause excitation of the genioglossus muscle. Stimulation of the tongue dorsum has an effect on other articulators as well, causing excitation of the masseter and lower orbicularis oris.

The tongue is also remarkably sensitive to touch. We can differentiate to points on the tongue tip separated by only about 1.5 mm. Another extremely sensitive region of the mouth is the periodontal ligament of the dental arch, which can sense movement as slight as

10 microns (if you have ever had a strawberry seed wedged between your teeth, you can verify this sensitivity). It is likely that this sensitivity is used to monitor production of dental consonants.

Velum

Early in the history of our field we found it tempting to treat the velum as a binary element: It was either opened or closed. We have since realized that it is unsafe to deal with such a complex structure in so simple a fashion. The velum is capable of a range of motion and rate of movement that, in the normally endowed individual, matches the needs of rapid speech and nonspeech functions.

The velum generally is closed for non-nasal speech, and this is the result of contraction of the levator veli palatini, a direct antagonist to the palatoglossus muscle. In speech, opening and closing of the velar port must occur precisely and rapidly, or the result will be hyper- or hyponasality. Failure to open the port will turn a 70 ms nasal phoneme into a voiced stop consonant, an unacceptable result. The soft palate opens and closes in coordination with the other articulators, thus avoiding the effect of nasal resonance on other phonemes (**assimilation**). In reality, some nasal assimilation is inevitable, acceptable, and in some geographic regions, dialectically appropriate.

Production of high-pressure consonants (such as fricatives and stops) requires greater velopharyngeal effort. To accomplish this seal, additional help is needed from the superior pharyngeal constrictor and uvular muscles. Even then, the pressures for speech are far less than those for, say, playing a wind instrument. Individuals may have difficulty avoiding nasal air escape when playing in the brass section but have perfectly normal speech.

The hard and soft palates are richly endowed with receptors that provide feedback concerning pressure, and it appears that these sensors facilitate or inhibit motor lingual activity. Indeed, the tensor veli palatini, palatoglossus, and levator veli palatini muscles have been found to have muscle spindles, and the input from these sensors may be important to initiation of the pharyngeal swallowing reflex (Kuehn, Templeton, & Maynard, 1990; Liss, 1990). In cats, when the soft palate is stimulated electrically, extrinsic tongue movement is inhibited. In contrast, when the hard palate is stimulated (as it would be by food crushed during oral preparation), the extrinsic lingual muscles are excited, producing a rhythmic movement of the tongue. Stretching the faucial pillars by pulling on the tongue or the pillars themselves inhibits the activity of the extrinsic tongue muscles as well. It appears that the interaction of the soft palate, fauces, and tongue is a well-organized and integrated system. Palatal, laryngeal, and pharyngeal stimulation activate protrusion of the tongue, whereas stimulation of the anterior oral region appears to stimulate retraction of the tongue.

Hypernasality refers to excessive, linguistically inappropriate nasal resonance arising from failure to adequately close the velopharyngeal port during non-nasal speech sound production. In contrast, hyponasality *refers to the absence of appropriately nasalized speech sounds, such that the velopharyngeal port is inadequately opened for the /n/, /m/, and /ŋ/ phonemes.*

To summarize, each of the articulators has both speech and non-speech functions which do not necessarily share the same patterns.

- The **lower lip** is much faster and stronger than the upper lip and responds reflexively to increases of pressure. This added responsiveness makes it quite effective at overcoming incidental **perturbations** while performing its assigned tasks.

- Movement of the **mandible** for speech is slight when compared with movement for chewing. In addition, the mandibular posture for speech is one of **sustained dynamic tension** between antagonists.

- The **tongue** is an extremely versatile organ, with the **extrinsic muscles** providing the major movement of the body, and the **intrinsic muscles** providing the shaping of the tongue.

- The **velum** must be maintained in a reasonably elevated position for most speech sounds, although it is capable of a range of movements.

Development of Articulatory Ability

The infant is faced with an enormous task during development. She begins life with no knowledge of the universe and with a motor system in which movement is governed by reflexes and out of her control. She will spend the next several years (perhaps the rest of her life!) making sense of the world around her and learning to manipulate her environment. Fortunately, she is born with an innate "desire" to acquire information and learn about her environment, and it appears that this drives the often-painful process of development.

The primitive human motor system is actually an extremely complex network of protective reflexes. Reflexes provide the means for an immature infant to respond to the environment in a stereotyped manner, without volition. This is not to argue that infants have no will, but rather to point out that they cannot express it voluntarily. If a breast touches the lips of an infant, the infant will orient to the breast and start sucking reflexively (you can stimulate this reflex with a stroke of your fingers). The infant does not need to think, "Gee, I'm hungry. I wonder if there is anything to eat around here?" Rather, nature has hard-wired the infant to meet its needs.

This reflexive condition results in what Langley and Lombardino (1991) refer to as "primitive mass patterns of movement." Movements are gross responses to environmental stimuli that help the infant meet its basic needs. Development is a process of gaining cortical control of the motor patterns for volitional purposes, and the development of the articulatory system has its roots in learning to walk.

The most pervasive postnatal experience an infant has is gravity. Always present, gravity provides the ultimate challenge to an infant who

Effects of Neuromuscular Disease on Velopharyngeal Function

A deficit associated with the velopharyngeal port can have significant effects on speech. In neuromuscular disorders, such as amyotrophic lateral sclerosis or multiple sclerosis, muscular weakness arises from damage to the myelin sheath surrounding the axons of motor neurons. When the weakness involves the muscles of the velum, the nasal cavity resonance is added to that of the oral cavity for non-nasal sounds. This "anti-resonance," as it is called, pulls energy out of the speech signal in the 1,500 Hz to 2,500 Hz range, causing a marked loss of clarity in the speech signal. Speech of the affected individual sounds muffled, monotone, and low in vocal intensity.

It is not uncommon for the speech-language pathologist to be the first person approached by an individual with early signs of neuromuscular disease. The velopharyngeal port requires constant elevation for non-nasal sounds and is an early indicator of progressive muscular weakness. An individual may come to the clinician with the complaint that people say his or her speech sounds muffled. Your oral-peripheral examination will reveal slow velar activity, and your referral to a physician will be most helpful to the client.

wants to experience a universe that is out of reach. Reflexive movement against gravity provides the child with information about the effects of movement. He can see his hands as he moves them and learns that there is a relationship between the sensation and the hands he sees. These are the essential elements of motor development: *reflexive response* to *environmental stimuli*, providing *feedback* to an intact *neuromotor system*. Motor development is a process of refining gross movements, and this refinement will occur **cephalo-caudally** (from head to tail) and **proximo-distally** (from medial structures to distal structures). The infant will develop gross mandibular movements before fine mandibular movements and will have head control before she develops trunk control. She will develop posterior tongue control before anterior tongue control. Four vital elements of basic motor control support later speech development: experience with gravity, flexor-extensor balance, trunk control, and differentiation.

During the reflexive period (roughly birth to six months), the infant's vestibular system is being stimulated by parental handling. Vestibular stimulation causes changes in muscle tone relative to gravity, setting the stage for the tonic activity of the postural muscles.

The baby begins life in a general state of flexion, and the advent of extension heralds an infant's ability to attend actively to her environment. When the newborn is placed on her stomach, her weight will shift to her face. When she is pulled up from a supine position by her hands, her head will flop back with no control. The three-month-old has a great deal of extensor balance and can now control her head when pulled from supine. She can now control head rotation to view her environment

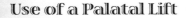

Use of a Palatal Lift

A **palatal lift prosthesis** is a device, typically anchored to the teeth, used to elevate the soft palate to more closely approximate the position of the velum for closure. The device looks like an orthodontic appliance with a projection in the back. This prosthesis is useful for individuals with muscular weakness, perhaps as a result of **hypoplasia** (inadequate muscle development) or a **neurogenic** condition (deficit arising from neurological cause).

when sitting, which requires little support. Soon her trunk muscles will be under sufficient control that she can rotate and reach for objects in her environment.

The combination of trunk stability and extensor-flexor balance gives her the tools for standing and walking—and talking. It is no surprise that the infant's speech begins to develop in concert with her locomotor skills. If you remember that the tongue is intimately related to the hyoid and larynx, you will realize that it is unreasonable to expect a child to control the complex, refined movements of the tongue until the trunk and neck muscles are stabilized.

Following stabilization, the infant must develop differential motor control. In the articulatory system, the manifestations of this control are evident in the rapidly increasing complexity of his speech production. The simple consonant-vowel (CV) syllable represents the most basic valving of the articulatory system. All the child must do to produce this syllable is begin phonation and open and close the mouth repeatedly. Tongue contact will approximate a velar or alveolar stop, or lip contact will produce a bilabial plosive. In any case, this infant has babbled, much to the delight of its parents!

The simple valving gives way to refined control of the tongue. With mandible stability accomplished, the child can begin the process of differentiating the tongue movements from those of the mandible. Following this, the infant differentiates tongue body and tip movements, as well as lateralization.

This development is hierarchical. The infant must balance muscle tone before being able to sit, and must sit before he can establish independent head and neck control. With control of neck muscles comes the freedom to move the mandible and tongue independently, and with that freedom comes the ability to differentially move the articulators.

Does this mean that a child with deficits of motor development will never develop speech? The answer, fortunately, is "no." The task is doubly difficult, however, and still depends on gaining the voluntary control and differentiation of those muscles. This is where you, the clinician, take your cue.

To summarize, the neonate depends on **reflexive responses** for protection and to meet his or her needs.

Phonological Development and Motor Control

Certainly the development of a child's phonology is a marvel. It should now be fairly clear that the maturation of the motor speech system governs, in large part, the speech sounds a child is capable of making. The stops (/p,t,k,b,d,g/) are present in the child's repertoire fairly early in development, although mastery will occur later than emergence. The reason for this is apparently motoric. A child of two or three years of age is quite capable of the basic "valving" gesture of opening and closing the mouth (/ba/), raising and lowering the tongue on the alveolar ridge (/da/), or near the velum (/ga/). However, controlled production of the stops requires the ability to differentiate labial, mandibular, and lingual movements, and thus mastery of the stops may occur as late as six years.

As the child develops greater motor control, he gains the ability to make graded movements with the tongue, so that he can sustain one articulator against the other with a constant pressure. The "raspberry" you hear in the preverbal child is very likely the precursor to the fricatives that will develop later. With graded control of lingual pressure comes the ability to make minute adjustments of an articulatory posture, such as those made with the dorsum of the tongue to differentiate /s/ and /ʃ/ through width of the tongue groove and tongue tip elevation.

- These primitive patterns gradually develop with **voluntary control patterns** to facilitate control of trunk, neck, and limbs.
- With this control comes the ability to make graded movements of the mandible and, subsequently, differentiated lingual movements.

Coordinated Articulation

Theories of motor control for speech have undergone a great deal of evolution, but are centered generally around the notions of locus of control, the need for consistency for the motor act, and task specification. Speech is arguably the most complex sequential motor task performed by humans. Consider the following hierarchical elements of speech, as implied by MacKay (1982).

Within the initial, **conceptual system**, we must first develop the proposition, or idea to be expressed, and that idea represents the sentence to be spoken. This idea or proposition must be mapped into a syntactical system to establish the language forms acceptable to match the concept, and appropriate words must be selected to match the syntax and to fit the proposition. Thus, if the idea "Tomorrow is Monday" is the chosen proposition, the syntax for that proposition must be selected, and the words chosen to fit the syntax and the proposition.

In the **phonological system**, syllable structure is parsed from the lexical selections. Phonological rules are applied to establish the correct phoneme combinations to meet the needs of the words chosen previously, and the individual features of those phonemes are parsed from the phonological specifications. Thus, at the phonological system level, the selected words ("Tomorrow is Monday") will be further broken into syllables, selected phonemes, and features for the phonemes. For instance, the /t/ in "tomorrow" will be defined as lingua-alveolar, stop, and voiceless. Notice that, throughout all of this, there has been no mention of muscles of articulation.

In the **muscle movement system**, muscles are activated to meet the needs of the feature selection process. The /t/ of the phonological system was broken into features, such as "lingua-alveolar," and this is now translated into movement of the muscles of the tongue that will produce that lingua-alveolar gesture (such as the superior longitudinal and genioglossus muscles).

Speaking assumes that we have developed an idea that we wish to express and that we somehow map that idea into muscle movements that change the three-dimensional space of the oral cavity. Those changes result in an acoustical output that is an acceptable representation of our goal.

In the early twentieth century, researchers recognized that learning sequential acts could be easily explained if one assumed that we linked a series of basic movements, like beads on a string. By this theory, the **associated chain theory**, the production of /t/ required only that the speaker learn all of the motor sequences leading up to elevation of the tongue to the alveolar ridge, and so forth. We could link a series of reflexive movements and entrain them in a sequential activation pattern. Once the motor act was learned, the speaker would forever be prepared to produce a word with /t/ in it. Lashley (1951) argued that the articulatory system is not a set of "sleeping" muscles waiting to be activated, but is rather a set of dynamic structures under continuous activation. In addition, the associative chain theories could not begin to account for variability in speech, much less the overlapping effect of one articulatory pattern on another (**coarticulation**). Future theories would have to account for the fluidity of speech production, the inherent variability of articulation based on context, and the ability of the articulators to achieve their phonetic target despite unpredictable alteration of the context of that production. Two major theoretical frameworks emerged from Lashley's concerns: the central control theory and the dynamic systems perspective.

Central Control Theory

The various forms of central control theory hold that there is a "master control" mechanism that dictates the muscle movements based on the linguistic goal. In the most extreme case, the command system would be oblivious to the state of the articulators at any moment and would administer the muscle commands without regard to articulator conditions of the moment. The beauty of such a model is the direct access that the motor system has to the language processor. Individual phonemes would be represented by a burst of neural excitation, so that the plan for a /t/ would be expertly executed with faithful precision. This provides a very nice solution to a major problem: The articulatory act for any phoneme requires precise activation of an overwhelming number of neurons and muscle fibers, and the activation must be accurate, timely, and result in correct movement. Thus, simply activating a program that your brain knows will produce a /t/ is much simpler than having to "micromanage" your articulatory system.

Clearly, feedback from sensors within the articulators and related structures, as well as of the auditory signal itself, had to be accounted for. Without feedback we would be unable to arrive at a production that was accurate and acceptable by our communicative partners. Fairbanks (1954) posed the earliest and most stringent of the **feedback theories**, holding that the brain commands the articulators to achieve a target, and that a mismatch between the feedback and the ideal results in correction of the output. Modification of articulation is driven by afferent information on an ongoing basis. In this view, the sensory system takes a dominant role in the production of speech.

The downside of these models is that they fail to account for the flexibility of the articulatory system in response to varying environmental conditions. If you pay attention to your tongue as you say the words "beat" and "toot," you will notice that the tongue is in two very different locations as it moves up for the final /t/, yet you are perfectly able to achieve both goals. Central control theories are forced to establish individual articulatory patterns to represent each allophone to accommodate this need—a very weighty proposition. Although the notions of central control remain robust and promising (e.g., MacKay, 1982), clearly there is a need to explain how we are able to articulate with such precision in the face of continuous variability.

Dynamic or Action Theory Models

As theorists worked to explain accurate and variable articulatory ability, the notion of **articulatory goals** evolved. The end product of muscle activity (and central control) was viewed as being a major determinant in execution. Saltzman (1986) viewed goal-related movement as composed of an **effector system**, a portion of which is the **terminal device**. The effector system would include the entire group of articulators involved in a given gesture, and the terminal device, or **end-effector**, is that portion of the effector system directly related to the articulatory goal (such as the dorsum of the tongue for articulation of the phoneme /i/). By differentiating these components, one can account for the problem of having to coordinate large numbers of muscle fibers in concert. From this point, one can view the articulatory effector system in a dynamic fashion. The components of the effector system are assigned the goal of the articulation, but are free to work within the degrees of freedom inherent in the system to accomplish the task. That is, no two acts are ever produced the same way twice, and yet there are definitely commonalities among motor acts. The dynamic models state that the commonality is that the motor act is accurately achieved within the bounds of variability, and the functional units of activation are groups of **coordinative structures**. Coordinative structures are functionally defined muscle groups which, when activated, contribute to achieving the goal at the terminal effector.

Trajectories, or movement paths, can be seen as targets of movement, and the structures involved in achieving a target are grouped as coordinative structures. If the movement is disturbed during execution, the coordinative structures are capable of altering their degree of activation to compensate for this "perturbation" without an altered central command. As an example, if you were to pick up a glass of milk, your target would be accurate movement of the glass rim to your lips.

Apraxia

Apraxia refers to a deficit in the programming of musculature for voluntary movement in absence of any muscular weakness or paralysis. There appear to be many types and subtypes of apraxia. **Limb apraxia** is identified as the inability to perform volitional gestures using the limbs. A patient with limb apraxia might reveal deficits in voluntarily using multiple objects to perform a sequence of acts upon request, such as making a sandwich. The act may be fluent, but the object is used inappropriately. The patient's ability to perform the act through imitation would be much less impaired.

A patient with **oral apraxia** might reveal difficulty programming the facial and lingual muscles for nonspeech acts. When this individual is asked to blow out a candle, she may experience a great deal of effortful groping in an attempt to find the right gesture with the lips in coordination with the outward flow of air. Often the oral apractic individual also has a verbal apraxia.

Verbal apraxia refers to a deficit in programming the articulators for speech sound production. The verbally apractic individual will make errors in correct articulation of the sounds of speech, although the errors vary widely from one attempt to another. The individual is aware of the error and will make frequent attempts at production, so that the flow of speech is greatly impeded. This patient will have more difficulty with multisyllabic than monosyllabic words, and semiautomatic speech (such as greetings) may be quite fluent.

By definition, apraxias occur without muscular weakness, although muscular weakness or paralysis may co-occur with the apraxia. Apraxias may arise from lesions to a variety of brain structures. Damage to the left hemisphere premotor region and insula of the cerebral cortex appears to have the greatest probability of producing apraxia, and the specific premotor region involved with speech is known as *Broca's area*. Damage to the supramarginal gyrus of the parietal lobe also may result in verbal apraxia, with the errors being more pure phonemic errors than those seen with damage in Broca's area, which will contain more distortions.

Unknown to you, the glass has a very heavy base. When you lift the glass, you expect it to be lighter than it is, so your muscular effort is less than if you had expected a heavier glass. If you depended on a central program to correct your movement, you might not reach your lips, and you probably would pour the milk down your shirt. As it is, your effector system adapts its activities to match the trajectory (table to lips), you add extra force, and your thirst is quenched. This ability to compensate is essential for speech production.

The **dynamic models** take into account the physical properties of the systems involved in articulation. Muscles and connective tissue have elastic properties that result in recoil, and dynamic models account for these variables in the equation. These models have more quickly accommodated the role of afferent information concerning the state of the musculature. According to Kelso and Ding (1993), there are many solutions to achieving any trajectory, and the relationship of the coordinative structures simply defines the solution from a given point of trajectory initiation to the point of termination.

Models of speech production also must somehow account for the fact that speech occurs at an extraordinarily rapid rate, and that, somehow, the articulatory system is very resistant to perturbation. We can accommodate a wide range of surprises in speech with no trouble at all. Dynamic models account for the dynamic aspects of the physical system required to achieve a specific target within the environment. If the articulatory command specifies an output product rather than a specific movement, the system retains the flexibility to adapt to changes in the environment.

These models attempt to account for many difficulties in articulation theory, not the least of which is **coarticulation** (the overlapping effect of one articulatory gesture on another). During running speech we will begin movement toward an articulatory posture well in advance of when it is needed *if* that activation does not interfere with the articulations preceding it. For example, pay attention to your lips when you say the words "see" and "sue." The /s/ in "see" is made with retracted lips, whereas the /s/ in "sue" is produced with rounded lips, both illustrating preparatory articulation. You will *not* see this effect in the word "booty," however. Try saying that word with your lips retracted for the /I/, and you will hear an unacceptable vowel production.

We are amazingly resilient in our articulatory abilities, and our resistance to **perturbation** (sudden, unexpected force applied to an articulator) supports the notion of functional synergies or coordinative structures. A functionally defined group of muscles and associated articulators are assigned a task (such as "close the lips"), but they have many different ways to accomplish the task. A perturbation or bite block reduces the number of ways available to accomplish the task, but as long as there is a solution, the articulators will find it.

To summarize, major theories of motor function approach the task from opposite directions.

- **Central control theories** postulate that a command for muscle movement originates in response to the linguistic needs.
- **Task dynamic theories** posit that the movement arises from the response by coordinated structures to an implicit trajectory.
- **Central control theories** account for the **linguistic dominance** of articulation for speech, while the **dynamic models** account for **variability** and **coarticulatory** effects.
- Both theories account for feedback in speech.

 CHAPTER SUMMARY

The **lower lip** is much faster and stronger than the **upper lip**, and responds reflexively to increases of pressure. Movement of the **mandible** for speech is slight when compared with movement for chewing. The mandibular posture for speech is one of sustained dynamic tension between antagonists. The **tongue** is versatile, with the extrinsic muscles providing the major movement of the body and the intrinsic muscles providing the shaping of the tongue. The **velum** must be maintained in a reasonably elevated position for most speech sounds, although it is capable of a range of movements.

Development of articulatory function involves gaining control of postural muscles that provide trunk **stability** and **differentiation** of muscle group function. **Reflexive responses** are protective and nurturant, and these primitive patterns gradually develop with **voluntary control** patterns to facilitate control of trunk, neck, and limbs, and finally differentiation for graded oral movement.

Complex speech production requires control of many parameters simultaneously. We use **sensory feedback** to learn articulator function in speech and probably use it for error control as well. **Central control theories** hold that the motor command for an articulation is driven by an articulatory configuration determined through consideration of linguistic elements. The motor command specifies the characteristics of muscle contraction without respect to speaking environment, but the theories cannot account for articulatory variability or the nearly infinite variety of speaking environments. **Dynamic theories** hold that **coordinative structures** interact to accomplish completion of a trajectory, and the theories accommodate the wide variability and flexibility of the articulatory system in speech.

▷ STUDY QUESTIONS

1. Identify the muscle that best fits the statement. (In some cases there is more than one muscle that fills the bill.)

   a. _____ Elevates tongue tip

   b. _____ Depresses tongue tip

   c. _____ Protrudes tongue

   d. _____ Retracts tongue

   e. _____ Elevates posterior tongue

   f. _____ Narrows tongue

   g. _____ Flattens tongue

   h. _____ Depresses velum

   i. _____ Constricts esophageal opening

   j. _____ Constricts upper pharynx

   k. _____ Elevates velum

2. The _____ (lower lip/upper lip) is faster and stronger than the _____ (lower lip/upper lip).

3. Motor control in the body develops from _____ (head/tail) to _____ (head/tail) and from _____ (proximal/distal) to _____ (proximal/distal).

4. The _____ theory of motor control would require the speaker to learn the sequences of motor acts required for articulation and to link these sequences of motor acts to form an articulatory gesture.

5. _____ is the overlapping effect of one articulatory gesture on another.

6. _____ theory holds that there is a "master control" mechanism that dictates the muscle movements based on the linguistic goal.

7. _____ theories generally see articulation as a process of achieving a goal through interaction of coordinative structures. Coordinative structures are muscle groups which, when activated, contribute to achievement of the goal at the terminal effector.

8. Tongue movement depends on the graceful balance of many muscles. Which of the muscles will be involved in elevation of the back of the tongue? As you think of this, ponder the muscles that must work as antagonists to help structures as well!

STUDY QUESTION ANSWERS

1. Identify the muscle that best fits the statement (In some cases there is more than one muscle that fills the bill.)
   a. <u>SUPERIOR LONGITUDINAL INTRINSIC</u> Elevates tongue tip
   b. <u>INFERIOR LONGITUDINAL INTRINSIC</u> Depresses tongue tip
   c. <u>GENIOGLOSSUS, POSTERIOR PORTION</u> Protrudes tongue
   d. <u>GENIOGLOSSUS, ANTERIOR PORTION; STYLOGLOSSUS</u> Retracts tongue
   e. <u>PALATOGLOSSUS</u> Elevates posterior tongue
   f. <u>TRANSVERSE INTRINSIC</u> Narrows tongue
   g. <u>VERTICAL INTRINSIC; GENIOGLOSSUS</u> Flattens tongue
   h. <u>PALATOGLOSSUS; PALATOPHARYNGEUS</u> Depresses velum
   i. <u>CRICOPHARYNGEUS</u> Constricts esophageal opening
   j. <u>SUPERIOR PHARYNGEAL CONSTRICTOR</u> Constricts upper pharynx
   k. <u>LEVATOR VELI PALATINI</u> Elevates velum
2. The <u>LOWER LIP</u> is faster and stronger than the <u>UPPER LIP</u>.
3. Motor control in the body develops from <u>HEAD</u> to <u>TAIL</u> and from <u>PROXIMAL</u> to <u>DISTAL</u>.
4. The <u>ASSOCIATED CHAIN</u> theory of motor control would require the speaker to learn the sequences of motor acts required for articulation and to link these sequences of motor acts to form an articulatory gesture.
5. <u>COARTICULATION</u> is the overlapping effect of one articulatory gesture on another.
6. <u>CENTRAL CONTROL</u> theory holds that there is a "master control" mechanism that dictates the muscle movements based upon the linguistic goal.
7. <u>TASK DYNAMIC</u> theories generally see articulation as a process of achieving a goal through interaction of coordinative structures. Coordinative structures are muscle groups which, when activated, contribute to achievement of the goal at the terminal effector.
8. Elevation of the posterior tongue requires active contraction of the palatoglossus, and perhaps the styloglossus, as well as the vertical intrinsic muscle. In addition, realize that the tongue is pulling against the soft palate to achieve elevation, because the palatoglossus is a velar depressor as well. When the palatoglossus contracts to elevate the tongue, the levator veli palatini must contract to keep the soft palate elevated.

 REFERENCES

Abbs, J. H., & Cole, K. J. (1991). Consideration of bulbar and suprabulbar afferent influences upon speech motor coordination and programming. In S. Grillner, B. Lindblom, J. Lubker, & A. Persson (Eds.), *Speech motor control* (pp. 159–186). Oxford: Pergamon Press.

Abrahams, P. H., McMinn, R. M. H., Hutchings, R. T., Sandy, C., & Mark, S. (2003). *McMinn's color atlas of human anatomy* (5th ed.). Philadelphia: Mosby.

Baken, R. J., & Orlikoff, R. F. (1999). *Clinical measurement of speech and voice* (2nd ed.). San Diego, CA: Singular Publishing Group.

Barlow, S. M., & Netsell, R. (1986). Differential fine force control of the upper and lower lips. *Journal of Speech and Hearing Research, 29,* 163–169.

Barlow, S. M., & Rath, E. M. (1985). Maximum voluntary closing forces in the upper and lower lips of humans. *Journal of Speech and Hearing Research, 28,* 373–376.

Basmajian, J. V. (1975). *Grant's method of anatomy.* Baltimore: Williams & Wilkins.

Bateman, H. E., & Mason, R. M. (1984). *Applied anatomy and physiology of the speech and hearing mechanism.* Springfield, IL: Charles C. Thomas.

Beck, E. W., Monson, H., & Groer, M. (1982). *Mosby's atlas of functional human anatomy.* St. Louis, MO: C. V. Mosby.

Bly, L. (1983). *The components of normal movement during the first year of life and abnormal motor movement.* Chicago: Neuro-Developmental Treatment Association.

Bly, L. (1994). *Motor skills acquisition in the first year.* Tucson, AZ: Therapy Skill Builders.

Bunton, K., & Weismer, G. (1994). Evaluation of a reiterant force-impulse task in the tongue. *Journal of Speech and Hearing Research, 37,* 1020–1031.

Chusid, J. G. (1985). *Correlative neuroanatomy and functional neurology* (17th ed.). Los Altos, CA: Lange Medical Publications.

DeNil, L. F., & Abbs, J. H (1991). Influence of speaking rate on the upper lip, lower lip, and jaw peak velocity sequencing during bilabial closing movements. *Journal of the Acoustical Society of America, 89*(2), 845–849.

Duffy, J. R. (1995). *Motor speech disorders.* St. Louis, MO: C. V. Mosby.

Ettema, S. L., & Kuehn, D. P. (1994). A quantitative histologic study of the normal human adult soft palate. *Journal of Speech and Hearing Research, 37,* 303–313.

Fairbanks, G. (1954). A theory of the speech mechanism as a servosystem. *Journal of Speech and Hearing Disorders, 19,* 133–139.

Flege, J. E. (1988). Anticipatory and carry-over nasal coarticulation in the speech of children and adults. *Journal of Speech and Hearing Research, 31,* 525–536.

Folkins, J. W., Linville, R. N., Garrett, J. D., & Brown, C. K. (1988). Interactions in the labial musculature during speech. *Journal of Speech and Hearing Research, 31,* 253–264.

Ganong, W. F. (2003). *Review of medical physiology* (21st ed.). New York: McGraw-Hill/Appleton & Lange.

Garcia-Colera, A., & Semjen, A. (1988). Distributed planning of movement sequences. *Journal of Motor Behavior, 20*(3), 341–367.

Gelb, H. (1985). *Clinical management of head, neck and TMJ pain and dysfunction.* Philadelphia: W. B. Saunders.

Goffman, L., & Smith, A. (1994). Motor unit territories in the human perioral musculature. *Journal of Speech and Hearing Research, 37,* 975–984.

Gracco, V. L. (1988). Timing factors in the coordination of speech movements. *Journal of Neuroscience, 8*(12), 4628–4639.

Gracco, V. L. (1994). Some organizational characteristics of speech movement control. *Journal of Speech and Hearing Research, 37,* 4–27.

Gracco, V. L., & Abbs, J. H. (1989). Sensorimotor characteristics of speech motor sequences. *Experimental Brain Research, 75,* 586–598.

Gray, H., Bannister, L. H., Berry, M. M., & Williams, P. L. (Eds.). (1995). *Gray's anatomy.* London: Churchill Livingstone.

Groher, M. E. (1984). *Dysphagia.* Boston: Butterworths.

Hall, P. K., Hardy, J. C., & LaVelle, W. E. (1990). A child with signs of developmental apraxia of speech with whom a palatal lift prosthesis was used to manage palatal dysfunction. *Journal of Speech and Hearing Disorders, 55,* 454–460.

Hellstrand, E. (1981). The neuromuscular system of the tongue. In S. Grillner, B. Lindblom, J. Lubker, & A. Persson (Eds.), *Speech motor control* (pp. 141–157). Oxford: Pergamon Press.

Horak, M. (1992). The utility of connectionism for motor learning: A reinterpretation of contextual interference in movement schemas. *Journal of Motor Behavior, 24*(1), 58–66.

Jordan, M. I. (1990). Motor learning and the degrees of freedom problem. In M. Jeannerod (Ed.), *Attention and performance XIII: Motor Representation and control.* Hillsdale, NJ: Lawrence Erlbaum.

Landgren, S., & Olsson, K. A. (1981). Oral mechanoreceptors. In S. Grillner, B. Lindblom, J. Lubker, & A. Persson (Eds.), *Speech motor control* (pp. 129–139). Oxford: Pergamon Press.

Kaplan, H. M. (1971). *Anatomy and physiology of speech.* New York: McGraw-Hill.

Katz, W. F., Kripke, C., & Tallal, P. (1991). Anticipatory coarticulation in the speech of adults and young children: acoustic, perceptual, and video data. *Journal of Speech and Hearing Research, 34,* 1222–1249.

Kelso, J. A., & Ding, M. (1993). Fluctuations, intermittency, and controllable chaos in biological coordination. In K. M. Newell & D. M. Corcos (Eds.), *Variability and motor control* (pp. 291–316). Champaign, IL: Human Kinetics.

Kelso, J. A. S., Tuller, B., Vatikiotis-Bateson, E., & Fowler, C. A. (1984). Functionally specific articulatory cooperation following jaw perturbations during speech: Evidence for coordinative structures. *Journal of Experimental Psychology: Perception and Performance, 19,* 812–832.

Kent, R. D. (1997). *The speech sciences.* San Diego, CA: Singular Publishing Group.

Kent, R. D., Kent, J. F., & Rosenbek, J. C. (1987). Maximum performance tests of speech production. *Journal of Speech and Hearing Disorders, 52,* 367–387.

Kuehn, D. P., Lemme, M. L., & Baumgartner, J. M. (1989). *Neural bases of speech, hearing, and language.* Boston: Little, Brown.

Kuehn, D. P., Templeton, P. J., & Maynard, J. A. (1990). Muscle spindles in the velopharyngeal musculature of humans. *Journal of Speech and Hearing Research, 33,* 488–493.

Landgren, S., & Olsson, K. A. (1981). Oral mechanoreceptors. In S. Grillner, B. Lindblom, J. Lubker, & A. Persson (Eds.), *Speech motor control* (pp. 129–139). Oxford: Pergamon Press.

Langley, M. B., & Lombardino, L. J. (1991). *Neurodevelopmental strategies for managing communication disorders in children with severe motor dysfunction.* Austin, TX: Pro-Ed.

Lashley, K. S. (1951). The problem of serial order in behavior. In L. A. Jerrers (Ed.), *Cerebral mechanisms in behavior* (pp. 506–528). New York: John Wiley.

Lieberman, P. (1977). *Speech physiology and acoustic phonetics: An introduction.* New York: Macmillan.

Liss, J. M. (1990). Muscle spindles in the human levator veli palatini and palatoglossus muscles. *Journal of Speech and Hearing Research, 33,* 736–746.

Logemann, J. (1983). *Evaluation and treatment of swallowing disorders.* Boston: College-Hill Press.

Love, R. J., Hagerman, E. L., & Taimi, E. G. (1980). Speech performance, dysphagia, and oral reflexes in cerebral palsy. *Journal of Speech and Hearing Disorders, 45,* 59–75.

MacKay, D. G. (1982). The problem of flexibility, fluency, and speed-accuracy trade-off in skilled behavior. *Psychological Review, 89,* 483–506.

McClean, M. (1973). Forward coarticulation of velar movement at marked junctural boundaries. *Journal of Speech and Hearing Research, 16,* 286–296.

McNeil, M. R., Weismer, G., Adams, S., & Mulligan, M. (1990). Oral structure nonspeech motor control in normal, dysarthric, aphasic, and apraxic speakers: isometric force and static position control. *Journal of Speech and Hearing Research, 33,* 255–268.

Møller, A. R. (2003). *Sensory systems: Anatomy and physiology.* New York: Academic Press.

Moore, C. A. (1993). Symmetry of mandibular muscle activity as an index of coordinative strategy. *Journal of Speech and Hearing Research, 36,* 1145–1157.

Moore, C. A., Smith, A., & Ringel, R. L. (1988). Task-specific organization of activity in human jaw muscles. *Journal of Speech and Hearing Research, 31,* 670–680.

Netsell, R. (1973). Speech physiology. In F. D. Minifie, T. J. Hixon, & F. Williams (Eds.), *Normal aspects of speech, hearing, and language.* Englewood Cliffs, NJ: Prentice-Hall.

Netter, F. H. (1997). *Atlas of human anatomy.* Los Angeles: Icon Learning Systems.

Rohen, J. W., Yokochi, C., Lutjen-Drecoll, E. L., & Romrell, L. J. (2002). *Color atlas of anatomy: A photographic study of the human body* (5th ed.). Philadelphia: Williams & Wilkins.

Rosenbaum, D. A., Kenny, S. B., & Derr, M. A. (1983). Hierarchical control of rapid movement sequences. *Journal of Experimental Psychology: Human Perception and Performance, 9*(1), 86–102.

Rosenbek, J. C., Robbins, J., Fishback, B., & Levine, R. L. (1991). Effects of thermal application on dysphagia after stroke. *Journal of Speech and Hearing Research,* 34, 1257–1268.

Rosse, C., Gaddum-Rosse, P., & Rosse, G. (1997). *Hollinshead's textbook of anatomy.* Philadelphia: Lippincott-Raven.

Saltzman, E. (1986). Task dynamic coordination of the speech articulators: A preliminary model. *Experimental brain research* (pp. 129–144). Berlin-Heidelberg: Springer-Verlag.

Schmidt, R. A. (1975). A schema theory of discrete motor skill learning. *Psychological Review, 82,* 225–260.

Shaffer, L. H. (1976). Intention and performance. *Psychological Review, 33*(5), 375–393.

Shriberg, L. D., & Kent, R. D. (2002). *Clinical phonetics* (3rd ed.). New York: Allyn & Bacon.

Small, A. M. (1973). Acoustics. In F. D. Minifie, T. J. Hixon, & F. Williams (Eds.), *Normal aspects of speech, hearing, and language.* Englewood Cliffs, NJ: Prentice-Hall.

Smith, A., McFarland, D. H., & Weber, C. M. (1986). Interactions between speech and finger movements: An exploration of the dynamic pattern perspective. *Journal of Speech and Hearing Research,* 29, 471–480.

Square-Storer, P., & Roy, E. A. (1989). The apraxias: Commonalities and distinctions. In P. Square-Storer (Ed.), *Acquired apraxia of speech in aphasic adults: Theoretical and clinical issues.* London: Taylor & Francis.

Weber, C. M., & Smith, A. (1987). Reflex responses in human jaw, lip, and tongue muscles elicited by mechanical stimulation. *Journal of Speech and Hearing Research,* 30, 70–79.

Westbury, J. R. (1988). Mandible and hyoid bone movements during speech. *Journal of Speech and Hearing Research,* 31, 405–416.

Wickens, J., Hyland, B., & Anson, G. (1994). Cortical cell assemblies: a possible mechanism for motor programs. *Journal of Motor Behavior, 26*(2), 66–82.

Wohlert, A. B., & Goffman, L. (1994). Human perioral muscle activation patterns. *Journal of Speech and Hearing Research, 37,* 1032–1040.

Zemlin, W. R. (1998). *Speech and hearing science: Anatomy and physiology* (4th ed.). Needham Heights, MA: Allyn & Bacon.

Zickefoose, W. (1989). *Techniques of oral myofunctional therapy.* Sacramento, CA: O.M.T. Materials, Inc.

CHAPTER 9

Physiology of Mastication and Deglutition

BIOLOGICAL FUNCTION

In Chapter 2 we introduced you to the concept of the relationship between biological and speech function in anatomy and physiology. Humans have done a marvelous job of taking the anatomical structures and their physiology and capitalizing on those functions for speech. In many ways the physiology of **mastication** (the process of preparing food for swallowing) and **deglutition** (the processes of swallowing) provides an exquisite view of those integrated systems we use so effortlessly in speech. As we discuss these very basic and fundamental processes, you will see that we must invoke the respiratory, phonatory, articulatory, and nervous systems. Further, keep an eye on the Clinical Notes we provide in boxes to see just how problematic it can be when the anatomy and physiology of *any one of these systems* is disrupted. As practicing speech-language pathologists, you may very likely be deeply involved in these processes, so we hope you will take this information to heart!

mastication: *the process of preparing food for swallowing*

deglutition: *the process of swallowing*

Introduction to Mastication and Deglutition

Mastication refers to the processes involved in food preparation, including moving unchewed food onto the grinding surface of the teeth, chewing it, and mixing it with saliva in preparation for swallowing. *Deglutition* refers to swallowing. These two biological processes require integration of lingual, velar, pharyngeal, and facial muscle movement (Chapter 8) with laryngeal adjustments (Chapters 5 and 6) and respiratory control (Chapters 2 and 3). Consider this: During the mature mastication and deglutition process, all muscles inserting into the orbicularis oris may be called into action to open, close, purse, and retract the lips as food is received. All intrinsic and extrinsic muscles of the tongue will be invoked to move the food into position for chewing and preparation of the **bolus** (either liquid or a mass of food) for swallowing. The velar elevators seal off the nasal cavity to prevent regurgitation, and the pharyngeal constrictors must contract in a highly predictable fashion to move the bolus down the pharynx and into the esophagus. With the addition of laryngeal elevation, we have just invoked more than 55 pairs of muscles whose timing and innervation patterns must be integrated through accurate activation of cranial and spinal nerves. All this for a snack!

As you ponder the biological processes associated with deglutition, please do not lose sight of the relationship between feeding and speech. We have long recognized that feeding skills are both preparatory and supportive of the speech act, and inadequate development of feeding reflects directly on speech development. In this chapter we will first discuss developmental and adult mastication and deglutition patterns, as related to the underlying anatomy and physiology, and then we will discuss the neuroanatomical underpinnings of these processes in an attempt to integrate this important function with its control mechanisms.

Anatomical and Physiological Developmental Issues

As we discussed in Chapter 8, maturation of the infant nervous system provides a stable trunk, neck, and head base upon which mastication and deglutition are developed. The maturation process of the physical and physiological systems sets an important stage for adult swallowing function.

At birth, the neonate is restricted to reflexive responses. The infant gains nutrition through the reflexive **rooting reflex**, which involves orienting toward the direction of tactile contact of the mouth region (**perioral region**). The full rooting response involves head rotation and mouth opening. Soft tactile contact with the inner margin of the lips will elicit the **sucking reflex**, which involves piston-like tongue protrusion and retraction in preparation for receiving food from the mother's breast.

Movements at this stage are gross and reflexive. The gross movements of the mandible during sucking will ultimately give way to refined movement of the mandible during speech. Tongue protrusion distal to the mouth during sucking will evolve into a sucking gesture that does not require tongue protrusion, as in sucking on a soda straw. The gross,

bolus: *ball of food or liquid to be swallowed*

rooting reflex: *reflexive response of infant to tactile stimulation of the cheek or lips; causes the infant to turn toward the stimulus and open his or her mouth*

perioral region: *region around the mouth*

sucking reflex: *reflex involving tongue protrusion and retraction in preparation for receipt of liquid; stimulated by contact to the upper lip*

piston-like swallow of an infant (to be discussed) gives way to a gracefully orchestrated mature swallow.

Figures 9-1 and 9-2 show the infant oral-pharyngeal structures as compared with those of the adult. If you look closely at these figures, you will realize that there are marked differences between these two systems. The infant's oral cavity is necessarily smaller, but notice also the location of the laryngeal structures and the magnitude of the velum relative to the pharynx. The larynx is markedly elevated at birth, but descends over the course of the first four years. The hyoid is elevated and relatively forward as compared with the adult, and there is no dentition in the neonate. The relatively larger velum and elevated larynx play a vital role in respiration and deglutition, as we shall see.

The sucking reflex is a critically important response. This reflex is elicited by tactile stimulation of the lips and perioral space, as well as through visual presentation of a food source in older infants. This reflex involves protrusion of the tongue with sufficient force to initiate flow of

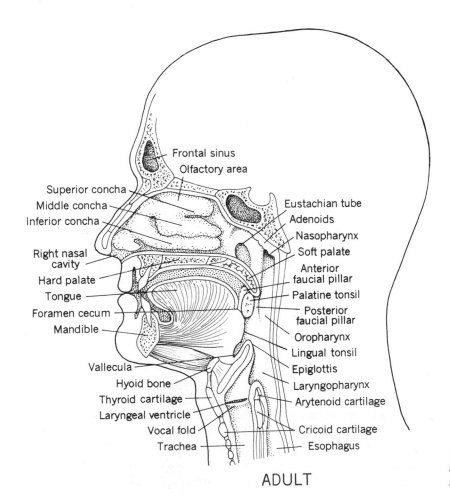

ADULT

Figure 9-1. Oral, pharyngeal, and laryngeal structure of an adult. (After Netter, 1976.)

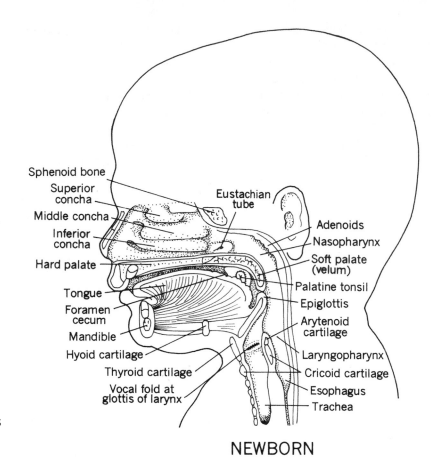

Labels on figure:
Sphenoid bone
Superior concha
Middle concha
Inferior concha
Hard palate
Tongue
Foramen cecum
Mandible
Hyoid cartilage
Thyroid cartilage
Vocal fold at glottis of larynx
Eustachian tube
Adenoids
Nasopharynx
Soft palate (velum)
Palatine tonsil
Epiglottis
Arytenoid cartilage
Laryngopharynx
Cricoid cartilage
Esophagus
Trachea

NEWBORN

Figure 9-2. The relationship between oral and velar structures in the neonate. (After Netter, 1976.)

milk from the breast. Repeated forward pumping of the tongue results in milk entering the oral cavity. After four or five thrusts of the tongue, a swallow is triggered, with the tongue base lowered to permit the milk bolus to enter the oropharynx during the next forward pumping action of the tongue. This swallow pattern is often referred to as an "immature" swallow pattern, which is perfectly appropriate for an infant.

This swallow pattern of the neonate is precisely supported by the anatomy of the infant. Take a look at Figure 9-3. You can see from this drawing that the velum of the infant "locks" into the space between the epiglottis and tongue at the location of the valleculae. This configuration seals off the infant's airway so that the bolus cannot enter the respiratory passageway. The infant breathes and swallows at the same time without interference.

This larynx-velum relationship is found in most mammals as well. The pharynx of quadrupeds (four-footed animals) is actually a simple extension of the oral cavity, and the ability to breathe while holding prey with one's mouth is critical to survival of predators. Further, prey animals are able to monitor their environment for dangers through the

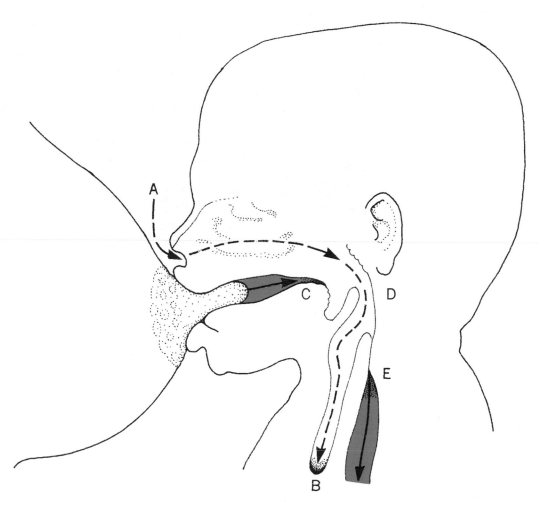

Figure 9-3. Oral, pharyngeal, and laryngeal structures of a neonate during sucking and swallowing. Note that the infant breathes through the nostrils (A), with unimpeded flow of air into the respiratory passageway (B). Milk from nursing flows around the posterior tongue (C) and through the pyriform sinus to the (D) esophagus (E). (After Netter, 1976.)

sense of smell while grazing (Netter, 1976). In humans, this ability is lost as the oral cavity increases in size, and as the hyoid and larynx drop to their adult positions. The adult pharynx serves as a passageway for both the respiratory and gastrointestinal systems, a clear incompatibility. The adult human swallow pattern compensates for this vulnerability by tightly closing and protecting the airway.

Around the sixth month, dentition begins erupting, and the infant is introduced to his or her first relatively solid food. The dentition blocks the anterior protrusion of the tongue, which supports retraction of the tongue during swallow. Further, dentition supports chewing and grinding movements, which strengthen the muscles of mastication. The mature swallow (to be described later) requires contraction of the masseter, temporalis, and medial pterygoid muscles to counteract the force of the tongue upon the roof of the mouth as the bolus is propelled backward. The immature swallow does not require this same degree of force, as the tongue does not push against the palate to force the bolus into the pharynx. The force directed onto the palate is critical for proper development of the dental arches and hard palate. If the muscles of mastication are not utilized during the transitional and mature swallow, the maxillary dental arch will collapse medially and a vaulted palate will develop (see Figure 7-29C). A cross-bite will develop, in which the upper dentition does not make proper contact with the lower dentition. This oral configuration will also result in an elongated and narrowed maxilla, giving the impression of a long and narrow face, classically referred to as the "mouth breather **facies**," because it is often associated with nasal obstruction that prohibits proper nasal respiration.

facies: *surface of a structure*

ORGANIZATIONAL PATTERNS OF MASTICATION AND DEGLUTITION

Mastication and deglutition in the adult consist of a sequence of four extremely well-orchestrated events or stages. These stages are the **oral preparatory stage** (**mastication**), **oral stage** (**propulsion of bolus**), **pharyngeal stage** (**pharyngeal swallow**), and **esophageal stage** (**esophageal transit**). We will discuss these stages in broad behavioral terms before discussing their underlying physiology.

oral preparatory stage: *the stage in which food is prepared for swallow*

oral stage: *the stage of swallow in which the bolus is transmitted to the pharynx*

pharyngeal stage: *the stage of swallow in which the bolus is transmitted to the esophagus; involves numerous physiological protective responses*

esophageal stage: *the stage of swallow in which food is transported from the upper esophageal region to the stomach*

Oral Preparatory Stage (Mastication)

In this stage, food is prepared for swallowing. To complete this task, a number of processes must occur at virtually the same time (Table 9-1). We should emphasize that although this may be a voluntary process, it can be performed automatically without conscious effort.

First, we introduce food into the mouth and keep it there by tightly occluding the lips. This lip seal demands that we breathe through the nose, so the tongue bunches up in back and the soft palate is pulled down to keep the food in the oral cavity.

The tongue cups in preparation for the input food. The food must be ground up so that it can easily pass through the esophagus for digestion, and this is performed by the coordinated activity of the muscles of mastication, as well as the lingual muscles. The tongue is in charge of keeping the food in the oral cavity, and it does so by effecting a seal along the alveolar ridge. As it holds the food in place, it may compress it against the hard palate, partially crushing it in preparation for the teeth. The tongue then begins moving the food onto the grinding surfaces of the teeth, pulling the food back into the oral cavity to be mixed

Table 9-1. Muscles of the oral preparation stage.

MUSCLE	FUNCTION	INNERVATION (CRANIAL NERVE)
Facial Muscles		
Orbicularis oris	Maintains oral seal	VII
Mentalis	Elevates lower lip	VII
Buccinator	Flattens cheeks	VII
Risorius	Flattens cheeks	VII
Mandibular Muscles		
Masseter	Elevates mandible	V
Temporalis	Elevates mandible; retracting, protruding	V
Medial pterygoid	Elevates mandible; lateral movement, grinding	V
Lateral pterygoid	Protruding, grinding	V
Tongue Muscles		
Mylohyoid	Elevates floor of mouth	V
Geniohyoid	Elevates hyoid; depresses mandible	XII
Digastric	Elevates hyoid; depresses mandible	V, XII
Superior longitudinal	Elevates tip; deviates tip	XII
Inferior longitudinal	Depresses tip; deviates tip	XII
Vertical	Cups and grooves tongue	XII
Genioglossus	Moves tongue body; cups tongue	XII
Styloglossus	Elevates posterior tongue	XII
Palatoglossus	Elevates posterior tongue	IX, X, XI
Soft Palate Muscles		
Palatoglossus	Depresses velum	IX, X, XI
Palatopharyngeus	Depresses velum	X, XI

with saliva, and then moving it back to the teeth for more of a work-up. The salivary glands (parotid, submandibular, and sublingual glands) secrete saliva into the oral cavity to help form the mass of food into a bolus for swallowing. The facial muscles of the buccal wall (risorius and buccinator) contract to keep the food from entering the lateral sulcus (between the gums and cheek wall).

Deficits of the Oral Preparatory Stage

Numerous problems arise when neuromuscular control of mastication is compromised. Loss of sensation and awareness, coupled with weak buccal musculature, can lead to pocketing of food in the lateral or anterior sulci. Weak muscles of mastication can cause inadequately chewed food; weak lingual muscles will result in poor mixture of saliva with the food, inadequate bolus production, and difficulty compressing the bolus onto the hard palate. If the muscles of the soft palate are compromised, the velum may not be fully depressed and the tongue may not be elevated in the back, permitting food to escape into the pharynx prior to initiation of the pharyngeal reflexes. This is life-threatening, because food entering the pharynx in the absence of the reflexive response may well reach the open airway. Aspiration pneumonia (pneumonia secondary to aspirated matter) is a constant concern for individuals with dysphagia (a disorder of swallowing).

This is quite a feat of coordination. To prove this to yourself, take a bite of a cracker and attend to the process. If you count the number of times you chew on the cracker, you will realize that you grind it between 15 and 30 times before you swallow any of it. As you introduce the cracker into your mouth, your tongue may push it up against the anterior hard palate to begin breaking it down. Your tongue then performs the dance of mastication, flicking in between the molars as your mandible lowers, then quickly moving out of the way before the jaw closes forcefully to continue grinding. Your tongue organizes the ground food onto its dorsum, mixes the food with saliva, and moves it back out to the teeth if the bolus does not meet your specification for "ready to swallow." The buccal musculature helps to keep the food out of the buccal cavity during oral preparation.

If you still question the grace of this process, try to remember the last time you bit your tongue, lip, or cheek. A snack of 10 crackers will invoke at least 600 oscillations of the mastication musculature, and a full meal clearly requires thousands of grinding gestures. Despite this, you can scarcely remember the last painful time your tongue and mandible failed the coordination test!

Oral Stage

When the bolus of food is finally ready to swallow, the **oral stage** of swallowing begins (see Table 9-2). When this point is reached, several processes must occur sequentially. The tongue base is elevated in the posterior during mastication, but now it drops down and pulls posteriorly. Mastication stops, and the anterior tongue elevates to the hard palate and squeezes the bolus back toward the faucial pillars. Contact

Table 9-2. Muscles of the oral stage required to propel the bolus into the oropharynx.

MUSCLE	FUNCTION	INNERVATION (CRANIAL NERVE)
Mandibular Muscles		
Masseter	Elevates mandible	V
Temporalis	Elevates mandible	V
Internal pterygoid	Elevates mandible	V
Tongue Muscles		
Mylohyoid	Elevates tongue and floor of mouth	V
Superior longitudinal	Elevates tip	XII
Vertical	Cups and grooves tongue	XII
Genioglossus	Moves tongue body; cups tongue	XII
Styloglossus	Elevates posterior tongue	XII
Palatoglossus	Elevates posterior tongue	IX, X, XI

Deficits of the Oral Stage

Deficits of the oral stage center around sensory and motor dysfunction. Weakened movements cause reduced **oral transit time** of the bolus toward the pharynx. With greater motor involvement, food may remain on the tongue or hard palate following transit.

In patients with oral-phase involvement, there is a tendency for the epiglottis to fail to invert over the laryngeal opening and to have limited elevation of the hyoid. Perlman, Grahack, and Booth (1992) found that individuals with such a deficit showed increased pooling of food or liquid within the valleculae.

Difficulty initiating a reflexive swallow may be the result of sensory deficit. Application of a cold stimulus to the anterior faucial pillars, coupled with instructions to attempt to swallow, is a time-honored method to assist these individuals in initiating a swallow, although ongoing clinical research is needed to determine its efficacy (Rosenbek, Robbins, Fishback, & Levine, 1991).

with the fauces, soft palate, or posterior tongue base appears to be the stimulus that triggers the reflexes of the pharyngeal stage. Logemann (1998) noted that this "trigger point" appears to change over the life of the adult, such that the geriatric swallow is triggered at a more posterior location.

oral transit time: *time required to move the bolus to the point of initiation of the pharyngeal stage of swallowing*

Pharyngeal Stage

The **pharyngeal stage** consists of a complex sequence of reflexively controlled events (see Table 9-3 and Figure 9-4). As the bolus reaches the region of the faucial pillars (or, alternately, the posterior base of the tongue near the valleculae in older individuals [Logemann, 1998]), the pharyngeal swallow response is initiated, beginning with elevation of the soft palate, which had been depressed. The oropharynx is now separated from the nasopharynx.

Respiration ceases reflexively at this point. With the velum elevated, the tongue retracted, and the lips sealed, both the oral and nasal outlets are closed so that air cannot escape or enter for respiration. More importantly, food is entering the pharynx, and the airway must be protected. To accomplish the protective function the vocal folds tightly adduct, followed by constriction of the false vocal folds and depression of the epiglottis via the aryepiglottic muscles and elevation of the larynx relative to the tongue.

With the airway sealed, the larynx moves up and forward as a unit. The hyoid bone is a palpable indication of laryngeal elevation, because we can feel it elevate and move forward in this stage. The epiglottis now descends to cover the laryngeal aditus, assisted by the aryepiglottic muscles. Simultaneously, the cricopharyngeus muscle of the inferior constrictor relaxes. This serves as the sphincter for the superior esophagus, and is referred to as the upper esophageal sphincter (UES). During respiration (i.e., when a person is not swallowing), the UES is continually contracted until the swallow is initiated. This tonic contraction of the cricopharyngeus keeps gastric contents from escaping into the laryngopharynx (**esophageal reflux**). Relaxing this muscle gives the bolus a place to go.

Food is propelled down the pharynx toward the esophagus by means of sequential contraction of the superior, middle, and inferior pharyngeal constrictors. As food is forced into the oropharynx, the posterior faucial pillars move medially, effectively channeling the bolus downward.

esophageal reflux: *esophageal regurgitation into the hypopharynx*

nasal regurgitation: *loss of food or liquid through the nose*

pharyngeal transit time: *the time required to move the bolus, measured from the beginning of pharyngeal swallow to the time the bolus enters the esophagus*

Deficits of the Pharyngeal Stage

Sensory and motor deficit can be dangerous at this stage of swallowing. Slowed velar elevation may result in **nasal regurgitation** (loss of food or liquid through the nose), while reduced sensation at the fauces, posterior tongue, pharyngeal wall, or soft palate may result in elevated threshold for trigger of the swallowing reflex. Reduced function of the pharyngeal constrictors may result in slowed **pharyngeal transit time** of the bolus, in which case the individual may prematurely reinitiate respiration. Weakened pharyngeal function may result in residue left in the valleculae. Failure of the hyoid and thyroid to elevate may result in loss of airway protection, so that food will fall into the larynx and be aspirated on reinflation of the lungs.

Table 9-3. Muscles of the pharyngeal stage required to propel the bolus toward the esophagus, elevate the larynx, and close the airway.

MUSCLE	FUNCTION	INNERVATION (CRANIAL NERVE)
Tongue Muscles		
Mylohyoid	Elevates hyoid and tongue	V
Geniohyoid	Elevates hyoid and larynx; depresses mandible	C-1
Digastricus	Elevates hyoid and larynx	V, XII
Genioglossus	Retracts tongue	XII
Styloglossus	Elevates posterior tongue	XII
Palatoglossus	Narrows fauces; elevates posterior tongue	IX, X, XI
Stylohyoid	Elevates hyoid and larynx	VII
Hyoglossus	Elevates hyoid	XII
Thyrohyoid	Elevates hyoid	XII
Superior longitudinal	Elevates tongue	XII
Inferior longitudinal	Depresses tongue	XII
Transverse	Flattens tongue	XII
Vertical	Narrows tongue	XII
Soft Palate Muscles		
Levator veli palatini	Elevates soft palate	X, XI
Tensor veli palatini	Dilates Eustachian tube	V
Musculus uvulae	Shortens soft palate	X, XI
Pharyngeal Muscles		
Palatopharyngeus	Constricts oropharynx to channel bolus	X, XI
Salpingopharyngeus	Elevates pharynx	XI
Stylopharyngeus	Raises larynx	IX
Cricopharyngeus	Relaxes esophageal orifice	X, XI
Middle constrictor	Narrows pharynx	X, XI
Inferior constrictor	Narrows pharynx	X, XI
Laryngeal Muscles		
Lateral cricoarytenoid	Adducts vocal folds	X
Transverse arytenoid	Adducts vocal folds	X
Oblique arytenoid	Adducts vocal folds	X
Aryepiglotticus	Retracts epiglottis; constricts aditus	X
Thyroepiglotticus	Dilates airway following swallow	X

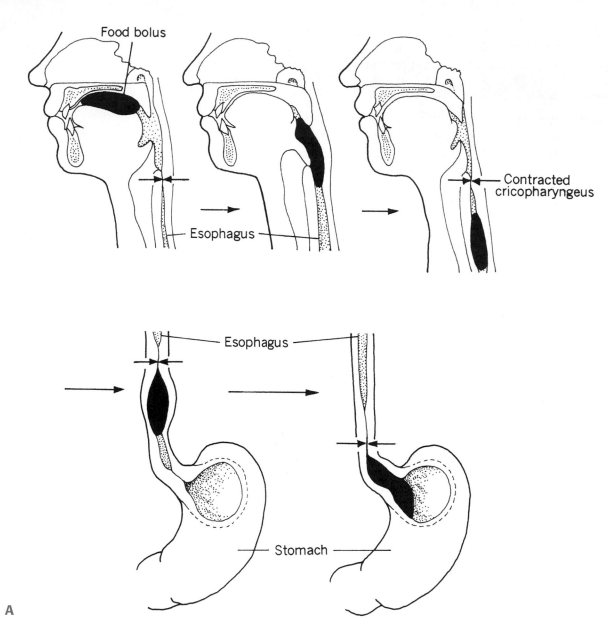

Figure 9-4. A. Stages of deglutition. (After Campbell, 1990.) *(continues)*

When the bolus reaches the laryngopharynx, it passes over the epiglottis. The bolus is divided into two roughly equal masses, passing to either side of the larynx, through the pyriform sinuses, to recombine at the esophageal entrance.

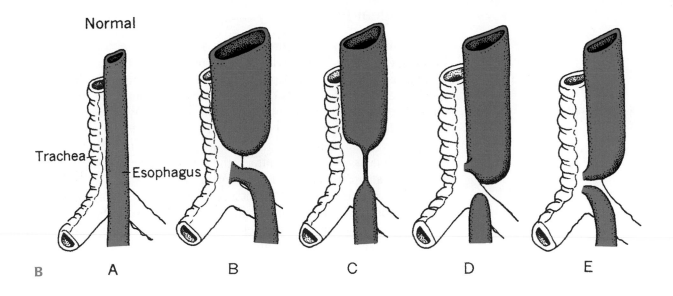

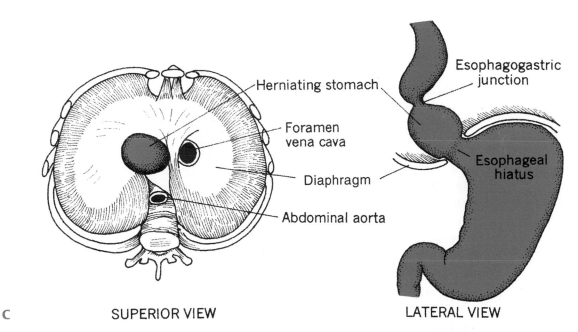

SUPERIOR VIEW　　　　　　　　**LATERAL VIEW**

Figure 9-4. *(continued)* **B.** Developmental malformations of the esophagus. A. Normal esophagus. B. Esophagus anastomosing with trachea. C. Esophageal stenosis. D. Esophageal discontinuity with tracheal porting. E. Esophageal fusing with trachea, resulting in esophageal porting. (Adapted from Newman and Randolph, 1990.) **C.** Herniation of stomach through esophageal hiatus of diaphragm. *Left:* View from above the diaphragm, showing herniation of stomach. *Right:* Lateral view. Note the position of the lower esophageal sphincter (esophagastric junction). (After Healy and Seybold, 1969, and Payne and Ellis, 1984.)

Esophageal Phase

The **esophageal phase** is purely reflexive and is not within voluntary control. This stage begins when the bolus reaches the orifice of the esophagus. The bolus is transported through the esophagus to the lower esophageal sphincter (LES) by means of segmental and inferiorly directed **peristaltic** (wavelike) contraction and gravity, arriving at the stomach for the process of digestion after 10 to 20 seconds of transit time. When the bolus enters the UES for transit to the stomach, the cricopharyngeus will again contract, the larynx and soft palate will be depressed, and respiration will begin again. In the normal swallow, respiration is suspended for only about a second. Reinitiation of respiration increases pressure in the laryngopharynx, and food at the laryngeal entryway will typically be blown clear and propelled to the esophagus, since most individuals exhale after swallowing.

peristaltic: *wavelike*

Pressures of Deglutition

You can think of the swallowing process as a series of manipulations of a bolus by muscles, but you can also think of swallowing in terms of

Deficits of the Esophageal Stage

Although the esophageal stage is not directly treated by the speech-language pathologist, a working knowledge of problems associated with it is certainly important. Gastroesophageal reflux disease (GERD) is significant and potentially life-threatening. You may have experienced "heartburn" at one time or another, but that burning feeling may have been the acids from your stomach (i.e., gastric region) being recycled into your esophagus or pharynx. In some individuals the lower esophageal sphincter relaxes, allowing gastric juices to enter the esophagus. If the upper sphincter is likewise weakened or flaccid, these acids may "reflow" ("reflux") into the pyriform sinus, assaulting the delicate pharyngeal tissue. If this occurs during the night while you are supine, the acid may flow into the airway, resulting in aspiration. (We know of one client with oral, pharyngeal, and esophageal dysphagia secondary to irradiation for cancer. Her pharyngeal dysphagia was being well controlled through treatment directed toward improving pharyngeal responses, and her esophageal reflux had been controlled surgically. The surgical procedure to prevent reflux failed and this patient was hospitalized with aspiration pneumonia.)

The stomach can herniate through the esophageal hiatus (see Figure 9-4C), which is termed a *hiatal hernia*. When this occurs, the lower esophageal sphincter may malfunction, allowing reflux into the esophagus. More rarely, a congenital malformation of the esophagus, such as stenosis (see Figure 9-4B), may cause a severe, life-threatening loss of nutrition in a newborn. Rare maldevelopment of the esophagus may even result in the esophageal contents directly entering the trachea.

manipulation of oral, pharyngeal, and esophageal pressures that in turn move the bolus. During the oral preparation stage, the oral and pharyngeal cavity pressures are equalized with atmospheric pressure, because of the open nasal airway. When entering the oral stage of the swallow, the soft palate tightly closes, separating the oropharynx and nasopharynx, and the tongue begins squeezing the bolus posteriorly. The positive pressure created by the movements of the tongue propels the bolus toward the oropharynx. The tongue makes contact with the posterior oropharynx, transferring the bolus into the pharynx with an additional pressure gradient. The pharyngeal walls compress the bolus, increasing pressure to prompt it toward the esophagus. Elevation of the larynx creates a relatively lower pressure at the esophageal entryway, and relaxation of the cricopharyngeus further increases the superior-inferior pressure gradient. The laryngeal entryway is tightly clamped to avoid confounding the pressures of deglutition with those of respiration, so that the bolus is naturally drawn to the area of lower pressure, the esophageal entrance. The cricopharyngeus contracts most forcefully during inspiration, thereby prohibiting inflation of the esophagus.

In summary, there are four stages of mastication and deglutition:

- In the **oral preparation stage**, food is introduced into the oral cavity, moved onto the molars for chewing, and mixed with saliva to form a concise bolus between the tongue and hard palate.

- In the **oral stage**, the bolus is moved back toward the oropharynx by the tongue.

- The **pharyngeal stage** begins when the bolus reaches the faucial pillars. The soft palate and larynx elevate, and the bolus is propelled through the pharynx to the esophageal sphincter, which has relaxed to receive the material. The epiglottis has dropped to partially cover the laryngeal opening, while the intrinsic musculature of the larynx has effected a tight seal to protect the airway. Food passes over the epiglottis and through the pyriform sinuses to the esophagus.

- The final, **esophageal stage** involves peristaltic movement of the bolus through the esophagus.

NEUROPHYSIOLOGICAL UNDERPINNINGS OF MASTICATION AND DEGLUTITION

It is critically important for the experience of eating to be pleasant and behaviorally reinforcing. Natural drives related to hunger bring you to the process of acquiring nutrition, but the food must be palatable for it to be consumed in sufficient quantities to properly nourish you. Further, there must be an adequate neuroanatomical substrate that supports the stages of swallowing. Let us discuss these substrates in turn, and then see how they integrate into the acts of mastication and deglutition.

Sensation Associated with Mastication and Deglutition

Numerous stimuli are critical for completion of the chewing, sucking, and swallowing (CSS) elements associated with mastication and deglutition. (For a thorough review of sensory systems, see Møller, 2003, Kandel, Schwartz, & Jessell, 2000.) Among these are gustatory (taste), tactile (touch), temperature (thermal), and pressure senses. Each plays a critical role in successful completion of the CSS routines. We will go into considerable detail in our discussion of these senses, but some of the material may become clear to you only upon studying the underlying neuroanatomy (Chapters 12 and 13).

Gustation

Gustation (taste) is a complex and critical component of CSS. Taste drives the desire to continue eating, which fulfills the nutritional requirements of the body. Taste receptors (or **taste buds**, or **taste cells**) consist of a class of sensor known as **chemoreceptors**, in that they respond when specific chemicals come in contact with them. Taste receptors are found interspersed within the epithelia of the tongue within **papillae**, or prominences (see Figure 9-5). An opening in the epithelium called the **taste pore** permits isolation of a sample of the tasted substance, which is held in place by **microvilli** (small hair-like fibers projecting from the taste cell into the taste pore).

If you examine Figure 7-36, you can see that the tongue is richly invested with papillae of various forms. The filiform papillae are the dominant papillary formation of the tongue. They appear as small threads on the surface of the tongue, are pink/gray in color, and make the dorsum of the tongue look rough. They include not only taste sensors but also mechanoreceptors to provide fine tactile sensory ability to the tongue, permitting fine discrimination of the bolus characteristics (discussed below). Fungiform papillae are bright red, and are found interspersed with filiform papillae on the tip and sides of the tongue. Vallate papillae are the large V-shaped formation of circles seen in the posterior dorsum of the tongue. There are typically a dozen or so of them on a tongue, and each has a "moat" surrounding it. Foliate papillae are sparsely present on the lateral margins of the tongue.

Taste is mediated by means of three cranial nerves. The VII facial nerve mediates the sense of taste from the anterior two-thirds of the tongue, specifically involving sweet and sour sensations (see Figure 9-6), while the IX glossopharyngeal nerve transmits primarily bitterness information from the posterior one-third of the tongue. Taste receptors of

taste buds (cells): *chemoreceptors for gustation*

chemoreceptors: *neural receptors that respond to specific chemical composition*

papillae: *prominences*

taste pore: *opening in lingual epithelium that houses taste cell*

microvilli: *small, hairlike fibers projecting from the taste cell into the taste pore*

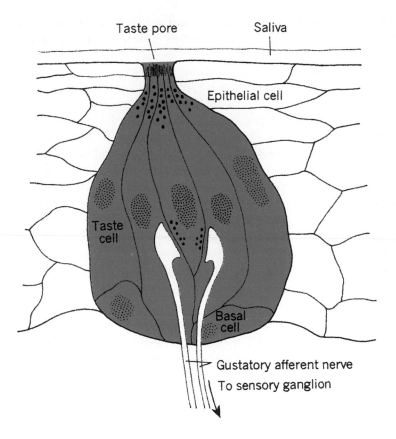

Figure 9-5. Taste sensor. (Adapted from Buck, 2000.)

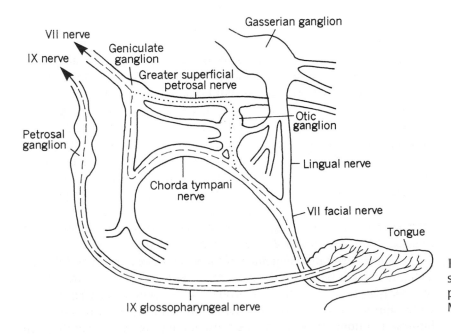

Figure 9-6. Innervation schematic for anterior and posterior tongue. (Adapted from Mountcastle, 1974.)

the palate are innervated by the VII facial nerve. Although not shown on Figure 9-6, taste receptors of the epiglottis and esophagus are innervated by the X vagus nerve.

Taste receptors are found on the tongue, epiglottis, pharynx, and esophageal entrance. Most tongue taste sensors are found in the moats surrounding the vallate papillae, as well as in the foliate and fungiform papillae. Although all types of taste receptors are found throughout the surface of the tongue (Kandel, Schwartz, & Jessell, 2000), receptors for bitter taste are concentrated on the posterior aspect of the tongue, while salt- and sour-sensitive receptors are found on the sides of the tongue. Receptors for sweet tastes are on the tongue tip. A fifth taste receptor, **umami**, appears to be processed by glutamate receptors on the tongue, and is represented perceptually as the taste of monosodium glutamate (Kandel, Schwartz, & Jessell, 2000).

Taste sense of the VII facial nerve is relayed through the geniculate ganglion to the solitary tract within the medulla, to terminate at the rostral and lateral aspects of the solitary tract nucleus gustatory region of the brainstem. Taste sensation from the IX glossopharyngeal nerve is mediated via the petrosal ganglion, and fibers also terminate in the solitary tract nucleus. Epiglottal and esophageal taste sense are transmitted via the X vagus nerve through the nodose ganglion, likewise to the solitary tract nucleus. This taste information is then relayed to the ventral posterior medial nucleus (VPMN) of the thalamus, which subsequently relays this information ipsilaterally to the anterior portion of the insula of the cerebral cortex. Figure 9-7 illustrates the taste pathways in humans.

Now examine Figure 9-8, which illustrates the relative contribution of each nerve to taste perception. First notice the relative magnitude of tastes mediated by each of the nerves (VII, IX, and X) relating to their locations. This information converges on the nucleus of the solitary tract (NST), and is then sent to the ventral posterior nucleus (VPN) of the thalamus. The sensation is subsequently transmitted to the primary sensory cortex (located in the postcentral gyrus of the cerebrum) and to the insular cortex of the frontal lobe (located in a fold of the cerebral cortex underlying the operculum), as well as the operculum overlying the insula. Taste and smell are probably integrated at the insula (Møller, 2003). Fibers from the insula project to the limbic system and the motor regions of the brainstem.

The NST also projects to the motor cortex, specifically to the region serving the tongue (see Figure 12-15B). This is important. Our nutritional needs govern our selection of sweet and umami tastes, as these indicate presence of carbohydrates (sweet) and protein (umami). Salt is also a necessary mineral, so we "crave" that taste as well. These tastes will elicit salivation, as well as ingestive responses, including tongue protrusion to receive the food, release of insulin, mastication, and deglutition. In contrast, bitter and sour tastes typify poisons, and they will

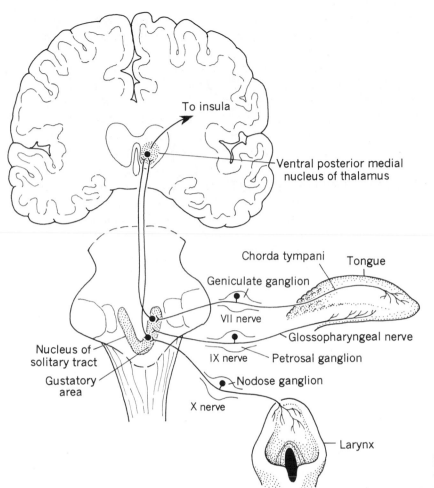

Figure 9-7. Pathways mediating the sensations of taste. (After Buck, 2000.)

often elicit protective responses that include gagging, coughing, apnea, and salivation (salivation in this case encapsulates the material and protects the oral cavity). Admittedly, we *do* eat sour and bitter foods, but notice next time you have a particularly bitter taste how you find it difficult to swallow, or at least become wary of it! This underscores a critically important point. Tastes can elicit motor responses that may or may not be under volitional (or even conscious) control. The gag response is a complex motor act involving elevation of the larynx and clamping of the vocal folds, elevation of the velum, and protrusion of the tongue. Coughing entails tightly closing the vocal folds, compressing the abdomen and thorax, and forcefully blowing the vocal folds apart. Now recognize that each of these responses has components of the swallow embedded within it, and you can see that deglutition is made up of a complex set of motor responses dictated by stimuli present in the oral and pharyngeal spaces.

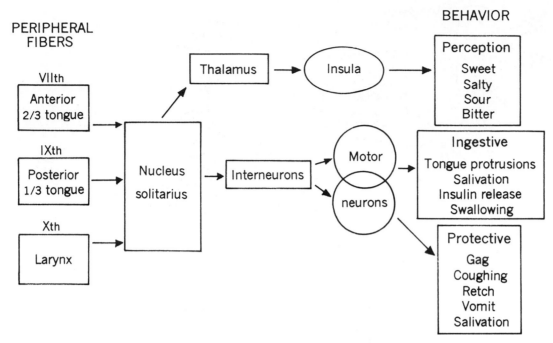

Figure 9-8. Schematic illustration of routing and response to taste within the nervous system. (After S. A. Simon & S. D. Roper [1993]. *Mechanisms of taste transduction.* Boca Raton, FL: CRC Press.)

Olfaction

Olfaction (the sense of smell) plays a vital role in appetite and taste. Molecules arising from food pass over olfactory chemoreceptors to increase the magnitude of the taste perception, a fact to which you can relate if you remember how "flat" your favorite food tasted when you had nasal congestion. In fact, if you tightly occlude your nares and blindly take a bite of apple and then a bite of onion, you will not be able to taste the difference!

Olfactory sensors arise from the olfactory bulb, and have the distinction of a short life and continual replacement. They last only about 60 days before being replaced by new sensors. Olfactory sensors are found within the epithelial lining of the upper posterior nasal cavity (see Figure 9-9). There are small cilia protruding from the olfactory sensor, similar to the microvilli of the taste cell. These cilia are highly specialized, in that they transduce the molecular stimulant into the perception of smell that is transmitted to the olfactory bulb located within the cranial space. Recent research has revealed that although the basic structure of the odor receptors on the cilia is similar for all olfactory sensors, the specific structure of the receptor varies slightly, so that more than 1,000 different odors are decoded by the olfactory system!

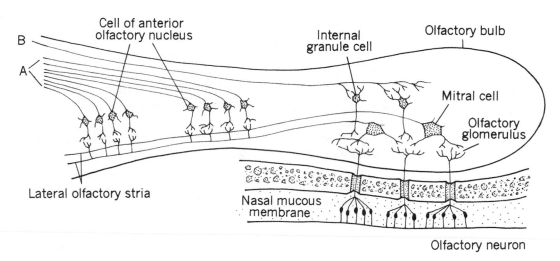

Figure 9-9. Detail of olfactory bulb.

After an odorant stimulates a specific receptor, information that the receptor has been activated is transmitted to the olfactory bulb, which resides within the braincase. More than 1,000 axons of sensory cells converge on a single olfactory interneuron (termed a **glomerulus**) in the olfactory bulb. This information is transmitted by means of the olfactory tract to the olfactory region of the cortex, which includes the amygdala, the anterior olfactory nucleus, the piriform cortex, the olfactory tubercle, and a portion of the entorhinal cortex. Information from some of these brain centers is routed through the thalamus, and subsequently relayed to the frontal lobe of the cerebral cortex, orbital region. Olfactory information from the amygdala is transmitted to the hypothalamus, while olfactory information from the entorhinal area terminates in the hippocampus within the temporal lobe. The functional implications are that olfaction arrives at the cerebral cortex through multiple pathways, including the thalamus, and that the information serves as a stimulus to emotion and motivation (amygdala), physiological responses (hypothalamus), and memory encoding (hippocampus). The information reaching the orbitofrontal region of the cerebral cortex appears to be involved in olfactory discrimination (i.e., conscious, discriminative processing of smell). Again, recognize that motor responses are readily mediated by reception of olfactory stimulation. Salivation arises from pleasant food odors, while gagging or even vomiting can be triggered by unpleasant odors.

Tactile Sense

The sense of touch is mediated by means of a number of **mechanoreceptors**, which are sensors that are sensitive to physical contact. Generally, sensors differ based on whether the epithelium contains hair or is

mechanoreceptors: *neural receptors designed to sense mechanical forces* hairless (**glabrous** skin). Glabrous skin of the hands contains "finger-prints" that are, in reality, the overlay for dense collections of mechanoreceptors. Touch receptors are broadly distributed about the body, and are differentiated based on the type of stimulus that causes them to respond (see Figure 9-10). Hairy skin receptors are less critical to our discussion of swallowing, as the epithelial lining of the oral and pharyngeal cavities are hairless.

Glabrous (hairless) skin contains **Meissner's corpuscles** and **Merkel disk receptors**. Meissner's corpuscles are physically coupled to the papilla in which they reside (similar to taste receptors), and respond to minute mechanical movement. Merkel disk receptors transmit the sense of pressure. Meissner's corpuscles adapt quickly to stimulation (that is, they stop responding after a brief period of sustained stimulation), whereas Merkel disk receptors respond for longer periods of time to sustained stimulation. Both of these receptors are found within the superficial layer of lingual epithelium. Both Meissner's corpuscles and Merkel disk receptors are found at the end of the papillary ridge. Deep

glabrous: *hairless*

Meissner's corpuscles: *superficial cutaneous mechanoreceptors for minute movement*

Merkel disk receptors: *superficial cutaneous mechanoreceptors for light pressure*

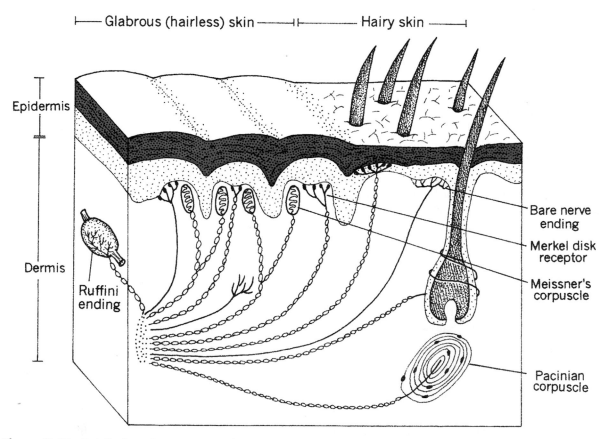

Figure 9-10. Detail of mechanoreceptors. (After detail of Gordon, Martin, and Jessell, 2000.)

cutaneous tissues contain **Pacinian corpuscles** and cells with the **Ruffini ending**. The Pacinian corpuscle is similar to the Meissner's corpuscle, and responds to rapid deep pressure to the outer epithelium. Ruffini endings sense stretch within the deep tissues, and are critical to our perception of the shape of objects perceived by touch. It is important to note that Meissner's corpuscles and Merkel disk receptors have small receptor fields, which means that their effective sensory area is more limited than those of the deeply embedded Ruffini endings and Pacinian corpuscles, which have larger receptive fields. Deep pressure has the potential to stimulate a larger field and greater array of sensors than light pressure, an issue that is important in treatment for dysphagia.

Vibration sense is a subclass of tactile sense. Vibration may be considered as either deep or superficial pressure, depending on the amplitude of the vibrator. In both cases vibration is sensed as individual deformation of tactile sensors. Pacinian corpuscles (deep pressure sensors) respond most efficiently to stimulation between 70 Hz and 500 Hz (best frequency = 280 Hz), whereas Meissner's corpuscles respond best between 10 Hz and 100 Hz, with a shallow best frequency of 50 Hz. (**Best frequency** refers to the frequency of vibration at which a sensor responds most effectively.) Though both of these receptors are rapidly adapting sensors, Pacinian corpuscles (deep receptors) have a markedly lower threshold to vibration than Meissner's corpuscles (superficial receptors). Rapidly adapting sensors have lower thresholds of stimulation than slowly adapting receptors, meaning that Meissner's and Pacinian corpuscles will respond to lower levels of stimulation than Ruffini endings and Merkel disk receptors.

The classic test for spatial density of receptors is through two-point discrimination, wherein an individual is provided a pressure of calibrated force by means of two probes. The distance between probes that can be perceived as two versus one stimulus is considered an index of the density of receptors for the structure. That is to say, if the two points are close enough together, they will both stimulate the same single receptor, giving the perception of a single contact point.

Thermal Receptors

Four classes of thermal stimulation are differentiated by human senses: warm, hot, cool, and cold. Thermal receptors are actually the same as pain sensors, in that they are bare nerve endings. While it is convenient to group pain and thermal sense, the reality is that thermal sensors are functionally different from pain sensors, with different nerve endings responding to these two broad classes of stimulation.

Thermal receptors differ from mechanoreceptors in a critical manner: Mechanoreceptors respond only when stimulated, whereas thermal receptors have a tonic, ongoing discharge. The individual receptors for each of the four classes of temperature have "best temperature" responses to which they respond. Cold sensors will increase their firing

Pacinian corpuscles: *deep cutaneous mechanoreceptors for deep pressure*

Ruffini endings: *deep cutaneous mechanoreceptors for tissue stretch*

response as the temperature of stimulation drops, even as the cool-sensitive sensors drop back to their basal firing rate. Thermal receptors apparently are most effective at identifying thermal stimulation that differs markedly from the ambient temperature of the skin. Thus, a slow increase or decrease in stimulus temperature will be more difficult to detect than a rapid change in temperature. At high temperatures, heat sensors cease firing and pain sensors fire instead. Thermal sense requires longer duration of stimulation for perception of the sensation, but the sensation is retained for longer periods of time.

Pain Sense (Nociception)

Pain sense is included in this discussion because of its importance in development of structural disorders of swallowing. As an example, structural defects such as oral or pharyngeal lesions (e.g., cold sores) can cause pain that can interfere with swallowing responses.

nociceptors: *pain sensors*

Nociceptors (pain sensors) respond directly to a noxious stimulus (e.g., chemical burn), to noxious molecules released by injured tissue (such as positive potassium ions, serotonin, and acetylcholine), to acidity caused by injury, or to direct contact with a traumatic source. Some nociceptors respond to mechanical trauma, while others respond to thermal stimulation. Most nociceptors respond to general destruction of tissue rather than to the specific quality of a stimulus, and the perception arising from stimulation of these receptors (termed *polymodal nociceptors*) is a burning sensation.

Muscle Stretch and Tension Sense

Muscle stretch is sensed by muscle spindle fibers, which consist of nuclear chain fibers and nuclear bag fibers within muscle tissue itself. Stretch receptors are found predominantly in larger muscles, such as the antigravity muscles of the legs, but are also found within oral musculature. The mandibular elevators (masseter, temporalis, and lateral and medial pterygoid muscles) are richly endowed with stretch receptors, as are the deep tongue fibers of the genioglossus and the palatoglossus muscles. Facial muscles are notably deficient in stretch receptors.

Muscle spindle fibers return a muscle to its original position following passive stretching. As an example, if you were to pull sharply down on your relaxed mandible, the mandible would quickly elevate thereafter, to the point that your teeth might make contact (depending

Nociceptors

Nociceptors produce the perception of pain when they are traumatized, such as in burning. The direct trauma to a nerve ending relays this information to higher centers so that you can withdraw from the painful stimulus. If the nerve ending is destroyed entirely, there will be no perception of pain; this is one indication of third-degree burn.

Mouth Breathing

Chronic mouth breathing is more than an unpleasant habit; it is at the root of facial malformation and hearing loss. Mouth breathing is attributed to hypertrophy of the tonsilar ring, prohibiting adequate nasal respiration. In children with this condition, the adenoids are frequently enlarged, blocking the nasal choanae and also the orifice of the Eustachian tube. Inadequate ventilation of the middle ear cavity may result in otitis media (inflammation of the middle ear cavity). Chronic otitis media is often associated with fluid in the middle ear (serous otitis media), a condition resulting in conductive hearing impairment.

The hypertrophy also makes mouth breathing mandatory. During normal nasal respiration, the tongue maintains fairly constant contact with the upper alveolar ridge and hard palate; but with the mouth open constantly for respiration, the tongue will exert little pressure there. Without that pressure, the dental arch will narrow and the palate will bulge upward to an extreme vault as the facial bones develop. With narrow dental arches, the permanent teeth will not have adequate space, so they become crowded and prone to caries (decay of bone or tooth). The narrowed maxillae will cause the upper lip to pull up, exposing the upper front teeth. The nasal cavity will become narrow, increasing the probability of later nasal obstruction. The look of "adenoid facies" includes an open mouth, narrow mandible, and dental crowding. When coupled with persistent conductive hearing loss, mouth breathing presents a sizable (yet generally preventable) deficit to the developing child.

on how relaxed you are and how low your threshold of stimulation is). This sensor system is designed to maintain a muscle at a preset length, so that the monitored muscle group contracts in response to passive stretching. The spindle function is normally inhibited during active contraction, although damage to the upper motor neuron can cause hyperactive stretch reflexes and spasticity (to be discussed in Chapters 12 and 13).

Muscle tension is sensed by Golgi tendon organs (GTOs), found within tendons and fascia. These organs respond to active contraction of muscles, and serve to inhibit the muscle spindle fibers.

Muscle tone is regulated partially through the interaction of muscle spindles and GTOs. **Muscle tone** refers to the perception of resistance to passive movement of a stretching. High tone of spasticity results from inadequately inhibited response from muscle spindle sensors, while low tone results from inadequate tonic stimulation, either from lower motor neuron disease or cerebellum lesion. Muscular rigidity arises from a basal ganglia lesion, and occurs as a result of co-contraction of agonists and antagonists. Reflexes may be normally elicited despite abnormally high muscle tone. High muscle tone resulting from muscle spindle disinhibition may result in clasp-knife response to passive stretching. In this response, there is initial resistance to a stretch that is released, apparently as a result of input from cutaneous sensors and nociceptors. Thus, it is possible that cutaneous, thermal, and pain sensors may be used to reduce or inhibit spastic responses in pathological conditions.

Mechanical deformation (touch and pressure), thermal sense, pain sense, and joint and tendon sense of the face and oral cavity are primarily mediated by the V trigeminal nerve, although the IX glossopharyngeal and X vagus also have pathways associated with these sensations (Møller, 2003).

Salivation Response

salivation: *production and release of saliva into the oral cavity*

Related to taste, smell, and noxious stimulation is the salivation response. **Salivation** (the production and release of saliva into the oral cavity) is not a sensory system, but rather a motor response. It is an essential and often-overlooked component of mastication and deglutition, and deserves attention in this discussion of normal function. Salivation is an essential component of taste, mastication, and deglutition. When saliva mixes with tasteless starch, the combination produces sugars that taste sweet and thus make the food more desirable.

Salivation is the product of three major glands: the parotid, submandibular, and sublingual. In addition, mucus-secreting accessory salivary glands are present throughout the oral cavity, embedded within the mucosa. These glands are activated by stimulation of taste receptors (anterior two-thirds of the tongue), mediated by the VII facial nerve via the nucleus solitarius of the dorsal pons (sublingual and submandibular glands) and IX glossopharyngeal nerve (parotid gland). This nucleus projects to the inferior and superior salivatory nuclei of the pons, which excites the salivary glands to secrete saliva.

The submandibular gland is found behind the free margin of the mylohyoid muscle, between the mylohyoid muscle and the submandibular fossa of the inner mandible. It extends as far posteriorly as the second molar, and extends forward as the submandibular duct (see Figure 9-11). The duct courses anteriorly and medially, opening into the oral cavity just lateral to the lingual frenulum.

The sublingual gland is above the mylohyoid muscle and medially placed. It is an elongated mass located in the floor of the mouth, with the right and left glands meeting in the front of the oral cavity. The visual manifestation of the gland is a ridge seen to follow the base of the tongue along the floor of the mouth, upon elevation of the tongue. The sublingual gland empties into the mouth through ducts within the sublingual fold. The parotid gland is located posterior to the mandibular ramus and superior to the sternocleidomastoid muscle, and secretions from it empty into the pharynx.

mucus: *thick, high-viscosity saliva*

Each of these glands has distinctly different secretions. The sublingual gland produces **mucus**, a high-viscosity (thick), protein-rich secretion that helps in formation of the bolus of food. Its ropey quality encapsulates food particles, permitting tongue action to prepare the food for propulsion to the pharynx.

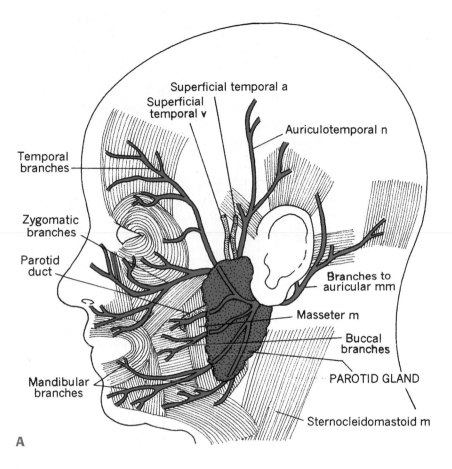

Superficial temporal a
Superficial temporal v
Auriculotemporal n
Temporal branches
Zygomatic branches
Parotid duct
Branches to auricular mm
Masseter m
Buccal branches
PAROTID GLAND
Mandibular branches
Sternocleidomastoid m

A

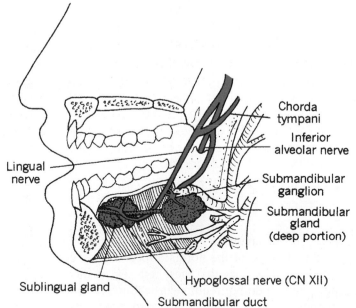

Chorda tympani
Inferior alveolar nerve
Submandibular ganglion
Submandibular gland (deep portion)
Lingual nerve
Sublingual gland
Hypoglossal nerve (CN XII)
Submandibular duct

B

Figure 9-11. Salivary glands and ducts. **A.** Parotid gland. **B.** Sublingual and submandibular glands. (After Liebgott, 2001.)

417

▶ **serous:** *thin, low-viscosity saliva*

The submandibular gland produces both **serous** and mucus secretions. Serous saliva has markedly lower viscosity (that is, it is thinner in consistency), and serves as a lubricant to the bolus. The posteriorly placed parotid gland produces only serous saliva, which is instrumental in active and rapid propulsion of the bolus into and through the pharynx.

Salivary flow is stimulated behaviorally by the sight, smell, and taste of food. The salivary glands produce as much as 1.2 liters of saliva per day, although the production is reduced to minute quantities during sleep.

In summary:

- **Gustation** (taste) is mediated by **chemoreceptors** that transmit information to the brain via the IX glossopharyngeal and VII facial nerves. Taste sensors are specialized for sweet, sour, salty, bitter, and umami sense.

- Taste sense determines whether a **bolus** is ingested or ejected from the oral cavity.

- **Olfaction** (the sense of smell) is mediated by chemoreceptors within the nasal mucosa.

- The sense of touch (**tactile** sense) is mediated by means of **mechanoreceptors** that respond to deep or shallow touch.

- Four classes of **thermal stimulation** are differentiated by human senses: warm, hot, cool, and cold.

- Pain sense (**nociception**) is a response to a noxious stimulus.

- Muscle **stretch** is sensed by muscle spindle fibers, and muscle **tension** is sensed by Golgi tendon organs (GTOs), found within tendons and fascia.

- Tactile sense, thermal sense, pain sense, and joint and tendon sense of the face and oral cavity are mediated by the V trigeminal, IX glossopharyngeal, and X vagus nerves.

- **Salivation** occurs as a result of stimulation of the salivary glands.

- The type of saliva varies by gland. The **sublingual gland** produces thick **mucus** secretions, the **submandibular gland** produces both thin **serous** and mucus secretions, and the **parotid gland** secretes only serous saliva.

REFLEXIVE CIRCUITS OF MASTICATION AND DEGLUTITION

The individual reflex circuits associated with mastication and deglutition are the building blocks for the normal processes associated with intake of food and drink. Recognize that these reflexes are mediated at the level of the brainstem and do not require cortical involvement. This does not imply that there is no cortical activity associated with CSS, but rather that the cortex is not essential. We have included **expulsive reflexes** here as well (gag, retch) because of their close association with the systems of mastication and deglutition. Most of the reflexes that we will discuss are controlled by circuitry within the phylogenetically old reticular formation of the brainstem (see Figure 9-12).

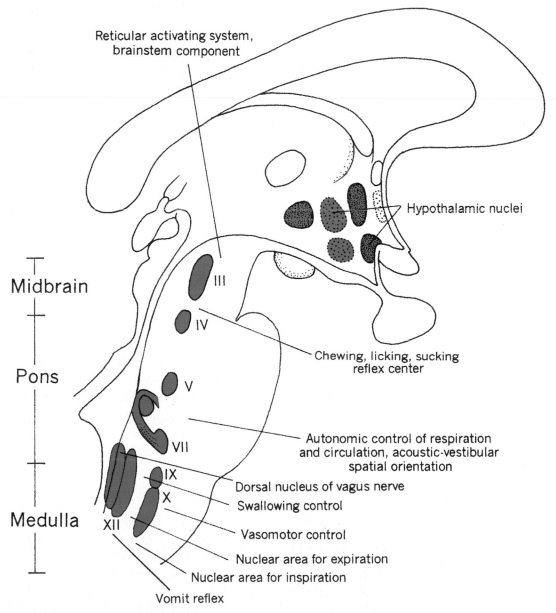

Figure 9-12. Cross-section of brainstem showing various reflex centers. (After Noback, Strominger, & Demarest, 1991.)

Chewing Reflex

Chewing is a complex reflex that can be triggered by deep pressure on the roof of the mouth, as when you bite a cracker. It involves alternating left-side and right-side contraction of the muscles of mandibular elevation (masseter and medial pterygoid muscles), such that a rotatory motion of the mandible is produced. The alternating contraction of these mandibular elevators is interspersed with depression of the mandible, which allows the lingual musculature to move the bolus onto and off of the molars. The chewing center is located within the midbrain, near the III oculomotor and IV trochlear nerve nuclei. This center is also involved in reflexive movements of the tongue for sucking and licking (Duus, 1998).

Rooting and Sucking Reflexes

The **rooting** and **sucking** reflexes—very functional for neonates and infants—rely on tactile stimulation of the perioral region. Lightly stroking the lips or cheek on one side will cause the infant's mouth to open and its head to turn toward the stimulus; this is termed the rooting reflex. Light contact within the inner margin of the lips will initiate a sucking response, which involves generating a labial seal (contraction of the upper and lower orbicularis oris), and alternately protruding and retracting the tongue. Tactile stimulation of the perioral region is mediated by the V trigeminal nerve, and central mediation of sucking is within the midbrain reticular formation.

Uvular (Palatal) Reflex

Uvular elevation occurs in response to excitation of the IX glossopharyngeal general visceral afferent (GVA) component (see Appendix G) by irritation. It appears to be mediated in a manner similar to the gag reflex (below), involving the palatal muscles innervated by the X vagus.

Gag (Pharyngeal) Reflex

The **gag reflex** is elicited by tactile stimulation of the faucial pillars, posterior pharyngeal wall, or posterior tongue near the lingual tonsils. Tactile stimulation (light or deep touch) of this region is mediated by the IX glossopharyngeal nerve GVA component. Dendrites convey sensation through the petrosal (inferior) and superior ganglia of IX glossopharyngeal to the solitary nucleus and solitary fasciculus of the medulla oblongata in the brainstem. Connection with the X vagus nerve via interneurons activates muscles of general visceral efferent (GVE) lineage, including abdominal muscles and muscles of the velum and pharynx, causing the soft palate to elevate and the pharynx to elevate and constrict. Note that,

Gag Reflex

The gag reflex is a useful response in that it helps us avoid aversive stimuli. If a person has a hyperactive gag reflex, perhaps as a result of neurological damage, there can be significant consequences to the health of that individual. A child with a hyperactive gag reflex may find tooth-brushing very aversive, and will often avoid hard foods because of their high stimulus value. (One of us once had a client whose gag reflex was elicited by contact with the lips!) Likewise, these children may tend to avoid making posterior sounds (i.e., are phonological "fronters"), because even contact of the tongue on the palate is aversive. Fortunately, you, as speech-language pathologists, will have the ability and knowledge to desensitize this gag reflex to help the person accommodate to physical contact in the oral cavity.

as mentioned earlier, the gag reflex can be elicited by taste, specifically mediated by the IX glossopharyngeal nerve, special visceral afferent (SVA) component.

Retch and Vomit Reflex

Retching is an involuntary attempt at vomiting. **Vomiting** refers to the oral expulsion of gastrointestinal contents. The retching reflex is a complex response mediated by noxious smells (I olfactory), tastes (IX glossopharyngeal), gastrointestinal distress (X vagus), vestibular dysfunction (VIII vestibulocochlear), or a even distressing visual or mental stimulation. Stimulation by one or more of these sensory systems apparently activates a retching center located near the swallow center in the reticular formation of the medulla oblongata, near the motor nuclei associated with the complex of responses associated with vomiting. The vomit response includes multiple simultaneous and/or synchronous reflexes, including occlusion of the airway by vocal fold adduction, extreme contraction of abdominal muscles, relaxation of the upper and lower esophageal sphincters, elevation of the larynx and velum, depression of the epiglottis, elevation of the pharynx, and tongue protrusion.

Cough Reflex

The **cough** reflex is typically initiated by noxious stimulation of the pharynx, larynx, or bronchial passageway. The GVA component of the vagus nerve transmits information concerning this stimulation to the nucleus solitarius of the medulla. Interneurons activate the expiration center of the medullary reticular formation, which causes the abdominal muscles to contract. The nucleus ambiguus, the motor nucleus of the X vagus, causes laryngeal adduction prior to exhalation, permitting sufficient subglottal pressure to be generated to dislodge the irritating substance from the airway.

Tongue Base Retraction and Elevation

Retraction of the tongue may be reflexively stimulated by pulling the tongue forward. This reflex is mediated by muscle spindle fibers within the genioglossus that are stretched when the tongue is pulled forward. Elevation of the posterior tongue may be stimulated by pushing down on the posterior tongue, thereby stretching the palatoglossus muscle, which also contains muscle spindles. Both of these reflexive responses are intrinsic localized responses of the XII hypoglossal (for genioglossus), XI accessory, and X vagus (for the palatoglossus) nerves.

Pain Reflex

While not technically a reflex associated with mastication or deglutition, the **pain withdrawal reflex** can have an effect on mastication and swallowing. You may remember the unpleasant sensation of having a lesion on your tongue or oral mucosa. When you masticate, you become very aware of the area and tend to avoid it if possible. This response represents a conscious version of the withdrawal response, a natural response to noxious stimuli. The classic withdrawal reflex involves rapid, total removal of a limb from a noxious stimulus, such as a hot stove. Oral and pharyngeal pain responses include removal of the noxious bolus (spicy or excessively hot food), either by expectoration or by swallowing.

Respiration Reflexes

Respiration occurs reflexively, but can be voluntarily controlled to a degree. A sensor system near the carotid sinus (the **carotid body**) responds to the quantity of oxygen and carbon dioxide in the blood, as well as to blood acidity. When oxygen levels decline below a specific criterion level, or when carbon dioxide and/or acidity increases beyond a specific level, a signal mediated by the IX glossopharyngeal nerve via the nucleus solitarius is relayed to the respiratory center, which increases the respiration rate. There are individual inspiratory and expiratory centers: excitation of inspiration inhibits expiratory musculature, and vice versa. Two respiratory centers are located in the lower medulla (the inspiratory and expiratory controls are separate).

In summary:
- **Chewing, sucking**, and **swallowing** are the product of numerous individual reflex patterns executed in synchronous sequence.
- The chewing reflex involves rotatory movement of the mandible, coordinated with movement of the bolus by the tongue.
- The **rooting reflex** involves orientation to light tactile stimulation of the cheek area, which causes the infant's head to turn toward the stimulus.

- The **sucking reflex** is elicited by soft contact with the inner margin of the lips, causing protrusion and retraction of the tongue, as well as closing of the lips.
- **Uvular elevation** occurs in response to tactile stimulation of the faucial pillars, lingual tonsils, or upper pharynx.
- The **gag reflex** is elicited by tactile stimulation of the faucial pillars, posterior faucial wall, or posterior tongue near the lingual tonsils. It results in termination of respiration and elevation of the larynx.
- The **retching** and **vomiting reflexes** are complex responses that are similar to the gag.
- The **cough reflex** involves laryngeal adduction, abdominal contraction to develop increased subglottal pressure, and forceful exhalation.
- The **pain withdrawal reflex** causes withdrawal from a noxious stimulus.
- **Respiration** occurs as a result of inadequate oxygenation of the blood or excessive carbon dioxide or blood acidity.

REEXAMINATION OF THE PATTERNS FOR MASTICATION AND DEGLUTITION

As mentioned earlier, the patterns associated with mastication and deglutition are governed by unconscious, automatic sensorimotor systems (see Figure 9-13). Again, this does not mean that the processes will not reach consciousness or that they cannot be controlled voluntarily (i.e., cortically), but rather that they spring from basic protective and nutritive reflexes. Let us examine the processes of mastication and deglutition from a brainstem control perspective.

Receipt of food by the tongue appears to have evolved from the basic tongue posture of the neonate. The infant sucking gesture involves three to four piston-like pumps followed by a protrusive (immature) swallow. During the suck cycles, the liquid is pooled on the tongue in preparation for swallowing, a gesture not unlike the tongue-dishing that occurs as adults and infants receive food into the mouth. Food is moved

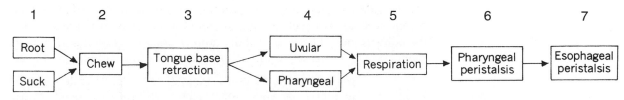

Figure 9-13. Schematic of sequential and simultaneous reflexes involved in mastication and deglutition.

from the tongue to the molars for chewing, processes that are governed by the chewing response of the midbrain, and is mixed with saliva, production of saliva is triggered by taste primarily on the anterior two-thirds of the tongue. Tactile sensation within the oral cavity provides feedback concerning the consistency, size, and shape of the bolus. The bolus is retained within the oral cavity with the aid of the buccal musculature and orbicularis oris.

When the consistency of the bolus is sensed to be adequate, the mature swallow is initiated. This process begins with retraction of the tongue base sufficient to cause the bolus to contact the fauces and/or soft palate. The palatal reflex is stimulated by contact of a foreign object with the fauces or pharynx, and causes the velum to elevate. The pharyngeal reflex is initiated by similar contact with the fauces, posterior tongue base, or valleculae by the bolus. In reality, the determination of whether these two reflexes result in ingestion or expulsion of the bolus depends on the nature of the stimulus (review Figure 9-7). Both noxious and benevolent stimuli result in elevation of the larynx and opening of the cricopharyngeus, but only noxious stimuli elicit abdominal contraction related to vomiting or retching. When the bolus is propelled posteriorly, the orbicularis oris, buccinator, risorius, masseter, temporalis, medial pterygoid, and superior constrictor are all contracted, which in turn pulls the superior constrictor forward by virtue of its attachment. If the bolus is "palatable," the middle and inferior constrictors will assist in ingestion, whereas an unpalatable bolus would stimulate an opposite response.

It is critical to understand that this complex gesture, which we regard as an ordinary, everyday function, is comprised of motor elements that have their roots in basic reflexive responses. This knowledge will allow you, as a therapist, to approach therapy of disordered swallow stages with a full view of the systems you are attempting to remediate.

◥ CHAPTER SUMMARY

Mastication and **deglutition** can be viewed behaviorally or as a system of reflexive responses. The behavioral stages of mastication and deglutition include the **oral preparatory**, **oral**, **pharyngeal**, and **esophageal stages**. In the oral preparation stage, food is introduced into the oral cavity, moved onto the molars for chewing, and mixed with saliva to form a concise bolus between the tongue and hard palate. In the oral stage, the bolus is moved back toward the oropharynx by the tongue. The pharyngeal stage begins when the bolus reaches the faucial pillars. The soft palate and larynx elevate, and the bolus is propelled through the pharynx to the esophageal sphincter, which has relaxed to receive the material. The epiglottis has dropped to partially cover the laryngeal opening, while the intrinsic musculature of the larynx has effected a tight seal to protect the airway. Food passes over the epiglottis and through the pyriform sinuses to the esophagus. The final, esophageal stage involves peristaltic movement of the bolus through the esophagus.

Sensory elements of mastication and deglutition are critical for elicitation of the muscular components of chewing and swallowing, as well as maintenance of the various qualities of these processes. **Gustation** (taste) is mediated by **chemoreceptors** that transmit information to the brain via the IX glossopharyngeal and VII facial nerves. **Taste sensors** are specialized for sweet, sour, salty, bitter, and umami sense. Taste sense determines whether a bolus is ingested or removed from the oral cavity. **Olfaction** (the sense of smell) is mediated by chemoreceptors within the nasal mucosa. The sense of touch (**tactile sense**) is mediated by mechanoreceptors that respond to deep or shallow touch. Four classes of thermal stimulation are differentiated by human senses: warm, hot, cool, and cold. Pain sense (**nociception**) is a response to a noxious stimulus, and acts as a protective response against inappropriate entry of foreign objects into the gastrointestinal system. Muscle stretch is sensed by **muscle spindle fibers**, and muscle tension is sensed by **Golgi tendon organs**, found within tendons and fascia. Tactile sense, thermal sense, pain sense, and joint and tendon sense of the face and oral cavity are mediated by the V trigeminal, IX glossopharyngeal, and X vagus nerves. **Salivation** occurs as a result of stimulation of the salivary glands. The type of saliva produced varies by gland: the **sublingual gland** produces thick mucus secretions, the **submandibular gland** produces both thin serous and mucus secretions, and the **parotid gland** secretes only serous saliva.

A neurophysiological view of CSS patterns reveals that chewing, sucking, and swallowing are the product of numerous individual reflex patterns executed in synchronous sequence. The **chewing reflex** involves rotatory movement of the mandible, coordinated with movement of the bolus by the tongue. The **rooting reflex** is oriented to light tactile stimulation of the cheek area, which causes the infant's head to turn toward the stimulus. The **sucking reflex** is elicited by soft contact with the inner margin of the lips, and causes protrusion and retraction of the tongue, as well as closing of the lips. The uvular elevation of the **palatal reflex** occurs in response to tactile stimulation of the faucial pillars, lingual tonsils, or upper pharynx. The **gag reflex** is elicited by tactile stimulation of the faucial pillars, posterior faucial wall, or posterior tongue near the lingual tonsils. It results in termination of respiration and elevation of the larynx. The **retching** and **vomiting reflexes** are complex responses similar to the gag. The **cough reflex** involves laryngeal adduction, abdominal contraction to develop increased subglottal pressure, and forceful exhalation. The **pain withdrawal reflex** causes withdrawal from a noxious stimulus. Respiration occurs as a result of inadequate oxygenation of the blood or excessive carbon dioxide or blood acidity.

STUDY QUESTIONS

1. _____ refers to the process of preparing food for swallowing.

2. _____ refers to the processing of swallowing

3. _____ refers to a "ball" of food or drink.

4. List five of the elements of the oral preparatory stage of mastication and deglutition.

    a. _____

    b. _____

    c. _____

    d. _____

    e. _____

5. List three of the elements of the oral stage of deglutition.

    a. _____

    b. _____

    c. _____

6. List seven of the critical elements of the pharyngeal stage of deglutition.

    a. _____

    b. _____

    c. _____

    d. _____

    e. _____

    f. _____

    g. _____

7. The _____ reflex involves orienting toward the direction of tactile stimulation of the cheek.

8. _____ refers to "mouth region."

9. The _____ reflex is elicited by soft contact with the lower lip, and results in tongue protrusion and retraction.

10. List three essential differences between the oral-pharyngeal anatomy and physiology of an infant and that of an adult.

    a. _____

    b. _____

    c. _____

11. T/F   The infant must coordinate respiration and swallowing, as milk and air share the same passageway during deglutition.

12. The _____ stage is the stage in which food is prepared for swallow.

13. The _____ stage is the stage of swallow involving oral transit of the bolus to the pharynx.

14. The _____ stage is the stage of swallow involving transit of the bolus to the esophagus, and includes numerous physiological protective responses.

15. The _____ stage is the stage of swallow in which food is transported from the upper esophageal region to the stomach.

16. _____ refers to wavelike action.

17. List three critical elements relative to the pressures of deglutition.
    a. _____
    b. _____
    c. _____

18. The acronym "CSS" refers to the words _____, _____, and _____.

19. _____ refers to the sense of taste.

20. _____ is the class of receptors that respond to chemical stimulation.

21. Taste from the anterior two-thirds of the tongue is mediated by the _____ cranial nerve (name and number).

22. Taste from the posterior one-third of the tongue is mediated by the _____ cranial nerve (name and number).

23. Taste from the epiglottis and esophagus is mediated by the _____ cranial nerve (name and number).

24. The taste of bitterness is predominantly transmitted by the _____ cranial nerve (name and number).

25. The taste of sweetness is predominantly mediated by the _____ cranial nerve (name and number).

26. The tastes of sourness and saltiness are predominantly mediated by the _____ cranial nerve (name and number).

27. _____ refers to the sense of smell.

28. _____ corpuscles respond to minute mechanical movement in the superficial epithelia.

29. _____ receptors transmit the sense of pressure within the superficial epithelia.

30. _____ respond to rapid deep pressure.

31. Cells with _____ endings sense stretch within the deep layers of the epithelium.

32. List the four classes of thermal receptors that mediate thermal events.

   a. _____

   b. _____

   c. _____

   d. _____

33. T/F   Thermal sensors and pain sensors share the same morphology.

34. _____ refers to the sense of pain.

35. Muscle stretch is sensed by _____.

36. T/F   Facial muscles have muscle spindles.

37. _____ sense muscle tension.

38. _____ refers to production and release of saliva into the oral cavity.

39. The parotid glands release _____ (type of saliva) into the posterior oral cavity and pharynx.

40. The sublingual glands release _____ (type of saliva) into the anterior oral cavity.

41. The _____ reflex involves rotary motion of the muscles of mastication.

42. The _____ reflex involves elevation of the soft palate.

43. The _____ reflex involves evacuation of the contents of the stomach.

44. The _____ reflex involves contracting the muscles of adduction and forcefully blowing them open to expel foreign matter from the respiratory passageway.

45. The _____ reflex involves retraction of the tongue.

STUDY QUESTION ANSWERS

1. MASTICATION refers to the process of preparing food for swallowing.
2. DEGLUTITION refers to the processing of swallowing
3. BOLUS refers to a "ball" of food or drink.
4. List five of the elements of the oral preparatory stage of mastication and deglutition.
   a. FOOD IS RECEIVED IN MOUTH
   b. FOOD IS MOVED ONTO MOLARS BY TONGUE
   c. FOOD IS MIXED WITH SALIVA
   d. FOOD IS FORMED INTO BOLUS
   e. FOOD IS REMOVED FROM BUCCAL CAVITY BY TONGUE ACTION
5. List three of the elements of the oral stage of deglutition.
   a. TONGUE TIP ELEVATES TO ALVEOLAR RIDGE
   b. BOLUS IS PROPELLED POSTERIORLY BY SQUEEZING ACTION
   c. BOLUS MAKES CONTACT WITH FAUCIAL PILLARS AND VELUM
6. List seven of the critical elements of the pharyngeal stage of deglutition.
   Answer could include any of the following:
   - BOLUS ENTERS OROPHARYNX
   - VELUM ELEVATES
   - LARYNX ELEVATES
   - VOCAL FOLDS ADDUCT
   - EPIGLOTTIS INVERTS TO PROTECT AIRWAY
   - TONGUE CONTACTS POSTERIOR PHARYNGEAL WALL
   - UPPER ESOPHAGEAL SPHINCTER OPENS
   - PHARYNX CONTRACTS WITH PERISTALTIC ACTION
7. The ROOTING reflex involves orienting toward the direction of tactile stimulation of the cheek.
8. PERIORAL refers to "mouth region."
9. The SUCKING reflex is elicited by soft contact with the lower lip, and results in tongue protrusion and retraction.
10. List three essential differences between the oral-pharyngeal anatomy and physiology of an infant and that of an adult.
    a. LARYNX IS ELEVATED IN INFANT
    b. TONGUE FILLS GREATER PROPORTION OF ORAL CAVITY
    c. INFANT IS MANDATORY MOUTH BREATHER
11. F   The infant must coordinate respiration and swallowing, as milk and air share the same passageway during deglutition.
12. The ORAL PREPARATORY stage is the stage in which food is prepared for swallow.
13. The ORAL stage is the stage of swallow involving oral transit of the bolus to the pharynx.
14. The PHARYNGEAL stage is the stage of swallow involving transit of the bolus to the esophagus, and includes numerous physiological protective responses.
15. The ESOPHAGEAL stage is the stage of swallow in which food is transported from the upper esophageal region to the stomach.
16. PERISTALSIS refers to wavelike action.

17. List three critical elements relative to the pressures of deglutition.
    a. <u>VELUM ELEVATES</u>
    b. <u>TONGUE AND LIPS FORM ORAL SEAL</u>
    c. <u>CRICOPHARYNGEUS OPENS AS LARYNX ELEVATES</u>

18. The acronym "CSS" refers to the words <u>CHEW</u>, <u>SUCK</u>, and <u>SWALLOW</u>.

19. <u>GUSTATION</u> refers to the sense of taste.

20. <u>CHEMORECEPTOR</u> is the class of receptors that respond to chemical stimulation.

21. Taste from the anterior two-thirds of the tongue is mediated by the <u>VII FACIAL</u> cranial nerve (name and number).

22. Taste from the posterior one-third of the tongue is mediated by the <u>IX GLOSSOPHARYNGEAL</u> cranial nerve (name and number).

23. Taste from the epiglottis and esophagus is mediated by the <u>X VAGUS</u> cranial nerve (name and number).

24. The taste of bitterness is predominantly transmitted by the <u>IX GLOSSOPHARYNGEAL</u> cranial nerve (name and number).

25. The taste of sweetness is predominantly mediated by the <u>VII FACIAL</u> cranial nerve (name and number).

26. The tastes of sourness and saltiness are predominantly mediated by the <u>VII FACIAL</u> cranial nerve (name and number).

27. <u>OLFACTION</u> refers to the sense of smell.

28. <u>MEISSNER'S</u> corpuscles respond to minute mechanical movement in the superficial epithelia.

29. <u>MERKEL DISK</u> receptors transmit the sense of pressure within the superficial epithelia.

30. <u>PACINIAN CORPUSCLES</u> respond to rapid deep pressure.

31. Cells with <u>RUFFINI</u> endings sense stretch within the deep layers of the epithelium.

32. There are four classes of thermal receptors, mediating the following classes of thermal events.
    a. <u>COOL</u>
    b. <u>COLD</u>
    c. <u>WARM</u>
    d. <u>HOT</u>

33. <u>T</u> Thermal sensors and pain sensors share the same morphology.

34. <u>NOCICEPTION</u> refers to the sense of pain.

35. Muscle stretch is sensed by <u>MUSCLE SPINDLES</u>.

36. <u>F</u> Facial muscles have muscle spindles.

37. <u>GOLGI TENDON ORGANS</u> sense muscle tension.

38. <u>SALIVATION</u> refers to production and release of saliva into the oral cavity.

39. The parotid glands release <u>SEROUS</u> (type of saliva) into the posterior oral cavity and pharynx.

40. The sublingual glands release <u>MUCUS</u> (type of saliva) into the anterior oral cavity.

41. The <u>CHEWING</u> reflex involves rotary motion of the muscles of mastication.

42. The <u>UVULAR</u> (<u>PALATAL</u>) reflex involves elevation of the soft palate.

43. The <u>VOMIT</u> reflex involves evacuation of the contents of the stomach.

44. The <u>COUGH</u> reflex involves contracting the muscles of adduction and forcefully blowing them open to expel foreign matter from the respiratory passageway.

45. The <u>TONGUE BASE RETRACTION</u> reflex involves retraction of the tongue.

REFERENCES

Basmajian, J. V. (1975). *Grant's method of anatomy.* Baltimore: Williams & Wilkins.

Bateman, H. E., & Mason, R. M. (1984). *Applied anatomy and physiology of the speech and hearing mechanism.* Springfield, IL: Charles C. Thomas.

Beck, E. W., Monson, H., & Groer, M. (1982). *Mosby's atlas of functional human anatomy.* St. Louis, MO: C. V. Mosby.

Behrman, R. E., Vaughan III, V. C. & Nelson, W. E. (Eds.). (1987). *Nelson textbook of pediatrics* (13th ed.). Philadelphia: W. B. Saunders.

Bhatnagar, S. C., & Andy, O. J. (2002). *Neuroscience for the study of communicative disorders* (2nd ed.). Baltimore: Williams & Wilkins.

Bly, L. (1983). *The components of normal movement during the first year of life and abnormal motor movement.* Chicago: Neuro-Developmental Treatment Association.

Bly, L. (1994). *Motor skills acquisition in the first year.* Tucson, AZ: Therapy Skill Builders.

Bowman, J. P. (1971). *The muscle spindle and neural control of the tongue.* Springfield, IL: Charles C. Thomas.

Buck, L. B. (2000). Smell and taste: The chemical senses. In E. R. Kandel, J. H. Schwartz, & T. M. Jessell (Eds.), *Principles of neural science* (4th ed.). New York: McGraw-Hill.

Campbell, N. A. (1990). *Biology.* Redwood City, CA: Benjamin/Cummings.

Carpenter, M. B. (1991). *Core text of neuroanatomy* (4th ed.). Baltimore: Williams & Wilkins.

Chusid, J. G. (1985). *Correlative neuroanatomy and functional neurology* (17th ed.). Los Altos, CA: Lange Medical Publications.

Cotman, C. W., & McGaugh, J. L. (1980). *Behavioral neuroscience.* New York: Academic Press.

Ganong, W. F. (2003). *Review of medical physiology* (21st ed.). New York: McGraw-Hill/Appleton & Lange.

Gardner, E. P., Martin, J. H., & Jessell, T. M. (2000). The bodily senses. In E. R. Kandel, J. H. Schwartz, & T. M. Jessell (Eds.), *Principles of neural science* (4th ed.). New York: McGraw-Hill.

Gosling, J. A., Harris, P. F., Humpherson, J. R., Whitmore, I., & Willan, P. L. T. (1985). *Atlas of human anatomy.* Philadelphia: J. B. Lippincott.

Gray, H., Bannister, L. H., Berry, M. M., & Williams, P. L. (1995). *Gray's anatomy.* London: Churchill Livingstone.

Grobler, N. J. (1977). *Textbook of clinical anatomy* (Vol. 1). Amsterdam: Elsevier Scientific.

Groher, M. E. (1997). *Dysphagia* (3rd ed.). St. Louis, MO: Butterworth-Heinemann

Healey, J. E., & Seybold, W. D. (1969). *A synopsis of clinical anatomy.* Philadelphia: W. B. Saunders.

Kahane, J. C., & Folkins, J. F. (1984). *Atlas of speech and hearing anatomy.* Columbus, OH: Charles E. Merrill.

Kandel, E. R., Schwartz, J. H., & Jessell, T. M. (2000). *Principles of neural science* (4th ed.). New York: McGraw-Hill.

Kuehn, D. P., Lemme, M. L., & Baumgartner, J. M. (1991). *Neural bases of speech, hearing, and language.* Boston: Little, Brown.

Kuehn, D. P., Templeton, P. J., & Maynard, J. A. (1990). Muscle spindles in the velopharyngeal musculature of humans. *Journal of Speech and Hearing Research, 33,* 488–493.

Landgren, S., & Olsson, K. A. (1981). Oral mechanoreceptors. In S. Grillner, B. Lindblom, J. Lubker, & A. Persson (Eds.), *Speech motor control* (pp. 129–139). Oxford: Pergamon Press.

Langley, L. L., Telford, I. R., & Christensen, J. B. (1969). *Dynamic anatomy and physiology.* New York: McGraw-Hill.

Langley, M. B., & Lombardino, L. J. (1991). *Neurodevelopmental strategies for managing communication disorders in children with severe motor dysfunction.* Austin, TX: Pro-Ed.

Liebgott, B. (2001). *The anatomical basis of dentistry* (2nd ed.). St. Louis, MO: Mosby.

Liss, J. M. (1990). Muscle spindles in the human levator veli palatini and palatoglossus muscles. *Journal of Speech and Hearing Research, 33,* 736–746.

Logemann, J. (1998). *Evaluation and treatment of swallowing disorders* (2nd ed.). Austin, TX: Pro-Ed.

Mackay, D. G. (1982). The problems of flexibility, fluency, and speed-accuracy trade-off in skilled behaviors. *Psychological Review, 89,* 483–506.

McMinn, R. M. H., Hutchings, R. T., & Logan, B. M. (1994). *Color atlas of head and neck anatomy.* London: Mosby-Wolfe.

Møller, A. R. (2003). *Sensory systems: Anatomy and physiology.* New York: Academic Press.

Mountcastle, V. B. (1974). *Medical physiology.* St. Louis, MO: Mosby.

Netter, F. (1976). *Clinical symposia: Development of the upper respiratory system.* Summit, NJ: CIBA Pharmaceutical Company.

Netter, F. H. (1983). *The CIBA collection of medical illustrations. Vol. 1. Nervous system. Part I. Anatomy and physiology.* West Caldwell, NJ: CIBA Pharmaceutical Company.

Netter, F. H. (1997). *Atlas of human anatomy.* Los Angeles: Icon Learning Systems.

Newman, K. D., & Randolph, J. (1990). Surgical problems of the esophagus in infants and children. In D. C. Sabiston & F. C. Spencer (Eds.), *Surgery of the chest* (5th ed., pp. 815–839). Philadelphia: W. B. Saunders.

Noback, C. R., Demarest, R. J., & Strominger, N. L. (1991). *The nervous system: Introduction and review.* Philadelphia: Williams & Wilkins.

Nolte, J. (2002). *The human brain* (5th ed.). St. Louis, MO: Mosby.

Payne, W. S., & Ellis, F. H., Jr. (1984). Esophagus and ciaphragmatic hernias. In S. I. Schwartz, G. T. Shires, F. C. Spencer, & E. H. Storer (Eds.), *Principles of surgery* (4th ed., pp. 1063–1112). New York: McGraw-Hill.

Perlman, A. L., Grayhack, J. P., & Booth, B. M. (1992). The relationship of vallecular residue to oral involvement, reduced hyoid elevation, and epiglottic function. *Journal of Speech and Hearing Research, 35,* 734–741.

Perlman, A. L., Luschei, E. S., & Du Mond, C. E. (1989). Electrical activity from the superior pharyngeal constrictor during reflexive and nonreflexive tasks. *Journal of Speech and Hearing Research, 32,* 749–754.

Perlman, A. L., & Schulze-Delrieu, K. (1997). *Deglutition and its disorders.* San Diego, CA: Singular Publishing Group.

Rademaker, A. W., Pauloski, B. R., Logemann, J. A., & Shanahan, T. K. (1994). Oropharyngeal swallow efficiency as a representative measure of swallowing function. *Journal of Speech and Hearing Research, 37,* 314–325.

Rohen, J. W., Yokochi, C., Lutjen-Drecoll, E., & Romrell, L. J. (2002). *Color atlas of anatomy* (5th ed.). Philadelphia: Williams & Wilkins.

Rosenbek, J. C., Robbins, J., Fishback, B., & Levine, R. L. (1991). Effects of thermal application on dysphagia after stroke. *Journal of Speech and Hearing Research, 34,* 1257–1268.

Rosse, C., Gaddum-Rosse, P., & Rosse, G. (1997). *Hollinshead's textbook of anatomy.* Philadelphia: Lippincott-Raven.

Snell, R. S. (1978). *Gross anatomy dissector.* Boston: Little, Brown.

Sonies, B. C. (1997). *Dysphagia. A continuum of care.* Gaithersburg, MD: Aspen.

Weber, C. M., & Smith, A. (1987). Reflex responses in human jaw, lip, and tongue muscles elicited by mechanical stimulation. *Journal of Speech and Hearing Research, 30,* 70–79.

Wickens, J., Hyland, B., & Anson, G. (1994). Cortical cell assemblies: A possible mechanism for motor programs. *Journal of Motor Behavior, 26*(2), 66–82.

Winans, S. S., Gilman, S., Manter, J. T., & Gatz, A. J. (2002). *Manter and Gatz's essentials of clinical neuroanatomy and neurophysiology* (10th ed.). Philadelphia: F. A. Davis.

Wohlert, A. B., & Goffman, L. (1994). Human perioral muscle activation patterns. *Journal of Speech and Hearing Research, 37*, 1032–1040.

Zemlin, W. R. (1998). *Speech and hearing science: Anatomy and physiology* (4th ed.). Needham Heights, MA: Allyn & Bacon.

CHAPTER 10

Anatomy of Hearing

It is a recurring theme that communication ability is superimposed on a physical system clearly designed for another function. The auditory system is the only system that has no other function besides communication. One might argue that our distant ancestors were more interested in the sounds that supported survival than those that arose from society, but nonetheless **audition** (the process associated with hearing) is an essential element of verbal communication.

The mechanisms of hearing are extraordinary in size and complexity. In this chapter we will discuss these structures. The next chapter will be devoted to the reasons these structures exist: the physiology of hearing.

THE STRUCTURES OF HEARING

The physical structures of the ear are deceptively simple, especially in light of their exquisite function. The ear is an energy **transducer**, which means that it converts acoustic energy into electrochemical energy. The details of these structures will set the stage for discussion of the transduction process in Chapter 11.

transducer: *L., trans, across + ducer, to lead*

We will talk about the ear in terms of the basic elements involved: the outer ear, middle ear, inner ear, and auditory pathways (see Figure 10-1).

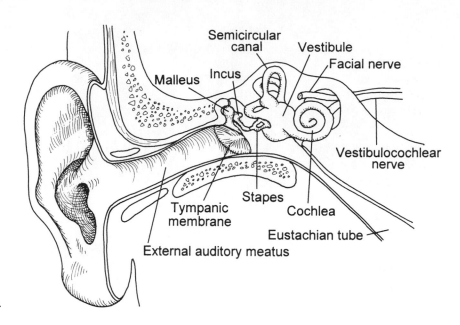

Figure 10-1. Schematic of frontal section revealing outer, middle, and inner ear structures.

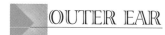OUTER EAR

pinna: *L., feather*

The outer ear is composed of two basic components with which you are quite familiar (Table 10-1). The **pinna** (or auricle) is the prominence we colloquially refer to as the ear, although it serves primarily as a collector of sound to be processed at deeper levels (e.g., the eardrum and cochlea). The structure of the pinna is provided by cartilage.

The pinna has several important functions, including aiding localization of sound in space and "capturing" sound energy. Landmarks of the pinna are important for a number of reasons, not the least of which is their diagnostic significance (see Figure 10-2). The **helix** forms the curled margin of the pinna, marking its most distal borders. A superior-posterior bulge on the helix is known as the **auricular tubercle** (or **Darwin's tubercle**). Immediately anterior to the helix is the **antihelix**, a similar fold of tissue marking the entrance to the concha. Between helix and antihelix is the **scaphoid fossa**. The antihelix bifurcates superiorly, producing the **crura anthelicis**, and the space between them forms the **triangular fossa** (**fossa triangularis**). The **cymba conchae** is the anterior extension of the helix marking the anterior entrance to the concha, and the **cavum conchae** is the deep portion of the concha. The **concha** (or **concha auriculae**) is the entrance to the ear canal, known as the **external auditory meatus** (abbreviated **EAM**; alternately **meatus acousticus externus**). A flap of epithelium-covered cartilage known as the **tragus** looks as if it could cover the entrance to the meatus (and probably did in an earlier version of the auditory mechanism). Superior to the tragus is the **tuberculum supratragicum**. Posterior and inferior to the tragus is

helix: *Gr., coil*

concha: *Gr., konche, shell*

tragus: *Gr., tragos, goat*

Table 10-1. Landmarks of the outer ear.

Auricle
  Helix
  Auricular tubercle (Darwin's tubercle)
  Antihelix
  Crura
  Crura anthelicis
  Triangular fossa
  Scaphoid fossa
  Concha
    Cymba conchae
    Cavum conchae
  Tragus
  Intertragic incisure
  Antitragus
  Lobule

External Auditory Meatus
  Cartilagenous meatus
  Osseous meatus
  Isthmus
  Tympanic membrane

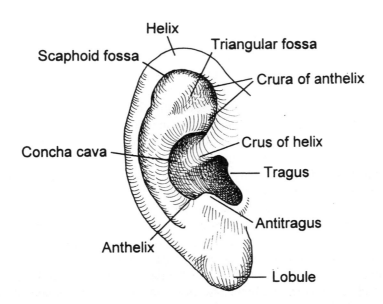

Figure 10-2. Landmarks of the auricle.

the **antitragus** (the region between tragus and antitragus is termed the **intertragic incisure** or **incisura intertragica**), and below the antitragus is the **lobule** or **lobe**.

If you palpate these structures on yourself, you will realize that the lobule is one of the few structures devoid of cartilage. The **auricular cartilage** is a unitary structure closely following the landmarks we have just described and covered with a layer of epithelial tissue invested with fine hairs that are useful for keeping insects and dirt out of the ear canal.

The **external auditory meatus** is approximately 7 mm in diameter and 2.5 cm long when measured from the depth of the concha, but you would add another 1.5 cm to its length if you chose to measure it from the tragus. This is, in reality, not a trivial matter: The EAM and conchae both contribute to hearing as resonating cavities, and determination of the resonant frequency depends in large part on the length of the cavity, as we shall see in Chapter 11.

The lateral third of the canal is comprised of cartilage and is about 8 mm long; the medial two-thirds is the bony meatus of the temporal bone. The EAM is S-shaped: If you were a fly walking toward the **ear drum** (**tympanic membrane**, abbreviated **TM**), you would start out hiking generally medially, forward, and up. At the juncture of the osseous and cartilaginous EAM, you would take a turn down as you made your approach. During your hike you would see two constrictions: The first marks the end of the cartilaginous portion and the beginning of the osseous EAM. The second constriction, termed the **isthmus**, is about 0.5 cm from the tympanic membrane itself. At the end of your hike you would run into the tympanic membrane, a thin trilaminar sheet of tissue that sits at an oblique angle in the EAM. The epithelial cover of the pinna continues into the EAM and serves as the outer layer of the tympanic membrane, to be discussed.

Because the adult ear canal takes a turn downward, you cannot see the medial end of the canal without some effort. If you were to look into the ear canal (you will have to manipulate the pinna and use a **speculum**, a device used to view cavities of the body), you would see that the outer third of the EAM is lined with hairs, and has **cerumen**, or "ear wax." These are both quite functional additions to the canal, as they trap insects and dirt, protecting the medial-most point of the outer ear, the tympanic membrane.

The tympanic membrane (TM) or ear drum marks the boundary between the outer and middle ears. It completely separates the two spaces, being an extremely thin three-layered sheet of tissue. The epithelial lining of the EAM continues as the external layer of the tympanic membrane, while the lining of the middle ear provides the inner layer. Sandwiched between these two delicate epithelial linings is a layer of fibrous tissue that provides structure for the tympanic membrane.

The tympanic membrane is approximately 55 mm² in area, and has a number of important landmarks (see Figure 10-3). If you take the time to view one of your friend's tympanic membranes (carefully), you will see the **umbo**, which is the most distal point of attachment of the inner tympanic membrane to one of the bones of the middle ear, the malleus.

isthmus: *Gr., isthmos, passageway*

speculum: *L., mirror*

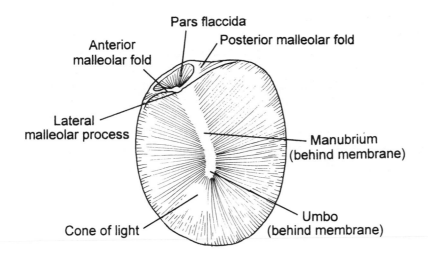

Figure 10-3. Left ear tympanic membrane, as viewed from the external auditory meatus.

Otitis Externa and Cerumen

The epithelial lining of the auricle and EAM is tightly bound to the cartilage and bone of these structures, and this accounts for the pain involved in any swelling of the tissue. **Otitis externa** refers to inflammation of the skin of the external ear. When tissue is inflamed, it responds with **edema** (swelling). If the epithelium is tightly bound to its underlying structure, as it is in the EAM and pinna, the swelling increases the tension on the epithelium, making it quite painful.

Otitis externa may result from bacterial infection following trauma or abrasion. Failure to clean probe tips and specula could result in transmission of the infection between clients. Otitis externa may also result from viral infection, including infection with herpes zoster virus. This painful infection may lead to facial paralysis or hearing loss if the facial or vestibulocochlear nerves are involved.

The EAM is invested with cilia and ceruminous glands, largely restricted to the cartilaginous portion of the canal. **Cerumen** (ear wax) is secreted by the glands into the ear canal, trapping insects and dirt that would otherwise threaten the tympanic membrane. Individuals with overly active ceruminous glands may find that the EAM becomes occluded, and removal of the cerumen may be required. Attempts to remove the cerumen by the individual using cotton swabs often results in cerumen and dirt being packed against the inferior boundary of the tympanic membrane, as the oblique angle forms a perfect "pocket" to catch the matter.

The interested student and budding audiologist would be well-advised to read the descriptions of these and other conditions provided by Martin (1981).

The tympanic membrane is particularly taut at this point, and the location inferior and anterior to this is referred to as the **cone of light** because it reflects the light of the audiologist's otoscope. You may be able to see the handle (or manubrium) of the malleus behind the tympanic

Malformations of the Pinna and EAM

If the pinna is subjected to trauma, as in that inflicted during the sport of boxing, the result can be permanent deformation of its structure. Trauma can cause hemorrhaging between the epithelium and cartilage, and, if left untreated, the resulting swelling may cause a permanent distortion.

Several congenital conditions may be manifest in the EAM and pinna. **Atresia**, or congenital absence of the EAM, may signal absence of middle ear structures as well. **Stenosis** or narrowing of the ear canal will reduce its ability to transmit sound to the middle ear structures. **Aplasia** of the pinna occurs when it fails to develop or does not develop completely. If the pinna is abnormally small, it is termed **microtia**. If something interferes with development, the pinnae may remain set low on the sides of the face.

A number of genetic syndromes are manifested in auricle anomalies. Children affected by branchio-oto-renal syndrome will often have cupped ears or microtia, in conjunction with stapes disconnection and conductive or sensorineural hearing loss. A high proportion of individuals with Down syndrome (Trisomy 21) will show microtia, often have small earlobes and helix malformation, and occasionally stenosis of the ear canal.

membrane, appearing as a streak on the membrane; if you are looking at the left tympanic membrane, the handle of the malleus will look like the hand of a clock pointing to the 1.

The tympanic membrane is slightly concave when viewed from the EAM, and the umbo is the most depressed portion of this concavity. Although most of the tympanic membrane is invested with fibrous tissue, the **pars flaccida** is not, and this "flaccid part" may be seen in the superior quadrant of the tympanic membrane. On either side of the pars flaccida is a recess, consisting of the **anterior** and **posterior malleolar folds**. These folds and the region at the cone of light are the result of the malleus pushing distally on the membrane, much as if you were to stretch an unfilled balloon and push it from behind. This tight binding between membrane and malleus permits ready transmission of acoustic energy from the tympanic membrane to the ossicular chain. If the tympanic membrane is particularly transparent, you may also be able to see the long process of the incus parallel to the lateral process of the malleus. In addition, the chorda tympani may sometimes be seen through the superior tympanic membrane.

In summary, the outer ear is composed of the pinna, the structure that serves primarily as a sound collector, and the **external auditory meatus** or ear canal.

- Landmarks of the pinna include the margin of the **auricle**, the **helix**, and the **auricular tubercle** on the helix.

Structure of the Tympanic Membrane

The tympanic membrane is a slightly oval structure, approximately 10 mm in diameter in the superior-inferior dimension. The anterior-posterior dimension is slightly smaller (about 9 mm in diameter), and the entire membrane is placed within the canal at a 55° angle with the floor. The circumference of the membrane is a fibrocartilaginous ring that fits into the **tympanic sulcus**, a groove in the temporal bone. The sulcus is incomplete in the superior aspect, accommodating the anterior and posterior malleolar folds.

The tympanic membrane is made up of three layers of tissue: the outer, intermediate, and inner layers. The **outer (cuticular) layer** is a continuation of the epithelial lining of the EAM and pinna.

The **intermediate (fibrous) layer** is made up of two parts: The superficial layer is composed of fibers that radiate out from the handle of the malleus to the periphery. The deep layer is made up of circular fibers that are found mostly in the periphery of the membrane. The **inner (mucous) layer** is continuous with the mucosa of the middle ear.

- The **cymba conchae** is the anterior extension of the helix and is the anterior entrance of the concha.
- The external auditory meatus has both osseous and cartilaginous parts.
- The distal, cartilaginous portion makes up one-third of the ear canal; the other two-thirds are housed in bone.
- At the terminus of the external auditory meatus is the tympanic membrane, the structure separating the outer and middle ears.

MIDDLE EAR

The middle ear is a small but extremely important space occupied by three of the smallest bones of the body. First, let us examine these bones and their attachments, and then discuss the landmarks of the cavity itself (Table 10-2).

Ossicles

The bones of the ear, known as the **ossicles**, include the malleus, incus, and stapes (see Figures 10-4 through 10-6). This **ossicular chain** of three articulated bones provides the means for transmission of acoustic energy impinging on the tympanic membrane to the inner ear. The **malleus** is the largest of the ossicles, providing the point of attachment with the tympanic membrane.

malleus: *L., hammer*

Table 10-2. Landmarks of the middle ear.

Ossicles
　Malleus
　　Manubrium (handle)
　　Head (caput)
　　Lateral process
　　Anterior process
　　Facet for incus
　　Ligaments
　　　Superior ligament
　　　Lateral ligament
　　　Anterior ligament
　Incus
　　Short process (crus breve)
　　Long process (crus longum)
　　Lenticular process
　　Facet for malleus
　　Superior ligament of incus
　　Posterior ligament of incus
　Stapes
　　Head (caput)
　　Neck
　　Posterior crus (crus posterius)
　　Anterior crus (crus anterius)
　　Base (footplate)

Muscles
　Stapedius muscle
　Tensor tympani muscle

Medial Wall
　Promontory
　　Oval window
　　Round window
　　Prominence of facial nerve
　Prominence of lateral semicircular canal
　Canal of tensor tympani

Anterior Wall
　Entrance of Eustachian tube

Posterior Wall
　Prominence of stapedial pyramid
　Origin of prominence of facial nerve
　Aditus to mastoid antrum

Floor

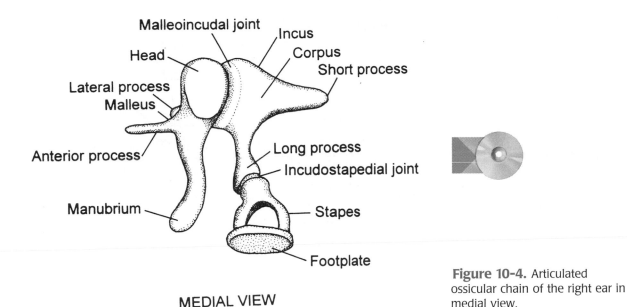

MEDIAL VIEW

Figure 10-4. Articulated ossicular chain of the right ear in medial view.

As you can see in Figure 10-5, the **handle** or **manubrium** of the malleus is a long process, separated from the **head** by a thin neck. The **anterior** and **lateral processes** provide points of attachment for ligaments, to be discussed. The manubrium attaches to the tympanic membrane along its length, terminating with the **lateral process**. This attachment

manubrium: *L., handle*

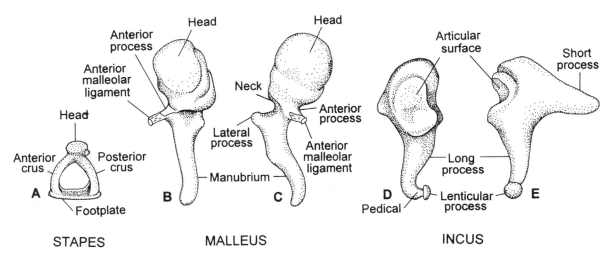

STAPES   MALLEUS   INCUS

Figure 10-5. Ossicles of the middle ear and their landmarks. A. Stapes landmarks. B. Posteromedial view of malleus. C. Anteromedial view of malleus. D. Anteromedial view of incus. E. Posteromedial view of incus. (Adapted from Comparative Anatomy of the Middle Ear by O. W. Henson, 1974, p. 95. In H. Autrum, R. Jung, W. R. Loewenstein, D. M. MackKay, & H. L. Teuber [Eds.], *Handbook of sensory physiology*.)

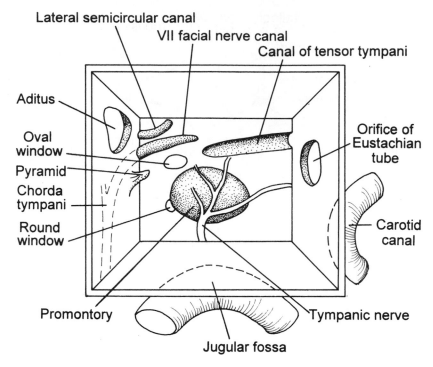

Lateral semicircular canal

VII facial nerve canal

Canal of tensor tympani

Aditus

Oval window

Pyramid

Chorda tympani

Round window

Orifice of Eustachian tube

Carotid canal

Promontory

Tympanic nerve

Jugular fossa

Figure 10-6. Schematic representation of the middle ear cavity of the right ear, as viewed from the external auditory meatus with tympanic membrane removed. (Redrawn by permission. From *Anatomy: A regional study of human structure*, 5th ed., by E. Gardner, D. J. Gray, & R. O'Rahilly, 1986, p. 623. Copyright 1986 by R. O'Rahilly. Philadelphia, PA: W. B. Saunders.)

of the lateral process with the tympanic membrane forms the anterior and posterior malleolar folds and the pars flaccida.

Examination of the malleus will reveal that the bulk of the bone is in the **head** (or **caput**) — not coincidentally the point of articulation with the incus. The head of the malleus protrudes into the epitympanic recess of the middle ear, to be discussed. Although the malleus is the largest of the ossicles, it is only 9 mm long and it weighs a mere 25 mg.

The **incus** (fancied to be shaped like an anvil) provides the intermediate communicating link of the ossicular chain. The **body** of the incus articulates with the head of the malleus by means of the **malleolar facet** in such a way that the **long process** of the incus is nearly parallel with the long process of the malleus; the body is nearly entirely within the epitympanic recess. The **short process** projects posteriorly, while the end of the long process bends medially, forming the **lenticular process** with which the stapes will articulate. Needless to say, this is not an accidental arrangement of nature, but we will reserve discussion of the benefits of this configuration for Chapter 11.

The incus weighs approximately 30 mg, and its longest process is approximately 7 mm. The malleus and incus articulate by means of a saddle joint, although it appears that movement at the joint is quite limited. Rather, the malleus and incus appear to move as a unit upon movement of the tympanic membrane.

incus: *L., anvil*

lenticular: *L., lenticularis, lens-like*

Otitis Media with Effusion

Serous (**secretory**) otitis media refers to any condition in which fluid accumulates in the middle ear cavity. The typical sequence is as follows: The Eustachian tube stops functioning properly, allowing the middle ear space to become anaerobic as tissue within the space absorbs the available oxygen. Parallel to this, the poorly functioning Eustachian tube may not allow equalization of pressure between the middle ear space and the environment. In either condition, a relatively negative pressure may ensue in the middle ear space, pulling serous fluid from the blood of the middle ear tissues (termed **transudation**). The negative air pressure may also stimulate secretion of mucus from the middle ear tissue. This state, termed **middle ear effusion**, creates a barrier to sound transmission, in that the movement of the tympanic membrane is greatly inhibited.

The **stapes**, or "stirrup," is the third bone of this chain. The **head** (**caput**) of the stapes articulates with the lenticular process of the incus, and the neck of the stapes bifurcates to become the crura. The arch formed by the **anterior** and **posterior crura** converges on the **footplate** or **base** of the stapes. The footplate of the stapes rests in the oval window of the temporal bone, held in place by the **annular ligament**. This is the smallest of the ossicles, weighing approximately 4 mg, with the area of the stapes being only about 3.5 mm. The articulation of the incus and stapes (the **incudostapedial joint**) is of the ball-and-socket type.

The ossicular chain is held in place by a series of strategically placed ligaments that suspend the ossicles from the walls of the middle ear cavity. The **superior ligament of the malleus** holds the head of the malleus within the epitympanic recess. An **anterior ligament of the malleus** binds the neck of the malleus to the anterior wall of the middle ear, and the **lateral ligament of the malleus** attaches the head of the malleus to the lateral wall. The **posterior ligament of the incus** suspends the incus by means of its short process, while a poorly formed **superior ligament of the incus** may be seen to bind the incus to the epitympanic recess.

▶ **stapes:** *L., stirrup*

Tympanic Muscles

- **Stapedius**
- **Tensor tympani**

Two important muscles of the middle ear are attached to the ossicles. These are the smallest muscles of the human body, appropriately so considering their attachment to the smallest bones (see Figure 10-5).

Stapedius

The **stapedius muscle**, approximately 6 mm long, is embedded in the bone of the posterior wall of the middle ear, with only its tendon emerging from the **pyramidal eminence** in the middle ear space. The muscle inserts into the posterior neck of the stapes, so that when it contracts the stapes is rotated posteriorly. Muscle spindles have been found in the stapedius muscle. Innervation of the stapedius is by means of the stapedial branch of the VII facial nerve.

Tensor Tympani

The **tensor tympani** is approximately 25 mm in length, arising from the anterior wall of the middle ear space, superior to the orifice of the Eustachian tube. As with the stapedius, only the tendon of the tensor tympani is found in the middle ear space; the muscle itself is housed in bone. The muscle originates from the cartilaginous part of the Eustachian tube, as well as from the greater wing of the sphenoid, coursing through the **canal for the tensor tympani** in the anterior wall of the middle ear. The tendon for the tensor tympani emerges from the canal, courses around a bony outcropping called the **trochleariform process** (alternately **cochleariform process**), and inserts into the upper manubrium malli. Contraction of this muscle pulls the malleus antero-medially, thereby reducing the range of movement of the tympanic membrane by placing indirect tension on it. Indeed, both the tensor tympani and the stapedius muscles stiffen the middle ear transmission system, thereby reducing transmission of acoustical information in the lower frequencies. That is, contraction of these muscles reduces the strength of the signal

Muscle:	Stapedius
Origin:	Posterior wall of middle ear space of temporal bone
Course:	Anteriorly
Insertion:	Posterior crus of stapes
Innervation:	VII facial nerve
Function:	Rotates footplate of stapes posteriorly, thereby stiffening ossicular chain

Muscle:	Tensor tympani
Origin:	Cartilaginous portion of Eustachian tube and greater wing of sphenoid
Course:	Posteriorly through canal for tensor tympani and around trochleariform process
Insertion:	Manubrium malli
Innervation:	V trigeminal nerve via the otic ganglion
Function:	Pulls malleus antero-medially and stiffens ossicular chain

Acoustic Reflex

The **acoustic reflex** (also known as the **stapedial reflex**) is a staple of the audiologist's diagnostic toolkit. The stapedius muscle applies a force on the footplate of the stapes that reduces the amplitude of excursion of the footplate, thereby reducing the sound pressure level reaching the cochlea. It is thought that this is a basic protective mechanism for the cochlea, as it is triggered by loud sounds, typically greater than 85 dB SPL. The acoustic reflex may also include response by the tensor tympani muscle.

The neural circuit for the acoustic reflex is such that stimulation of either ear results in response by both ears, although attenuation of the signal by the ipsilateral ear is stronger than the attenuation in the contralateral ear. As outlined by Møller (1983), a stimulus entering the right ear is transduced by the right cochlea, right ventral cochlear nucleus, and right medial superior olive, consecutively. The right medial superior olive communicates with both the right- and left-side nuclei of the VII facial and V trigeminal nerves, so that the appropriate stimulus triggers a response in stapedius muscles on both left and right sides.

reaching the cochlea, potentially protecting it from damage due to high signal intensity. Unfortunately, the protective function is compromised, in that the stiffening of the ossicular chain provides little barrier to transmission of the high-frequency sound so dominant in modern industrial societies. Innervation of the tensor tympani is by the V trigeminal nerve via the otic ganglion.

The arrangement of these ligament and muscle attachments is critical to function of the middle ear. As we shall see in Chapter 11, the attachments of the ossicles provide the precise "tuning" necessary to support vibration while prohibiting continued oscillation.

Landmarks of the Middle Ear

The middle ear space is invested with numerous landmarks of importance in the study of auditory function. Figure 10-6 is a schematic of the right middle ear represented as a box, to help our discussion.

Medial Wall

Four landmarks related to the cochlea and vestibular system lie immediately medial to the space. The **oval window** (**fenestra vestibuli**; **fenestra ovalis**) in which the footplate of the stapes is embedded lies in the superior-posterior aspect, and below that point is the **round window** (**fenestra cochlea**; **fenestra rotunda**), an opening sealed by the **secondary tympanic membrane** and marking the entrance into the scala tympani of the cochlea. Between these two is the **promontory**, a bulge

fenestra: *L., window*

created by the basal turn of the cochlea. Immediately above the oval window is the prominence of the **lateral semicircular canal** of the vestibular mechanism, to be discussed. In addition to these landmarks, you can see a portion of the canal within which the tensor tympani is housed, and from which its tendon emerges, as well as the **prominence of the facial nerve**.

Anterior Wall

Examination of the anterior wall reveals the **entrance to the Eustachian tube**, and within that wall the internal carotid artery courses. The canal for the tensor tympani arises from the medial-most aspect of this wall, marked by the trochleariform process, as mentioned previously (see Figure 10-6).

The **Eustachian tube** (also known as the **pharyngotympanic tube** or **auditory tube**) was discussed previously in Chapter 7. This important structure provides the sole means of bringing oxygen to the middle ear space (**aeration**), a crucial process for maintaining equilibrium between the middle ear and atmospheric pressure. The Eustachian tube is about 36 mm in length, coursing anteriorly and medially on its way to the nasopharynx. The bony portion of the Eustachian tube (approximately 12 mm in length) terminates at the juncture of the petrous and squamous parts of the temporal bone. The cartilaginous Eustachian tube is twice as long as the bony tube, and in cross-section is seen to be incomplete along the entire inferior aspect. That is, the Eustachian tube is capable of expanding by pulling the inferior margins away from each other, a function performed by the tensor veli palatini, discussed in Chapter 7.

Posterior Wall and Floor

On the posterior wall is the **prominence of the stapedial pyramid** (**pyramidal eminence**) from which the tendon of the stapedius arises en route to the neck of the stapes. The **aditus to the mastoid antrum** opens into the epitympanic recess of the mastoid antrum. Within the posterior wall courses the chorda tympani, and the VII facial nerve prominence may be seen to continue on the medial wall.

Beneath the floor of the middle ear cavity lies the jugular bulb. **Mastoid air cells** comprising much of the mastoid process may extend to the floor of the middle ear cavity. Infection of the middle ear space may result in subsequent infection of the mastoid air cells, sometimes requiring mastoidectomy.

In summary, the middle ear cavity houses the important middle ear ossicles, and has a number of important landmarks.

- The **malleus** is the largest of the ossicles, providing the point of attachment with the tympanic membrane.

- The **incus** provides the intermediate communicating link of the ossicular chain, and the **stapes** is the third bone of this chain.

- The ossicular chain is held in place by a series of important ligaments: the **superior**, **anterior**, and **lateral ligaments of the malleus**, and the **posterior** and **superior ligaments of the incus**.

- The **stapedius muscle** inserts into the posterior neck of the stapes and pulls the stapes posteriorly.

- The **tensor tympani** muscle inserts into the upper manubrium malli, and pulls the malleus antero-medially.

- Landmarks of the medial wall of the middle ear cavity include the **oval window**, the **round window**, the **promontory** of the cochlea, and the **prominence of the facial nerve**.

- The anterior wall houses the entrance to the **Eustachian tube**, and the posterior wall houses the **prominence of the stapedial pyramid**.

 ## INNER EAR

The inner ear houses the sensors for balance (the vestibular system) and hearing (the cochlea) (see Table 10-3). The entryway to the cochlea is termed the **vestibule**.

Examination of Figure 10-7 will help in this preliminary discussion of the inner ear. Depicted in this figure is the **osseous** or **bony** labyrinth, representing the cavities (tunnels) within which the inner ear structures (the **membranous labyrinth**) are housed.

The osseous labyrinth is made up of the entryway to the labyrinth, the vestibule, the semicircular canals, and the osseous cochlear canal.

labyrinth: *Gr., labyrinthos, maze*

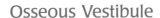 ## Osseous Vestibule

The oval window is within the lateral wall of the **vestibule**, anterior to the semicircular canals and posterior to the cochlea. The vestibule is marked by three prominent recesses, the spherical, cochlear, and elliptical recesses. The **spherical recess** of the medial wall contains minute perforations termed the **macula cribrosa media**, passages through which portions of the vestibular nerve pass to the saccule of the membranous labyrinth. The **cochlear recess** provides similar communication between the vestibule and the basal end of the cochlear duct. The **elliptical recess** is similarly perforated, providing communication between the utricle it houses and the ampullae of the superior and lateral semicircular canals, to be discussed.

Table 10-3. Landmarks of the inner ear.

Vestibule
  Saccule
  Utricle
  Macula
  Otolithic membrane
  Stereocilia
  Kinocilium
  Ductus reunien
  Endolymphatic duct

Semicircular canals
  Lateral semicircular canal
  Anterior vertical semicircular canal
  Posterior vertical semicircular canal
  Ampulla
  Crista ampularis
  Stereocilia
  Kinocilium

Cochlea
  Scala vestibuli
  Scala tympani
  Scala media (cochlear duct)
    Reissner's membrane
    Basilar membrane
    Spiral ligament
    Stria vascularis
    Organ of Corti
      Inner and outer hair cells
      Deiter's cells
      Tunnel of Corti
      Spiral limbus
      Inner spiral sulcus
      Tectorial membrane
      Reticular lamina
      Hensen's cells
      Cells of Claudius
      Rods of Corti

Osseous spiral lamina
  Habenula perforata

Helicotrema

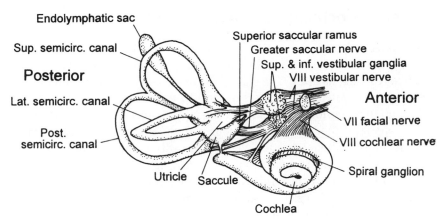

Figure 10-7. The membranous labyrinth, revealing components of the inner ear.

Osseous Semicircular Canals

The osseous semicircular canals house the sense organs for movement of the body in space. These consist of the **anterior** (anterior vertical; superior), **posterior** (posterior vertical), and **horizontal** (lateral) **semicircular canals**, the name describing the orientation of each canal. You can envision the canals as a series of three rings attached to a ball (the vestibule), and lying behind and above that ball. Each ring is in a plane at right angles to one other ring, so that the interaction of the three permits the brain to code three-dimensional space. The semicircular canals all open onto the vestibule by means of apertures, although the vertical canals (anterior and posterior semicircular canals) share an aperture, the **crus commune**. Near the opening to the vestibule in each canal is an enlargement that houses the ampulla, to be discussed.

The anterior vertical canal is oriented so that it senses movement in a plane roughly perpendicular to the length of the temporal bone. The anterior end of the canal houses the ampulla; the other end combines with the nonampulated end of the posterior vertical canal at the crus commune.

The posterior vertical semicircular canal is oriented roughly parallel to the length of the temporal bone. Its ampulla is housed in the lower crus, entering the vestibule below the oval window.

The lateral (horizontal) semicircular canal senses movement roughly in the transverse plane of the body. Its ampulated end enters the vestibule near that of the anterior semicircular canal, above the level of the oval window.

Binaural orientation of the two semicircular canals is such that the anterior semicircular canal of one ear is parallel to the posterior canal of the other. The horizontal canals lie in the same plane, but the ampullae are in mirror-image locations. This horizontal orientation of the canal helps your brain differentiate rotatory movement toward the left versus right.

Osseous Cochlear Labyrinth

The osseous labyrinth has the appearance of a coiled snail shell. It coils out from a base near the vestibule, wrapping around itself 2¾ times before reaching its **apex**. The core of the osseous labyrinth, the **modiolus**, is finely perforated bone: Fibers of the VIII vestibulocochlear nerve pass through these perforations en route to ganglion cells within the modiolus. The core of the modiolus is continuous with the **internal auditory meatus** of the temporal bone, through which the vestibulocochlear nerve passes.

modiolus: *L., hub*

The labyrinth is divided into two incomplete chambers, the **scala vestibuli** and the **scala tympani**, by an incomplete bony shelf protruding from the modiolus, the **osseous spiral lamina**. This very important structure forms the point of attachment for the scala media, which houses the sensory organ for hearing. The osseous spiral lamina becomes progressively smaller approaching the apex, such that the space between it and the opposite wall of the labyrinth increases. At the apex the two chambers formed by the incomplete lamina become hooklike (hence the name **hamulus**), forming the **helicotrema**, the region through which the scala tympani and scala vestibuli will communicate in life.

The osseous labyrinth has three prominent openings. The **round window** (**foramen rotunde**) provides communication between the scala tympani and the middle ear. The oval window, within which the stapes is placed, permits communication between the scala vestibuli and the middle ear space. The **cochlear canaliculus** or **cochlear aqueduct** is a minute opening between the scala tympani in the region of the round window and the subarachnoid space of the cranial cavity. It is hypothesized that **perilymph**, the fluid that fills the scala vestibuli and scala tympani, passes through this duct, although this has not been demonstrated.

In summary, the inner ear houses the sensors for balance (the vestibular system) and hearing (the cochlea).

- The entryway to these structures is termed the **vestibule**.
- The **osseous labyrinth** is made up of the entryway to the labyrinth, the vestibule, the semicircular canals, and the osseous cochlear canal.
- The osseous labyrinth has the appearance of a coiled snail shell.
- The labyrinth is divided into two incomplete chambers, the **scala vestibuli** and the **scala tympani**, by the **osseous spiral lamina**, an incomplete bony shelf protruding from the modiolus.
- The **round window** provides communication between the scala tympani and the middle ear.
- The **oval window** permits communication between the scala vestibuli and the middle ear space.
- The **cochlear aqueduct** connects the upper duct and the subarachnoid space.

Membranous Labyrinth

The structure of the membranous labyrinth parallels that of the bony labyrinth. First, orient yourself to the oval window, recognizing its link to the stapes of the middle ear. Beneath it, but not quite visible, is the round window. The **vestibule** or entryway to the inner ear is a space shared by the sense organ of hearing, the cochlea, and the sense organs of balance, the semicircular canals. The same fluid flows through all of the membranous labyrinth, making balance and hearing intimately related in both function and pathology. Let us examine the sensory components of the inner ear (see Figure 10-8).

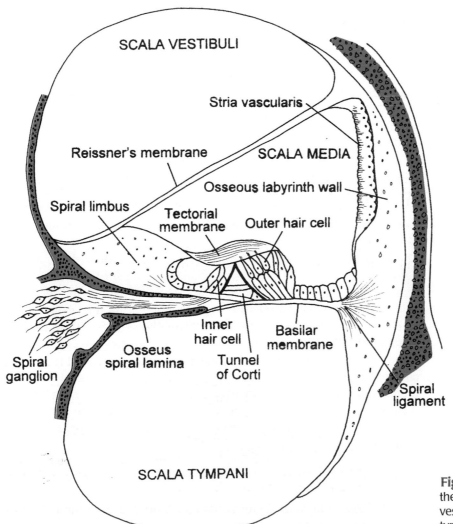

Figure 10-8. Cross-section of the cochlea, revealing scala vestibuli, scala media, and scala tympani.

Vestibular System

The **membranous labyrinth** can be thought of as a fluid-filled sac that rests within the cavity of the osseous labyrinth. This sac does not completely fill the labyrinth, but rather forms an additional space within the already fluid-filled region. The duct forms only a small portion of the labyrinth and contains fluid of a slightly different composition from that of the region surrounding the duct. This fluid in the cochlear duct is termed **endolymph**.

In the vestibular system, the membranous labyrinth houses the vestibular organ. As you will recall, the **ampulla** is the expanded region of the semicircular canals near one opening to the vestibule. Each ampulla houses a **crista ampularis**, over which a cupola lies. The crista is the receptor organ for movement, being made up of ciliated receptor cells and a supporting membrane. From each of the 6,000 receptor cells protrude approximately 50 **stereocilia**, minute hairs that sense movement in fluid, and one **kinocilium**. A **cupola** overlays the crista ampularis such that the cilia are embedded within the cupola.

Within the vestibule lie the **utricle** and **saccule**, housing for the otolithic organs of the vestibular system. The utricular **macula** is the sensory organ, which is endowed with hair cells and cilia. It is covered by the **otolithic membrane**, which is invested with crystals (**otoliths**). The saccule lies near the scala vestibuli in the vestibule, and is similarly endowed with macula and otolithic membrane. The saccule and utricle communicate by means of the **endolymphatic duct**, which is embedded in the dura mater. The saccule communicates with the cochlea by means of the minute **ductus reuniens**.

Cochlear Duct

The membranous labyrinth of the cochlea, the **cochlear duct**, resides between the scala vestibuli and tympani, making up the intermediate **scala media**. This structure houses the sensory apparatus for hearing.

A cross-section through the region of the scala media reveals its extraordinary structure, as shown in Figure 10-9. Note first the osseous spiral lamina, discussed previously. This shelf courses the extent of the osseous labyrinth, forming the major point of attachment for the cochlear duct. Again, looking at Figure 10-8, you can see **Reissner's membrane**, an extremely thin separation between the perilymph of the scala vestibuli and the endolymph of the scala media. One end is continuous with the **stria vascularis**, highly vascularized tissue that is firmly attached to the **spiral ligament**.

The **basilar membrane** forms the "floor" of the scala media, separating the scala media and scala tympani. It is on this membrane that the organ of hearing is found.

The **organ of Corti** is grossly similar to the design of the vestibular organs. There are four rows of hair cells resting on a bed of Deiters' cells

---

crista: *L., crest*

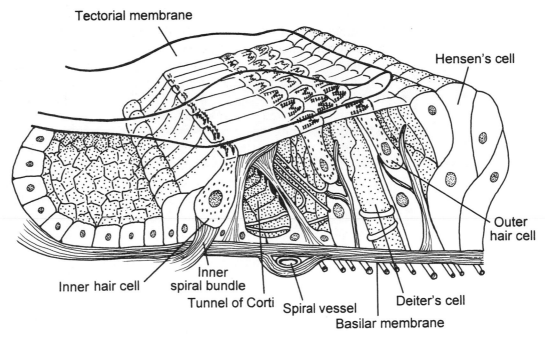

Figure 10-9. Landmarks and structures of the organ of Corti.

for support. The outer three rows of hair cells, known as **outer hair cells**, are separated from the single row of **inner hair cells** by the **tunnel of Corti**, the product of **pillar cells of Corti**. The superior surface of the outer hair cells and the phalangeal processes of Deiters' cells form a matrix termed the *reticular lamina*, through which the cilia protrude.

On the modiolar side of the cochlear duct is found the **spiral limbus**, from which arises the **tectorial membrane**. The tectorial membrane overlays the hair cells, and has functional significance in the processing of acoustic stimuli. The outer hair cells are clearly embedded in this membrane, but the inner hair cells do not make physical contact with the tectorial membrane, although its proximity to the hair cells is an important contributor to hair cell excitation, as will be discussed.

Inner and outer hair cells differ markedly in number. The hair cells on the modiolar side of the tunnel of Corti are termed the **inner hair cells** (IHC) (see Figure 10-10). The 3,500 inner hair cells form a single row stretching from the base to apex. The upper surface of each hair cell is graced with a series of approximately 50 **stereocilia** forming a slight "U" pattern opened toward the modiolar side. There are three rows of outer hair cells, broadening to four rows in the apical end, and numbering approximately 12,000. As with the inner cells, the stereocilia protrude from the surface of each outer hair cell, but with a "W" or "V" pattern formed by approximately 150 stereocilia. In both inner and outer hair cells, the stereocilia for a given cell are graduated in length, so that

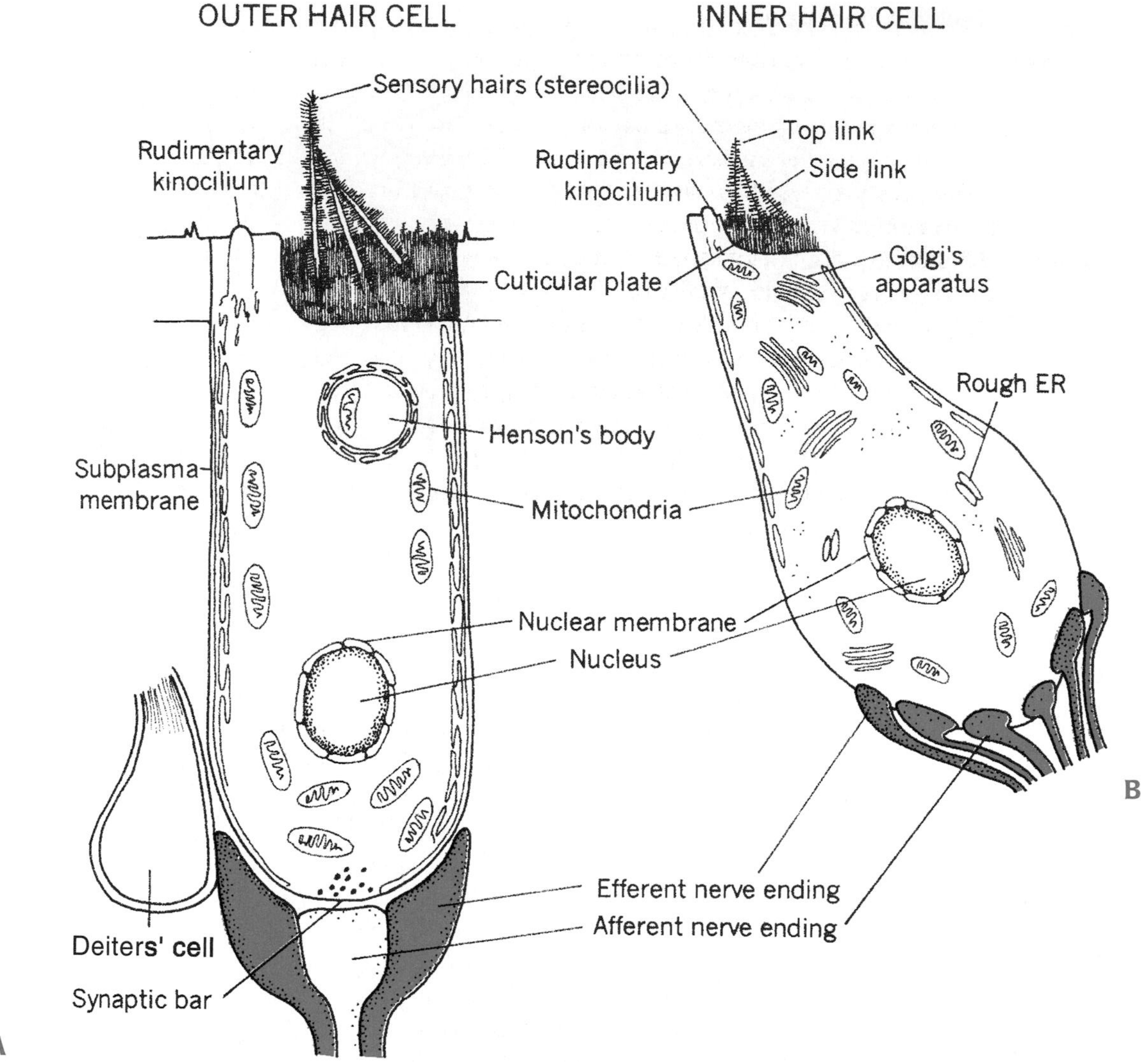

OUTER HAIR CELL   INNER HAIR CELL

Figure 10-10. Details of hair cells. **A.** Outer hair cell. **B.** Inner hair cell. Note presence of both afferent and efferent fibers innervating both types of sensory cells. (Adapted from D. J. Lim, 1986, Effects of noise and ototoxic drugs at the cellular level in the cochlea.)

the longer cilia are distal to the modiolar side. The cilia of a hair cell are all connected by thin, filamentous links. Shorter cilia are connected to the taller cilia by "tip links," and cilia are also linked laterally, thus ensuring that movement of one cilia involves disturbance of adjacent cilia on a hair cell. Stereocilia found in the apex are longer than those found in the base.

The morphology of the hair cells differs markedly. The inner hair cells are teardrop or gourd shaped, with a broad base and narrowed neck. The outer hair cells, in contrast, are shaped like a test tube. Inner hair cells are embedded in a matrix of inner phalangeal cells for support, while outer hair cells are nested in outer phalangeal cells of Deiters. Phalangeal processes apparently replace hair cells lost through acoustic trauma, thereby maintaining the delicate cuticular plate.

Innervation Pattern of the Organ of Corti

The hair cells of the cochlea receive both afferent and efferent innervation, as discussed in Chapter 13. The pattern of innervation is strikingly different between outer and inner hair cells.

Afferent Innervation.   As shown in Figure 10-11 each inner hair cell is connected to as many as 10 VIII nerve fibers, referred to as "many-to-one" innervation. In contrast, each outer hair cell shares its innervation with 10 other outer hair cells, all being innervated by the same VIII nerve fiber ("one-to-many" innervation).

VIII nerve fibers consist of Type I fibers (large, myelinated fibers) and Type II fibers (small, both myelinated and unmyelinated fibers). Type I fibers, making up 95% of the VIII nerve, apparently innervate the inner hair cells, whereas the unmyelinated Type II fibers innervate the outer hair cells. Type I fibers innervating hair cells course medially through the habenula perforata, after which point myelin will be found on the fiber. Most of the Type II outer hair cell fibers course medially to the habenula perforata as the inner radial bundle. A small portion of Type II fibers course within the tunnel of Corti apically to join with the outer spiral bundle. The outer spiral bundle fibers innervating the outer hair cells contain both afferent and efferent fibers, to be discussed.

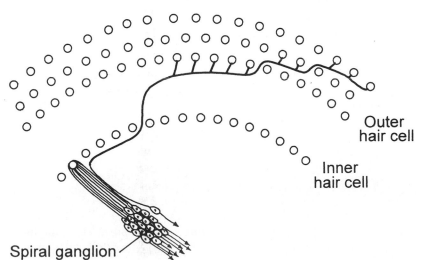

Figure 10-11. Innervation scheme of organ of Corti. Note that many nerve fibers innervate each inner hair cell, while many outer hair cells are innervated by one nerve fiber. (Adapted from The Afferent Innervation of the Cochlea, by H. Spoendlin, 1978, p. 28.

Efferent innervation. As discussed in Chapter 12, the efferent innervation of the outer hair cell is inhibitory, reducing the afferent activity caused by hair cell stimulation. The **olivocochlear bundle** is comprised of about 1,600 fibers, consisting of the **crossed olivocochlear bundle** (**COCB**) and the **uncrossed olivocochlear bundle** (**UCOB**). The COCB arises from a region near the medial superior olive of the olivary complex, descends to the fourth ventricle where the majority of the fibers decussate, and proceed to innervate the outer hair cells. The UCOB originates near the **lateral superior olive** of the olivary complex and courses primarily ipsilaterally to the inner hair cells of the cochlea. Activation of the olivocochlear bundle appears to be controllable through cortical activity, and assists in detection of a signal within a background of noise.

In summary:

- The **membranous labyrinth** can be thought of as a fluid-filled sac that rests within the cavity of the osseous labyrinth and is filled with **endolymph**.
- In the vestibular system, the membranous labyrinth houses the vestibular organ.
- The **ampulla** is the expanded region of the semicircular canals containing the **crista ampularis**. Within the vestibule lie the **utricle** and **saccule**.
- The membranous labyrinth of the cochlea resides between the scala vestibuli and tympani, making up the intermediate **scala media**.
- **Reissner's membrane** forms the upper boundary of the scala media, and the basilar membrane forms the floor.
- The **organ of Corti** has four rows of hair cells resting on a bed of Deiters' cells for support.
- The **outer hair cells** are separated from the **inner hair cell** row by the **tunnel of Corti**.
- The upper surface of each hair cell is graced with a series of **stereocilia**.
- Each inner hair cell is connected with as many as 10 VIII nerve fibers, and each outer hair cell shares its innervation with 10 other outer hair cells, all being innervated by the same VIII nerve fiber.

◤ CHAPTER SUMMARY

The **outer ear** is composed of the **pinna** and the **external auditory meatus**. Landmarks of the pinna include the margin of the **auricle**, the **helix**, and the **auricular tubercle** on the helix. The external auditory meatus has both osseous and cartilaginous parts: The cartilaginous portion makes up one-third of the ear canal, while the other two-thirds are housed in bone. At the terminus of the external auditory meatus is the **tympanic membrane**, the structure separating the outer and middle ears.

The **middle ear cavity** houses the middle ear **ossicles**. The **malleus** is the largest of the ossicles, providing the point of attachment with the tympanic membrane. The **incus** provides the intermediate communicating link of the ossicular chain, and the **stapes** is the third bone of this chain. The ossicular chain is held in place by a series of important **ligaments**. The **stapedius muscle** inserts into the posterior neck of the stapes and pulls the stapes posteriorly; the **tensor tympani** muscle inserts into the upper manubrium malli, pulling the malleus anteromedially. Landmarks of the medial wall of the middle ear cavity include the **oval window**, the **round window**, the **promontory** of the cochlea, and the **prominence of the facial nerve**. The anterior wall houses the entrance to the **Eustachian tube**, and the posterior wall houses the **prominence of the stapedial pyramid**.

The **inner ear** houses the sense mechanism for balance (the **vestibular system**) and hearing (the **cochlea**). The entryway to these structures is termed the **vestibule**. The **osseous labyrinth** is made up of the entryway to the labyrinth, the **vestibule**, the **semicircular canals**, and the **osseous cochlear canal**. It has the appearance of a coiled snail shell, and is divided into two incomplete chambers, the **scala vestibuli** and the **scala tympani**, by the **osseous spiral lamina**, an incomplete bony shelf protruding from the **modiolus**. The **round window** provides communication between the **scala tympani** and the middle ear. The **oval window** permits communication between the scala vestibuli and the middle ear space. The **cochlear aqueduct** connects the upper duct and the subarachnoid space.

The **membranous labyrinth** can be thought of as a fluid-filled sac that rests within the cavity of the osseous labyrinth and is filled with **endolymph**. In the vestibular system, the membranous labyrinth houses the vestibular organ. The **ampulla** is the expanded region of the semicircular canals containing the **crista ampularis**. Within the vestibule lie the **utricle** and **saccule**. The membranous labyrinth of the cochlea resides between the scala vestibuli and the scala tympani, making up the intermediate **scala media**. **Reissner's membrane** forms the distal boundary of the scala media, and the basilar membrane forms the proximal boundary. The **organ of Corti** has four rows of hair cells resting on a bed of Deiters' cells for support. The **outer hair cells** are separated from the row of **inner hair cells** by the **tunnel of Corti**. The upper surface of each hair cell is graced with a series of **stereocilia**. Each inner hair cell innervates as many as 10 VIII nerve fibers, while each outer hair cell shares its innervation with 10 other outer hair cells, all being innervated by the same VIII nerve fiber.

◤ STUDY QUESTIONS

1. The ear is a _____, in that it converts acoustical energy into an electrochemical energy.

2. The _____ serves the function of sound collector.

3. The _____ meatus is a conduit for sound reaching the tympanic membrane.

4. The _____ meatus is a conduit for the VIII nerve fibers coursing to the brainstem.

5. The tympanic membrane (or eardrum) is made up of _____ layers of tissue.

6. The outer layer of the tympanic membrane is continuous with the _____.

7. The _____ layer of the tympanic membrane is made up primarily of radiating fibers.

8. The _____ is a landmark produced by the most distal part of the manubrium malli.

9. The _____ is the bone of the middle ear directly attached to the tympanic membrane.

10. The _____ is the bone of the middle ear directly communicating with the oval window.

11. The _____ of the malleus attaches to the tympanic membrane.

12. The _____ of the stapes articulates with the oval window.

13. The _____ muscle pulls the stapes posteriorly.

14. The _____ muscle pulls the malleus antero-medially.

15. The entryway to the cochlea and vestibular system is via the space known as the _____.

16. The _____ is the system of cavities within bone that houses the membranous labyrinth.

17. The scala _____ and scala _____ are incomplete spaces within the osseous labyrinth.

18. The _____ window provides communication between the scala tympani and the middle ear.

19. The _____ window permits communication between the scala vestibuli and the middle ear space.

20. The _____ is a fluid-filled sac attached to the walls of the osseous labyrinth, and is filled with endolymph.

21. _____ membrane separates the scala vestibuli and the scala media; the membrane separates the scala media from the scala tympani.

22. There is/are _____ row(s) of outer hair cells and _____ row(s) of inner hair cells.

23. The _____ separates the outer and inner hair cells.

24. The hair cells are innervated by the _____ nerve.

24. Microsurgery procedures have advanced rapidly in recent years, permitting rearticulation of ossicles that have become disarticulated. Considering how well protected the ossicles are, what could cause them to become disarticulated?

STUDY QUESTION ANSWERS

1. The ear is a TRANSDUCER , in that it converts acoustical energy into an electrochemical energy.

2. The OUTER EAR serves the function of sound collector.

3. The EXTERNAL AUDITORY meatus is a conduit for sound reaching the tympanic membrane.

4. The INTERNAL AUDITORY meatus is a conduit for the VIII nerve fibers coursing to the brainstem.

5. The tympanic membrane (or eardrum) is made up of THREE layers of tissue.

6. The outer layer of the tympanic membrane is continuous with the EPITHELIUM OF THE EXTERNAL AUDITORY MEATUS .

7. The INTERMEDIATE layer of the tympanic membrane is made up primarily of radiating fibers.

8. The UMBO is a landmark produced by the most distal part of the manubrium malli.

9. The MALLEUS is the bone of the middle ear directly attached to the tympanic membrane.

10. The STAPES is the bone of the middle ear directly communicating with the oval window.

11. The MANUBRIUM of the malleus attaches to the tympanic membrane.

12. The FOOTPLATE of the stapes articulates with the oval window.

13. The STAPEDIUS muscle pulls the stapes posteriorly.

14. The TENSOR TYMPANI muscle pulls the malleus antero-medially.

15. The entryway to the cochlea and vestibular system is via the space known as the VESTIBULE .

16. The OSSEOUS LABYRINTH is the system of cavities within bone that houses the membranous labyrinth.

17. The scala VESTIBULI and scala TYMPANI are incomplete spaces within the osseous labyrinth.

18. The ROUND window provides communication between the scala tympani and the middle ear.

19. The OVAL window permits communication between the scala vestibuli and the middle ear space.

20. The MEMBRANOUS LABYRINTH is a fluid-filled sac attached to the walls of the osseous labyrinth, and is filled with endolymph.

21. REISSNER'S membrane separates the scala vestibuli and the scala media; the BASILAR membrane separates the scala media from the scala tympani.

22. There is/are THREE rows of outer hair cells and ONE row of inner hair cells.

23. The TUNNEL OF CORTI separates the outer and inner hair cells.

24. The hair cells are innervated by the VIII VESTIBULOCOCHLEAR nerve.

25. As with any other body structure, the ossicles are subject to trauma. A frequent cause of disarticulation of the ossicles is head trauma that involves the temporal bone (this may also cause a perilymph fistula, which is a tear in the basilar or Reissner's membrane that allows perilymph and endolymph to mingle). Another cause of disarticulation is noise or high-pressure trauma: The high-pressure forces associated with explosions can easily cause disarticulation.

REFERENCES

Altschuler, R. A., Bobbin, R. P., & Hoffman, D. W. (1986). *Neurology of hearing: The cochlea.* New York: Raven Press.

Anson, B. J., & Donaldson, J. R. (1973). *Surgical anatomy of the temporal bone and ear.* Philadelphia: W. B. Saunders.

Beck, E. W., Monson, H., & Groer, M. (1982). *Mosby's atlas of functional human anatomy.* St. Louis, MO: C. V. Mosby.

Carpenter, M. B. (1991). *Core text of neuroanatomy* (4th ed.). Baltimore: Williams & Wilkins.

Cazals, Y., Demany, L., & Horner, K. (1991). *Auditory physiology and perception.* Oxford: Pergamon Press.

Chusid, J. G. (1985). *Correlative neuroanatomy and functional neurology* (17th ed.). Los Altos, CA: Lange Medical Publications.

Cianfrone, G., & Grandori, F. (1985). Cochlear mechanics and otoacoustic emissions. *Scandinavian Audiology* (suppl. 25).

Dallos, P. (1973). *The auditory periphery.* New York: Academic Press.

Duifhuis, H., Horst, J. W., van Dijk, P., & van Netten, S. M. (1993). *Biophysics of hair cell sensory systems.* Singapore: World Scientific.

Durrant, J. D., & Lovrinic, J. H. (1995). *Bases of hearing science* (3rd ed.). Baltimore: Williams & Wilkins.

Engstrom, H., Ades, H. W., & Andersson, A. (1966). *Structural pattern of the organ of corti.* Baltimore: Williams & Wilkins.

Gardner, E., Gray, D. J., & O'Rahilly, R. (1986). *Anatomy: A regional study of human structure* (5th ed.). Philadelphia: W. B. Saunders.

Gelfand, S. A. (2001). *Hearing.* New York: Thiene Medical Publishers.

Gray, H., Bannister, L. H., Berry, M. M., & Williams, P. L. (Eds.). (1995). *Gray's anatomy.* London: Churchill Livingstone.

Green, D. (1976). *An introduction to hearing.* Hillsdale, NJ: Lawrence Erlbaum Associates.

Gulick, W. L. (1971). *Hearing physiology and psychophysics.* New York: Oxford University Press.

Henson, O. W. (1974). Comparative anatomy of the middle ear. In H. Autrum, R. Jung, W. R. Loewenstein, D. M. MacKay, & H. L. Teuber (Eds.), *Handbook of sensory physiology* (pp. 40–110). New York: Springer-Verlag.

Kandel, E. R., Schwartz, J. H., & Jessell, T. M. (2000). *Principles of neural science* (4th ed.). New York: McGraw Hill.

Kiang, N. Y-S. (1965). *Discharge patterns of single fibers in the cat's auditory nerve.* Cambridge, MA: The M.I.T. Press.

Kuehn, D. P., Lemme, M. L., & Baumgartner, J. M. (1991). *Neural bases of speech, hearing, and language.* Boston: Little, Brown.

Lewis, E. R., Leverenz, E. L., & Bialek, W. S. (1985). *The vertebrate inner ear.* Boca Raton, FL: CRC Press.

Lim, D. J. (1980). Cochlear anatomy related to cochlear micromechanics: A review. *Journal of the Acoustical Society of America, 67*(5), 1686–1695.

Lim, D. J. (1986). Effects of noise and ototoxic drugs at the cellular level in the cochlea. *American Journal of Otolaryngology, 7,* 73–99.

Martin, F. N. (1981). *Medical audiology.* Englewood Cliffs, NJ: Prentice-Hall.

Minifie, F. D., Hixon, T. J., & Williams, F. (Eds.). (1992). *Normal aspects of speech, hearing, and language.* Englewood Cliffs, NJ: Prentice-Hall.

Møller, A. R. (1973). *Basic mechanisms of hearing.* New York: Academic Press.

Møller, A. R. (1983). *Auditory physiology.* New York: Academic Press.

Møller, A. R. (2003). *Sensory systems: Anatomy and physiology.* New York: Academic Press.

Netter, F. H. (1997). *Atlas of human anatomy.* Los Angeles: Icon Learning Systems.

Parkins, C. W., & Anderson, S. W. (1983). Cochlear prostheses. *Annals of the New York Academy of Sciences, 405.*

Pickles, J. O. (1988). *An introduction to the physiology of hearing* (2nd ed.). London: Academic Press.

Rohen, J. W., Yokochi, C., Lutjen-Drecoll, E., & Romrell, L. J. (2002). *Color atlas of anatomy* (5th ed.). Philadelphia: Williams & Wilkins.

Rosse, C., & Gaddum-Rosse, P. (1997). *Hollinshead's textbook of anatomy* (5th ed.). Philadelphia: Lippincott-Raven.

Rossing, T. D. (1990). *The science of sound.* Reading, MA: Addison-Wesley.

Spoendlin, H. (1978). The afferent innervation of the cochlea. In R. F. Naunton & C. Fernandez (Eds.), *Evoked electrical activity in the auditory nervous system.* New York: Academic Press.

Syka, J., & Masterton, R. B. (1988). *Auditory pathway structure and function.* New York: Plenum Press.

Tobias, J. V., & Schubert, E. D. (1983). *Hearing research and theory* (Vol. 2). New York: Academic Press.

von Békésy, G. (1960). *Experiments in hearing.* New York: McGraw-Hill.

Williams, P. L., Bannister, L. H., Berry, M. M., Collins, P., Dyson, M., Dussek, J. E., & Ferguson, M. W. J. (1995). *Gray's anatomy* (38th ed.). New York: Churchill Livingstone.

Wilson, J. P., & Kemp, D. T. (1989). *Cochlear mechanisms: Structure, function, and models.* New York: Plenum Press.

Yost, W. A. (2000). *Fundamentals of hearing: An introduction* (4th ed.). New York: Academic Press.

Zemlin, W. R. (1998). *Speech and hearing science: Anatomy and physiology* (4th ed.). Needham Heights, MA: Allyn & Bacon.

CHAPTER 11
Auditory Physiology

The auditory mechanism is responsible for processing the acoustic signal of speech. Auditory stimuli can arrive at the tympanic membrane with an amazingly wide range of sound pressures, from the whisper of a leaf blowing in the breeze to the pressures associated with painfully loud sound. Likewise, the human auditory mechanism has a frequency range of approximately 10 octaves, spanning 20 to 20,000 Hz. Within these broad requirements are much finer tasks, including differentiating small increments in frequency and intensity. Even beyond these tasks are the everyday requirements of listening to a signal embedded in a background of noise and listening to extremely rapid sequences of sounds. The beauty of the auditory system is that it performs all of these tasks and more with breathtaking ease. This chapter cannot provide a thorough examination of all aspects of auditory physiology, but we hope it will show you why audiologists are so excited by their field.

The field of audiology owes a great deal to the extraordinary scientist Georg von Békésy, whose work resulted in a Nobel Prize. Von Békésy (1960) performed exceedingly intricate measurements on the auditory mechanism, and was at times forced to create tools where none existed. We will refer frequently to his work, which defined the basic function of the middle and inner ears, as we discuss the basic physiological principles involved in transmission of an acoustic stimulus to a form that is

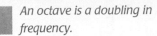

An octave is a doubling in frequency.

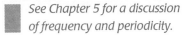

See Chapter 5 for a discussion of frequency and periodicity.

465

interpretable by the brain. The organizing principle to keep in mind is this: The outer ear collects sound and "shapes" its frequency components somewhat; the middle ear matches the airborne acoustic signal with the fluid medium of the cochlea; the inner ear performs temporal and spectral analysis on the ongoing acoustical signal; the auditory pathway conveys and further processes that signal. The cerebral cortex interprets the signal.

OUTER EAR

The outer ear can be seen primarily as a collector of sound. The pinna, with its ridges, grooves, and dished-out regions, is an excellent funnel for information directed toward the head from the front or side, although less effective for sound arising from behind the head.

Indeed, the crevices and crannies of the pinna are functional. If you have blown across the lip of a soda bottle and produced a tone, you know that cavities have characteristics that make them particularly responsive to specific frequencies. When a tube or bottle is **excited** by an input stimulus, it will tend to select energy at its resonant frequency, while tending to reject energy at frequencies other than the resonant frequency. The result is **selective enhancement** of certain frequencies (see Figure 11-1).

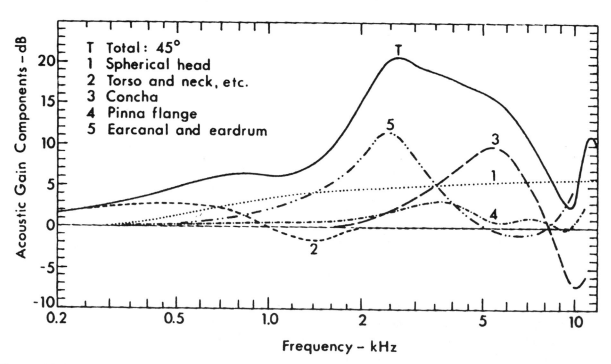

Figure 11-1. Effect of various landmarks of the outer ear upon the input acoustic signal. (Reprinted by permission from "The External Ear," by E. A. G. Shaw, 1974, p. 95. In W. D. Keidel & W. E. Neff [Eds.] *Handbook of sensory physiology.*)

Because the outer ear has no active (moveable) elements, it can have only a passive effect on the input stimulus. The pinna acts as a "sound funnel," focusing acoustic energy into the external auditory meatus, and the external auditory meatus funnels sound to the tympanic membrane. Both of these structures, however, have shapes that boost the relative strength of the signal through resonance, with the result being relatively enhanced signal intensity between 1,500 Hz and 8,000 Hz.

As can be seen in Figure 11-1, the components of the pinna contribute a relatively small amount to the overall gain as compared with that of the external auditory meatus. Nonetheless, the contribution of the entire system results in a net gain reaching 20 dB at approximately 2,000 Hz.

MIDDLE EAR FUNCTION

As you remember, the primary structures of the middle ear are the tympanic membrane, the ossicles, and the entry to the cochlea, the oval window. These are the players in one of the most important evolutionary dramas of the auditory mechanism.

If you can recall a dreamy summer day at the swimming pool, you may also remember that it was almost impossible to communicate vocally with someone in that pool *if the person was submerged.* When you tried to yell at your friend from above the water, nearly all of the sound energy of your speech reflected off the surface of the water.

The cochlea is a fluid-filled cavity, and were it not for the presence of the middle ear mechanism, talking to each other would be like trying to talk to someone under water: *The sound energy would reflect off the oval window because of the vast differences in the liquid and gaseous media of perilymph and air.* Somewhere in our evolution a mechanism arose to improve our plight.

The middle ear mechanism is designed to increase the pressure arriving at the cochlea, thereby overcoming the resistance to flow of energy, termed **impedance**. You will recall from Chapter 3 that **pressure = force/area**. That is, to increase pressure, you must either increase the force or decrease the area over which the force is being exerted. The middle ear mechanism uses the latter as the primary means of matching the impedance of the outer and inner ears. That is, the primary function of the middle ear is to match the impedance of two conductive systems, the outer ear and the cochlea.

The first mechanism of impedance matching is achieved through the area function of the tympanic membrane and oval windows. As mentioned earlier, pressure can be increased by decreasing the area over which force is distributed: A lightweight individual in a spike heel can do much more damage to floor tiles than a piano mover in sneakers. The tympanic membrane has an effective area of about 55 mm^2, while the area of the oval window is about 3.2 mm^2, making the tympanic membrane

17 times larger, depending on species size. Sound energy reaching the tympanic membrane is "funneled" to the much smaller area of the oval window, so there is a gain of 17:1, which translates to an increase of about 25 dB.

The second impedance-matching function is achieved by a lever difference. The length of the manubrium is approximately 9 mm, while that of the long process of the stapes is about 7 mm, giving an overall gain of about 1.2. The lever effect arising from this gain is nearly 2 dB.

A third effect arises from the buckling of the tympanic membrane. As it moves in response to sound, the tympanic membrane buckles somewhat, such that the arm of the malleus moves a shorter distance than the surface of the tympanic membrane. This results in a reduction in velocity of the malleus, with a resulting increase of force that provides a 4 to 6 dB increase in effective signal.

Combined, the area, lever, and buckling effects result in a signal gain of about 31 dB, from tympanic membrane to cochlea, depending on the stimulus frequency. Again, were the middle ear removed, a signal entering the external auditory meatus would have to be 31 dB more intense to be heard. This middle ear transformer action is very important to audition, and any process that reduces the effectiveness of this function (such as otitis media, otosclerosis, or glomus tumors) can have a serious impact on conduction of sound to the inner ear.

In summary, the outer and middle ears serve as funneling and impedance-matching devices.

- The **pinna** funnels acoustical information to the **external auditory meatus** and aids in **localization** of sound in space.
- The **resonant frequencies** of the pinna and external auditory meatus are those of important components of the speech signal, between 1,500 and 8,000 Hz.
- Resistance to flow of energy is termed **impedance**.
- The middle ear mechanism is an **impedance-matching device**, increasing the pressure of a signal arriving at the cochlea.
- The **area ratio** between the tympanic membrane and the oval window provides a 25 dB gain.
- The **lever advantage** of the ossicles provides a 2 dB gain.
- The buckling effect provides a 4–6 dB gain.

INNER EAR FUNCTION

Vestibular Mechanism

The semicircular canals are uniquely designed to respond to rotatory movement of the body. By virtue of their orientation, each canal is at right angles to one other canal, so that all movements of the head can be mapped by combinations of outputs of the sensory components, the cristae ampulares. Activation of the sensory element arises from inertia: As your head rotates, the fluid in the semicircular canals tends to remain in the same location. The result of this is that the cilia are stimulated by relative movement of the fluid during rotation. The utricle and saccule sense acceleration of the head during body or head tilting, rather than rotation. Taken together, the vestibular mechanisms provide the major input to the proprioceptive system serving the sense of one's body in space. This information is integrated with joint sense, muscle spindle afferents, and visual input to form the perception of body position.

Auditory Mechanism: Mechanical Events

One simply must be awed by the cochlea. This structure would neatly fit on the eraser of a pencil, and the fluid within it would be but a drop on your table top. The structures are astoundingly small and delicate, and yet this mechanism, given some reasonable care, can serve a lifetime of hearing without appreciable degeneration. Admittedly, the high-impact noise of modern society takes a rapid toll on such a delicate mechanism, but that is another story. Let us examine what is arguably the most amazing sensory system of the human body, the cochlea.

As we mentioned in the introduction to this chapter, the inner ear is responsible for performing spectral and temporal acoustic analyses of the incoming acoustical signal. By **spectral analysis**, we refer to the process of extracting or defining the various frequency components of a given signal. You will recall from our discussion in the End Note of Chapter 6 that frequency and intensity of vibration define the psychological correlates of "pitch" and "loudness." The cochlea is specifically designed to sort out the frequency components of an incoming signal, determine their amplitude, and even identify basic temporal aspects of that signal. This provides the first level of auditory processing of an acoustic signal. Subsequent processing occurs as the signal works its way rapidly along the auditory pathway, ultimately to the brain. To get a notion of how this happens, we need to consider the input to the cochlea.

As you remember, sound is a disturbance in air. The airborne disturbance causes the tympanic membrane to move, and that movement is translated to the oval window. When the tympanic membrane moves inward, the stapes footplate in the oval window also moves in; and when the tympanic membrane moves out, so does the footplate. This movement is a direct analog to the compressions and rarefactions of sound, so that, for the most part, the complexities of sound are directly translated to the cochlear fluid medial to the stapes footplate.

When the stapes compresses the perilymph of the scala vestibuli, Reissner's membrane is distended toward the scala media, and the basilar membrane is distended toward the scala tympani. That is, a compression in the fluid of the scala vestibuli is translated directly to the basilar membrane. You will remember that the frequency of a sound is determined by the number of oscillations or vibrations per second. In this case, it is the number of oscillations of the tympanic membrane-ossicle-footplate combination: A 100 Hz signal results in the footplate moving inward and outward 100 times per second, and that periodic vibration is translated to the basilar membrane, where it initiates a wave action known as the **traveling wave**.

Georg von Békésy discovered that the basilar membrane is particularly well designed to support wave action that directly corresponds to the frequency of vibration of the input sound. Specifically, when high-frequency sounds impinge on the inner ear, they cause vibration of the basilar membrane closer to the vestibule, the basal end of the cochlea. Low-frequency sounds result in a long traveling wave that reaches toward the apex, covering a greater distance along the basilar membrane. In this way, the traveling wave separates out the frequency components of complex sounds, because high-frequency sounds are processed in basal regions, whereas low-frequency sounds are processed nearer the apex. When a sound has both high- and low-frequency components, those components are separated out and processed at their respective portions of the basilar membrane (see Figure 11-2).

If you have experienced an ocean beach, you will be familiar with wave action. Waves roll in from the ocean and swell to a large amplitude as they break on the beach. Although the analogy is not perfect, it may help you to recognize the driving force behind differentiating frequency components: The point of maximum amplitude excursion of the traveling wave on the basilar membrane is the primary point of neural excitation of the hair cells within the organ of Corti. Said another way, the traveling wave moves along the basilar membrane, growing and swelling as it travels, until it reaches a point of maximum growth. The wave very quickly damps down after that point, so there is only one truly *strong* point of disturbance from the traveling wave (see Figure 11-3). In this manner, the low-frequency sound discussed earlier will cause the traveling wave to "break" closer to the apex, and that place of maximum disturbance determines the frequency information that is transmitted to the brain.

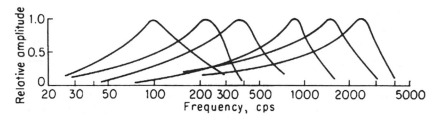

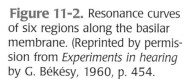

Figure 11-2. Resonance curves of six regions along the basilar membrane. (Reprinted by permission from *Experiments in hearing* by G. Békésy, 1960, p. 454.

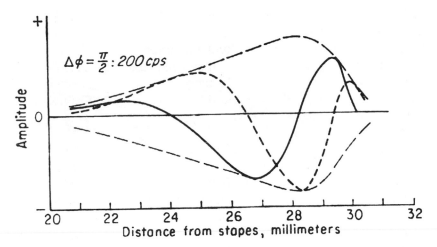

$\Delta\phi = \frac{\pi}{2} : 200\,cps$

Figure 11-3. Vibratory pattern of the basilar membrane at two points within a cycle of vibration. Input stimulation is 200 Hz signal. (Reprinted by permission from *Experiments in hearing* by G. Békésy, 1960, p. 462.

Our understanding of the mechanism that determines *where* the point of maximum amplitude excursion occurs is another of von Békésy's legacies. Von Békésy fashioned instruments from exotic materials such as pig bristles to measure the stiffness of the basilar membrane. As stiffness increases, the natural frequency of vibration of a body increases. See the software auditory physiology lessons to test the effects of stiffness on the traveling wave. Von Békésy's pig bristle experiments revealed that the basal end of the basilar membrane is stiffer than the apical end, and that the stiffness decreases in a graded fashion from base to apex. (In fact, the cochlear duct is flaccid at its most apical end, where it is not connected to the bony labyrinth, to form the helicotrema.) In addition, we know that as mass of a structure increases, its resonant frequency decreases. The basilar membrane becomes increasingly more massive, from base to apex. Finally, the basilar membrane becomes progressively wider from base to apex. These three components—graded stiffness, graded mass, graded width—combine to make the basilar membrane an excellent frequency analyzer. Verification of the importance of these resonance characteristics is provided by the fact that the traveling wave can be stimulated in the absence of the middle ear mechanism (as in bone conduction testing of an individual without middle ear ossicles). No matter how the traveling wave is initiated, it *always* travels from base to apex, because of the impedance gradient of the basilar membrane.

Excitation of the hair cells occurs as the result of several interacting variables. First, the cilia of the outer hair cells are embedded within the tectorial membrane (see Figure 11-4). As the traveling wave moves along the basilar membrane, the hair cells are displaced relative to the tectorial membrane. This produces a **shearing action** that is, of course, greatest at the point of maximum perturbation of the basilar membrane.

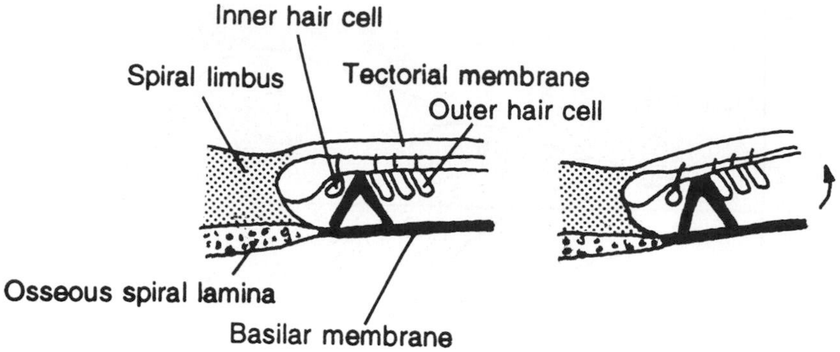

Figure 11-4. Schematic representation of shearing action of basilar membrane-tectorial membrane relationship. (From view and data of Davis, 1958.)

Tonndorf (1958) and later Møller (1973) and Dallos (1973) described another mechanism that helps to explain how the inner hair cells are excited. Recall that the inner hair cells are not embedded in the tectorial membrane, so they are not subjected to the same forces as the outer hair cells. Further, their placement closer to the osseous spiral lamina gives them reduced opportunity to capitilize on shear. Rather, it appears that the inner hair cells depend on fluid movement of the endolymph to excite them. As the traveling wave moves along the basilar membrane, it effectively slides past the fluid molecules. Put another way, the fluid moves relative to the hair cell. The cilia are displaced by the fluid movement, just as grass in a river bed is drawn by the fluid flow. If you invoke the Bernoulli principle studied in Chapter 6, you will see the final stage of excitation. At the point of maximum excursion, the basilar membrane is "humped" up, essentially protruding into the fluid stream. The Bernoulli principle states that at the constriction, velocity of fluid flow will increase. This disturbance at the point of maximum excitation causes a turbulence, which produces eddies or swirls of fluid molecules. In this way, the fluid is more turbulent at the point of maximum excitation, meaning that the hair cells are more likely to be excited at that point than at other, less turbulent locations.

Stimulation of the hair cell presents a paradox, however. A hair cell is stimulated when the cilia are bent in a direction away from the modiolus, but the traveling wave produces a disturbance that is apically directed along the length of the basilar membrane, at right angles to the pattern that excites the hair cell. This dilemma is easy to resolve, however. Remember that the basilar membrane is anchored to the spiral lamina. When the traveling wave perturbs the basilar membrane, the shearing action on the cilia is produced in the medial-proximal dimension because of the hingelike function of the lamina. Because of the nature of the traveling wave, the primary shear at the peak of the traveling wave is radial, as described, whereas the shear apical to the maximum of the wave is longitudinal, a direction that does not stimulate the hair cell (see Figure 11-5).

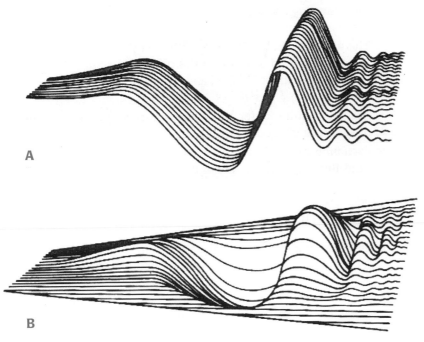

A

B

Figure 11-5. Traveling wave patterns. **A.** Pattern of oscillation in absence of lateral restraints. **B.** Pattern of vibration arising from stimulation, but accounting for lateral attachment of basilar membrane. (Reprinted with permission from "Shearing Motion in Scala Media of Cochlear Models" by J. Tonndorf, 1960, p. 241. *Journal of the Acoustical Society of America*, *32*(5). Copyright 1960, Acoustical Society of America.)

The hingelike arrangement of the basilar membrane and spiral limbus place the outer hair cells in a position to be activated by a lower level stimulus than the inner hair cells. Thus, it appears that, at least for intensities less than 40 dB SPL, the outer hair cells are an important mechanism for coding intensity, although the inner hair cells are essential for frequency coding. Loss of outer hair cells does not result in complete loss of hearing, but rather elevation of the threshold of audition.

In summary, basic cochlear function is awe-inspiring for a number of reasons:

- The inner ear is responsible for performing **spectral** (frequency) and **temporal acoustic analyses** of the incoming acoustical signal.
- Movement of the tympanic membrane is translated into analogous movement of the stapes footplate and the fluid in the scala vestibuli.
- Compression in the fluid of the scala vestibuli is translated directly to the basilar membrane, and the disturbance at the basilar membrane initiates the **traveling wave**.
- The cochlea has a **tonotopic arrangement**, with high-frequency sounds resolved at the base and low-frequency sounds processed at the apex.
- The point of **maximum excursion** of the basilar membrane determines the frequency information transmitted to the brain.

- The traveling wave quickly **damps** after reaching its point of maximum excursion.
- The frequency analysis ability of the basilar membrane is determined by graded **stiffness**, **thickness**, and **width**. The basilar membrane is stiffer, thinner, and narrower at the base than at the apex.
- Excitation of the **outer hair cells** occurs primarily as the result of **shearing effect** on the cilia.
- Excitation of the **inner hair cells** is produced by the effect of **fluid flow** and **turbulence** of endolymph.

Electrical Events

The cochlea is both a spectrum analyzer and a transducer. The mechanical properties of the organ of Corti and its components provide spectral analysis, and the stimulation of hair cells permits the mechanical energy arriving at the cochlea in the form of movement of the stapes footplate to be converted into electrochemical energy. As with any other neural component of the nervous system, the hair cells are designed to transmit information. When the basilar membrane is displaced toward the scala vestibuli, the hair cells are activated, whereas when the basilar membrane is displaced toward the scala tympani, electrical activity of the hair cell is inhibited. Stimulation of the hair cells results in four electrical potentials.

Resting Potentials

The **resting** or **standing potentials** are those voltage potential differences that can be measured from the cochlea at rest. Ions do not travel between the endolymphatic region (scala media) and those of perilymph (scala tympani and scala vestibuli), and there are cochlear potential differences among those spaces. The scala vestibuli is slightly more positive than the scala tympani (about +5 mV), but the scala media is considerably more positive (about +80 mV). That is, the scala media has a constant positive potential (the **endocochlear potential**) relative to the scala tympani and scala vestibuli. There is evidence that the strong positive potential arises from active ion pumping by the stria vascularis (Pickles, 1988), and this notion is supported by evidence that the endocochlear potential is not found in the vestibular system endolymph. Another resting potential, the **intracellular resting potential**, is found within the hair cells. The potential difference between the endolymph and the intercellular potential of the hair cell is −70 mV relative to the endolymph, giving a very large 150 mV difference between the hair cells and the surrounding fluid.

Potentials Arising from Stimulation

Stimulation of the hair cells results in generation of a number of potentials, although not all of them are thought to be important in auditory processing. The **cochlear microphonic** was once thought to be the "prime mover" of cochlear activity, and for good reason. Wever and Bray (1930) found that the cochlear microphonic recorded from a living cat's cochlea directly followed the speech signal (see Figure 11-6). It was felt that the potential was "microphonic" (like a microphone), directly responding to the input signal. They were correct at first blush: The potential *does* directly follow the movement of the basilar membrane, and it appears to be generated by the outer hair cells or current changes at the reticular lamina in the vicinity of the outer hair cells. Although microelectrode recording of inner hair cell intracellular potentials shows an alternating current (AC) potential, the potential is not large enough to account for the microphonic. In any case, the cochlear microphonic is an AC potential that follows the movement of the input signal as it impinges upon the basilar membrane.

The **summating potential** is a sustained, direct current (DC) shift in the endocochlear potential that occurs upon stimulation of the organ of Corti by sound (see Figure 11-6). The inner hair cells are depolarized when stimulated by sound, and that results in reduced intracellular potential (a less negative potential). This potential difference between the hair cell and the endolymph may produce the summating potential. It is seen as a DC shift in electrical output that is maintained as long as an auditory stimulus is presented to the ear.

The **whole-nerve action potential** (also known as the **compound action potential**), abbreviated AP, arises directly from stimulation of a large number of hair cells simultaneously, eliciting nearly simultaneous individual action potentials in the VIII nerve, as discussed in Chapter 10.

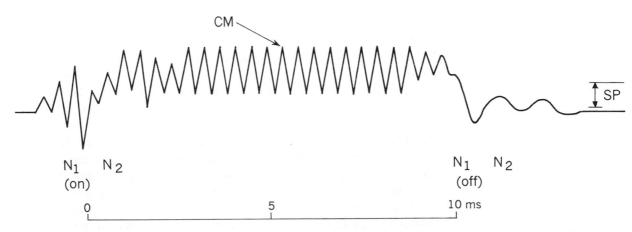

Figure 11-6. Response to tone burst, as measured from the scala tympani. (Modified from Pickles, 1988.)

Measured extracochlearly, the whole-nerve action potential represents the sum of action potentials generated by stimulation of the hair cells. It is best elicited using clicks with broad spectral content rather than tones, although tones certainly can be used. The AP has two major negative components, N_1 and N_2, and amplitude of the AP increases as sound stimulus intensity increases. The individual action potential arising from stimulation of an individual VIII nerve fiber tells a very important story at the microscopic level. Looking at single-unit (single VIII nerve fiber) responses reveals that the cochlear mechanism has an extraordinarily fine ability to differentiate frequency components (frequency specificity), and by processing data from large number of individual fibers we can learn a great deal about coding of simple and complex stimuli by the auditory nervous system.

In summary, when the basilar membrane is displaced toward the scala vestibuli, the hair cells are activated, resulting in **electrical potentials.**

- **Resting** or **standing potentials** are those voltage potential differences that can be measured from the cochlea at rest.
- The scala vestibuli is 5 mV more positive than the scala tympani, but the scala media is 80 mV more positive.
- The **intracellular resting potential** within the hair cell reveals a potential difference between the endolymph and the hair cell of –70 mV, giving a 150 mV difference between the hair cells and the surrounding fluid.
- Stimulus-related potentials include the alternating current **cochlear microphonic** generated by the outer hair cells; the **summating potential**, a direct current shift in the endocochlear potential; and the **whole-nerve action potential**, arising directly from stimulation of a large number of hair cells simultaneously.

Neural Responses

There are two basic types of VIII nerve neurons: **low spontaneous rate** (high-threshold) and **high spontaneous rate** (low-threshold) fibers. High-threshold neurons require a higher level of stimulation to fire, respond to the higher end of our auditory range of signal intensity, and have little or no random background firing noise. Low-threshold fibers, in contrast, respond at very low signal intensities and display random firing even when no stimulus is present. Thus, it appears that the low-threshold neurons may be a mechanism for hearing sound at near-threshold levels, whereas high-threshold fibers may pick up where the low-threshold fibers stop, as the signal increases.

The background "chatter" of random firing poses some problems for examining neuron response, however. The task of neurophysiologists is to identify neuron responses related to a specific stimulus and to separate them from the background noise of random firing. Two basic techniques have evolved to manage that problem, and both have provided important clues to neural function. Let us look at these techniques and the results of their application.

Post-Stimulus Time (PST) Histograms

Histograms are a convenient method of looking at data that occur over time. When you are taking an anatomy exam, you know that the whole class does not finish at the same time. Rather, the first person may finish after 40 minutes, the next one at 43 minutes, then a couple more at 44 minutes, and so on. If you were interested in the *modal* finishing time for an exam, you could plot the elapsed test-taking time for each person in the form of a bar graph (**histogram**) and identify the point at which the greatest number of people got up to leave at the same time. You can also look at the response time of neurons the same way. Auditory physiologists record bursts of electrical activity of single neurons and plot their response. Because they know when the stimulus was presented (just as your instructor knows when the test started), the researcher can plot the responses relative to the onset of the stimulus—hence, post-stimulus histogram.

Because neurons are all-or-none devices, every unit response is equal to the next in intensity and duration. Thus, the only way neurons can provide differential response is in rate of firing. Single-unit neural information is conveyed in the timing of its response. If you were to record the spike-rate activity of a neuron that is firing randomly, in the absence of a stimulus, there would be no real dominant mode of activity; rather, the neural response would spread fairly evenly over the entire recording period. If you were to record that activity in response to a tonal stimulus, you would get a response more like that of Figure 11-7. When an VIII nerve fiber responds to tonal stimulation, there is an initial burst of strong activity, followed by a decline to a plateau of discharge over the duration of the tone. When the tone is terminated, the response of the

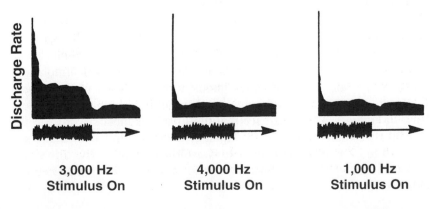

Figure 11-7. Schematic representation of post-stimulus time histogram for 3,000 Hz, 4,000 Hz, and 1,000 Hz tones, as recorded from a nerve fiber with a characteristic frequency of 3,000 Hz.

fiber drops to below baseline levels, rising up to the baseline "noise" level after recovery.

This fairly straightforward post-stimulus time histogram has provided us with very important verification of the **frequency specificity**, the ability of the cochlea to differentiate different spectral components of a signal. Figure 11-7 displays a hypothetical array of spike rate PST histograms generated for the same neuron under different stimulus conditions. In this case, we have placed an electrode on a fiber serving the area of the cochlea in which 3,000 Hz signals are processed. Look at the responses. When we deliver a 3,000 Hz signal, the fiber has a strong response shortly after onset, with the characteristic plateau until the tone ends. Now see what happens when we present a 4,000 Hz signal. The response is *much* weaker to that stimulation, as it is to that of the 1,000 Hz signal. As you know from the traveling wave theory, signals above 3,000 Hz will not cause much disturbance on the basilar membrane at the 3,000 Hz point. Likewise, the traveling wave must necessarily pass through the region of our electrode on its way to the 1,000 Hz point (toward the apex, or low-frequency region), but the traveling wave has not gained much amplitude at that point so there is not much excitation. In other words, if we record the firing rate of a neuron, we can get a fair estimate of its **characteristic** or **best frequency**. The characteristic frequency (CF) of a neuron is the frequency to which it responds best. In the case shown in Figure 11-7, the CF of the neuron we were recording was 3,000 Hz.

One goal of auditory physiology is to explain humans' extraordinary ability to discriminate signals in the frequency domain. Researchers who study auditory perceptual abilities as they relate to the physical mechanism (**psychoacousticians**) have found that, in general, humans can discriminate change in frequency of signals of about 2%. (Recognize that this gross generalization ignores differences in signal intensity, variations based on different stimulus frequency, signal duration, etc.) That is, if a 100 Hz tone is presented, you can hear the difference between it and a 102 Hz tone, an increase of 2%. The challenge to physiologists was to identify how the cochlea could produce such fine discriminations.

Figure 11-8 shows a "tuning curve" for a single-unit recording. A tuning curve is basically a composite of the responses of a single fiber at each frequency of presentation. For instance, researchers placed an electrode on a neuron and presented different frequencies of stimulation. They then recorded the stimulus intensity at which the neuron began to fire in response to the stimulus (its threshold) and plotted that intensity. In Figure 11-8, you can see that the fiber was most sensitive to the 10,000 Hz signal. As the signal frequency decreased to 8,000 Hz the signal had to be of greater intensity to cause the neuron to fire. The signal at 5,000 Hz had to be 60 dB stronger than that at the CF for that neuron, 10,000 Hz.

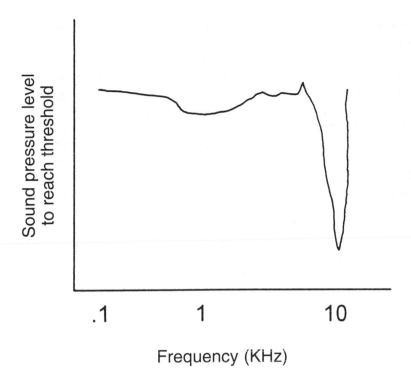

Figure 11-8. Schematic representation of tuning curve for VIII nerve fiber with characteristic frequency of 10,000 Hz.

Frequency (KHz)

.1   1   10

Sound pressure level to reach threshold

This tuning curve is a measure of neural specificity in one sense, but probably as much a measure of basilar membrane response. The electrode is, in effect, measuring the activity at one point on the basilar membrane (10,000 Hz, near the base) and activity farther up the cochlea toward the apex has less and less effect on the neuron we are recording. *The sharper the tuning curve, the greater the frequency specificity of the basilar membrane.* Indeed, when Khanna and Leonard (1982) compared the tuning curves of the basilar membrane and the auditory nerve, they found that the two curves were quite similar. That is, the basilar membrane is a very finely tuned filter capable of fine differentiation.

What happens when the stimulation to the cochlea is more complex than a simple sinusoid? For instance, if a tone complex including 500 Hz, 1,000 Hz, 1,500 Hz, and 2,000 Hz were presented to the ear, how would the cochlea and VIII nerve respond? Essentially, the nerve fibers with characteristic frequencies of the stimulus components (i.e., 500 Hz, 1,000 Hz, etc.) will respond, whereas those fibers at other frequencies (i.e., 510 Hz, 511 Hz, 512 Hz, etc.) without direct stimulation will take much more stimulation to fire. You will notice that we judiciously avoided 505 Hz in our list of off-stimulus CF, because that difference is probably not discriminable. That is, the cochlea generally cannot differentiate a difference smaller than that, so the fibers at 502 Hz would respond the same as those at 500 Hz. To the brain, those two frequencies are indiscriminable.

The PST histogram provides excellent support for the **Place Theory of Hearing**, stating that frequency resolution of the cochlea occurs as a result of place of stimulation by the traveling wave. The tonotopic array of the cochlea is clearly relayed to the auditory nervous system in the form of individual nerve fiber activation.

Firing rate is also used to encode **intensity of the stimulation** (see Figure 11-9). As the intensity of stimulation increases, rate of firing increases, up to a point. Because neurons are limited by the refractory period, they typically cannot fire more than once per millisecond. The dynamic range for intensity that can be encoded in rate of firing is on the order of 30 to 40 dB, far too low for encoding of intensity. We are capable of differentiating a much greater range of intensities than this. Recall that different neurons have different thresholds of response (low- and high-threshold neurons). Apparently intensity is coded by using both types of neurons: Low-threshold neurons can process low-intensity signals, while high-threshold neurons carry the load of higher intensity sound. Taken together, they account for the dynamic range of hearing for intensity. Evidence from Kiang, Liberman, Sewell, and Guinan (1986) reveals that outer hair cells (OHCs) augment the function of the inner hair cells in frequency discrimination, as evidenced by a marked loss of tuning curve sharpness when the OHCs are traumatized.

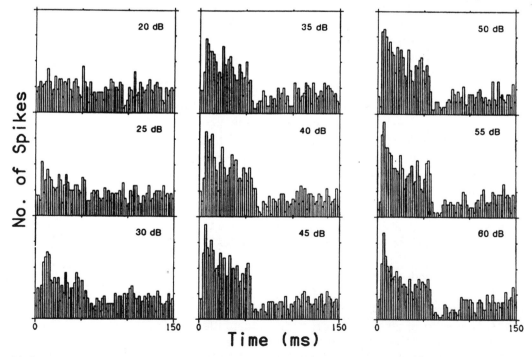

Figure 11-9. Effect of signal intensity upon firing rate. (Reprinted by permission of Lippincott-Raven from "Basic Response Properties of Auditory Nerve Fibers" by E. Javel, 1986, p. 216. In R. A. Altschuler, R. P. Bobbin, & D. W. Hoffman [Eds.]. *Neurobiology of hearing: The cochlea.* New York: Raven Press.)

The efferent system of the auditory mechanism has the effect of reducing neural response. When the crossed-olivocochlear and uncrossed-olivocochlear bundles are stimulated, the firing rate of neurons innervated by them is reduced dramatically. This has the effect of reducing response to unwanted information, perhaps permitting the nervous system to "focus" on a desired signal while damping the response to noise. The efferent system also appears to have a role in frequency discrimination.

Interspike Interval (ISI) and Period Histograms

Although rate histograms reveal a great deal about how the cochlea and VIII nerve respond to sound, **interspike interval (ISI) histograms** provide details of the temporal structure of the VIII nerve response. With ISI histograms, the interval between successive firings of a neuron is measured and recorded. Figures 11-10 and 11-11 show "phase-locking" of a neuron to stimulation. The stimulus is a 812 Hz tone, and the period of vibration associated with a 812 Hz tone is approximately 1.2 ms. If you

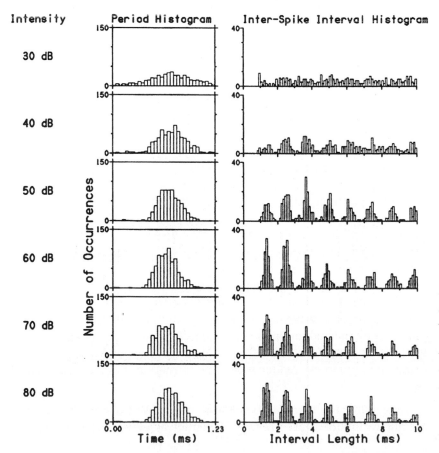

Figure 11-10. Period and interstimulus histograms presented at 10 dB steps. Characteristic frequency of the fiber was 812 Hz. (Reprinted by permission of Lippincott-Raven from "Basic Response Properties of Auditory Nerve Fibers" by E. Javel, 1986, p. 218. In R. A. Altschuler, R. P. Bobbin, & D. W. Hoffman [Eds.]. *Neurobiology of hearing: The cochlea.* New York: Raven Press.)

Response from single neuron

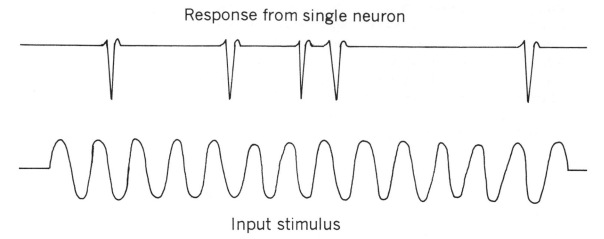

Input stimulus

Figure 11-11. Relationship between neuron response (lower trace) and signal phase (upper trace). (Modified from Yost, 2000.)

look closely at the response, you will recognize that the interval between the spikes of the histogram is 1.2 ms, the period of the tone. **Phase-locking** refers to the quality of a neuron wherein it responds to the period of the stimulus, in this case 1.2 ms. Because a neuron requires 1 ms to recover from depolarization, we should not expect to see phase-locking to signals above 1,000 Hz (Period = 1 ms), but we do see it. Phase-locking is seen in signals up to 5,000 Hz, although this does not mean that the basic physiology of neural excitation should be redefined. The VIII nerve fiber responds to the phase of the signal, but not necessarily to *every* cycle of vibration. As you can see in Figure 11-11, a fiber will respond when it is capable of responding, and it will respond at whole-number multiples of the period of excitation.

One can reorganize the interval histogram data by examining a period histogram. A **period histogram** displays the point in the cycle of vibration at which firing occurs (Figure 11-10). In this manner, the degree of phase-locking is represented in the major peak of the figure. As the signal increases, the histogram becomes more peaked, representing a greater degree of phase-locking.

It is clear from the interval and period histograms that temporal information of the waveform is preserved and potentially transmitted to the brain by the auditory nervous system. It appears that both place and temporal information are used in the coding of acoustical information, extracting important redundancy of information from the acoustical signal.

In summary, there are two basic types of VIII nerve neurons, and specific techniques have been developed for assessing their function.

- **High-threshold neurons** require a higher intensity and encompass the higher end of our auditory range of signal intensity.
- **Low-threshold fibers** respond at very low signal levels and display random firing even when no stimulus is present.
- Low-threshold neurons may process near-threshold sounds, whereas high-threshold fibers process higher level sounds.
- **Frequency specificity** is the ability of the cochlea to differentiate the spectral components of a signal.
- **Post-stimulus time histograms** are plots of neural response relative to the onset of a stimulus.
- The **characteristic** or **best frequency** of a neuron is the frequency to which it responds best.
- A **tuning curve** is a composite of the responses of a single fiber at each frequency of presentation.
- The sharper the tuning curve, the greater the frequency specificity of the basilar membrane.
- The **tonotopic array** of the cochlea is clearly relayed to the auditory nervous system in the form of individual nerve fiber activation.
- As the intensity of stimulation increases, **rate of firing** increases.
- When the **crossed-olivocochlear** and **uncrossed-olivocochlear bundles** are stimulated, the firing rate of neurons innervated by them is reduced dramatically.
- **Interspike interval histograms** record the interval between successive firings of a neuron, revealing phase-locking of neurons to stimulus period.

Auditory Pathway Responses

The cochlea and VIII nerve represent only the first stage of information extraction of the auditory signal. Temporal and tonotopically arrayed information is passed to progressively higher centers for further extraction of information (see Figure 11-12).

Cochlear Nucleus

At the first way-station in the auditory pathway, the cochlear nucleus (CN), tonotopic representation is readily observable in tuning curves. There is evidence that significant signal processing occurs at this level of the brainstem.

Pfeiffer (1966) demonstrated at least six different neural responses to auditory stimulation, in contrast to the single-unit response seen at the

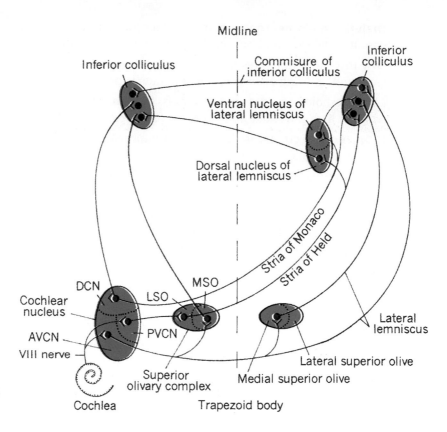

Figure 11-12. Schematic representation of auditory pathway in humans. (After Møller, 2003.)

VIII nerve level (see Figure 11-13). **Primary-like** responses are the firing patterns that most resemble VIII nerve responses. Some neurons exhibit **onset** responses, in which there is an initial response to onset of a stimulus, followed by silence. **Chopper** responses do not seem to be related to stimulus frequency, but appear to respond with a periodic, chopped temporal pattern as long as a tone is present. **Pausers**, found in the dorsal cochlear nucleus, take a little longer to respond than other neurons: If the signal is of higher intensity, the pauser has an initial on-response, is quiet, and then responds with a low-level firing rate throughout stimulation. **Buildup** neurons slowly increase in firing rate through the initial stages of firing.

These complex responses reflect not only different cell types within the cochlear nucleus, but also interactions among neurons. Although these responses may all be seen in different neurons in response to the same tonal stimulus, it would be unwise to assume that they are *simply* responses to stimulation. They are most certainly the result of complex interaction and neural processing.

Superior Olivary Complex

The superior olivary complex (SOC) is the first site of binaural interaction, receiving information from the cochlear nuclei of both ears, and is

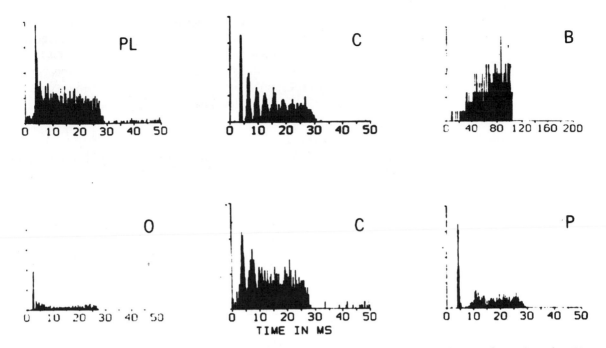

Figure 11-13. Peristimulus time histograms showing response characteristics of cochlear nucleus. Note that PL = Primary Like; O = Onset type; C = Chopper type; B = Buildup type; P = Pauser type. (Reprinted with permission from "The Use of Intracellular Techniques in the Study of the Cochlear Nucleus" by W. S. Rhode, 1985, p. 321. *Journal of the Acoustical Society of America, 78*(1). Copyright 1985 by Acoustical Society of America.)

specialized for localization of sound in space. Two basic responses occur within the SOC. **Contralateral stimulation** (stimulation of the ear opposite the side of the SOC being studied) by high-frequency information results in excitation with the **lateral superior olive** (LSO, or S-segment) that is directly related to stimulus intensity. These so-called **E-E** (excitatory-excitatory) responses provide a means of comparing the intensity of a signal on one side of the head with that on the other side. In the **medial superior olive** (MSO), when low-frequency tones are presented, an **E-I** (excitatory-inhibitory) response occurs, wherein contralateral input excites neurons and **ipsilateral stimulation** causes inhibition of neurons. Said another way, a low-frequency signal arriving at the left ear causes excitation of the right-side MSO, while inhibiting the left-side MSO. In addition, some cells in the MSO respond to a **characteristic delay** in arrival time, so that the MSO detects minute changes in arrival time of a sound between the two ears. This **interaural phase (time) difference** is the primary mechanism for localization of low-frequency sounds in space; the **interaural intensity difference** is the primary means of localization of high-frequency sound in space. The neurons responding to specific characteristics or features of the stimulus are termed **feature detectors**. That is, they respond to specific features of the stimulus (e.g., interaural phase differences), extract that information from the signal, and convey the results of analysis to the cerebral cortex. In this way the complex acoustic signal can be broken into some subset of characteristics. Indeed, the different responses at the cochlear nucleus (e.g., pauser, onset-response, etc.) most likely represent the second level of feature extraction, the first level being at the cochlea.

Inferior Colliculus

The inferior colliculus (IC) receives bilateral innervation from the LSO, as well as indirect input from the cochlear nucleus via the lateral lemniscus. A wide range of responses is apparent at the inferior colliculus, including neurons with sharp frequency tuning curves, inhibitory responses, onset and pauser responses, and intensity-sensitive units. Some neurons are sensitive to interaural time and intensity differences, apparently used in localization function similar to the SOC. It appears that the inferior colliculus may be the site at which frequency information from the cochlear nucleus discarded through localization processing at the SOC can be recombined with phase and intensity information.

Medial Geniculate Body

The medial geniculate body (MGB) is a relay of the thalamus, the final sensory way-station of the brainstem. The ventral portion of the MGB projects directly to the primary auditory reception area of the temporal lobe, the medial portion projects to other regions of the temporal lobe, and the dorsal portion projects information to association regions of the cerebrum. Although a distinct tonotopic arrangement is apparent even at this level, a complex interaction of response types is also apparent. Surprisingly, these include neurons responsive to minute interaural intensity differences, much as the SOC and IC demonstrate.

Cerebral Cortex

The cerebral cortex receives input primarily from the contralateral ear via the ipsilateral MGB. A full tonotopic map is found at the primary reception area of the temporal lobe, Heschl's gyrus. In addition, the auditory reception area is organized in columns, with each column having similar CFs, but different tuning curve widths. Further, different neurons within the columns respond to different stimulus parameters, such as frequency up-glides, down-glides, intensity up- and intensity down-glides, and so on. It is clear that the neurons of the cerebral cortex use the ipsilateral and contralateral temporal and spectral information extracted at earlier processing stages for identification of the features of speech. For example, neurons that are sensitive to frequency up-glides would be very useful in encoding information concerning formant frequency transitions, whereas the vocal fundamental frequency would be readily coded by the temporal information arising from the phase-locking at the cochlear level and presented, intact, to the cortex.

To summarize, the auditory nervous system is a complex processor of sound that defies simplistic description. The audiologist and speech-language pathologist must recognize that this most astounding of the sensory systems provides the raw material for development of speech and language.

Temporal and tonotopically arrayed information is passed to progressively higher centers for further extraction of information.

- At the **cochlear nucleus**, tonotopic representation is readily observable in **tuning curves**.
- **Primary-like** responses are the firing patterns that most resemble VIII nerve responses.
- **Onset** responses are those in which there is an initial response to onset of a stimulus followed by silence.
- **Chopper** responses do not appear related to stimulus frequency, but have a periodic, chopped temporal pattern as long as a tone is present.
- **Pausers** take longer to respond than other neurons, having an initial on-response for strong stimuli.
- **Buildup responses** slowly increase in firing rate through the initial stages of depolarization.
- The superior olivary complex (SOC) is the primary site of **localization** of sound in space.
- **Contralateral stimulation** of the SOC by high-frequency information results in excitation related to stimulus intensity.
- **Low-frequency stimuli** presented binaurally to the SOC result in interaural time difference detection.
- A wide array of responses is seen at the **inferior colliculus** (IC), including inhibitory responses, onset and pauser responses, intensity-sensitive units, interaural time-sensitive and intensity-sensitive neurons.
- The **medial geniculate body** (MGB) is a relay of the thalamus.
- The **cerebral cortex** receives input primarily from the contralateral ear via the ipsilateral MGB.
- A full **tonotopic map** on the cortex may be seen at the primary reception area, Heschl's gyrus.
- The **auditory reception area** is organized in columns, with each column having a similar CF.
- Different neurons within the columns respond to different stimulus parameters, such as frequency up-glides, down-glides, intensity up- and down-glides, and so on.

CHAPTER SUMMARY

The outer and middle ears serve as funneling and impedance-matching devices. The **pinna** funnels acoustical information to the **external auditory meatus** and aids in **localization** of sound in space. Resistance to flow of energy is termed **impedance**. The middle ear mechanism is an **impedance-matching device**, increasing the pressure of a signal arriving at the cochlea. The **area ratio** between the tympanic membrane and the oval window provides a significant gain in output over input, and the **lever advantage** of the ossicles provides a smaller gain. The **buckling** effect grants another 4 to 6 dB gain.

The inner ear is responsible for performing **spectral** (frequency) and **temporal acoustic analyses** of the incoming acoustical signal. Movement of the tympanic membrane is translated into parallel movement of the stapes footplate and the fluid in the scala vestibuli. Movement of the fluid of the scala vestibuli is translated directly to the basilar membrane, and the disturbance at the basilar membrane causes the initiation of the **traveling wave**. The cochlea has a **tonotopic arrangement**, with high-frequency sounds resolved at the base and low-frequency sounds processed toward the apex. The point of **maximum displacement** of the basilar membrane determines the frequency information transmitted to the brain. The traveling wave quickly **damps** after reaching its point of maximum displacement. The frequency analysis ability of the basilar membrane is determined by graded **stiffness**, **thickness**, and **width**. The basilar membrane is stiffer, thinner, and narrower at the base than at the apex. Excitation of the **outer hair cells** occurs primarily as the result of **shearing effect** on the cilia. Excitation of the **inner hair cells** is produced by the effect of **fluid flow** and **turbulence** of endolymph.

When the basilar membrane is displaced upward, the hair cells are activated, resulting in **electrical potentials**. **Resting** or **standing potentials** are those voltage potential differences that can be measured from the cochlea at rest. The scala vestibuli is 5 mV more positive than the scala tympani, but the scala media is 80 mV more positive. The **intracellular resting potential** in the hair cells reveals a negative potential difference between the endolymph and the hair cell of 70 mV, giving a 150 mV difference between the hair cells and the surrounding fluid. Stimulus-related potentials include the alternating current **cochlear microphonic**, generated by the outer hair cells; the **summating potential**, a direct current shift in the endocochlear potential; and the **whole-nerve action potential**, arising directly from stimulation of a large number of hair cells simultaneously.

There are two basic types of VIII nerve neurons, and specific techniques have been developed for assessing their function. **High-threshold** neurons require a higher intensity for response and encompass the higher end of our auditory range of signal intensity. **Low-threshold** fibers respond at very low signal levels and display random firing even when no stimulus is present. Low-threshold neurons may process near-threshold sounds, whereas high-threshold fibers process higher-level sounds. **Frequency specificity** is the ability of the cochlea to differentiate the various spectral components of a signal. **Post-stimulus time histograms** are plots of neural response relative to the onset of a stimulus. The **characteristic** or **best frequency** of a neuron is the frequency to which it responds best. A **tuning curve** is a composite of the responses of a single fiber at each frequency of presentation. The sharper the tuning curve, the greater the frequency specificity of the basilar membrane. The **tonotopic array** of the cochlea is clearly maintained within the auditory nervous system in the form of individual nerve fiber activation. As the **intensity** of stimulation increases, **rate of firing** increases. When the **crossed-olivocochlear** and **uncrossed-olivocochlear bundles** are stimulated, the firing rate of neurons innervated by them is reduced dramatically. **Interspike interval histograms** record the interval between successive firings of a neuron, revealing **phase-locking** of neurons to stimulus period.

Temporal and tonotopically arrayed information progresses to higher centers for further extraction of information. The **cochlear nucleus** reveals tonotopic representation, with a wide variety of neuron responses. **Primary-like** responses most resemble VIII nerve firing, **onset** responses show an initial response to onset of a stimulus followed by silence, and **chopper** responses show a periodic, chopped temporal pattern as long as a tone is present. **Pauser responses** take longer to respond than other neurons. **Buildup responses** slowly increase in firing rate through the initial stages of firing.

The **superior olivary complex** is the primary site of localization of sound in space. **Contralateral stimulation** of the SOC by high-frequency information results in excitation related to **stimulus intensity**. Low-frequency stimuli presented binaurally to the SOC result in **interaural time difference** detection. A wide array of responses is seen at the **inferior colliculus**, including neuron inhibitory responses, onset and pauser responses, intensity-sensitive units, interaural time- and intensity-sensitive neurons. The **medial geniculate body** is a relay of the thalamus. The **cerebral cortex** receives input primarily from the contralateral ear via the ipsilateral MGB. A full tonotopic map on the cortex may be seen at the primary reception area. The auditory reception area is organized in columns, with each column having a similar characteristic frequency. Different neurons within the columns respond to different stimulus parameters, such as frequency up-glides, down-glides, intensity up- and down-glides, and so on.

STUDY QUESTIONS

1. The _____ of the outer ear is important for localization of sound in space.

2. Resistance to flow of energy is termed _____.

3. The area ratio between the tympanic membrane and the oval window provides a _____ dB gain, and the lever advantage gives a _____ dB gain.

4. The cochlea performs both _____ analysis and _____ analysis.

5. Compression in the fluid of the scala vestibuli is translated directly to the basilar membrane, and the disturbance at the basilar membrane causes the initiation of a _____ wave.

6. High-frequency sounds are resolved at the base of the cochlea, with progressively lower sounds processed at progressively higher positions on the cochlea. This array is termed _____.

7. The frequency analysis ability of the basilar membrane is determined by graded _____, _____, and _____.

8. At the apex, the basilar membrane is thinner/thicker (circle one) than at the base.

9. At the apex, the basilar membrane is wider/narrower (circle one) than at the base.

10. T/F   The cilia of the outer hair cells are embedded in the tectorial membrane.

11. T/F   The cilia of the inner hair cells are embedded in the tectorial membrane.

12. T/F   The scala vestibuli is 5 mV more positive than the scala tympani, but the scala media is 80 mV more positive.

13. The _____ arises directly from stimulation of a large number of hair cells simultaneously.

14. _____ neurons require a higher intensity and encompass the higher end of our auditory range of signal intensity, whereas _____ neurons respond at very low signal levels and display random firing even when no stimulus is present.

15. _____ refers to the ability of the cochlea to differentiate the various spectral components of a signal.

16. The _____ frequency of a neuron is the frequency to which it responds best.

17. Tuning curves are composites of the responses of a single fiber at each frequency of presentation. The sharper the tuning curve, the greater the _____ of the basilar membrane.

18. Rate of firing of neurons increases as the _____ increases.

19. Stimulation of the _____ bundle and the _____ bundle reduces the firing rate of neurons innervated by them.

20. _____ are those firing patterns that most resemble VIII nerve responses.

21. The _____ is the primary site of localization of sound in space.

22. Comparative anatomy provides insight into function. What changes in the cochlea would you predict when comparing the cochlea of a human with that of a mammal that used ultra-high-frequency sound to echolocate, such as a fruit bat? What changes would you predict that you would find when comparing an elephant's cochlea with that of a human?

STUDY QUESTION ANSWERS

1. The PINNA of the outer ear is important for localization of sound in space.
2. Resistance to flow of energy is termed IMPEDANCE.
3. The area ratio between the tympanic membrane and the oval window provides a 25 dB gain, and the lever advantage gives a 2 dB gain.
4. The cochlea performs both SPECTRAL analysis and TEMPORAL analysis.
5. Compression in the fluid of the scala vestibuli is translated directly to the basilar membrane, and the disturbance at the basilar membrane causes the initiation of a TRAVELING wave.
6. High-frequency sounds are resolved at the base of the cochlea, with progressively lower sounds processed at progressively higher positions on the cochlea. This array is termed TONOTOPIC.
7. The frequency analysis ability of the basilar membrane is determined by graded WIDTH, STIFFNESS, and THICKNESS.
8. At the apex, the basilar membrane is THICKER than at the base.
9. At the apex, the basilar membrane is WIDER than at the base.
10. T   The cilia of the outer hair cells are embedded in the tectorial membrane.
11. F   The cilia of the inner hair cells are embedded in the tectorial membrane.
12. T   The scala vestibuli is 5 mV more positive than the scala tympani, but the scala media is 80 mV more positive.
13. The WHOLE-NERVE ACTION POTENTIAL arises directly from stimulation of a large number of hair cells simultaneously.
14. HIGH-THRESHOLD neurons require a higher intensity and encompass the higher end of our auditory range of signal intensity, whereas LOW-THRESHOLD neurons respond at very low signal levels and display random firing even when no stimulus is present.

15. <u>FREQUENCY SPECIFICITY</u> refers to the ability of the cochlea to differentiate the various spectral components of a signal.

16. The <u>CHARACTERISTIC</u> frequency of a neuron is the frequency to which it responds best.

17. Tuning curves are composites of the responses of a single fiber at each frequency of presentation. The sharper the tuning curve, the greater the <u>FREQUENCY SPECIFICITY</u> of the basilar membrane.

18. Rate of firing of neurons increases as the <u>INTENSITY</u> increases.

19. Stimulation of the <u>CROSSED-OLIVOCOCHLEAR</u> bundle and the <u>UNCROSSED-OLIVOCOCHLEAR</u> bundle reduces the firing rate of neurons innervated by them.

20. <u>PRIMARY-LIKE</u> are those firing patterns that most resemble VIII nerve responses.

21. The <u>SUPERIOR OLIVARY COMPLEX</u> is the primary site of localization of sound in space.

22. The fruit bat cochlea is, naturally enough, smaller than that of the human. In addition, the cochlea of the bat is extremely sensitive to ultra-high frequencies (above human range of hearing), because high-frequency sounds are more efficient for echolocation. Elephants, in contrast, have larger cochleas than humans. They process sounds that are lower than those we can hear!

 # REFERENCES

Altschuler, R. A., Bobbin, R. P., & Hoffman, D. W. (1986). *Neurobiology of hearing: The cochlea.* New York: Raven Press.

Anson, B. J., & Donaldson, J. R. (1973). *Surgical anatomy of the temporal bone and ear.* Philadelphia: W. B. Saunders.

Békésy, G. (1960). *Experiments in hearing.* New York: McGraw-Hill.

Bhatnagar, S. C., & Andy, O. J. (2002). *Neuroscience for the study of communicative disorders* (2nd ed.). Baltimore: Williams & Wilkins.

Carpenter, M. B. (1991). *Core text of neuroanatomy* (4th ed.). Baltimore: Williams & Wilkins.

Cazals, Y., Demany, L., & Horner, K. (1991). *Auditory physiology and perception.* Oxford: Pergamon Press.

Chusid, J. G. (1985). *Correlative neuroanatomy and functional neurology* (17th ed.). Los Altos, CA: Lange Medical Publications.

Cianfrone, G., & Grandori, F. (1985). Cochlear mechanics and otoacoustic emissions. *Scandinavian Audiology* (Suppl. 25).

Dallos, P. (1973). *The auditory periphery.* New York: Academic Press.

Dallos, P., Billone, M. C., Durrant, J. D., Wang, C-Y., & Raynor, S. (1972). Cochlear inner and outer hair cells: Functional differences. *Science, 177,* 356–358.

Davis, H. (1958). Transmission and transduction in the cochlea. *Laryngoscope, 68,* 359–382.

Duifhuis, H., Horst, J. W., van Dijk, P., & van Netten, S. M. (1993). *Biophysics of hair cell sensory systems.* Singapore: World Scientific.

Durrant, J. D., & Lovrinic, J. H. (1995). *Bases of hearing science* (3rd ed.). Baltimore: Williams & Wilkins.

Engstrom, H., Ades, H. W., & Andersson, A. (1966). *Structural pattern of the organ of Corti.* Baltimore: Williams & Wilkins.

Gelfand, S. A. (1990). *Hearing.* New York: Marcel Dekker.

Gelfand, S. A. (2001). *Essentials of audiology* (2nd ed.). New York: Thieme Medical Publishers.

Gray, H., Bannister, L. H., Berry, M. M., & Williams, P. L. (Eds.). (1995). *Gray's anatomy.* London: Churchill Livingstone.

Green, D. (1976). *An introduction to hearing.* Hillsdale, NJ: Lawrence Erlbaum Associates.

Gulick, W. L. (1971). *Hearing physiology and psychophysics.* New York: Oxford University Press.

Javel, E. (1986). Basic response properties of auditory nerve fibers. In R. A. Altschuler, R. P. Bobbin, & D. W. Hoffman (Eds.), *Neurobiology of hearing: The cochlea* (pp. 213–245). New York: Raven Press.

Kandel, E. R., Schwartz, J. H., & Jessell, T. M. (2000). *Principles of neural science* (4th ed.). New York: McGraw-Hill.

Khanna, S. M., & Leonard, D. G. B. (1982). Basilar membrane tuning in the cochlea. *Science, 215,* 305–306.

Kiang, N. Y-S. (1965). *Discharge patterns of single fibers in the cat's auditory nerve.* Cambridge, MA: The M.I.T. Press.

Kiang, N. Y-S., Liberman, M. C., Sewell, W. F., & Guinan, J. J. (1986). Single unit clues to cochlear mechanisms. *Hearing Research, 22,* 171–182.

Kuehn, D. P., Lemme, M. L., & Baumgartner, J. M. (1991). *Neural bases of speech, hearing, and language.* Boston: Little, Brown.

Lewis, E. R., Leverenz, E. L., & Bialek, W. S. (1985). *The vertebrate inner ear.* Boca Raton, FL: CRC Press, Inc.

Martin, F. N. (1981). *Medical audiology.* Englewood Cliffs, NJ: Prentice-Hall.

Møller, A. R. (1973). *Basic mechanisms of hearing.* New York: Academic Press.

Møller, A. R. (1983). *Auditory physiology.* New York: Academic Press.

Møller, A. R. (2003). *Sensory systems: Anatomy and physiology.* New York: Academic Press.

Parkins, C. W., & Anderson, S. W. (1983). Cochlear prostheses. *Annals of the New York Academy of Sciences, 405.*

Pfeiffer, R. R. (1966). Classification of response patterns of spike discharges for units in the cochlear nucleus: Tone-burst stimulation. *Experimental Brain Research, 1,* 220–235.

Pickles, J. O. (1988). *An introduction to the physiology of hearing* (2nd ed.). London: Academic Press.

Rhode, W. W. (1985). The use of intracellular techniques in the study of the cochlear nucleus. *Journal of the Acoustical Society of America, 78,* 320–327.

Rossing, T. D. (2001). *The science of sound.* Reading, MA: Addison-Wesley.

Ryan, A., & Dallos, P. (1976). Physiology of the inner ear. In J. L. Northern, (Ed.), *Hearing disorders* (pp. 89–101). Boston, MA: Little, Brown.

Shaw, E. A. G. (1974). The external ear. In W. D. Keidel & W. D. Neff (Eds.), *Handbook of sensory physiology* (pp. 455–490). New York: Springer-Verlag.

Syka, J., & Masterton, R. B. (1988). *Auditory pathway structure and function.* New York: Plenum Press.

Tobias, J. V., & Schubert, E. D. (1983). *Hearing research and theory* (Vol. 2). New York: Academic Press.

Tonndorf, J. (1958). The hydrodynamic origin of aural harmonics in the cochlea. *Annals of Otology, 67,* 754–774.

Tonndorf, J. (1960). Shearing motion in scala media of cochlear models. *Journal of the Acoustical Society of America, 32*(5), 238–244.

Wever, E. G., & Bray, C. W. (1930). Action currents in the auditory nerve in response to acoustical stimulation. *Proceedings of the National Academy of Science, 16,* 344–350.

Wilson, J. P., & Kemp, D. T. (1989). *Cochlear mechanisms: Structure, function, and models.* New York: Plenum Press.

Winans, S. S., Gilman, S., Manter, J. T., & Gatz, A. J. (2002). *Manter and Gatz's essentials of clinical neuroanatomy and neurophysiology* (10th ed.). Philadelphia: F. A. Davis.

Yost, W. A. (2000). *Fundamentals of hearing: An introduction* (4th ed.). New York: Academic Press.

Yost, W. A., &. Nielsen, D. W. (1977). *Fundamentals of hearing: An introduction.* New York: Holt, Rinehart & Winston.

Zemlin, W. R. (1998). *Speech and hearing science: Anatomy and physiology* (4th ed.). Needham Heights, MA: Allyn & Bacon.

CHAPTER 12
Neuroanatomy

There is nothing in nature so awe-inspiring as the nervous system. Despite centuries of study, humans have only begun to gain understanding of this extraordinarily complex system. There are approximately 100 billion neurons in the nervous system, and each of these neurons may communicate directly with as many as 2,000 other neurons, providing at least 1 trillion points of communication. As before, we will discuss both the structure and function of this system.

OVERVIEW

During our discussion of human anatomy associated with speech and language, we have been quite concerned with voluntary musculature and the supporting framework associated with it. Communication *is*, by and large, voluntary. Nonetheless, the term *voluntary* takes on new meanings when seen in the context of automaticity and background. **Automaticity** refers to development of patterns of responses that no longer require highly specific motor control, but rather are relegated to automated patterns. **Background** activity is the muscular contraction that supports action or movement, providing the form against which voluntary movement is placed. Voluntary activities are generally considered to be conscious activities, but they are, in reality, largely automated responses. To prove this to yourself, try washing the dishes and actually thinking about the act of dishwashing. The movements and responses to this act are so automated that you probably feel you do them "without thinking." In fact, your brain receives more than 40,000 signals from body sensors per second (including information about soap suds and water temperature), but you need not respond to all of it, because your brain will monitor and alert you to dangers. You can think about other things while your hands do the dishes.

Speech capitalizes on similar automaticity, as you can see in your ability to easily speak while riding a bike or while walking. You no more think of every movement of the extraordinary number of muscles contracting for the simple speech act than you do during dishwashing. This changes when the mechanism changes, however. When your mouth is numb from the dentist's anesthesia, you become very aware of your lack of feedback from that system, and inaccurate speech results. When an individual suffers a cerebrovascular accident, the result is often a loss of previously attained automaticity in speech. When a child is born with **developmental apraxia of speech**, a condition that limits the ability of a child to plan articulatory function, achieving automaticity may be a lifelong struggle.

Automatic functions are supported by a background **tonicity**, a partial contraction of musculature to maintain muscle tone. All action occurs within an environment, and the environment of your musculature is the tonic contraction of supporting muscles. As you extend your arm to reach for a coffee cup, the action of the fingers of your hand to grasp the object is supported by the rotation of your shoulder and the extension of your arm. Without these background support movements, the act of grasping would not occur in the graceful, fluid manner to which you are accustomed. Your body works as a unit to meet your needs.

Voluntary functions are the domain of the **cerebral cortex** or **cerebrum**, a new structure by evolutionary standards that makes up the bulk of the human brain. It is the seat of consciousness, and sensory information that does not reach the level of the cerebrum does not reach consciousness. The cerebrum also is the source of voluntary movement, although many lower brain centers are involved in execution of commands initiated by the cerebrum (see Figure 12-1).

Movement requires coordination, and that is the responsibility of the **cerebellum**. Information from peripheral sensors is coordinated with the motor plan of the cerebrum to provide the body with the ability to make finely tuned motor gestures. The output from the cerebrum is modified by the **basal ganglia**, a group of nuclei (cell bodies) with functional unity deeply involved in background movement.

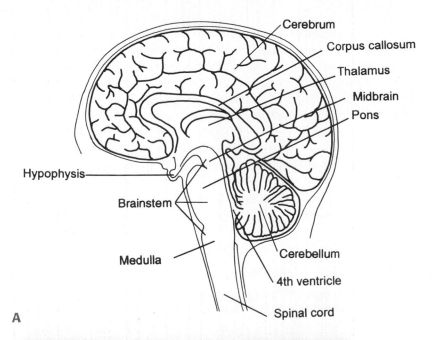

A

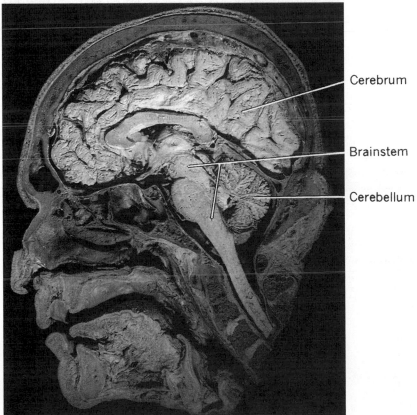

B

Figure 12-1. A. Medial view of cerebrum, brainstem, and cerebellum. **B.** Sagittal section showing relationship among cerebrum, cerebellum, and brainstem.

497

Motor commands are conveyed to the periphery for execution by neural pathways termed **nerves** or **tracts**. Sensory pathways transmit information concerning the status of the body and its environment to the brain for evaluation. This information permits the cerebrum and lower centers to act on changing conditions to protect the systems of the body and to adjust to the body's environment. For instance, information that tells your brain that it is cold outside will be transmitted to the cerebrum and hypothalamus—the result will be shivering and goosebumps, as well as a conscious effort to retrieve your ski parka from the car.

The brain can only communicate with its environment through sensors and effectors (see Tables 12-1 and 12-2). Sensors are the means by which your nervous system translates information concerning the

Table 12-1. Classes of sensation.

SUPERFICIAL SENSES	DEEP SENSES
Temperature	Muscle length and tension
Pain	Joint
Touch	Proprioception
	Muscle pain
	Pressure
	Vibration

Table 12-2. Sense, sensor, and stimulation.

SENSE	SENSOR TYPE	STIMULUS
Pain	Nerve ending	Aversive stimulation
Temperature	Thermosensor	Heat and cold
Mechanical stimulation	Pacinian corpuscle	Light and deep pressure
	Pacinian corpuscle	Vibration
	Golgi tendon organ	Joint sense
	Muscle spindle	Muscle stretch
Kinesthetic sense	Labyrinthine (vestibular) hair cells	Motion of body
Vision	Photoreceptors	Light stimulation
Olfactory	Chemoreceptors	Chemical stimulation
Audition	Labyrinthine (cochlear) hair cells	Acoustical stimulation
Gustatory	Chemoreceptors	Chemical stimulation

internal and external environment into a form that is useable by the brain, while effectors are the means by which your body responds to changing conditions. Broadly speaking, **superficial sensation** (temperature, pain, touch) is sensation arising from stimulation of the surface of the body. **Deep sensation** includes muscle tension, muscle length, joint position sense, muscle pain, pressure, and vibration. **Combined sensation** integrates both multiple senses to process stimulation. This involves integration of many pieces of sensory information to determine a quality, such as **stereognosis** (the ability to recognize the form of an object through touch).

Within each of these broad classes are specific types of sensation. **Somatic sense** is that sensation related to pain, thermal sensation (temperature sense), and mechanical stimulation. Mechanical stimulation takes the form of light and deep pressure, vibration (which is actually pressure that is perceived to change over time), and changes in joints and muscles, particularly stretch. **Kinesthetic sense** or *kinesthesia* is the sense of the body in motion. **Special senses** are those designed to **transduce** (change one form of energy into another) specific exteroceptive information. For example, in the **visual sense**, light from external sources is transduced into electrochemical energy by the photoreceptors of the retina; in **hearing**, acoustical disturbances in the air are transduced by the hair cells of the cochlea. Other special senses are **olfaction** (sense of smell), **tactile sense** (sense of touch), and **gustation** (sense of taste).

Sensor types vary by the stimulus to which they respond. Sensors communicate with the nervous system by means of dendritic connection with bipolar first-order sensory neurons. Axons of these first-order neurons **synapse** or make neurochemical connection within the central nervous system. A graded **generator potential** arises from adequate stimulation of the sensor, and adequate stimulation will cause generation of an action potential.

Receptors may be mechanoreceptors, chemoreceptors, photoreceptors, or thermoreceptors. **Mechanoreceptors** respond to physical distortion of tissue. Pressure on the skin, for example, will result in distension of **Pacinian corpuscles**, whereas hair follicles have mechanoreceptors to let you know that something has disturbed your hair. **Muscle spindle** and **Golgi tendon organs** and the **labyrinthine hair receptors** of the inner ear are also mechanoreceptors. In contrast, olfaction (smell) and gustation (taste) are mediated by **chemoreceptors** because they depend on contact with molecules of the target substance. Visual stimulation by light is transduced by highly specialized **photoreceptors**, and temperature sense arises from **thermoreceptors**. Visual and auditory sensors are also termed **teleceptors** because their respective light and sound stimuli arise from a source that does not touch the body (olfactory sense is stimulated directly by molecules of the material being sensed).

Another way to categorize receptors is by the region of the body receiving stimulation. **Interoceptors** monitor events within the body, such as distention of the lungs during inspiration or blood acidity. **Exteroceptors** respond to stimuli outside of the body, such as tactile stimulation, audition, and vision. Contact receptors are exteroceptors that respond to stimuli that touch the body (e.g., tactile, pain, deep and light pressure, temperature). **Proprioceptors** are sensors that monitor change in a body's position or the position of its parts, and these include muscle and joint sensors, such as muscle spindles and Golgi tendon organs. Vestibular sense falls into this category because it provides information about the body's position in space.

Despite our rich communicative ability, we can *only* know our environment by means of the sensory receptors of our skin, muscles, tendons, eyes, ears, and so forth. Without sensation, a perfectly functioning brain would be worthless as a communicating system. Likewise, communication *requires* some sort of muscular activity or glandular secretion. The absence of *all* motor activity would signal the end of communication. Fortunately, the extraordinary number of sensors in the human body permits us to use alternate pathways for receiving communication (e.g., **tactile** or touch communication) or for passing information to another person (e.g., use of eye-blink code). We are rarely completely cut off from communication with others. Let us now examine the components of this system.

 ## DIVISIONS OF THE NERVOUS SYSTEM

The **nervous system** can be viewed and categorized in a number of ways. It is important to develop a framework for discussion of this system, lest the volume of components become overwhelming. In the overview we discussed an informal **functional** view of nervous system organization, assessing the components in terms of their relationship to the systems of communication. We can view the nervous system as being composed of two major components (central nervous system and peripheral nervous system), or as having two major functions (somatic nervous system and autonomic nervous system). We can also view the nervous system in developmental terms, differentiating based on embryonic structures.

Central Nervous System/Peripheral Nervous System

The nervous system may be divided anatomically into central and peripheral nervous systems (see Table 12-3). The **central nervous system (CNS)** includes the brain (cerebrum, cerebellum, subcortical structures, brainstem) and spinal cord. The **peripheral nervous system (PNS)** con-

Table 12-3. Divisions of the nervous system from anatomical and physiological perspectives.

Anatomical Divisions of Nervous System:

Central Nervous System: Cerebrum, cerebellum, brainstem, spinal cord, thalamus, subthalamus, basal ganglia, etc.

Peripheral Nervous System: Spinal nerves, cranial nerves, sensors

Functional Divisions of Nervous System:

Autonomic Nervous System: Involuntary bodily function

Sympathetic nervous system: Expends energy (e.g., vasoconstriction when frightened)

Parasympathetic nervous system: Conserves energy (e.g., vasodilation upon removal of feared stimulation)

Somatic Nervous System: Voluntary bodily function

sists of the 12 pairs of cranial nerves and 31 pairs of spinal nerves, as well as the sensory receptors. All of the CNS components are housed within bone (skull or vertebral column), whereas most of the PNS components are outside of bone. We will spend a great deal of time within this organizational structure as we discuss the anatomy of the nervous system.

Autonomic/Somatic Nervous Systems

A functional view of the nervous system categorizes the brain into autonomic and somatic nervous systems (see Table 12-3). The **autonomic nervous system (ANS)** governs involuntary activities of the visceral muscles or **viscera**, including glandular secretions, heart function, digestive function, and so forth. You have little control over what happens to that triple chili cheeseburger once you make the commitment to eat it, although you will admit that occasionally you are *aware* of the digestive process.

The ANS may be further divided into two subsystems. The subsystem that responds to stimulation through energy expenditure is called the **sympathetic system** or **thoracolumbar system,** and the system that counters these responses is known as the **parasympathetic system** or **craniosacral system**. You feel the result of the sympathetic system when you have a close call in an automobile or hear a sudden, loud noise. Sympathetic responses include **vasoconstriction** (constriction of blood vessels), increase in blood pressure, dilation of pupils, cardiac acceleration, and "goosebumps." If you attend for a few more seconds, you will notice the glandular secretion of sweat under your arms. All of these fall into the category of "flight, fight, or fright" responses. Your body dumps the hormone norepinephrine into your system to provide you with a means of responding to danger, although the speed of modern emergencies such as automobile accidents clearly outstrips the rate of sympathetic responses (wear your seatbelt).

You may be less aware of the parasympathetic system response. This system is responsible for counteracting the effects of this preparatory act, because extraordinary muscular activity requires extraordinary energy. Parasympathetic responses include slowing of the heart rate, reduction of blood pressure, and pupillary constriction.

The central nervous system component of the ANS arises from the prefrontal region of the cerebral cortex, as well as from the hypothalamus, thalamus, hippocampus, brainstem, cerebellum, and spinal cord. The viscera are connected to these loci of control by means of **afferent** (ascending, typically sensory) and **efferent** (descending, typically motor) tracts.

The peripheral nervous system components of the ANS include paired **sympathetic trunk ganglia** running parallel and in close proximity to the vertebral column, **plexuses** (networks of nerves), and **ganglia** (groups of cell bodies having functional unity and lying outside the CNS).

The **somatic nervous system** (voluntary component) is of major importance to the discipline of speech pathology. This system involves the aspects of bodily function that are under our conscious and voluntary control, including control of all skeletal or **somatic muscles**. CNS control of muscles arises largely from the precentral region of the cerebral cortex, with neural impulses conveyed through descending motor tracts of the brainstem and spinal cord. Communication with the cranial nerves of the brainstem and with the spinal nerves of the spinal cord permits activation of the periphery of the body. Likewise, the sensory component of the somatic nervous system monitors information about the function of the skeletal muscles, their environment, and other "nonvisceral" activities.

The motor component of the somatic system may be subdivided into **pyramidal** and **extrapyramidal** systems, although defining all of the anatomical correlates of this functional division is difficult. The pyramidal system arises from pyramidal cells of the motor strip of the cerebral cortex and is largely responsible for initiation of voluntary motor acts. The extrapyramidal system also arises from the cerebral cortex (mostly from the premotor region of the frontal lobe), but is responsible for the background tone and movement supporting the primary acts. The extrapyramidal system is referred to as the **indirect system**, projecting to the basal ganglia and reticular formation.

There is one more important way of categorizing structures within the nervous system, and it is developmental in nature. The anatomical and developmental organizations overlap, and both sets of terminology are often used together.

> **afferent:** *L., ad ferre, to carry toward*
>
> **efferent:** *L., ex ferre, to carry away from*
>
> **somatic:** *Gr., soma, body*

Development Divisions

During the fourth week of embryonic development, the brain (**encephalon**) is composed of the **prosencephalon** (forebrain), **mesencephalon** (midbrain), and **rhombencephalon** (hindbrain). As the encephalon develops, further differentiation results in the telencephalon, rhinencephalon, diencephalon, metencephalon, and myelencephalon (see Table 12-4). The telencephalon refers to the "extended" or "telescoped" brain, and includes the cerebral hemispheres, the white matter immediately beneath it, the basal ganglia, and the olfactory tract. The rhinencephalon refers to structures within the telencephalon. The name arises from the relationship of the structures to olfaction. These are parts of the brain that developed early in our evolution, and include the olfactory bulb, tract, and striae; pyriform area; intermediate olfactory area; paraterminal area; hippocampal

Phylogeny refers to the evolution of a species, whereas ontogeny is the development of an individual organism. The statement that "Ontogeny recapitulates phylogeny" refers to the notion that structures that are phylogenetically oldest tend to emerge earliest in the developing organism, while later evolutionary additions, such as the cerebral cortex, will emerge later in development.

Table 12-4. Development and elements of the encephalon.

DEVELOPMENT OF ENCEPHALON	
Prosencephalon	Telencephalon (including rhinencephalon) Diencephalon
Mesencephalon	Mesencephalon
Rhombencephalon	Metencephalon Myelencephalon
COMPONENTS OF LEVELS OF THE ENCEPHALON	
Telencephalon	Cerebral hemispheres Basal ganglia Olfactory tract Rhinencephalon Lateral ventricle, part of third ventricle
Diencephalon	Thalamus Hypothalamus Pituitary gland (hypophysis) Optic tract Third ventricle
Mesencephalon	Midbrain Cerebral aqueduct Cerebral peduncles Corpora quadrigemina
Metencephalon	Pons Cerebellum Portion of fourth ventricle
Myelencephalon	Medulla oblongata Portion of fourth ventricle and central canal

telencephalon: *Gr., telos enkephalos, end or distant brain*

 rhinencephalon: *Gr., rhis enkephalos, nose brain*

formation; and fornix. The **diencephalon** is the next descending level, and includes the thalamus, hypothalamus, pituitary gland (hypophysis), and optic tract. The mesencephalon is the midbrain of the brainstem, and the **metencephalon** includes the pons and cerebellum. The **myelencephalon** refers to the medulla oblongata, the lowest level of the encephalon. The term **bulb** or **bulbar** refers technically to the pons and medulla, but is nearly always used to refer to the entire brainstem, including the midbrain.

Let us examine the nervous system, beginning with the building block of the nervous system. The basic units of the nervous system are neurons, from which all larger structures are composed.

ANATOMY OF THE CNS AND PNS

While it is an understatement to say that the CNS is extremely complex, it may be a comfort to realize that there is a common denominator to all the structures of the nervous system: All structures are made up of neurons. Functionally, the smallest organizational unit of the nervous system is also the neuron, followed in complexity by the spinal arc reflex, and higher reflexes (see Table 12-5). The brainstem provides the next

Table 12-5. Hierarchical order of complexity for structures of the nervous system.

STRUCTURE	FUNCTION
Glial cells	Nutrients to neurons, support, phagocytosis, myelin
Neuron	Communicating tissue
Reflexes	Subconscious response to environmental stimuli
Ganglia/nuclei	Aggregates of cell bodies with functional unity
Tracts	Aggregates of axons that transmit functionally united information; spinal cord
Structures of brainstem	Aggregates of ganglia, nuclei, and tracts that mediate high-level reflexes and mediate execution of cortical commands
Diencephalon	Aggregates of nuclei and tracts that mediate sensory information arriving at cerebrum and provide basic autonomic responses for body maintenance
Cerebellum	Aggregates of nuclei, specialized neurons, and tracts that integrate somatic and special sensory information with motor planning and command for coordinated movement
Cerebrum	All conscious sensory awareness and conscious motor function, including perception, awareness, motor planning and preparation, cognitive function, attention, decision-making, voluntary motor inhibition, language function, speech function

level of complexity, followed by subcortical structures and the cerebellum, and finally the most complex aggregate of tissue, the cerebral cortex. Let us begin with discussion of the most basic component of the nervous system, the neuron.

Neurons

Overview

The nervous system is comprised of the communicating elements, **neurons**, and support tissue, **glia** or **glial cells**. Neurons (nerve cells) are the functional building blocks of the nervous system and are unique among tissue types in that they are *communicating* tissue. Their function is to transmit information. Recently, however, the glial cell has come under close scrutiny and it looks as if its original role as a support system for neurons grossly understates its function. Some scientists have demonstrated that without glial cells the neurons would be virtually incapable of storing information in long-term memory. For now we will report the known support function of glial cells, but you may want to glimpse the future by reading Fields (2004).

The general structure of most neurons includes the **soma** or cell body; a **dendrite**, which transmits information toward the soma; and an axon, which transmits information away from the soma (see Table 12-6 and Figure 12-2).

Neurons respond to stimulation, and the neuron's response is the mechanism for transmitting information through the nervous system. A neuron can have one of two types of response: excitation or inhibition. **Excitation** refers to stimulation that causes an increase of activity of the

Table 12-6. Basic components of the neuron.

COMPONENT	FUNCTION
Dendrite	Receptor region
Soma	Contains metabolic organelles
Axon	Transmits information from neuron
Hillock	Generator site for action potential
Myelin sheath	Insulator of axon
Schwann cells	Form myelin in PNS
Oligodendrocytes	Form myelin in CNS
Nodes of Ranvier	Permit saltatory conduction
Telodendria	Processes from axon
Terminal end boutons	Contain synaptic vesicles
Neurotransmitter	Substance that facilitates synapse
Synaptic cleft	Region between pre- and postsynaptic neurons

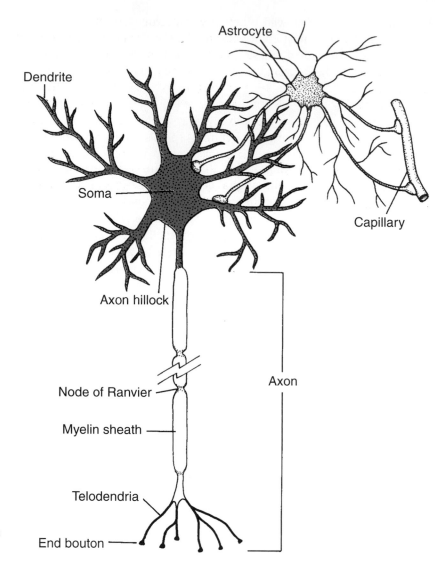

Dendrite

Astrocyte

Soma

Capillary

Axon hillock

Node of Ranvier

Axon

Myelin sheath

Telodendria

End bouton

Figure 12-2. Schematic of basic elements of a neuron. Note that the astrocyte is a glial cell that supports transport of nutrients to the neuron while shielding it from toxins via the blood-brain barrier.

tissue stimulated. That is, if a neuron is stimulated it will increase its activity in response. It is as if you were at a traffic signal in your car, and when the light changed the person behind you honked. Your response to this stimulation is to take off from the light (excitation). **Inhibition**, in contrast, refers to stimulation of a neuron that reduces the neuron's output. That is, when a neuron is inhibited, it will reduce its activity. Again, using the traffic analogy, if you hear a siren while at the traffic light, you know that there is an emergency vehicle coming. The siren inhibits your activity, and you decide *not to move* because of that stimulation. That is an inhibitory response. Neurons with excitatory responses give an active output when stimulated, whereas those with inhibitory responses *stop* responding when they are stimulated.

Morphology Characteristics. There are several important landmarks of the neuron (see Figure 12-3). A neuron may have many dendrites, often referred to as the "dendritic tree" because it looks "bushy," but the neuron will typically have only one axon. The **axon hillock** is the junction of the axon and the soma. Many axons are covered with a white fatty wrapping called the **myelin sheath**. Myelin is made up of **Schwann cells** in the PNS and of **oligodendrocytes** in the CNS, but in both cases myelin serves a very important function: It speeds up neural conduction. This means that axons (fibers) that have myelin wrapping around them are capable of conducting impulses at a much greater rate than those that do not have myelin. This will be very important when you study diseases that destroy the myelin, such as multiple sclerosis and amyotrophic lateral sclerosis.

Myelin is segmented, so that it looks a little like a series of hot dog buns linked together. The areas between the myelinated segments are known as **nodes of Ranvier**, and we shall see that these are important in conduction as well. If you follow the axon to its end point, you will see **telodendria**, which are long, thin projections. The telodendria have **terminal (end) boutons** (or **buttons**), and within the boutons are **synaptic vesicles**. Synaptic vesicles contain a special chemical known as

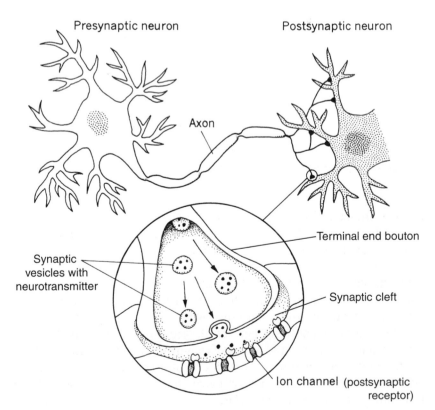

Figure 12-3. Schematic of elements of synapse. Note that the synapse consists of the terminal end bouton, synaptic cleft, and postsynaptic receptor sites.

neurotransmitter substance (or simply "neurotransmitter"). **Neurotransmitters** are compounds that are responsible for activating the next neuron in a chain of neurons. As we will discuss later on, neurotransmitter is released into the gap between two neurons (the **synaptic cleft**), and that causes the next neuron in the chain to be activated. The boutons also contain **mitochondria**, organelles responsible for energy generation and protein development. Groups of cell bodies appear gray and are referred to as **gray matter**, while **white matter** refers to myelin.

The **synapse** deserves special discussion. When a neuron is sufficiently stimulated, the axon discharges neurotransmitter into the synaptic cleft. The neurotransmitter is a lot like the key to your door: The neurotransmitter released into the synaptic cleft is the one to which the adjacent neuron responds. If some other class of neurotransmitter makes its way into that synaptic region, it will have no effect upon the adjacent neuron. This lock-and-key arrangement lets neurons have specific effects on some neurons while not affecting others.

We speak of the neurons in a chain as being either presynaptic or postsynaptic. **Presynaptic neurons** are those "upstream" from the synapse, and are the ones that stimulate the **postsynaptic neurons** (the ones following the synapse). This makes sense when you realize that information passes in only one direction from a neuron: information enters generally at the dendrite and exits at the axon.

Neurotransmitter released into the synaptic cleft stimulates **receptor sites** on the postsynaptic neuron. When the postsynaptic neuron is stimulated, ion channels in its membrane open up and allow ions to enter, and this leads to a discharge or "firing" of that neuron as well. Dendrites are the typical location for synapse on the receiving neurons, and these synapses are called **axodendritic synapses**. Synapse may also occur on the soma: These are called **axosomatic synapses** and are usually inhibitory. If synapse occurs on the axons of the postsynaptic neuron, it is called an **axoaxonic synapse** (see Figure 12-4), and these synapses tend to be modulatory in nature. Sometimes an axon stimulates a neuron secondarily on its way to the synapse with another neuron, and this is referred to as **en passant** ("in passing") synapse. Two other less common synapse formations are **somatosomatic synapse**, in which the soma of a neuron synapses with the soma of another neuron, and **dendrodendritic synapse**, in which communication is between two dendrites.

Synapse is a noun, but is often used as a verb, indicating the action of communication between two neurons.

Morphological Differences between Neurons. There are several types or *forms* of neurons distributed throughout the nervous system. **Monopolar (unipolar) neurons** are those with a single, bifurcating process arising from the soma (see Figure 12-5). Neurons with two processes are called **bipolar neurons**, and **multipolar neurons** will have more than two processes. Sensory neurons are generally monopolar or pseudomonopolar. The exception is neurons that transmit information about smell (**olfaction**), hearing (**audition**), and vestibular senses: these are bipolar.

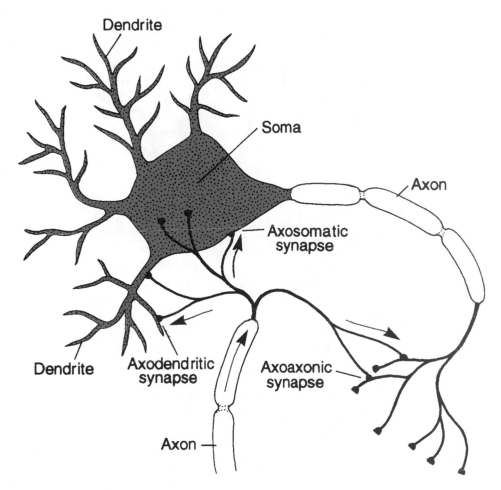

Dendrite

Soma

Axon

Axosomatic
synapse

Dendrite

Axodendritic
synapse

Axoaxonic
synapse

Axon

A

Figure 12-4. A. Types of synapses, including axodendritic (excitatory), axosomatic (inhibitory), and axoaxonal (modulatory). *(continues)*

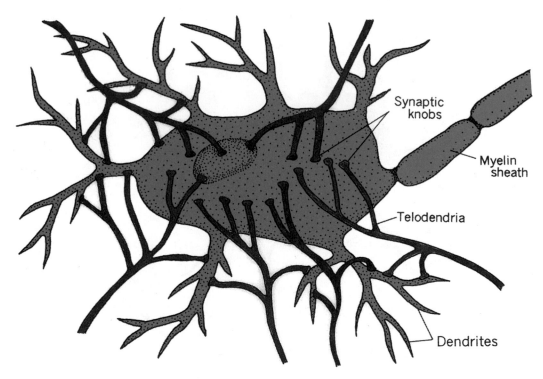

Synaptic knobs

Myelin sheath

Telodendria

Dendrites

B

Figure 12-4. *(continued)* **B.** Illustration of excitatory and inhibitory synapses on a postsynaptic neuron. Note that excitatory axons synapse on the dendrite, while inhibitory axons synapse at the cell body.

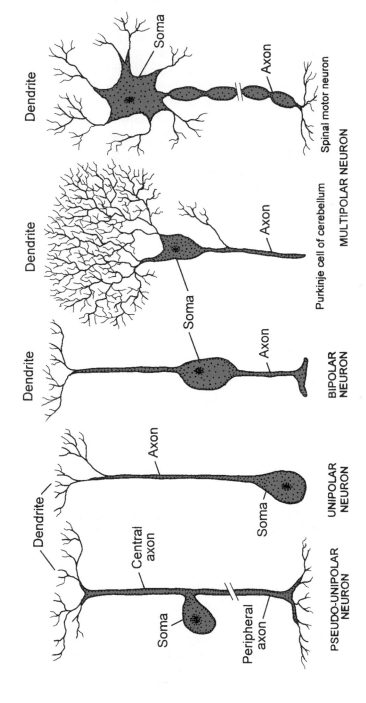

Figure 12-5. Types of neurons. Pseudo-unipolar and unipolar neurons are primarily somatic afferent neurons, while bipolar neurons mediate special senses. Multipolar neurons, which are primarily efferent, include pyramidal cells, spinal motor neurons, and Purkinje cells of the cerebellum.

Dendrite

Soma

Axon

Spinal motor neuron

MULTIPOLAR NEURON

Dendrite

Axon

Purkinje cell of cerebellum

Soma

Dendrite

Soma

Axon

BIPOLAR NEURON

Dendrite

Axon

Soma

UNIPOLAR NEURON

Central axon

Soma

Peripheral axon

PSEUDO-UNIPOLAR NEURON

Glial cells make up the majority of the brain tissue, providing support and nutrients to the neurons. **Astrocytes** appear to be largely structural, separating neurons from each other and adhering to capillaries. They appear to play a role in supplying nutrients to neurons. **Oligodendrocytes** are glial cells that make up the CNS myelin, and **Schwann cells** are glia constituting the myelin of the PNS. While technically not neurons, glial cells are an important component of the nervous system tissue. Astrocytes provide the primary support for neurons, aid in suspension of neurons, and transport nutrients from the capillary supply. They also provide the important **blood-brain barrier**, a membranous filter system that prohibits some toxins from passing from the cerebrovascular system to neurons.

Yet another type of glial cell, **microglia**, performs the housekeeping process known as *phagocytosis*. Microglia scavenge necrotic tissue formed by a lesion in the nervous system. Astrocytes will assist by forming scarring around necrotic tissue, effectively isolating it from the rest of the brain tissue.

Neuroscience is now taking a very hard look at the role of astrocytes. We have long known that they had an important role in support of neurons, including nutrient delivery, but only recently has evidence emerged to indicate that glial cells are critical to creation of long-term memory.

Functional Differences between Neurons. There are *functional* differences between neurons as well. **Interneurons** make up the largest class of neurons in the brain. The job of interneurons is to provide communication between other neurons, and interneurons do not exit the central nervous system. Another type of neuron is the **motor neuron**. Motor neurons are efferent in nature, and they are typically bipolar neurons that activate muscular or glandular response. These neurons usually have long axons that are myelinated. Motor neurons are further differentiated based on size, **conduction velocity** (how fast they can conduct an impulse), and degree of myelination. Generally speaking, a neuron with a wider axon and thicker myelin will have more rapid conduction of neural impulses.

Neuronal fibers are classified in terms of conduction velocity as being A, B, or C class fibers. The A and B fibers are myelinated. The **A fibers** are further broken down, based on conduction velocity, into **alpha, beta, gamma,** and **delta fibers** (see Table 12-7). **Alpha motor neurons** have high conduction velocities (between 50 and 120 m/s) and innervate the majority of skeletal muscle, called **extrafusal muscle fibers**. Slower-velocity **gamma motor neurons** innervate **intrafusal muscle fibers** within the **muscle spindle**, the sensory apparatus responsible for maintaining muscle length. Thus, alpha motor neurons activate the prime movers of the motor act; gamma motor neurons are responsible for maintaining muscle tone and muscle readiness for the motor act.

Table 12-7. Type A, B, and C sensory and motor fibers*.

FIBER CLASS	VELOCITY (m/s)	MOTOR FUNCTION	SENSORY FUNCTION
A-Alpha	50–120	Large alpha motor neurons innervating extrafusal muscle	
Ia	120		Primary muscle spindle afferents
Ib	120		Golgi tendon organs; pressure receptors
Beta			
II	70		Muscle spindle secondary afferents; touch and pressure
Gamma	40	Intrafusal muscle of spindle	
Delta			
III	15		Touch, pressure pain, coolness
B	14	Smooth muscle	
C	2	Smooth muscle	
IV	2		Pain and warmth

*Data from Winans, Gilman, Manter, & Gatz, 2002.

Sensory alpha fibers are identified by a Roman numeral and a lower-case letter (**type Ia, Ib, II, III, or IV fibers**), reflecting a different classification scheme. The **Ia** neurons are the **primary afferent fibers** from the muscle spindle, while the **Ib** neurons send sensory information generated at the **Golgi tendon organs**, sensors that respond to stretching of the tendon. Type **II** afferent fibers are secondary muscle spindle afferents of the beta class, and convey information from touch and pressure receptors. The type **III** afferent fibers are delta class, conducting pain, pressure, touch, and coolness sensation. Type **IV** fibers convey pain and warmth sense. Again, some sensory neurons are essential for movement, and these include types Ia, Ib, and II. Types III and IV are important for transmitting other body senses (pain, temperature, pressure) but are not essential to movement.

In summary, the **nervous system** is a complex, hierarchical structure made up of **neurons**.

- Many **motor functions** become automated through practice.
- **Voluntary movement**, **sensory awareness**, and **cognitive function** are the domain of the **cerebral cortex**, although we are capable of sensation and response without consciousness.

- The communication links of the nervous system are **spinal nerves**, **cranial nerves**, and **tracts** of the **brainstem** and **spinal cord**.
- The nervous system may be divided functionally as **autonomic** and **somatic nervous systems** serving involuntary and voluntary functions.
- It may be divided anatomically as **central** and **peripheral nervous systems** as well.
- **Developmental divisions** separate the brain into **prosencephalon** (which is further divided into telencephalon and diencephalon), the **mesencephalon** or midbrain, and the **rhombencephalon**, which includes the metencephalon and myelencephalon.
- **Neurons** are widely varied in morphology, but may be broadly categorized as **monopolor**, **bipolar**, or **multipolar**.
- Neurons communicate through **synapse** by means of **neurotransmitter** substance, and the response by the postsynaptic neuron may be **excitatory** or **inhibitory**.
- The size and type of axon is related to conduction of neural impulse.
- **Glial cells** provide the fatty sheath for **myelinated axons**, as well as support structure for neurons.

Anatomy of the Cerebrum

The cerebrum is the mostly highly evolved and organized structure of the human body. This is the largest structure of the nervous system, weighing approximately three pounds and made up of billions of neurons. The cerebrum is divided into grossly similar left and right hemispheres, and is wrapped by three meningeal linings that protect and support the massive structure of the brain. We will discuss those meningeal linings first, and then introduce you to the most important structure of your body.

Meningeal Linings

The central nervous system is invested with a triple-layer meningeal lining serving important protective and nutritive functions. There are three meningeal linings covering the brain. The **dura mater** is a bilayered, tough lining, which is the most superficial of the meningeal linings (see Figure 12-6). The dura mater itself is made up of two layers that are tightly bound together. The outer layer is more inelastic than the inner layer, and meningeal arteries course through this layer. While the layers making up the dura mater are bound together, the potential space superficial to the dura mater is called the **epidural space**, a term that will gain meaning when discussing vascular lesions that can release blood into

dura mater: *L., tough mother*

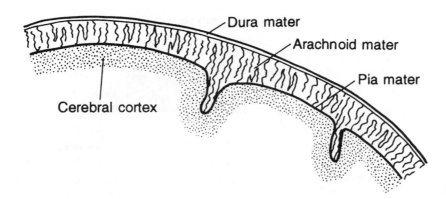

Dura mater

Arachnoid mater

Pia mater

Cerebral cortex

Figure 12-6. Schematic of the meningeal linings of the brain.

areas of the brain (e.g., *epidural hematoma* is a hemorrhagic release of blood into the space between the two layers of the dura mater).

The **arachnoid mater** is a covering through which many blood vessels for the brain pass. The arachnoid lining is a lacey, spiderlike structure separating the dura mater from the innermost meningeal lining, the **pia mater**. The pia mater is a thin, membranous covering that closely follows the contour of the brain. The major arteries and veins serving the surface of the brain course within this layer.

The function of the meningeal linings is to protect the brain, holding structures in place during movement and providing support for those structures. To provide this protection, the linings must conform to the structure of the brain. As part of this support, the dura mater takes on four major infoldings. These infoldings of the dura separate major structures of the brain, providing some isolation. The four infoldings are the falx cerebri, falx cerebelli, tentorium cerebelli, and diaphragma sella. The falx cerebri and falx cerebelli are sagittal dividers, separating left and right structures of the brain, while the tentorium cerebelli and diaphragma sella separate brain structures by means of a transversely posed membrane.

The **falx cerebri** separates the two cerebral hemispheres with a vertical sheath of dura, running from the crista galli of the ethmoid to the tentorium cerebelli. The falx cerebri completely separates the two hemispheres down to the level of the corpus callosum (to be discussed). The **falx cerebelli** performs the same function for the cerebellum, separating the left and right cerebellar hemispheres for protection and isolation (see Figure 12-7).

The **tentorium cerebelli** is a horizontal dural shelf at the base of the skull that divides the cranium into superior (cerebral) and inferior (cerebellar) regions. The **diaphragma sella** forms a boundary between the pituitary gland and the hypothalamus and optic chiasm. The dura mater encircles the cranial nerves as they exit the brainstem. Because of its placement, the tentorium cerebelli supports the cerebrum and keeps

arachnoid mater: *L., spider mother; so called because this structure looks like a spiderweb*

pia mater: *L., pious mother; so named because of its gentle but faithful attachment to the cerebral cortex*

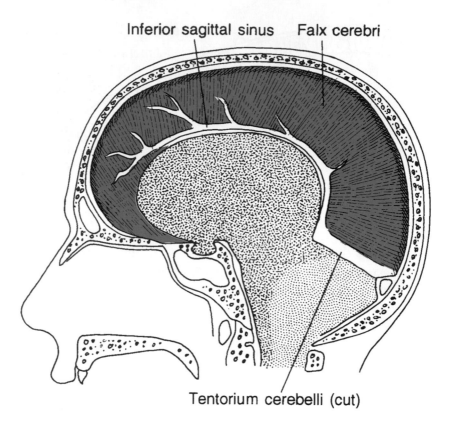

Inferior sagittal sinus   Falx cerebri

Tentorium cerebelli (cut)

Figure 12-7. The falx cerebri separates the left and right cerebral hemispheres. The tentorium cerebelli separates the cerebellum from the cerebrum. The falx cerebelli (not shown) separates the cerebellar hemispheres.

its mass from compressing the cerebellum and brainstem, as would most certainly happen if the dural lining was absent. The dural shelves can be liabilities when trauma results in **subdural hematoma**, a release of blood through hemorrhage beneath the dura that can push on the cerebrum, causing the temporal lobe to herniate under the tentorium. Subdural hematoma may also cause a life-threatening herniation of the brainstem into the foramen magnum.

There are meningeal linings of the spinal cord as well, paralleling the structure and function of the cerebral meninges. At the foramen magnum the meningeal linings are continuous with the **spinal meningeal linings**. The spinal meninges are broadly similar to those of the brain, with some exceptions. The dura of the brain adheres to the bone, but the dura of the spinal cord does not adhere to the vertebrae. As with the brain meninges, cerebrospinal fluid flows through the subarachnoid space. Likewise, the pia mater closely follows the surface of the spinal cord, but serves an anchoring function as well. The cord is attached to the dura by means of 22 pairs of **denticulate ligaments** arising from the pia. The dura extends laterally to encapsulate the dorsal root ganglion. At the inferior cord, the pia is continuous with the filum terminale, which is attached to the first segment of the coccyx (see Figure 12-8).

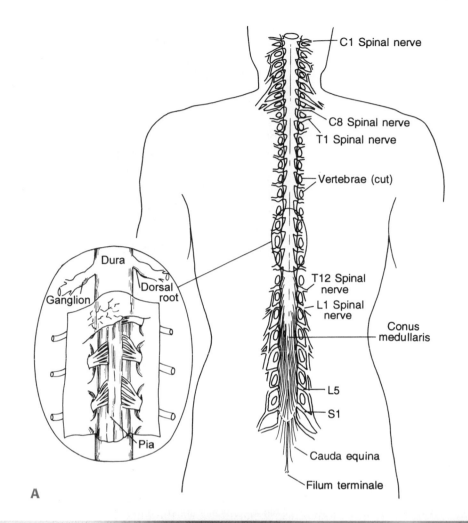

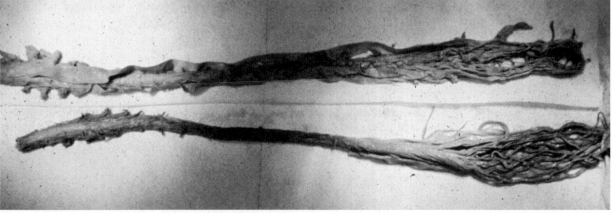

Figure 12-8. A. Spinal cord and emerging spinal nerves. Note the inset showing the meningeal linings of the spinal cord. **B.** Photograph of excised spinal cords. *(continues)*

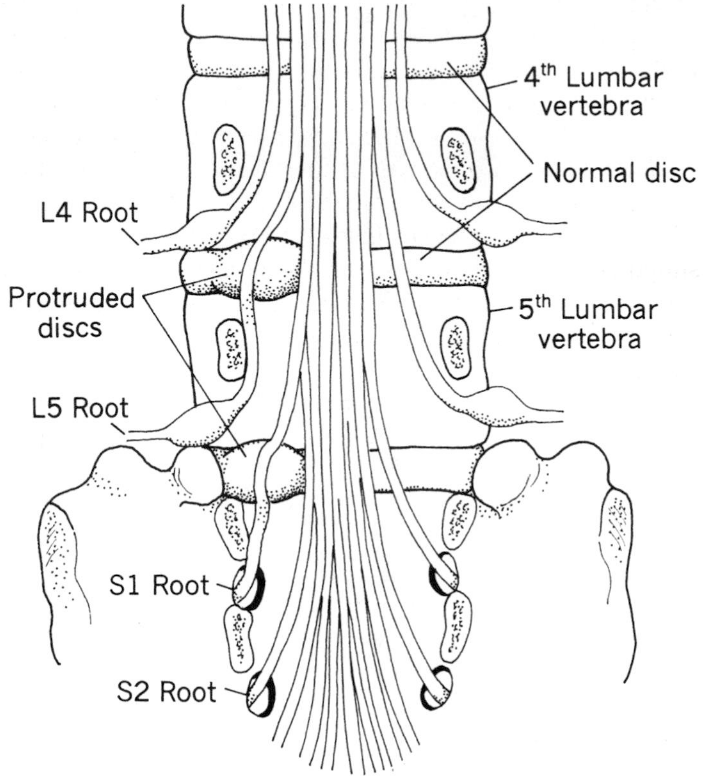

Figure 12-8. *(continued)*
C. Illustration of herniated vertebral disc and subsequent compression of spinal nerves L4 and L5.

C

Labels on figure:
- 4th Lumbar vertebra
- Normal disc
- L4 Root
- Protruded discs
- L5 Root
- 5th Lumbar vertebra
- S1 Root
- S2 Root

Hematoma

A **hematoma** is a pooling of blood, typically arising from breakage of a blood vessel. **Subdural hematoma** involves intracranial bleeding beneath the dura mater caused by rupture of cortical arteries or veins, usually as a result of trauma to the head. Pressure from the pooling blood displaces the brain, shifting and compressing the brainstem, forcing the temporal lobe under the tentorium cerebelli, and compressing cerebral arteries. This critically dangerous condition may not be immediately recognized, because it may take several hours before pooling blood compresses the brain sufficiently to produce symptoms such as reduced consciousness, hemiparesis, pupillary dilation, and other symptoms associated with compressed cranial nerves. **Epidural hematoma**, hematoma occurring above the dura mater, may result in a patient being initially lucid, but displaying progressively decreasing levels of consciousness, reflecting compression of the brain.

Hematomas are characterized by location of insult. **Frontal epidural hematomas** arise from blows to the frontal bone and may result in personality changes. **Posterior fossa epidural hematomas** arise from blows to the back of the head, producing visual and coordination deficits.

Together, the meningeal linings provide an excellent means of nurturing and protecting the CNS structures. The dura is a tough structure that provides a barrier between the bone of the skull and the delicate neural tissue, and to which blood vessels can be anchored as they pass to the cerebrum. The delicate pia mater completely envelopes the cerebrum, supporting the blood vessels as they serve the surface of the brain. Between the dura and pia is the arachnoid lining, through which a cushioning fluid, cerebrospinal fluid, flows (to be discussed). A similar network supports the spinal cord within the vertebral column. Thus, the meninges support the brain, separate major structures, and maintain the brain in its fluid suspension. In this manner the brain is able to overcome many otherwise dangerous shocks from external acceleration, such as those experienced during falls or blunt trauma. You may wish to read the Clinical Note on "An Ounce of Prevention" for a brief discussion of what happens when these protective measures are not enough.

The Ventricles and Cerebrospinal Fluid

The central nervous system is bathed in **cerebrospinal fluid (CSF)**, which provides a cushion for the delicate and dense neural tissue as well as some nutrient delivery and waste removal. Examining the system of ventricles and canals through which the cerebrospinal fluid flows will help you as we describe the cerebral cortex and subcortical structures. You will want to refer to Figure 12-9 for this discussion.

The ventricles of the brain are spaces within the brain through which cerebrospinal fluid flows. They are cavities that are, in reality, remnants of the embryonic neural tube. The system of ventricles consists

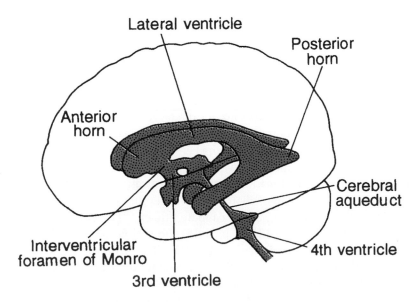

Figure 12-9. Ventricles of the brain.

An Ounce of Prevention

Should you choose to work in a trauma center, a significant portion of your caseload will arise from traumatic brain injury (TBI). TBI is one of the leading causes of death in individuals under 24 years of age, with transportation-related brain injury far exceeding all other causes (falls, assaults, sport, firearms). The addition of seat and lap belts to automobiles has resulted in a reduction of death in automobile accidents arising from brain injury by nearly 50%. Unfortunately, use of alcohol is related to reduced seatbelt use and increased death due to head injury during accidents. Mandatory use of helmets has reduced the frequency of brain injury in motorcycle accidents by 20 to 50% and up to 85% for bicycle riders.

Gunshot wounds to the head result in most deaths attributable to firearms, and handguns are involved in more than 60% of homicides. More than 40,000 people in the United States are killed by firearms annually. While laws that restrict access to firearms are hotly debated as a constitutional issue, the ability to eliminate accidental firearm deaths through trigger lock systems could greatly reduce the carnage that occurs in the United States, a country in which nearly 50% of the households have firearms. You will want to refer to Mackay, Chapman, and Morgan (1997) for an extremely thorough review of causes and treatment in TBI.

of four cavities: The right lateral ventricle, the left lateral ventricle, the 3rd ventricle, and the 4th ventricle. Within each ventricle is a **choroid plexus**, an aggregate of tissue that produces cerebrospinal fluid. While all ventricles produce CSF, the plexuses of the lateral ventricles produce the bulk of the fluid. The cavities are ideally suited to act as buffers for the delicate brain tissue. If you remember the discussion of the meningeal linings, you will recall that the cerebrum is supported by the tough dura and delicate pia, and that CSF flows between these two linings within the arachnoid space. That CSF buffers the cerebral hemispheres and structures from sudden movements of the head (accelerations), and the addition of CSF within the brain by means of ventricles further buoys up the brain against trauma.

The paired **lateral ventricles** are the largest of the ventricles, composed of four spaces bounded superiorly by the corpus callosum and extending into each of the lobes of the cerebrum. They are shaped somewhat like horseshoes opened toward the front, but with posterior horns attached. The **anterior horn** projects into the frontal lobe to the genu of the corpus callosum. The medial wall is the septum pellucidum, and the inferior margin is the head of the caudate nucleus. The **central portion**, located within the parietal lobe, includes the region between the **interventricular foramen of Monro** and the splenium, with the superior border being the corpus callosum, the medial boundary being the septum pellucidum, and the inferior being portions of the caudate nucleus. The **posterior** or **occipital horn** extends into the occipital lobe to a tapered termination, with its superior and lateral surfaces being the corpus callosum. The **inferior horn** extends into the temporal lobe, curving down behind the thalamus to terminate blindly behind the temporal pole. The hippocampus marks the lower margin of the inferior horn. The lateral ventricles communicate with the 3rd ventricle via the interventricular foramen of Monro.

The **3rd ventricle** is the unpaired medial cavity between the left and right thalami and hypothalami. The roof of the 3rd ventricle is the tela choroidea, and the ventricle extends inferiorly to the level of the optic chiasm. The prominent **interthalamic adhesion** (massa intermedia or intermediate mass) bridges the ventricle, connecting the two thalami. The CSF of the lateral ventricle passes into the 3rd ventricle by means of left and right interventricular foramina.

The **4th ventricle** is shaped roughly like a diamond, projecting upward from the central canal of the spinal cord and lower medulla. This ventricle is difficult to envision because it is the space between the brainstem and cerebellum. One must remove the cerebellum to see the 4th ventricle. The floor of the 4th ventricle is the junction of the pons and the medulla, and the cerebellum forms the roof and posterior margin. The 4th ventricle has three openings or **apertures**. The **median aperture (foramen of Magendie)** and the paired left and right **lateral apertures (foramina of Luschka)** permit CSF to flow into the subarachnoid space behind the brainstem and beneath the cerebellum, to be described.

Circulation of CSF. CSF is the clear, fluid product of the choroid plexus in each of the ventricles. It provides an excellent cushion to protect the brain against trauma and also serves a transport function, as mentioned previously. The volume of CSF in the nervous system is approximately 125 ml, which is replenished every seven hours. The fluid is under a constant pressure that changes with body position, and life-threatening conditions can develop should something occlude the pathway for CSF.

Circulation of CSF begins in each of the lateral ventricles, coursing through the interventricular foramina of Monro to the 3rd ventricle. From there, the fluid flows through the minute cerebral aqueduct to the 4th ventricle, where it drains into the subarachnoid space through the foramina of Luschka and Magendie to the cerebellomedullary cistern beneath the cerebellum and freely circulates around the brain and spinal cord. CSF then can course around the cerebellum and cerebrum to exit through the arachnoid granulation in sinuses of the dura mater and be absorbed by the venous system. Alternately, the CSF will course downward through the foramen magnum and subarachnoid space around the spinal cord.

In summary, the **cerebral cortex** is protected from physical insult by **cerebrospinal fluid** and the **meningeal linings**, the **dura**, **pia**, and **arachnoid mater**.

- The meninges provide support for delicate neural and vascular tissue, with the dura dividing into regions that correspond to the regions of the brain supported.
- The **spinal meningeal linings** similarly protect the spinal cord from movement trauma.
- Cerebrospinal fluid originating within the **ventricles** of the brain and circulating around the spinal cord cushions these structures from trauma associated with rapid acceleration.

Cerebrum

Layers of Cerebrum.   The **cerebrum** consists of two **cerebral hemispheres** or roughly equal halves of the brain (see Figure 12-10). The term **cortex** actually means "bark," referring to the bark or outer surface of a tree, and the cerebral cortex is the outer surface of the brain. The cortex is between two and four mm thick, being comprised of six cell layers.

The layers of the cerebrum consist of two basic cell types: pyramidal and nonpyramidal cells. **Pyramidal cells** are large, pyramid-shaped cells that are involved in motor function. Pyramidal cells are oriented so that the apex of the pyramid is directed toward the surface of the cortex, with the base directed medially. A single apical dendrite projects through cortex layers toward the surface, while multiple basal dendrites course laterally through the layer in which the cell body resides. Axons of pyramidal cells typically project to the white matter beneath the cortex or beyond, although they will have branches within the cortex itself.

Nonpyramidal cells are small and often stellate (star-shaped), and are involved in sensory function or intercommunication between brain regions. Their axons typically project only a short distance, either within a cortex layer or adjacent layers. Functionally, these nonpyramidal cells connect local regions, while pyramidal cells project to more distant regions, as will be discussed later.

The outermost layer of the cerebral cortex consists mostly of glial cells and axons from neurons of succeeding layers. The second and third layers consist of small and large pyramidal cells, respectively, and are thus highly involved in motor function. The fourth layer receives sensory input from the thalamus and consists of nonpyramidal cells, while the fifth layer is made up of large pyramidal cells that project to motor centers beyond the cerebrum (basal ganglia, brainstem, spinal cord). The sixth layer also consists of pyramidal cells, although these project to the thalamus.

The layers have varying densities within the cerebrum, corresponding to the dominant function for a specific region. For instance, the pyramidal layers will be thickest in the areas of the cortex responsible for motor function, while the granular layers will be most richly represented in the areas of the brain that process predominantly sensory input.

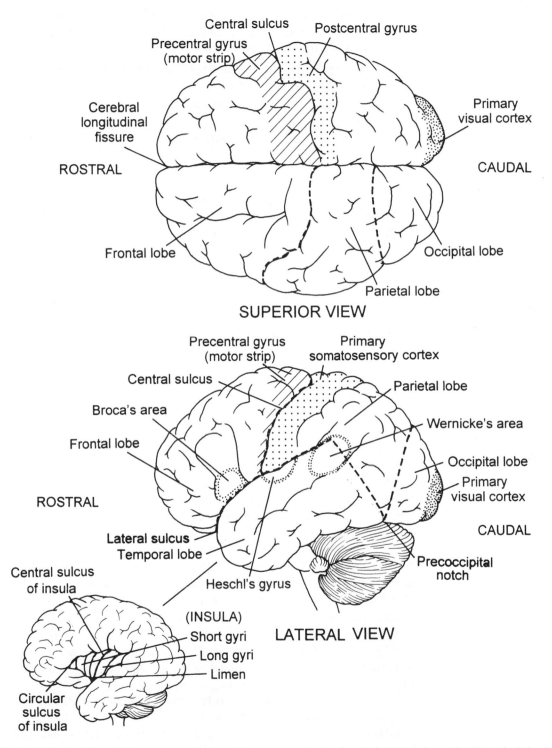

Figure 12-10. Major landmarks of the cerebrum as seen from above and from the side. Note that the insular cortex (insula, bottom left) is typically hidden from view.

For example, the region of primary motor output (the motor strip, to be discussed) has extremely rich representation of the fifth layer, with a very thin layer four, while the primary sensory areas have a rich layer four with few cells in the pyramidal layers. Areas involved in association of sensory and motor functions will have representation of both sensory and motor layers.

Much of our early knowledge concerning the cell structure of the cortical layers arose from the work of Korbinian Brodmann in the early part of the twentieth century (Kandel, 1991). His microscopic examination of the cerebral cortex revealed the dominant cell types of the cortical layers, and his keen analysis showed that localized areas of the brain were dominated by specific cell types, as discussed above. From his work came what has become known as the "Brodmann map" of the cerebrum (see Figure 12-11), a tool that remains a mainstay for navigating the regions of the cerebrum. Brodmann's observations proved to be quite important, and his notation has served many decades of neuroscience study. You will want to refer to this figure as we discuss landmarks of the superficial cortex.

Landmarks of Cerebrum.   The **cerebral longitudinal fissure** (also known as the **superior longitudinal fissure** and the **interhemispheric fissure**) separates the left and right cerebral hemispheres, as can be seen in Figure 12-10 and the photograph in Figure 12-12. You will remember from our discussion of the meningeal linings that the falx cerebri runs between the two hemispheres through this space. The cerebral longitudinal fissure completely separates the hemispheres down to the level of the corpus callosum, a major group of fibers providing communication between the two hemispheres, as will be discussed. Within the cerebral longitudinal fissure reside the anterior cerebral artery and its collaterals, to be discussed.

As you can also see in the photograph of Figure 12-12, the surface of the brain is quite convoluted. Early in development the cerebral cortex has few of these furrows and bulges, but as the brain growth outstrips the skull growth the cerebral cortex doubles in on itself. The result of this is greatly increased surface area, translating into more "neural horsepower." You can think of the surface as a topographical map with mountains and valleys. The mountains (**convolutions**) in this case are called **gyri** (singular, **gyrus**) and the infolding valleys that separate the gyri are called **sulci** (singular, **sulcus**). If the groove is deeper and more pronounced, it is termed a **fissure**. These sulci, fissures, and gyri provide the major landmarks for navigating the cerebral cortex.

We divide the cerebral cortex into six lobes. Four of them are reasonably easy to see and are named after the bones with which they are associated (see Figures 12-12 and 12–13), but two of these lobes (insular and limbic) require some thought and imagination. The six lobes are the frontal, parietal, occipital, temporal, insular, and limbic lobes.

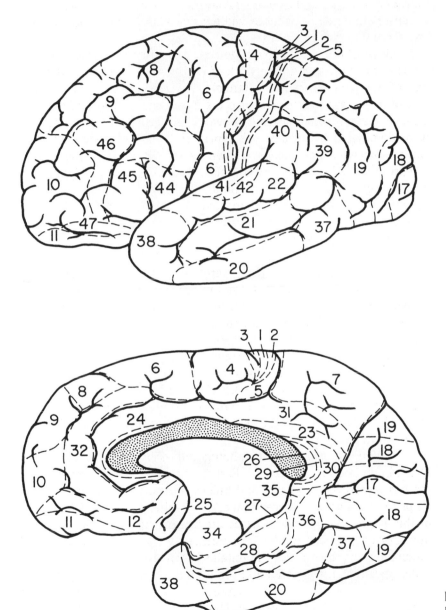

Figure 12-11. Brodmann map of lateral and medial cerebrum.

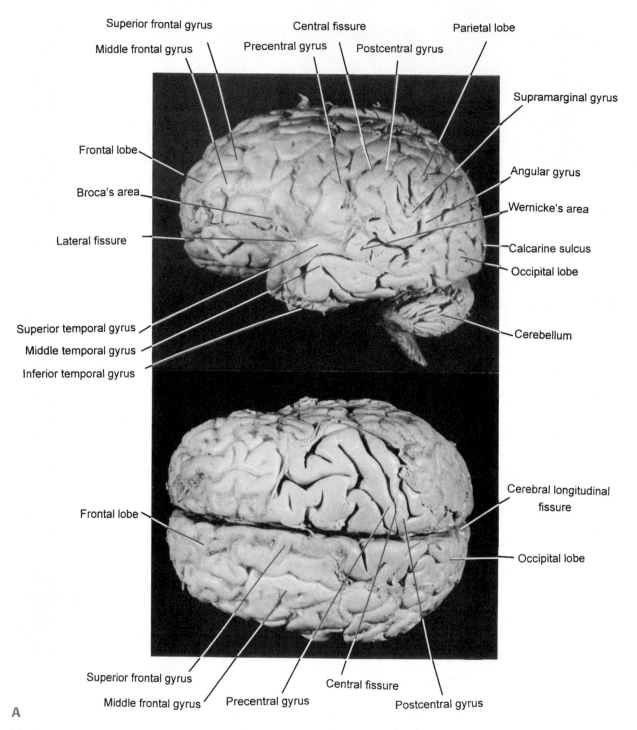

Figure 12-12. A. Lateral (upper) and superior (lower) views of cerebral cortex. Note that the pia mater may be seen in portions of both photographs. *(continues)*

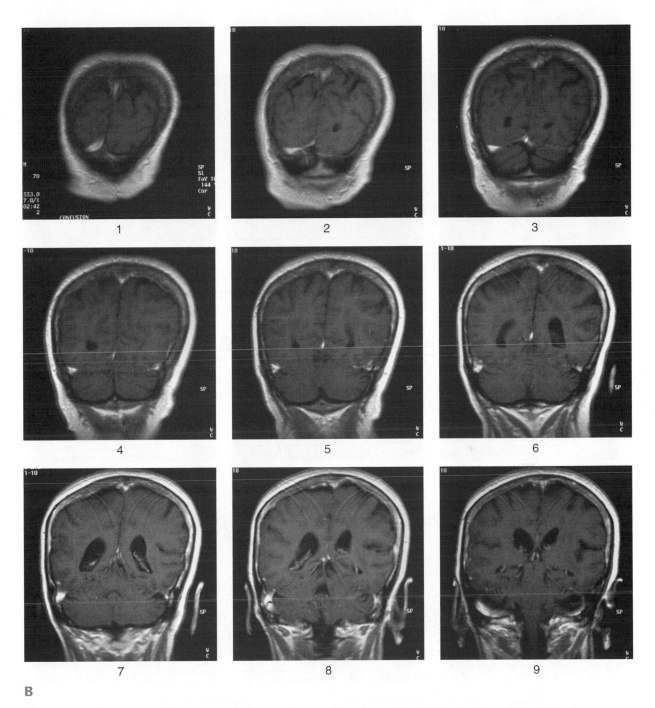

Figure 12-12. *(continued)* **B.** Magnetic resonance image of head, revealing brain structures. Note that a tumor emerges in the 12th slice, appearing lighter (denser) than the surrounding tissue. Note key to slice location in lower corner. *(continues)*

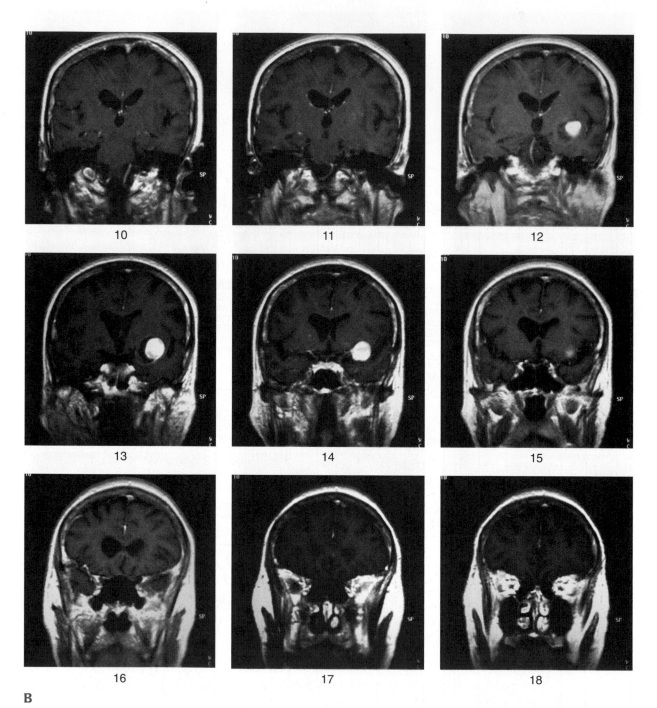

10	11	12
13	14	15
16	17	18

B

Figure 12-12. B. *(continued)*

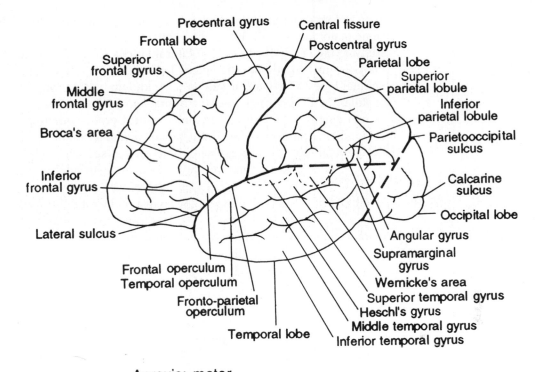

A

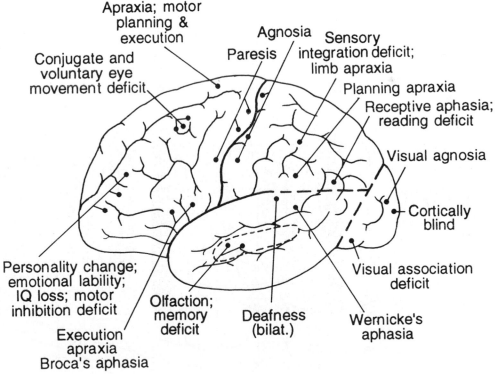

B

Figure 12-13. A. Landmarks of the left cerebral hemisphere. **B.** Effects upon function of lesion at different cerebral locations.

Before differentiating the lobes of the brain, it will help to identify some major landmarks. Two prominent sulci serve as benchmarks in our study of the cerebral cortex. The **lateral sulcus** (also known as the **Sylvian fissure**) divides the temporal lobe from the frontal and anterior parietal lobes. The **central sulcus** (also known as the **Rolandic sulcus** or **Rolandic fissure**) separates the frontal and parietal lobes entirely. The central sulcus is the very prominent vertical groove running from the cerebral longitudinal fissure to the lateral sulcus, terminating in the inferior parietal lobe. As you can see in the sagittal section of Figure 12-14, this sulcus does not extend far down the medial surface.

Frontal Lobe. The frontal lobe is the largest of the lobes, making up one-third of the cortex (see Figure 12-13). This lobe predominates in planning, initiation, and inhibition of voluntary motion, as well as cognitive function, as we shall see in Chapter 13. The frontal lobe is the anterior-most portion of the cortex, and is bounded posteriorly by the central sulcus. The inferior boundary is the lateral sulcus, and the medial boundary is the longitudinal fissure.

Three gyri run parallel to the longitudinal fissure in the frontal lobe. The **superior frontal gyrus** borders the longitudinal fissure and is

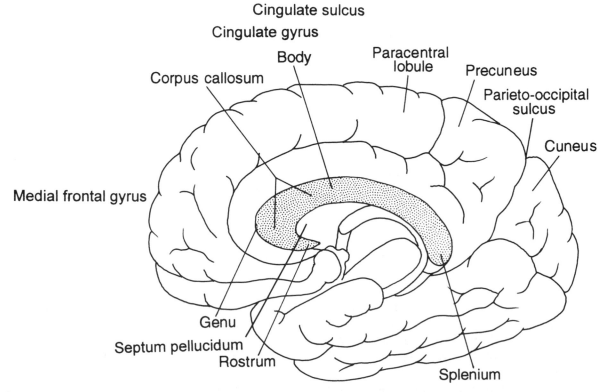

Figure 12-14. Medial surface of the cerebral cortex.

separated from the **middle frontal gyrus** by the **superior frontal sulcus**. The **inferior frontal gyrus** includes an extremely important region known as the **pars opercularis** or simply the **frontal operculum** (see Figure 12-13). This area overlies one of the "hidden lobes," the insular cortex. More importantly, the frontal operculum is more commonly referred to as **Broca's area**, an extremely important region for speech motor planning within the dominant hemisphere, as will be discussed in Chapter 13. Another important region of the inferior frontal gyrus is the **pars orbitale** or **orbital region**, the region of the inferior frontal gyrus overlying the eyes. The pars orbitale and anterior regions of the upper frontal lobe are associated with memory, emotion, motor inhibition, and intellect.

Another important landmark of the frontal lobe is the **precentral gyrus** or **motor strip**. It is anterior to the central sulcus (thus the name "*pre*-central"), and is the site of initiation of voluntary motor movement. Anterior to the motor strip is the premotor region, generally involved in motor planning. This region includes portions of the superior, middle, and inferior frontal lobes, but is indicated functionally as area 6 on the Brodmann map. The upper and medial portions of area 6 are called the **supplementary motor area (SMA)**. Axons from the motor strip and the supplementary motor areas give rise to the corticospinal and corticobulbar tracts, the major motor tracts of voluntary movement on the side of the body opposite to the area of the cortex giving the command. That is, a command arising from the left hemisphere to move the little finger will cause the finger of the right hand to twitch. We will discuss the mechanism for this **contralateral innervation** when we discuss the pathways of the brain.

The areas of the motor strip serving regions of the body have been well mapped. As you can see from Figure 12-15, different regions of the motor strip serve different regions of the body. The face, head, and laryngeal regions are on the far lateral edge, while the leg, thigh, and thorax are represented on the more medial surface of the superior cortex. If you compare this with the location of Broca's area on the side view of the hemisphere in Figure 12-13, you will see that these two regions are in close proximity. That is to say, you should begin to recognize that the area for motor function for the speech mechanisms (larynx, lips, facial muscles, muscles of mastication) is immediately adjacent to Broca's area, the region responsible for planning the motor act for speech. We will say more about the organization of this region in Chapter 13.

Parietal Lobe. Look at the parietal lobe in Figure 12-13. The parietal lobe is the primary reception site for somatic (body) sense. That is, all senses that reach consciousness terminate within the parietal lobe. The anterior boundary of the parietal lobe is the central sulcus, and the inferior boundary is the lateral sulcus. To define the posterior boundary, one must identify the **parieto-occipital sulcus** and draw an imaginary line to the **preoccipital notch**.

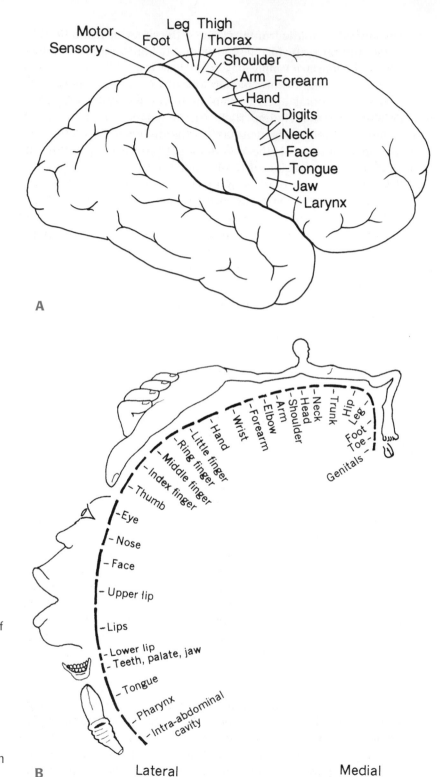

A

homunculus: *L., little man*

Figure 12-15. A. Right hemisphere, displaying regions of motor strip governing activation of specific muscle groups. **B. Homunculus** revealing areas of representation on the motor strip. Note that this represents a frontal section through the cerebral cortex. Size of structure drawn represents the degree of neural representation of the given structure (i.e., neural density).

B

Lateral   Medial

The **postcentral gyrus** is the sensory counterpart to the motor strip. The motor strip is the site of motor output, and the postcentral gyrus is the primary site of sensory input. This area receives somatic sensation from various body regions. Remember that motor function is spatially arrayed along the motor strip: The same is true for the postcentral gyrus. The distribution of sensory function by body region is quite close to that of the motor strip. Virtually all somesthetic sensation that reaches consciousness will terminate in this region, although the sensation from the left part of the body is projected to the right hemisphere.

Posterior to the postcentral gyrus is the **postcentral sulcus**, providing the anterior margin for the **superior** and **inferior parietal lobules**, separated by the **intraparietal sulcus**. The inferior parietal lobule is an important cortical **association area**, integrating information related to vision (from the occipital lobe), audition (from the temporal lobe), and somatic sense (from the parietal lobe). This inferior lobule is also quite important. It is divided into the **supramarginal** and **angular gyri**. The angular gyrus is particularly important in (but not solely responsible for) comprehension of written material. The supramarginal gyrus is involved in motor planning for speech.

Temporal Lobe. Find the temporal lobe on Figure 12-13. The temporal lobe is the site of auditory reception and is extraordinarily important for auditory and receptive language processing. It is bordered by the lateral sulcus medially, projecting back to the parietal and occipital lobes posteriorly.

The **superior temporal gyrus** runs posteriorly to the angular gyrus of the parietal lobe, and is separated from the **middle temporal gyrus** by the **superior temporal sulcus**. The superior temporal gyrus is of profound importance in both speech-language pathology and audiology. If you look at the upper surface of the superior temporal lobe (area 41) you will see **Heschl's gyrus**, the location of the brain to which all auditory information is projected. The region actually includes a portion of the medial surface of the temporal lobe. Lateral to Heschl's gyrus is area 42, a higher-order processing region for auditory stimulation. The posterior portion of the superior temporal gyrus is the functionally defined region known as **Wernicke's area**. Damage to this area of the dominant hemisphere results in disturbances of spoken language decoding, often profound. The middle temporal gyrus and inferior temporal gyrus are regions of higher-level processing. The inferior temporal gyrus lies within the middle fossa of the skull.

Occipital Lobe. Identify the occipital lobe on Figure 12-13. The occipital lobe is the posterior limit of the brain. The occipital lobe is the region responsible for receiving visual stimulation, as well as some of the higher-level visual processing. The occipital lobe rests on the tentorium cerebelli discussed previously, with its anterior margin being the parieto-occipital sulcus. The regions surrounding the **calcarine sulcus** are the

cuneus: *L., wedge*

insula: *L., island*

primary reception areas for visual information. The calcarine sulcus and **parieto-occipital sulcus** mark the boundaries of the wedge-shaped cuneus. Lateral to the calcarine sulcus is the **lingual gyrus**.

Insula.   Find the insular cortex on Figure 12-10. The insular cortex, or **island of Reil**, is located deep to a region of the cerebrum known as the operculum. The operculum consists of regions of the temporal lobe (medial areas 38, 41, 42), parietal lobe (inferior areas 1, 2, 3, and 40), and frontal lobes (areas 44, 45, and inferior 6) along the lateral sulcus. These regions, which overlie the insular cortex, are known as the **temporal operculum**, **fronto-parietal operculum**, and **frontal operculum**.
    To see the insular cortex, one would have to pull the temporal lobe laterally and lift up the frontal and parietal opercula. Upon doing that, you would see the **circular sulcus** that surrounds the insula, deep in the lateral sulcus. The **central sulcus of the insula** divides the insula into anterior short gyri and a single posterior long gyrus.

Limbic Lobe.   The limbic lobe is not an anatomically distinct region, but one arising from functional relationships associated with motivation, sex drive, emotional behavior, and affect. The limbic lobe includes the uncus (formed by the amygdala), parahippocampal gyrus, cingulate gyrus, and olfactory bulb and tract, as well as the hippocampal formation and the dentate gyrus, structures we shall discuss again (see Figure 12-16).

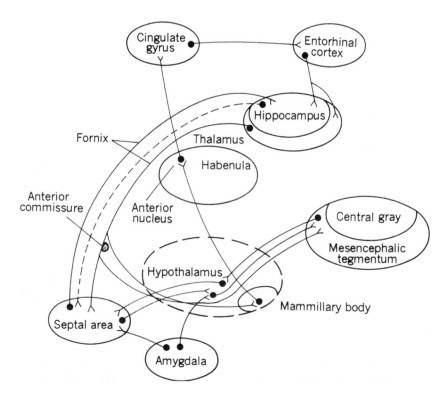

Figure 12-16. Schematic of components of the limbic system. (Modified from Carpenter, 1991.)

To summarize, the **cerebrum** is divided into two grossly similar, mirror-image **hemispheres** that are connected by means of the massive **corpus callosum**.

- The **gyri** and **sulci** of the hemispheres provide important landmarks for lobes and other regions of the cerebrum.
- The **temporal lobe** is the site of **auditory reception** and **Wernicke's area**.
- The temporal lobe is the prominent lateral lobe separated from the parietal and frontal lobes by the **lateral fissure**.
- The anterior-most region is the **frontal lobe**, the site of most voluntary **motor activation** and the important speech region known as **Broca's area**.
- Adjacent to the frontal lobe is the **parietal lobe**, the region of **somatic sensory reception**.
- The **occipital lobe** is the most posterior of the regions, and is the site of **visual input** to the cerebrum.
- The **insular lobe** is revealed by deflecting the temporal lobe and lies deep in the **lateral sulcus**.
- The **operculum** overlies the insula, and the functionally defined **limbic lobe** includes the **cingulate gyrus**, **uncus**, **parahippocampal gyrus**, and other deep structures.

Medial Surface of Cerebral Cortex

Viewing a sagittal section of the brain reveals a number of extremely important landmarks. As you can see from Figure 12-14, the **corpus callosum** (literally, "large body") is the large, dominating structure immediately inferior to the cerebral gray matter. The corpus callosum is the "information superhighway" of the brain. It provides communication concerning sensation and memory among the diverse regions of the two hemispheres by means of myelinated fibers. That is to say, any information arising in the left postcentral gyrus will be potentially shared by the right postcentral gyrus, so that each hemisphere "knows" what the other one knows.

corpus callosum: *L., large (or hard) body*

The corpus callosum makes up the roof of the lateral ventricles and the floor of the cerebral longitudinal fissure. The corpus callosum is divided into four major regions: rostrum, genu, body, and splenium. Fibers that course from one hemisphere to the other through the **genu** serve the anterior frontal lobes. Fibers of the posterior frontal lobes and parietal lobes course through the **body** (or **trunk**) of the corpus callosum. Information from the temporal and occipital lobes passes from one hemisphere to the other by means of the **splenium**.

genu: *L., knee*

Now look at the paracentral lobule in Figure 12-14. The **paracentral lobule** is in the superior aspect of the medial cortex. This landmark is the reflected union of the precentral and postcentral gyri of the frontal and parietal lobes, respectively. Posterior to the paracentral lobule is the **precuneus**, which is separated from the **cuneus** by the **parieto-occipital sulcus**. The **cingulate gyrus**, a major structure of the limbic system, dominates the region immediately superior to the corpus callosum.

Inferior Surface of Cerebral Cortex

Figure 12-17 shows the inferior cerebral cortex. The anterior portion is the **orbital surface** of the frontal lobe, so called because it is above the eyes and optic pathways. You can also see the inferior surface of the temporal lobe. In the posterior aspect is the inferior surface of the occipital lobe. Let us look at some of the landmarks of that region.

The **olfactory sulcus** is superior to the olfactory tract and bulb. As we will discuss, the olfactory mechanisms relay information concerning smell from the sensors within the nasal mucosa to the brain. The

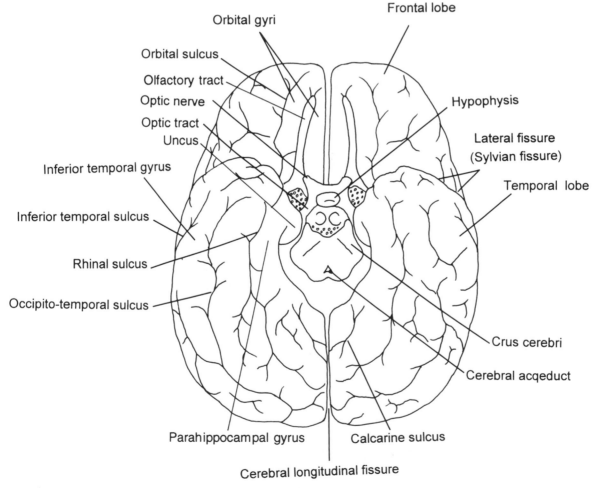

Figure 12-17. Inferior surface of the cerebral cortex.

parahippocampal gyrus is the medial-most portion of the cerebral cortex. This gyrus and the prominence known as the **uncus** combine with the lateral olfactory stria to make up the primary olfactory cortex, also known as the **pyriform lobe**. Within the parahippocampal gyrus is the important **hippocampus**, a structure deeply involved in memory.

From this view you can also see the undersurface of the inferior temporal gyrus and the calcarine sulcus of the occipital lobe. Visible also is the splenium of the corpus callosum, as well as the cerebral aqueduct, discussed with ventricles. Note also the pituitary gland or **hypophysis**, an important structure for autonomic regulation mediated by the hypothalamus.

Myelinated Fibers

The gray matter of the cortex is made up predominantly of neuron bodies, while the **white matter** of the brain represents myelinated axon fibers. These fibers make up the communication link among the neurons, and without them there would be no neural function. In diseases that cause **demyelination** of the fibers, dysfunction of the areas served is virtually guaranteed.

There are three basic types of fibers: projection fibers, association fibers, and commissural fibers.

Projection Fibers. The tracts running to and from the cortex to the brainstem and the spinal cord are made up of **projection fibers**. Projection fibers connect the cortex with distant locations. The **corona radiata** is a mass of projection fibers running from and to the cortex (see Figure 12-18). It condenses as it courses down, forming an "L" shape as it reaches a location known as the **internal capsule**. The **anterior limb** of

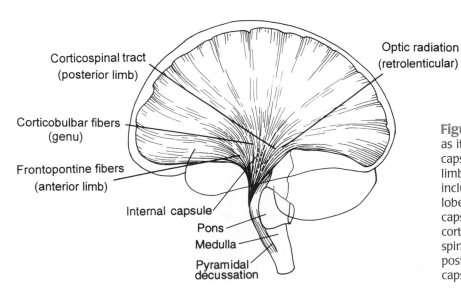

Figure 12-18. Corona radiata as it passes through the internal capsule. Note that the anterior limb of the internal capsule includes fibers from the frontal lobe, and the genu of the internal capsule includes fibers of the corticobulbar tract. The corticospinal tract passes through the posterior limb of the internal capsule.

Corticospinal tract (posterior limb)

Optic radiation (retrolenticular)

Corticobulbar fibers (genu)

Frontopontine fibers (anterior limb)

Internal capsule

Pons

Medulla

Pyramidal decussation

the internal capsule separates the caudate nucleus and the putamen of the basal ganglia, and serves the frontal lobe. The **posterior limb** includes the **optic radiation**, which is a group of fibers projecting to the calcarine sulcus for vision. Nearly all of the *afferent* fibers within the corona radiata arise from the thalamus, the major sensory relay of the brain. The point of juncture of the anterior and posterior limbs is called the **genu**. *Efferent* fibers from the cortex make up the motor tracts. We will discuss these tracts shortly.

Association Fibers. The second group of fibers consists of **association fibers**. Association fibers provide communication between regions of the same hemisphere. That is, association fibers may connect the superior temporal gyrus with the middle temporal gyrus within the left hemisphere.

There are both long and short association fibers. **Short association fibers** connect neurons of one gyrus to the next, traversing the sulcus. The **long association fibers** interconnect the lobes of the brain within the same hemisphere. The **uncinate fasciculus** connects the orbital portion, inferior, and middle frontal gyri with the anterior temporal lobe. The extremely important **arcuate fasciculus** permits the superior and middle frontal gyri to communicate with the temporal, parietal, and occipital lobes. A lesion of the arcuate fasciculus can result in **conduction aphasia**, in which expressive and receptive language remain essentially intact but the individual remains unable to repeat information presented auditorily. The **cingulum**, the white matter of the **cingulate gyrus**, connects the frontal and parietal lobes with the parahippocampal gyrus and temporal lobe.

Commissural Fibers. The third group of fibers is the **commissural fibers**. The corpus callosum is the major group of commissural fibers. Commissural fibers run from one location on a hemisphere to the corresponding

Amyotrophic Lateral Sclerosis

There are a number of **demyelinating diseases**, conditions that cause degeneration of the brain myelin. **Amyotrophic lateral sclerosis**, a form of motor neuron disease, is a progressive, demyelinating condition of unknown etiology with a typical course of two to five years from date of diagnosis to death. Patients, typically in their fourth to fifth decade of life, experience initial weakness in a limb, with fatigue and cramping. As the disease progresses, limb function is lost, although sensory function typically is retained. Motor symptoms indicate both upper and lower motor neuron degeneration, thereby sometimes producing symptoms of spasticity alternating with flaccidity. As the myelin deteriorates, it is replaced with a sclerosis or a covering of hardened tissue that markedly increases neural conduction time. In the later stages of the disease, the patient experiences difficulty with respiration, requiring alteration of posture to accommodate reduced ability to work against gravity. The patient eventually will experience dysphagia and paralysis of the muscles of speech while retaining full cognitive function.

location on the other hemisphere, such as from the supramarginal gyrus of the left parietal lobe to the supramarginal gyrus of the right parietal lobe. We have already discussed one of the groups of commissural fibers, the corpus callosum. Another important group of fibers makes up the **anterior commissure**. The anterior commissure crosses between hemispheres to connect the right and left olfactory areas, as well as portions of the inferior and middle temporal gyri.

Anatomy of the Subcortex

Basal Ganglia. The basal ganglia (or basal nuclei) are a group of cell bodies intimately related to control of background movement and initiation of movement patterns. The ganglia included under the broader term of basal ganglia include the **caudate nucleus** (including head, body, and tail), the **putamen**, and the **globus pallidus**. Some consider the **amygdaloid body** (or **amygdala**) to be part of the basal ganglia, but it is generally included within the limbic system. Functionally, the **subthalamic nuclei** and **substantia nigra** may be included as well, because of their central role in basal ganglia activity.

Visualizing the basal ganglia is somewhat of a challenge. The relationship of the parts may be seen in Figure 12-19. The **head of the caudate**

> **caudate nucleus:** *L., caudatus, tail*

> **putamen:** *L., shell*

> **globus pallidus:** *L., white (or pale) globe*

> **amygdaloid body:** *L., amygdalinus, almond*

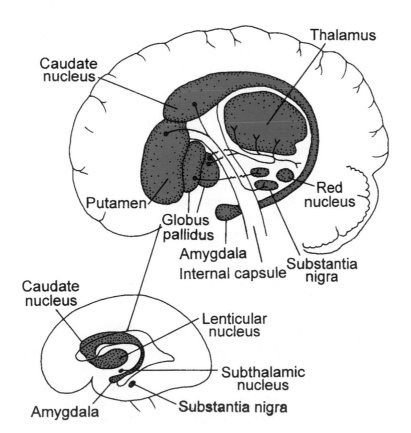

Figure 12-19. The basal ganglia consist of the caudate nucleus, amygdala, globus pallidus, and putamen. The basal ganglia are shown in relation to the other subcortical structures, including the diencephalic thalamus and hypothalamus, as well as the red nucleus and substantia nigra.

nucleus is anteriorly placed, the **body** courses up and back, and the **tail** curves down. The **amygdaloid body** is adjacent to the tail, but does not fuse with it. The **globus pallidus** and **putamen** attach to and reflect back on the caudate body.

The combination of globus pallidus and putamen is referred to as the **lentiform** or **lenticular nucleus** because their combined nuclei are lens-shaped. The putamen and caudate nucleus together are referred to as the **striatum**. The **corpus striatum** includes the striatum (putamen and caudate) and globus pallidus. (The corona radiata forming the internal capsule perforates the caudate and putamen, giving a striped appearance—hence the term "striated body.")

Within the brain, the lentiform nucleus (globus pallidus and putamen) is lateral to the internal capsule, and the caudate is medial to the internal capsule. The head of the caudate protrudes into the anterior horn of the lateral ventricle. The body makes up a portion of the floor of the lateral ventricle and is lateral to the superior thalamus. The amygdaloid body lies in the roof of the inferior horn of the lateral ventricle. Lesions to the basal ganglia result in extrapyramidal dysfunction, including hyperkinetic and hypokinetic dysarthrias.

lentiform nucleus: *L., lentis, lens*

corpus striatum: *L., striped body*

Hippocampal Formation. The hippocampal formation is strongly implicated in memory function, and is part of the rhinencephalon. It communicates with the hypothalamus, which is related to visceral function and emotion, and to portions of the temporal lobe associated with memory function. As you can see from Figure 12-20, the hippocampal formation includes the parahippocampal gyrus and makes up a portion of the floor of the inferior horn of the lateral ventricle.

The **pes hippocampus** ("foot of the hippocampus") is the anterior projection of the hippocampus, and the **fimbria** of hippocampus is a medial layer of white fibers that are continuous with the fornix. The **fornix** is a near-circle of myelinated fibers terminating in the **mammillary body**, and provides most of the communication between the hippocampus and the hypothalamus. It contains commissural fibers that permit communication with the opposite hippocampus.

The **dentate gyrus** (dentate fascia) lies between the fimbria of the hippocampus and the parahippocampal gyrus, and continues as the indusium griseum. The **indusium griseum** is a layer of cell bodies that overlies the corpus callosum and becomes continuous with the cingulate gyrus.

pes hippocampus: *L., foot of hippocampus*

fimbria: *L., fringe*

fornix: *L., arch*

mammillary body: *L., mamillia, nipple*

dentate: *L., referring to tooth; notched; toothlike*

Diencephalic Structures. The diencephalon is composed of the thalamus, epithalamus, hypothalamus, and subthalamus. This is a small and compact region.

Thalamus. The paired thalami are the largest structures of the diencephalon and are the final, common relay for sensory information

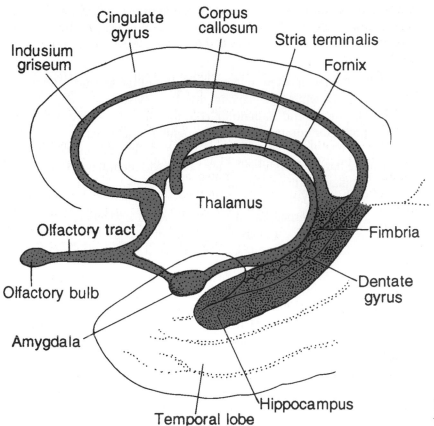

Figure 12-20. Orientation of the hippocampal formation.

directed toward the cerebral cortex. All sensation, with the exception of olfaction, passes through the thalamus, making it an exceedingly important region of the brain. Of those sensations, only pain (and possibly temperature) sense is consciously perceived at the thalamus, but pain cannot be localized without cortical function.

The **reticular activating system** that arises from the thalamus is the functional system responsible for arousing the cortex, and perhaps for focusing cortical regions to heightened awareness. In addition, the thalamus is the primary bridge for information from the cerebellum and globus pallidus to the motor portion of the cerebral cortex. Each of the nuclei that communicate with a cortical region also receives efferent, corticothalamic projections from the same region.

The thalami form a portion of the lateral walls of the 3rd ventricle, and are separated from the globus pallidus and putamen by the internal capsule. Fibers from the thalamus project to the cortex via the internal capsule and corona radiata. The thalamus is composed of 26 nuclei in 3 regions defined by the internal medullary lamina.

Thalamic nuclei may be organized into functional categories. **Specific thalamic nuclei** communicate with specific regions of the cerebral cortex. **Association nuclei** communicate with association areas of the cortex. **Subcortical nuclei** have no direct communication with the cerebral cortex.

Epithalamus. The most prominent structures of the epithalamus include the pineal body, which is a gland involved in development of gonads, the **habenular nuclei** and **habenular commissure**, the **striae medularis**, and the **posterior commissure**. The habenular nuclei receive input from the septum, hypothalamus, brainstem, raphe nuclei, and ventral tegmental area via the habenulopeduncular tract and stria medullaris. Connections with the thalamus, hypothalamus, and septal area from the habenular nuclei are via the habenulopeduncular tract (fasciculus retroflexus), terminating in the interpeduncular nucleus, which projects to those structures. The posterior commissure consists of decussating fibers of the superior colliculi, nuclei associated with visual reflexes.

Subthalamus. The major landmark of the subthalamus is the **subthalamic nucleus**, a lentiform structure on the inner surface of the internal capsule. Many fibers project through the subthalamus en route to the thalamus. The subthalamus receives input from the globus pallidus and the motor cortex and is involved in control of striated muscle. Lesions to it have been known to produce the violent, uncontrolled flailing movements of arms and legs known as **ballism**. Unilateral lesion produces **hemiballism** of the contralateral side.

Hypothalamus. The hypothalamus makes up the floor of the 3rd ventricle. Although it is comprised of numerous nuclei, it is generally divided into preoptic, mammillary, and tuberal regions (see Figure 12-21). The hypothalamus provides the organizational structure for the **limbic system**. Through interaction with the other components of this system (cingulate gyrus, septal area, parahippocampal gyrus, amygdala, and hippocampal formation), the hypothalamus regulates reproductive behavior and physiology, desire or perception of need for food and water, perception of satiation, control of digestive processes, and metabolic functions (including maintenance of water balance and body temperature). Damage to the hypothalamus can result in loss of appropriate autonomic responses, such as heart rate acceleration and sweating, shivering when cold, or even moving to a warmer environment when cold. Damage to the **satiety center** will result in voracious eating, whereas damage to the **feeding center** will result in starvation and dehydration. This structure is involved in the behavioral manifestations associated with emotion (tearing, heart rate acceleration, sweating, gooseflesh, flushing, mouth dryness), although it is assumed that cortical function is an important intermediary in normal emotional response.

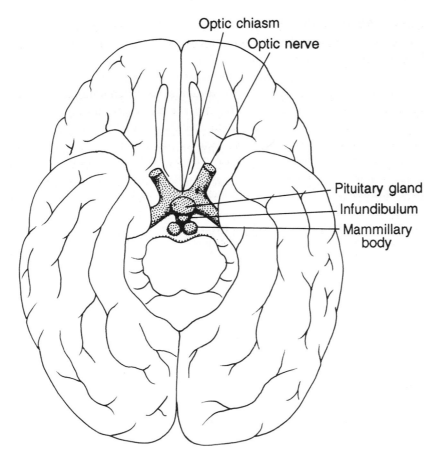

Figure 12-21. Structures of the hypothalamus visible from an inferior view.

In summary, the structures underlying the cerebral cortex are vital to modification of information arriving at or leaving the cerebral cortex.

- The **basal ganglia** are subcortical structures involved in control of **movement**, while the **hippocampal formation** of the inferior temporal lobe is deeply implicated in **memory** function.

- The **thalamus** of the **diencephalon** is the final relay for **somatic sensation** directed toward the cerebrum, and for other diencephalic structures.

- The **subthalamus** interacts with the globus pallidus to control **movement**, and the **hypothalamus** controls many bodily functions and desires.

- The regions of the cerebral cortex are interconnected by means of a complex network of **projection fibers**, connecting the cortex with other structures; **association fibers**, which connect regions of the same hemisphere; and **commissural fibers**, which provide communication between corresponding regions of the two hemispheres.

Cerebrovascular System

Although the brain makes up only 2% of the body weight, it consumes an enormous 20% of the oxygen transported by the vascular system to meet the high metabolic requirements of nervous tissue. The vascular system of the brain (the **cerebrovascular system**) maintains the constant circulation required by the nervous system. Disruption of this supply for even a few seconds will begin cellular changes in neurons, and longer vascular deprivation results in devastating effects.

The vascular supply of the brain arises from the carotid and vertebral branches, both of which originate from the aorta. The **carotid division** arises from left and right **internal carotid arteries** which enter the brain lateral to the optic chiasm. The internal carotid arteries give rise to the **anterior** and **middle cerebral arteries**.

The anterior cerebral artery courses along the superior surface of the corpus callosum within the medial longitudinal fissure (see Figure 12-22). It branches to supply the medial surface of the frontal and parietal lobes, corpus callosum, basal ganglia, and the anterior limb of the internal capsule.

The middle cerebral artery courses laterally along the inferior surface of the brain and through the lateral (Sylvian) fissure. It provides blood to the lateral surface of the hemispheres, including the temporal lobe, motor strip, Broca's area, Wernicke's area, sensory reception regions, and association areas. One branch of the middle cerebral artery serves the basal ganglia and internal capsule.

The **vertebral division** arises from the vertebral arteries that ascend on the anterior surface of the medulla oblongata. The vertebral artery branches, forming the descending **anterior** and **posterior spinal arteries**. The left and right vertebral arteries continue to ascend the ventral surface of the brainstem, joining at the superior medulla to form the **basilar artery**. The **superior cerebellar** and **anterior inferior cerebellar arteries** branch from the basilar artery to serve those locations of the cerebellum. (The **posterior inferior cerebellar artery** arises from the vertebral artery prior to this branching.) At the superior ventral pons, the basilar artery divides to become the left and right **posterior cerebral arteries**.

The posterior cerebral artery serves the inferior temporal and occipital lobes, the medial occipital lobe and primary visual cortex, upper midbrain, diencephalon, and cerebellum.

Circle of Willis. The cerebrovascular system of the brain contains many redundancies to ensure constant blood supply to the brain. The most prominent of these is the **circle of Willis**, a series of **anastomoses** (points of communication between arteries) that completely encircles the optic chiasm. If you will look again at Figure 12-22, you can see that the anterior cerebral arteries are connected by means of the **anterior communicating artery**, and the **posterior communicating artery** con-

Neuroanatomy **545**

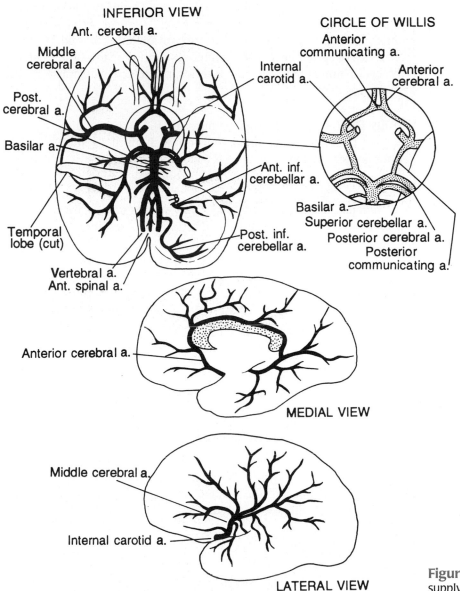

Figure 12-22. Major vascular supply of the cerebral cortex.

nects the middle cerebral artery with the posterior cerebral artery. This connects the vertebral and carotid systems, helps equalize locally high or low blood pressure, and promotes equal distribution of blood.

The anterior and posterior spinal arteries supply the spinal cord. The single anterior spinal artery descends in the anterior medial fissure of the spinal cord, giving off **radicular arteries** that serve the anterior spinal cord and anterior funiculus. The left and right posterior spinal arteries descend in similar fashion, also giving off radicular arteries.

Blood from the posterior spinal arteries serves the posterior funiculi and posterior horns, while that of the anterior spinal artery serves the anterior spinal cord. Radicular arteries from anterior and posterior arteries serve spinal nerves. Anastomoses with the vertebral, posterior intercostal, lumbar, and sacral arteries provide a safeguard against vascular accident.

Venous Drainage. The blood supply for the brain requires a return route for blood that has circulated and exchanged its nutrients. The **venous system** is the system of blood vessels called *veins* which provide the means of draining carbon-dioxide–laden blood to the lungs for reoxygenation.

Venous drainage is accomplished by means of a series of superficial and deep cisterns. Superficial drainage empties into the superior sagittal sinus and transverse sinus. Deep drainage is by means of the inferior sagittal sinus, the straight sinus, transverse sinuses, and the sigmoid sinus. Blood returns to the general bloodstream by means of the jugular veins, and spinal cord drainage is by means of radicular veins.

Obstruction of the cerebrovascular supply typically occurs in one of two ways. A **thrombus** is a foreign body (such as a clot of blood or bubble of air) that obstructs a blood vessel, and that obstruction is called a **thrombosis**. If the thrombus breaks loose from its site of formation and floats through the bloodstream, it becomes an **embolus**, or floating clot. An **embolism** is an obstruction of a blood vessel by that foreign body brought to the point of occlusion by blood flow. **Aneurysm** is a dilation or ballooning of a blood vessel due to weak walls. When an intracranial aneurysm ruptures, the blood is released into the space surrounding the brain, in most cases, because most aneurysms occur in arteries rather than capillaries. The pressure associated with both development of the ballooning aneurysm and the sudden release of blood into the cranial cavity is life-threatening, with sites of neural damage being related to the location of the rupture.

Occlusion of the anterior cerebral artery is infrequent, but may result in hemiplegia, loss of some sensory function, and personality change. Occlusion of the middle cerebral artery is the most common and can result in severe disability because of the critical nature of the areas served. In addition to severe unilateral or bilateral motor and sensory deficit, left-hemisphere damage to Broca's area, Wernicke's area, and association areas may produce profound aphasia. Posterior cerebral artery occlusion produces variable deficit that may include memory dysfunction.

In summary, the **cerebrovascular system** is the literal lifeblood of the brain.

- The **anterior cerebral arteries** serve the medial surfaces of the brain, while the **middle cerebral artery** serves the lateral cortex, including the temporal lobe, motor strip, Wernicke's area, and much of the parietal lobe.

- The **vertebral arteries** branch to form the anterior and posterior spinal arteries, with ascending components serving the ventral brainstem.

- The **basilar artery** gives rise to the **superior** and **anterior inferior cerebellar arteries** to serve the cerebellum, while the **posterior inferior cerebellar artery** arises from the **vertebral artery**.

- The basilar artery divides to become the **posterior cerebral arteries**, serving the inferior temporal and occipital lobes, upper midbrain, and diencephalon.

- The **circle of Willis** is a series of communicating arteries that provides redundant pathways for blood flow to regions of the cerebral cortex, equalizing pressure and flow of blood.

- Obstruction of the blood supply is always critical. A foreign body within the blood vessel (**thrombus**) creates an obstruction to blood flow (**thrombosis**), or becomes an **embolus** when released into the bloodstream.

- An **aneurysm** is a ballooning of a blood vessel, and rupture of an aneurysm results in blood being released into the region of the brain.

- The **middle cerebral artery** is the most common site of occlusion; the result may be significant language and speech deficit if the occlusion involves the dominant cerebral hemisphere.

Cerebellum

The cerebellum is the largest component of the hindbrain, resting within the posterior cranial fossa, immediately inferior to the posterior cerebral cortex. The cerebellum is responsible for coordinating motor commands with sensory inputs to control movement, and it communicates with the brainstem, spinal cord, and cerebral cortex by means of superior, middle, and inferior cerebellar peduncles.

From behind, one can see that the cerebellum is composed of two hemispheres and is prominently invested with horizontal grooves. As you can see from the posterior view of Figure 12-23, the **primary fissure** separates the cerebellar **cortex** into two lobes (by the way, you now realize that the term "cortex" is not specific to the cerebral cortex). The **anterior lobe** is often referred to as the *superior lobe*, and the **middle lobe** is known also as the *inferior lobe*. The vermis separates the two hemispheres and aids in defining the **intermediate** and **lateral** cerebellar regions of the posterior surface.

vermis: *L., worm*

To view the cerebellum from the front, one must remove it from the brainstem. The anterior surface reveals the third lobe of the cerebellum, the **flocculonodular lobe**, made up of the right and left **flocculi** and

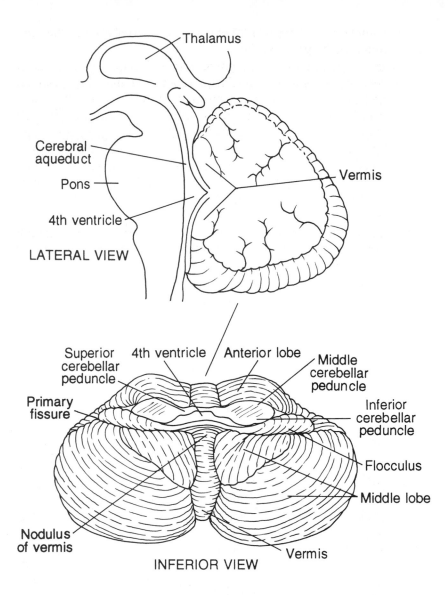

Figure 12-23. Cerebellum as seen in sagittal section and from beneath.

paleocerebellum: *Gr., paleo, old cerebellum*

neocerebellum: *Gr., neo, new cerebellum*

central **nodulus**. The prominent **middle cerebellar peduncle** is between the **superior** and **inferior cerebellar peduncles**.

The cerebellum may be divided functionally into three regions. The flocculonodular lobe is functionally referred to as the **vestibulocerebellum** (or **archicerebellum**), while the **spinocerebellum** (or **paleocerebellum**) is the anterior lobe and the portion of the posterior lobe associated with the arm and leg. The posterior lobes and the intermediate vermis make up the **neocerebellum** (or **pontocerebellum**).

The inner cerebellum is faintly reminiscent of the cerebral cortex. The outer cortex is a dense array of neurons, and beneath this is a mass of white communicating axons. At the center of the white fibers is a series of nuclei serving as relays between the cerebellum and the communicating regions of the body.

The cerebellar cortex is composed of three layers, the outer **molecular layer**, the intermediate **Purkinje layer**, and the deep **granular layer** (see Figure 12-24). The outer molecular layer contains **Golgi, basket**, and **stellate cells**, and the intermediate layer contains **Purkinje cells**. Purkinje cells are large neurons forming the boundary between the molecular and granular layers of the cortex. Axons of the 15 million Purkinje cells project to the central cerebellar nuclei. Excitation of a Purkinje cell causes inhibition of the nucleus with which it communicates. Golgi cells project their dendrites into the molecular layer and their axons into the granular layer. Their soma receive input from both climbing fibers and Purkinje cells, and the axons synapse with granule cell dendrites. Basket cells and stellate cells arborize to communicate with Purkinje cells.

Climbing fibers arising from the inferior olivary nuclei pass through the inner granular layer to communicate with the Purkinje cells. These fibers are strongly excitatory to Purkinje cells. Granule cells within this

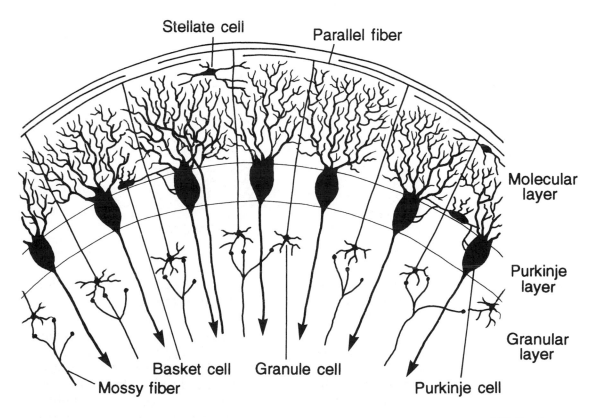

Figure 12-24. Cellular layers of the cerebellar cortex.

inner layer project axons to the outer layer where they divide into a "T" form. The branches course at roughly right angles to the base of the axon, synapsing with the dendritic arborization of the Purkinje cells. Activation of these granule cells excites basket and stellate cells but inhibits Purkinje cells. Projections from noncerebellar regions (spinal cord, brainstem, cerebral cortex) terminate in mossy fibers.

There are four pairs of nuclei within the cerebellum, all of which receive input from the Purkinje cells of the cortex (see Figure 12-25). The **dentate nucleus** has the appearance of a serrated sac, opening medially. Projections from this nucleus route through the superior cerebellar peduncle to synapse in the ventrolateral nucleus of the thalamus and from there ascend to the cerebral cortex by means of thalamocortical fibers. The **emboliform** and **globose nuclei** (collectively referred to as the **nucleus interpositus**) project to the red nucleus, providing input to

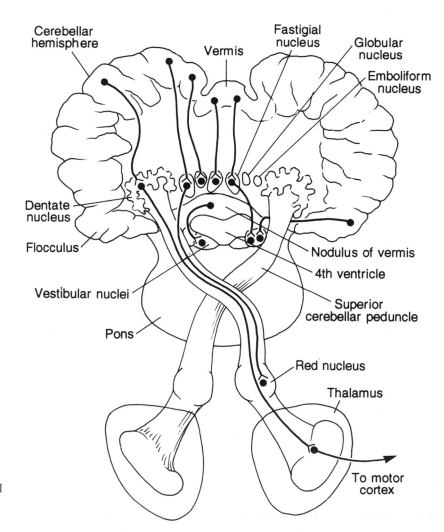

Figure 12-25. Schematic of cerebellar nuclei and interaction between cerebellum and cerebral cortex. (After view of Poritsky, 1992.)

the rubrospinal tract. The **fastigial nucleus** communicates with the vestibular nuclei of the brainstem, the reticular formation of the pons and medulla, and the inferior olive.

Tracts of the Cerebellum.   The **dorsal spinocerebellar tract** communicates sensation of temperature, proprioception (muscle spindle), and touch from the lower body and legs to the ipsilateral cerebellum. Afferents arise from the nucleus dorsalis (Clarke's column) in the spinal cord and project to both the anterior and posterior lobes of the cerebellum. The **cuneocerebellar tract** serves the same function for the arms and upper trunk, originating in the external cuneate nucleus of the cervical region and entering the cerebellum through the inferior cerebellar peduncle.

The **ventral spinocerebellar tract** transmits proprioception information (Golgi tendon organs) and pain sense from the legs and lower trunk to the ipsilateral cerebellar cortex. Fibers decussate within the spinal cord, ascend, enter through the superior cerebellar peduncle, and then decussate again to project to the cortex. The **rostral spinocerebellar tract** is the cervical parallel of the ventral spinocerebellar tract, serving the upper trunk and arm region.

Pontocerebellar fibers from the pontine nuclei provide the greatest input to the cerebellum as they cross midline and ascend as the middle cerebellar peduncle to terminate as mossy fibers. **Olivocerebellar fibers** from the inferior olivary and medial accessory olivary nucleus of the medulla project to the contralateral cerebellum, terminating as climbing fibers. The olive receives input from the spinal cord, cerebral cortex, and red nucleus, as well as visual information. All other tracts of the cerebellum terminate on mossy fibers. The **vestibulocerebellar** tract provides input from the vestibular nuclei to the flocculonodular lobe via the inferior peduncles.

The **corticopontine** projection is an important feedback system for control of voluntary movement. Projections from parietal, occipital, temporal, and frontal lobes (including the motor cortex) synapse on the pontine nuclei, projecting via pontocerebellar fibers to the opposite cerebellar cortex. The mossy fiber terminations synapse with granule cells, the branches of which synapse with Purkinje cell dendrites. The Purkinje cells synapse with the dentate nucleus, which projects back to the cerebellar cortex as well as to the motor cortex of the cerebrum via the superior cerebellar peduncle and thalamus. In this way the command for voluntary movement can be modified relative to body position, muscle tension, muscle movement, and so on.

Cerebellar Peduncles.   The superior cerebellar peduncle (brachium conjunctivum) arises in the anterior cerebellar hemisphere, coursing through the lateral wall of the 4th ventricle to decussate within the pons at the level of the inferior colliculi. Many tracts are served by this peduncle. **Dentatothalamic** fibers arise from the dentate nucleus and synapse in the opposite red nucleus and thalamus. The ventral spinocerebellar tract ascends within this peduncle, and fibers from the fastigial nucleus descend in conjunction with this peduncle as they course to the lateral vestibular nucleus. The **middle cerebellar peduncle** (brachium pontis) is made up of fibers projecting from the contralateral pontine nuclei. The **inferior cerebellar peduncle** (restiform body) communicates input from the spinocerebellar tracts to the cerebellum, exiting the brainstem at the upper medulla.

Cerebellar Function. Cerebellar function may be reasonably partitioned according to the portions of the cerebellum. The flocculonodular lobe (archicerebellum) is the oldest component and is responsible for orientation of the body in space. It receives input from the vestibular nuclei of the brainstem. Damage to this portion of the cerebellum will result in trunk ataxia, staggering, and generally reduced response to motion (as in reduced vestibular responses or motion sickness).

The newer anterior (superior) lobe (the paleocerebellum) exerts moderating control over antigravity muscles. Damage can result in increased stretch reflexes of support musculature. The "young" posterior (inferior) lobe (neocerebellum) is responsible for stopping or damping movements, especially those of the hands. Damage to this lobe will result in problems with fine movements, dysmetria (inability to control the range of movement), tremor associated with voluntary movement, and trouble with performing alternating movement tasks (such as oral diadochokinetic tasks). One can see gait deficits and hypotonia as well.

The cerebellum is a vital "silent partner" in integration of body movement with the internal and external environment of the body. Although it is incapable of initiating movement, it is intimately related to control of the rate and range of movement, as well as the force with which that movement is executed.

To summarize, the **cerebellum** is responsible for **coordinating motor commands** with sensory inputs, communicating with the brainstem, cerebrum, and spinal cord.

- The cerebellum is divided into **anterior**, **middle**, and **flocculonodular lobes**, and communicates with the rest of the nervous system via the **superior**, **middle**, and **inferior cerebral peduncles**.
- The **flocculonodular** lobe coordinates position in space via the **vestibular nuclei**.
- The **anterior lobe** coordinates **postural adjustment** against gravity, and the **posterior lobe** mediates **fine motor** adjustments.
- The **cerebellar cortex** consists of an **outer molecular layer**, a **Purkinje layer**, and a deep **granular layer**.
- The **Golgi**, **basket**, **stellate**, and **Purkinje cells** are responsible for coordinating input received from the nervous system.

Four pairs of nuclei are found in the cerebellum.

- The sacklike **dentate nucleus** projects output through the **superior cerebellar peduncle** to the **red nucleus**, **thalamus**, and ultimately the **cerebral cortex**.
- The **emboliform** and **globose nuclei** project to the **inferior olive** via the **red nucleus**, with information ultimately reaching the **contralateral cerebellar hemisphere**.
- The **fastigial nucleus** communicates with the **vestibular nuclei**.

Several tracts provide conduit to and from the cerebellum.

- The **dorsal spinocerebellar** and **cuneocerebellar tracts** communicate proprioception (muscle spindle), temperature, and touch sense from the lower and upper body to the cerebellum.
- The **ventral spinocerebellar** and **rostral spinocerebellar tracts** mediate ipsilateral proprioceptive information (Golgi tendon organ) and pain sense from the lower and upper body.
- The **olivocerebellar tract** mediates information received at the olivary complex from the spinal cord, cerebral cortex, red nucleus, and visual and cutaneous senses, and provides communication between cerebellar hemispheres.
- The **superior cerebellar peduncle** enters the pons at the level of the inferior colliculi, serving the dentate nucleus, red nucleus, and thalamus.
- The **middle cerebellar peduncle** consists of projections from the pontine nuclei, and the **inferior cerebellar peduncle** receives input from the spinocerebellar tracts, exiting at the upper medulla.

Anatomy of the Brainstem

The brainstem consists of the medulla oblongata, pons, and midbrain. The brainstem reflects an intermediate stage of organization, between the simple reflexive responses seen at the level of the spinal cord and the exquisitely complex responses generated by the cerebral cortex. Cranial nerves and their nuclei arise from the brainstem, and basic bodily functions for life are maintained here. We will work from the superficial to deep structures of the brainstem. It will help to refer to Figures 12-26 through 12-28 as we do this.

Superficial Brainstem Landmarks

Viewing the brainstem "from the outside" provides useful hints as to the structures housed within it. This is a good time to take a tour of the external form of this amazing part of the brain, before examining the internal structures. To do this, let us work from the lower reaches of the brainstem (medulla oblongata) to the upper portion (midbrain).

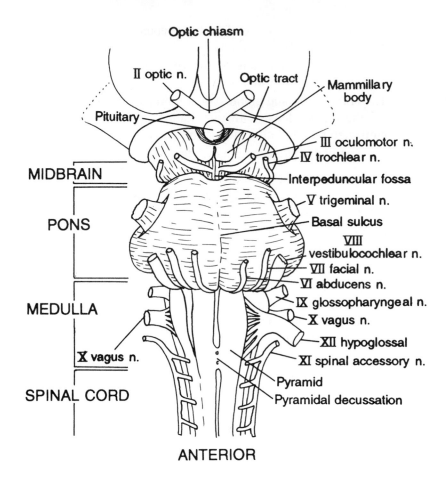

Optic chiasm

II optic n.

Optic tract

Mammillary body

Pituitary

III oculomotor n.

IV trochlear n.

MIDBRAIN

Interpeduncular fossa

V trigeminal n.

PONS

Basal sulcus

VIII vestibulocochlear n.

VII facial n.

VI abducens n.

IX glossopharyngeal n.

MEDULLA

X vagus n.

XII hypoglossal

X vagus n.

XI spinal accessory n.

Pyramid

Pyramidal decussation

SPINAL CORD

ANTERIOR

Figure 12-26. Anterior view of brainstem.

Superficial Medulla Oblongata. The **medulla oblongata**, or medulla, is the inferior-most segment of the brainstem. It looks like an enlargement of the upper spinal cord, and is about 2.5 cm long and 1 cm in diameter. This is a small-but-mighty structure: Damage to the medulla is imminently life-threatening.

Take a look at Figure 12-26 as we begin our discussion of the medulla. The **anterior (ventral) median fissure** of the spinal cord (to be discussed) continues through the medulla. There is an interruption in it, however, that marks a very important point for us. If you can find the **pyramidal decussation**, you will see the point within the medulla at which fibers of the corticospinal tract cross from one side to the other. That is, most of the axons carrying motor commands from the left hemisphere cross to the right side of the medulla to continue down through the spinal cord on the right side, and this is where that happens. The significance of this won't be lost on you if you remember meeting an individual with left-hemisphere stroke who had right-side hemiparesis. That is, unilateral paralysis signals a neuropathology on the side opposite the

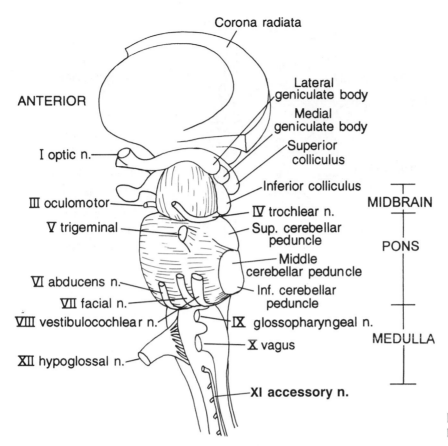

Figure 12-27. Lateral view of brainstem.

lesion. The point of decussation marks the lower border of the medulla, roughly at the level of the foramen magnum.

Now look at Figure 12-27 for a side view of the medulla. This is a good time to remind you that we are just looking at the external brain-stem, and that there are myriad structures within it that have a great impact on function. For instance, the sides of the medulla are marked by two prominent sulci. The **ventrolateral sulcus** marks the lateral margin of the pyramid, and is also the groove from which the **XII hypoglossal nerve** exits the medulla to innervate the muscles of the tongue (to be discussed). The **dorsolateral sulcus** is the groove from which the **XI accessory**, **X vagus**, and **IX glossopharyngeal nerves** exit. You can see from Figure 12-27 the spinal portion of the XI accessory nerve arising from the C2 through C5 spinal segments. If you recall Chapter 8 and the discussion of the auditory pathway, you may remember the inferior olivary complex. The **olive** is the bulge between the ventrolateral and dorsolateral sulci, caused by the **inferior olivary nuclear complex**, which consists of nuclei serving to localize sound in space.

Now let us look at the posterior surface of the medulla. In Figure 12-28, the cerebellum has been removed, revealing the 4th ventricle. As

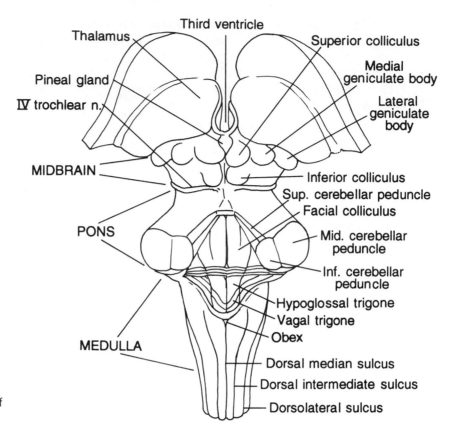

Figure 12-28. Posterior view of brainstem.

you recall, the ventricles provide a means for cerebrospinal fluid to be produced and to circulate through the central nervous system, and the 4th ventricle is the last of the series of ventricles. The 4th ventricle is the space between the cerebellum and brainstem, and by removing the cerebellum we can see several structures on the ventricle (dorsal) side of the brainstem that are otherwise hidden from view.

On Figure 12-28 you can see that the inferior-most point on the ventricle is the obex. The obex is a point that marks the beginning of a region known as the calamus scriptorius, so named because it looks like the point of a calligraphy pen. Lateral to the obex is the **clava** or **gracilis tubercle**, a bulge caused by the **nucleus gracilis**. As you shall see, one of the important afferent pathways is the fasciculus gracilis, and it terminates in the brainstem at the nucleus gracilis. To the side and a little above the clava is the **cuneate tubercle**, which is the prominence that marks the end point of the fasciculus cuneatus, to be discussed. Information concerning touch pressure, vibration, muscle stretch, and tension from the upper and lower extremities terminates at these two locations in the brainstem. As you can well imagine, focal damage to this region would affect sensation for the entire body.

The calamus scriptorius includes the **vagal trigone**, a bulge marking the dorsal vagal nucleus of the X vagus nerve, as well as the **hypoglossal trigone**, a prominence caused by the XII hypoglossal nucleus. You will remember the importance of the vagus nerve for phonation, because this is the nerve responsible for adducting, abducting, tensing, and relaxing the vocal folds (and so much more). You will also remember that the hypoglossal nerve activates the tongue muscles. A little reflection is all that is needed to realize the importance of the medulla for speech!

Superficial Pons.   The pons is above the medulla, serving as the "bridge" between medulla and midbrain, as well as to the cerebellum. The significant anterior bulge of the pons is an obvious landmark for this structure. The pons is the site of four cranial nerve nuclei, and is the origin of the middle and superior cerebellar peduncles, as we mentioned earlier. These peduncles serve as "superhighways" for communication with the cerebellum. At the junction of the medulla and the pons, the inferior cerebellar peduncle has expanded in diameter to its maximum and is entering the cerebellum.

Look once again at Figure 12-26. The anterior pons is marked by a prominent band of transverse fibers that provide communication between the cerebellum and the pons, the **pontocerebellar tract**. The **basal sulcus** is a prominent anterior landmark, because it marks the course of the vital basilar artery. The VI abducens nerve exits at the inferior border of the pons, from the **inferior pontine sulcus**. As you will learn, this nerve is important for rotating the eye outward, and a deficit in that ability serves as an indication to neurologists of the location of a lesion of the brainstem.

Now let us look at the lateral surface of the pons (Figure 12-27). You can see the middle **cerebellar peduncle (brachia pontis)**, which is the intermediate communicating attachment of the pons to the cerebellum. You may remember from your audiology coursework that one of the important functions of an audiologist is to help diagnose cerebellopontine angle tumors. The **cerebellopontine angle** is the space created by the cerebellum, the middle cerebellar peduncle, and the medulla oblongata. The VII facial and VIII vestibulocochlear nerves emerge from the cerebellopontine angle, so tumors at this location will cause sensorineural hearing loss, as well as facial paralysis. Also you will notice that the V trigeminal nerve exits the pons from the middle cerebellar peduncle of the lateral pons. You will recall that the trigeminal nerve is responsible for facial sensation and activation of the muscles of mastication.

The surface of the posterior pons marks the upper limit of the 4th ventricle. As can be seen in Figure 12-28, the **superior cerebellar peduncles (brachia conjunctiva)** form the upper lateral surface of the 4th ventricle, and the **superior** and **inferior medullary veli** and cerebellum provide the superior border. On either side of the median sulcus is a paired **facial colliculus**. The facial colliculus represents the location

colliculi: *L., mounds*

of the nucleus of the VI abducens nerve, as well as the place where the fibers of the VII cross that nucleus.

Superficial Midbrain. The superior-most structure of the brainstem is the midbrain. As you can see in Figure 12-26, the lower anterior surface of the midbrain is dominated by the prominent paired **crus cerebri**. These crura represent the **cerebral peduncles**, which house the communicating pathways leading to and from the cerebrum. Again, if you stop and think about it, a lesion to a small area in the midbrain could have devastating effects on the function of the entire body, because all of the motor fibers must pass through this crus.

Between the cerebral peduncles is an indentation known as the **interpeduncular fossa**. The III oculomotor nerve exits from this fossa, at the juncture between the pons and midbrain. The **optic tracts**, an extension of the optic nerve, course around the crus cerebri following the decussation at the **optic chiasm**. Once again, problems in visual function following stroke provide vital information to the neurologist about the site of a lesion, as we will discuss shortly.

Now turn your attention to the posterior midbrain (Figure 12-28). The posterior midbrain is the **tectum**. The tectum is behind the cerebral aqueduct, which is the upper extension of the 4th ventricle. There are four important landmarks on the tectum, known as the corpora quadrigemina. The corpora quadrigemina (literally "four bodies") are made up of the **superior** and **inferior colliculi**. As shown in this figure, the IV trochlear nerve emerges near the inferior colliculus and courses around the crus cerebri.

▶ **corpora quadrigemina:**
L., body of four parts

Deep Structure of Brainstem

An examination of the deep structure of the brainstem requires some patience and a good imagination. Similar to the spinal cord, the brainstem is organized vertically. It is made up of columnar nuclei and tracts that serve the periphery, spinal cord, cerebral, cerebellar, and subcortical structures. Referring to Figure 12-29 may help you with orientation as we discuss the brainstem. We will once again take you from the medulla to the level of the midbrain, this time looking at the deep structures of the brainstem.

Deep Structures of Medulla Oblongata. The deep structure of the medulla represents an expansion on developments that started in the spinal cord (see Figure 12-30). At the lowest regions of the medulla, the central canal makes a good reference point. This canal expands in the upper medulla to become the lower part of the 4th ventricle. Surrounding this canal is a zone of **central gray matter** containing nuclei, which expands to the **reticular formation**. The reticular formation is an important mass of nuclei that spans the medulla, pons, and midbrain. It is a composite of brainstem nuclei, forming the "oldest" part of the brain-

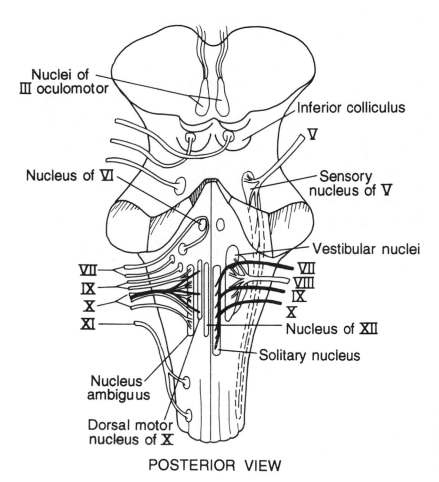

Nuclei of
III oculomotor

Inferior colliculus

V

Nucleus of VI

Sensory
nucleus of V

Vestibular nuclei

VII
IX
X
XI

VII
VIII
IX
X

Nucleus of XII

Solitary nucleus

Nucleus
ambiguus

Dorsal motor
nucleus of X

POSTERIOR VIEW

Figure 12-29. Posterior view of brainstem revealing orientation of major nuclei and cranial nerves supplied by those nuclei. (From views of Carpenter, 1991.)

stem and representing our first evolutionary effort at complex processing. This formation begins above the level of the decussation of the pyramids, and makes up the central structure of the brainstem. The reticular formation is extraordinarily important for life function, as it contains nuclei associated with respiration and maintenance of blood pressure.

At this lower level you can also see the **decussation of the pyramids**. As mentioned earlier, the pyramids represent the bundle of fibers that forms the corticospinal tracts. You will remember that the corticospinal tract is responsible for activation of skeletal muscle of the extremities, and commands to move those muscles arise from the cerebrum. Look again at Figure 12-25 to remind you that the pyramidal decussation is a visible blur on the anterior surface of the medulla. At the decussation, the fibers divide into **lateral** and **anterior corticospinal tracts**: The lateral tract forms after the fibers cross the midline, and the much smaller anterior tract is made up of uncrossed nerve fibers. This is also a good time to remember that motor commands originating in the

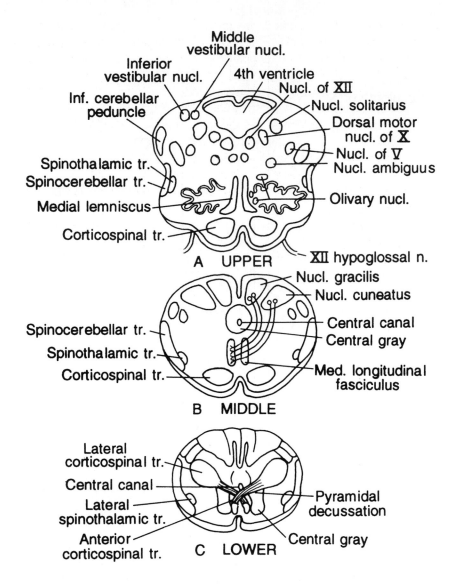

Figure 12-30. Low, mid, and upper medulla levels in a transverse schematic view.

left cerebrum activate muscles on the right side of the body. This decussation is the manifestation of that.

Looking again at Figure 12-30, you can see that the prominent fasciculus gracilis and cuneatus and their nuclei are in the posterior medulla. Information concerning kinesthetic sense, muscle stretch, and proprioceptive sense arrives from the lower body to the **accessory cuneate nucleus**. That information is relayed to the cerebellum by means of the **cuneocerebellar tract** passing through the inferior cerebellar peduncle. Also in the posterior portion of the medulla are the trigeminal nerve nucleus and the spinal tract of the trigeminal.

The complexity of the upper medulla reflects the importance of this region (upper portion of Figure 12-30). The corticospinal tract arising from the cerebrum has yet to divide into anterior and lateral components, so it appears as a single pathway. The central canal has now expanded to become the 4th ventricle. Lateral to the hypoglossal and dorsal vagal nuclei is the **nucleus solitarius**, an important nucleus of the X vagus nerve. The **hypoglossal nucleus** gives rise to the XII hypoglossal nerve, and the IX glossopharyngeal, X vagus, and XI accessory nerves arise from the **nucleus ambiguus**, dorsal vagal nucleus, and solitary tract nucleus. We will discuss these cranial nerves in detail.

You can quickly find the **inferior olivary complex** in the antero-lateral aspect of the medulla as a structure looking like an intestine doubled over on itself. A number of fibers from this complex decussate and enter the cerebellum via the inferior cerebellar peduncle. Parts of this structure take on the appearance of a bag with a drawstring (the **principal inferior olivary nucleus**), and axons from the nuclei within the complex decussate at the **median raphe** to ascend to the cerebellum as the major component of the inferior cerebellar peduncle. The lateral medulla is dominated by the inferior cerebellar peduncle, with the trigeminal spinal tract and nucleus medial to it. The nucleus ambiguus may be seen in the anterolateral medulla, marking the anterior boundary of the reticular formation.

Look closely at the posterior margin of the upper medulla and you can see the **medial** and **inferior vestibular nuclei**. You may remember these from your audiology course, because they are important nuclei associated with knowing and maintaining one's position in space (vestibular sense). Projections from the vestibular portion of the VIII vestibulocochlear nerve reach these nuclei. If you can locate the lateral spinothalamic tracts, you can identify the region that carries pain and touch information from the spine to the thalamus.

Clearly, a lesion to the medulla would have devastating impact on all motor and sensory function. We have just mentioned the nuclei associated with balance, motor function for the larynx, respiration, cardiac function, movement of the tongue and muscles of mastication, as well as pathways mediating the vestibular sense, all motor function in the periphery, and all sensations that reach the cerebrum or cerebellum. Take just an instant to realize that all of these extraordinarily important functions and processes are housed within an area about the size of the first joint of your thumb. Once again, ponder the danger associated with a lesion to this region, and we promise to tell you a story with a surprisingly happy ending related to a brainstem stroke.

Deep Structures of the Pons. The pons is classically divided into two parts: the posterior **tegmentum** and the anterior **basilar portion**. Look at Figures 12-31 and 12-32 as we discuss the pons.

First, let us examine the basilar (anterior) portion of the pons. Orient yourself by finding the corticospinal and corticobulbar tracts. At the level of the lower pons, the tracts are beginning to become organized

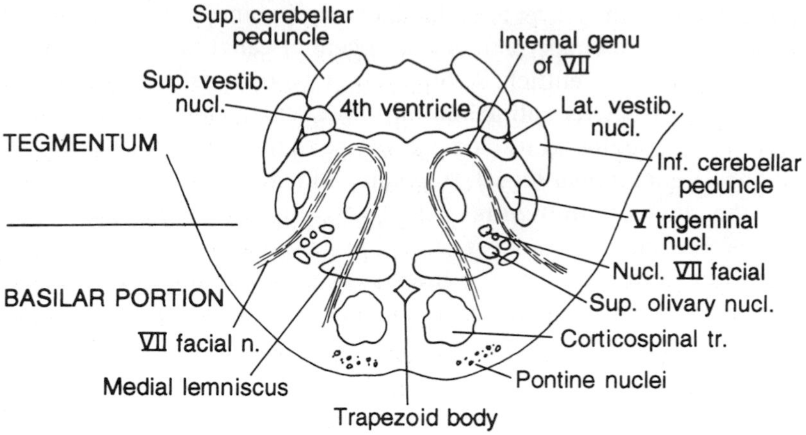

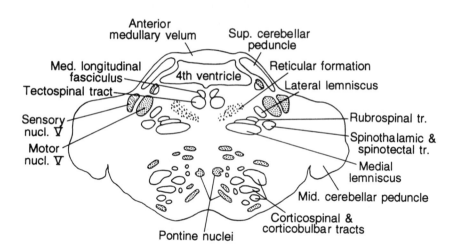

Figure 12-31. Schematic of a transverse section through the pons.

Figure 12-32. Schematic of middle pons; transverse section.

for their medulla decussation and course through the spine. At higher levels of the pons, you would see that the tracts are less well defined and more diffusely distributed. Near these tracts are the **pontine nuclei**. The pontine nuclei are important because they receive input from the cerebrum and spinal cord, with that information being relayed to the cerebellum. That information is relayed by means of the axons of the pontine nuclei that make up the pontocerebellar tract. This tract ascends to the cerebellum as the middle cerebellar peduncle. The transmission of information from the cerebrum to the pontine nuclei and pontocerebellar tract is an extremely important conduit between the cerebrum and cerebellum.

Locate the **medial lemniscus** on Figure 12-31. The lemniscal pathway begins to coalesce within the medulla, becoming the medial lemniscus within the pons. This is an important pathway for somatic (body) sense.

In the section on spinal cord anatomy we will discuss the medial longitudinal fasciculus (MLF), which is responsible for maintenance of flexor tone. Most of the ascending fibers of the MLF shown in Figure 12-32 arise from the vestibular nuclei and project to muscles of the eye for regulation of eye movement with relation to head position in space. Note the relationship between the vestibular nuclei (Figure 12-31) and the MLF (Figure 12-32) and you will see the important interaction between the vestibular system and ocular tracking: Without the vital information from the vestibular system, the eyes would interpret every movement as external to the body. As it is, the vestibular system can notify the visual system of how the head is moving (for instance, bumping up and down on a country road) so that the ocular muscles can adjust for these changes in head position.

You will also certainly remember that we discussed the vestibular nuclei as being part of the medulla. In reality, only the inferior vestibular nucleus is within the medulla: The lateral and superior vestibular nuclei are shown in Figure 12-31, although the medial vestibular nucleus is not visible in this view. Another center of the auditory system, the **trapezoid body**, is a mass of small nuclei and fibers seen at this level. The trapezoid body is a relay within the auditory pathway. Lateral and posterior to the trapezoid body is the **superior olivary complex**, containing auditory relays associated with localization of sound in space, as well as with the efferent component of the auditory pathway. We discuss this further in Chapter 13.

The posterior **pontine tegmentum** is actually a continuation of the reticular formation of the medulla. Projections from the reticular formation ascend to the thalamus and hypothalamus. As you can see from Figure 12-31, the tegmentum houses nuclei for cranial nerves V, VI, VII, as well as relays of the VIII. To remind you, within this small space are the control centers for mastication, ocular abduction, facial musculature, and portions of the auditory pathway. The ventral pons is made up largely of fibers of the corticospinal, corticobulbar, and corticopontine tracts. At this level those fibers are less compactly bundled than they are at the level of the medulla. Notice that the motor nucleus of the VII facial nerve is found near the superior olive. Axons from the facial nucleus course around the nucleus of the VI abducens nerve at the **internal genu** before exiting the brainstem.

If you examine the basilar portion of the pons in Figure 12-32, you can see that the corticospinal tract is broken into small bundles, as mentioned previously. Fibers of the **corticopontine tract** (not shown) course with the corticospinal tract but synapse with the pontine nuclei, which surround the corticospinal tract. Axons of these nuclei decussate to make up the middle cerebellar peduncle. The superior cerebellar peduncle of the tegmental region is dorsal to the nuclei of the trigeminal nerve. The superior cerebellar peduncle forms the lateral margin of the 4th ventricle, and the anterior medullary velum forms the roof of the ventricle, as mentioned earlier.

Deep Structures of Midbrain. Look at Figure 12-33 as we discuss the midbrain. The midbrain may be divided into three areas: the posterior **tectum** (also known as the *quadrigeminal plate*); the medial **tegmentum**, which is a continuation of the pontine tegmentum; and the **crus cerebri**, the prominent anterior structure.

In the posterior midbrain, the tectum is dominated by the **inferior colliculus**, an important auditory relay. This nucleus receives input from the lateral lemniscus, and those fibers encapsulate it. Within the tegmentum you can see the decussation of the superior cerebellar peduncle (tegmental decussation). Remember that the crus cerebri are the efferent pathways from the cerebrum serving the body. Included within the crus cerebri are the corticobulbar and corticospinal tracts, and the **fronto-**

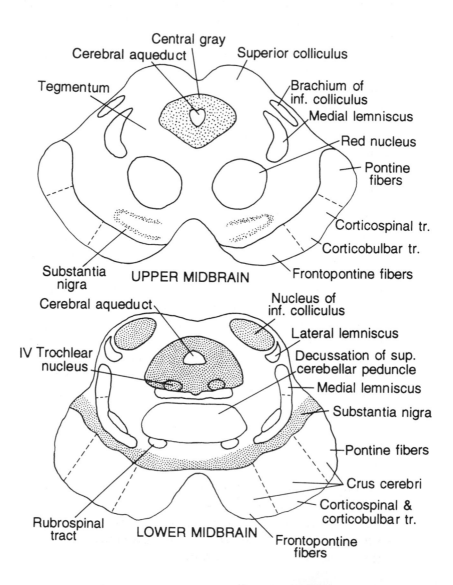

Figure 12-33. Schematic of upper and lower midbrain.

pontine fibers that will terminate in the pons. Between the crus cerebri and tegmentum is the **substantia nigra**, a dark brown mass of cells that manufactures dopamine, a neurotransmitter essential for normal movement. Destruction of this substance results in Parkinson's disease, a debilitating neuromuscular disease.

The **cerebral aqueduct** is an extremely narrow tube connecting the 4th ventricle with the 3rd ventricle, as previously discussed. Surrounding it is a mass of cells known as the **periaqueductal** or **central gray**, where the nucleus of the IV trochlear nerve can be found.

The **superior colliculus** can be found in the superior midbrain within the tectum. This nucleus receives input from the cerebral cortex, optic tract, inferior colliculus, and the spinal cord and appears to be responsible for eye and head movements relative to visual stimuli. Perhaps as a result of the inferior colliculus connection, it may also serve as a point of integration of auditory localization and visual orientation.

Also within the tegmentum lies the massive **red nucleus**. The red nucleus receives input from the cerebral cortex and cerebellum, and gives rise to the **rubrospinal tract**. Input from the red nucleus is from the cerebellum and cerebral cortex, and it is an important component of flexor control. Near the red nucleus is the **Edinger-Westphal nucleus**, controlling accommodation of the eye to light by the iris. Also medially placed is the III oculomotor nerve nucleus. The dorsolaterally placed **medial geniculate body** is actually a nucleus of the thalamus, and is the final subcortical relay of the auditory pathway.

In summary:

- The **brainstem** is divided into **medulla, pons,** and **midbrain**. It is more highly organized than the spinal cord, mediating higher-level body function such as vestibular responses.

- The **medulla** contains the important **pyramidal decussation**, the point at which the motor commands originating in one hemisphere of the cerebral cortex cross to serve the opposite side of the body. The **IX, X, XI,** and **XII cranial nerves** emerge at the level of the medulla, and the **inferior cerebellar peduncle** arises there. The **4th ventricle enlargement** is a prominent brainstem landmark in cross-section. The **pons** contains the **superior** and **middle cerebellar peduncles**, as well as four cranial nerve nuclei, the **V, VI, VII,** and **VIII** nerves.

- The **midbrain** contains the important **cerebral peduncles** and gives rise to the **III** and **IV cranial nerves**.

- The deep structure of the brainstem reflects the level of the brainstem's phylogenetic development.

- At the **decussation** of the pyramids, the **descending corticospinal tract** has condensed from the less structured form at higher levels to a well-organized tract.

- The **reticular formation** is a phylogenetically old set of nuclei essential for life function.
- In the rostral medulla, the expansion to accommodate the **4th ventricle** is apparent, marking a clear divergence from the minute central canal of the spinal cord and lower medulla.
- The levels of the pons and midbrain set the stage for communication with the higher levels of the brain, including the cerebellum and cerebrum.
- This communication link permits not only complex motor acts, but also consciousness, awareness, and volitional acts.

Cranial Nerves

Working knowledge of the cranial nerves is vital to the speech-language pathologist or audiologist. You may wish to refer to Appendixes F and G as we discuss them. Although not all cranial nerves are involved with speech or hearing, knowledge of cranial nerves is of great assistance in assessment.

Cranial Nerve Classification

Cranial nerves are referred to by name, number, or both. By convention, roman numerals are used when discussing cranial nerves, and the number represents inverse height in the brainstem. Cranial nerves I through IV are found at the level of the midbrain, V through VIII are pons-level cranials, and IX through XII are found in the medulla. When we discussed the spinal cord, we pointed out that the nuclei of sensory neurons resided in dorsal root ganglia and that their axons entered the spinal cord for synapse. This pattern is followed in the brainstem as well, where axons of sensory nuclei enter the brainstem for synapse and motor nuclei are within the brainstem.

Unlike spinal nerves, cranial nerves are differentiated based upon seven defining characteristics or categories. Cranial nerve functions are divided into *general* and *special*, with areas of service being *somatic* and *visceral*. Nerves can be efferent, afferent, or mixed efferent/afferent as well. Thus, you will see the notation *general somatic afferent* for one component of the V trigeminal nerve that combines all three functional categories.

General somatic afferent nerves (GSA) are sensory nerves involved in communicating the sensory information from skin, muscles, and joints, including pain, temperature, mechanical stimulation of skin, length and tension of muscle, and movement and position of joints. That is, GSA nerves provide general information about body function, and this information usually reaches consciousness (although the fact that this information reaches the level of consciousness does not necessarily mean that you attend to it). **Special somatic afferent nerves (SSA)**, in contrast, serve the special body senses such as vision and hearing. **General visceral afferent nerves (GVA)** transmit sensory information from receptors in visceral structures, such as the digestive tract; this information only infrequently reaches conscious levels. **Special visceral afferent nerves (SVA)** provide information from the special visceral senses of taste and smell.

Efferent nerves follow parallel form. **General visceral efferent nerves (GVE)** are the autonomic efferent fibers serving viscera and glands. **General somatic efferent nerves (GSE)** provide innervation of skeletal muscle and are quite important for speech production. The "wild cards" in this mixture are the **special visceral efferent nerves (SVE),** which are involved with innervation of striated muscle of branchial arch origin, including the larynx, pharynx, soft palate, face, and muscles of mastication.

Specific Cranial Nerves

I Olfactory Nerve (SVA)

The olfactory nerve is not a true cranial nerve because it reaches the brain without passing through the thalamus first. This *special visceral afferent* nerve mediates the sense of smell (olfaction), which developed quite early in our phylogenetic development. The olfactory sensors are embedded in the epithelium of the nasal cavity, including the superior conchae and the septum.

Dendrites of the bipolar cells that make up this nerve pass superiorly through the cribriform plate of the ethmoid bone to enter one of the paired **olfactory bulbs**, the nuclei of the nerve that resides within the cranium, at the base of the brain (see Figure 12-34). The olfactory nerve divides into medial and lateral branches. The lateral branches communicate with the olfactory cortex, which is made up of the pyriform lobe and hippocampal formation.

Damage to the I Olfactory Nerve

Trauma to the nasal region can result in loss of cerebrospinal fluid through the nose (**cerebrospinal fluid rhinorrhea**), which alternately becomes a route for **meningeal infection** (infection of the meningeal linings of the brain). The most common trauma resulting in **anosmia** (loss of sense of smell and taste) is an injury involving frontal impact, probably as a result of damage to the sensory apparatus itself, especially as a result of shearing forces applied to the nerve at the cribriform plate.

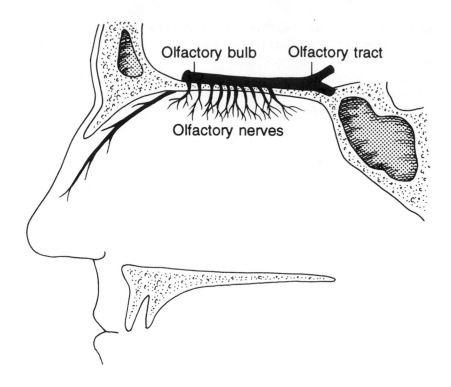

Figure 12-34. Olfactory bulb, nerves, and tract.

II Optic Nerve (SSA)

Although not technically related to speech, hearing, or language, the optic nerve provides valuable clinical insight into the extent of damage due to cerebrovascular accident. The optic nerve is the *special somatic afferent* component associated with the visual system. Motor function of the eye is accommodated through other nerves.

The retinal cells receive stimulation from light, and output from the rod and cone cells of the retina (first-order neurons) is relayed to bipolar cells and modified by horizontal interneuron cells (second-order neurons). The output of these cells is transmitted by alterations of membrane potential, but in the absence of an action potential. The result of this complex process of inhibition and excitation is transmitted to the dendrite of the bipolar ganglion cells of the optic nerve (third-order neurons) whose cell bodies lie in the **lateral geniculate body (LGB)**, a nucleus of the thalamus.

Visual information can take three different paths following synapse at the LGB (Mackay, Chapman, & Morgan, 1997). Eighty percent of information passes from the retina to the lateral geniculate body, and then to the calcarine sulcus. It is thought that this pathway is involved in spatial discrimination and form analysis. Information used for motor response passes from the retina to the thalamus and subsequently to the cerebrum, while the final pathway passes to the brainstem to mediate reflexes associated with vision, such as the pupillary responses to light. See the Clinical Note on this cranial nerve for an interesting insight into the different responses that can be manifested as a result of damage to one component of this pathway.

The paired optic nerves converge on the **optic chiasm**. There information from the medial half of the retina decussates, whereas information from the lateral half of each retina remains uncrossed (see Figure 12-35). Crossed and uncrossed information passes through the **optic tract** to the LGB. Dendrites of fourth-order neurons synapse and course via the **optic radiation** (geniculostriate projection) to the occipital lobe (Brodmann's area 17), the primary receptive area of the cerebral cortex. Branches from the LGB course to the **superior colliculus** of the midbrain, an apparent point of interaction between visual and auditory information received at the inferior colliculus and the relay involved in orienting to visual stimuli. The image from the retina is neurally projected onto the occipital lobe, inverted from the real-world object it represents.

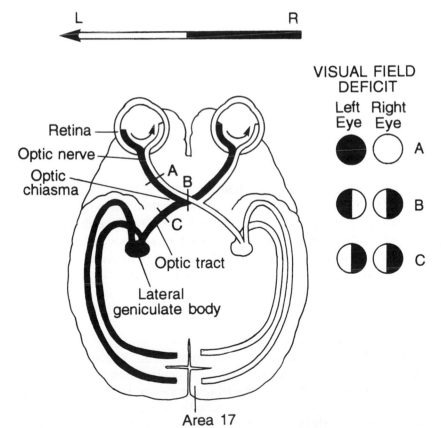

Figure 12-35. Representation of the visual pathway and effect of site of lesion. A cut in the optic nerve at point A would eliminate both left and right visual fields of the left eye. A lesion at point B would cause loss of information from the right and left temporal fields (heteronymous bitemporal hemianopsia). A lesion at point C on the optic tract will result in loss of information from the right visual field of both eyes (homonymous hemianopsia).

Lesions of the II Optic Nerve and Tract

Function provides a window on the site of a lesion. In the visual system, the degree of visual **cut** or loss will give clues as to the location of damage to the nerve or tract. Figure 12-35 illustrates the pathway, with reference to a visual image presented to the eyes. The image will reverse as it passes through the lens, so that it is inverted both vertically and horizontally when projected upon the retina.

Information is sensed and transduced such that light reaching the medial portion of the retina (area nearest the nose) crosses at the chiasm, while that on the lateral portion of the retina (near the temples) remains ipsilateral. Thus, light from the left **visual field** strikes the left medial and right lateral retinae, combining in the right hemisphere of the brain. Likewise, information from the right visual field strikes the right medial and left lateral retinae, and courses to the left cerebral hemisphere. In this manner, left visual field enters the right hemisphere, and right visual field enters the left hemisphere.

Difficulties occur when part of the pathway is damaged. Definition of an individual's visual impairment is always with reference to damage to the visual field. If a lesion to the optic tract occurs behind the optic chiasm, the result will be loss of vision of the opposite field. Right optic tract damage will result in loss of left visual field, as in point C on the figure. This is referred to as left **homonymous** ("having the same name," or more appropriately, same side) **hemianopia** (blindness in half of the field of vision).

A lesion arising at the chiasm (point B), such as a tumor compressing the nerve, will result in loss of decussating information. In this case, the right eye will lose right visual field and the left eye will lose the left visual field. This is termed **heteronymous** (different side) **bitemporal** (affecting both temporal regions) **hemianopia**. A patient with a chiasm lesion may also lose olfaction, because of the close proximity of the olfactory nerve.

Traumatic injury to the optic nerve and tract can have devastating and seemingly paradoxical effects. A blow to the region of the eyebrow frequently results in unilateral optic neuropathy by compressing the optic nerve at the optic canal. Visual impairment resulting from trauma may also arise from occipital lobe damage, resulting in cortical blindness or inability to process higher-level visual information. Because of the separate pathways mediating visuo-spatial information and movement, cortical blindness arising from trauma or cerebrovascular accident may leave the individual responsive to moving visual stimulation due to sparing of the retinal-thalamic-cortical pathway associated with oculomotor function (see Mackay, Chapman, & Morgan, 1997).

III Oculomotor Nerve (GSE, GVE)

The III oculomotor is comprised of two components. The *general somatic efferent* component serves the extrinsic ocular muscles ipsilaterally, including the superior levator palpebrae; superior, medial, and inferior rectus muscles; and inferior oblique muscle. The only ocular muscles not innervated by the III oculomotor nerves are the superior oblique and lateral rectus muscles (see Figure 12-36). The oculomotor nuclei are found

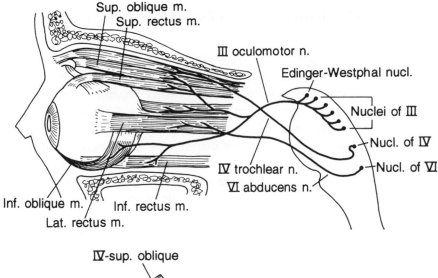

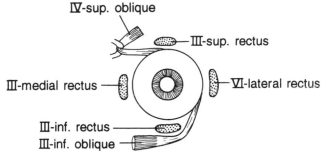

Figure 12-36. Schematic of III oculomotor, IV trochlear, and VI abducens nerve and muscle innervated.

within the midbrain at the level of the superior colliculus, an important relay for the visual system. Axons from the nuclei course through the red nucleus and medial to the cerebral peduncles, exiting the brainstem to differentiate into inferior and superior branches. Activation of muscles served by the oculomotor nucleus results in the eye being turned up and out (temporally), inward (nasally), or down and out.

The *general visceral efferent* component arising from the Edinger-Westphal (accessory oculomotor) nucleus provides light and accommodation reflexes associated with pupil constriction and focus. The nuclei reside ventral to the cerebral aqueduct, emerge medial to the cerebral peduncle, and pass into the orbit via the superior orbital fissure.

IV Trochlear Nerve (GSE)

The IV trochlear is broadly classed as a *general somatic efferent* nerve. It arises from the trochlear nucleus of the midbrain, and innervates the ipsilateral superior oblique muscle of the eye, which turns the eye down and slightly out. Fibers of the trochlear nerve course around the cerebral peduncles and enter the orbit.

Lesion to the III Oculomotor, IV Trochlear, and VI Abducens Nerves

These three nerves provide motor control of the eye, eyelid, and iris. The III oculomotor nerve passes near the circle of Willis and is subject to compression from tumors, aneurysms, or hemorrhage. It serves the muscles responsible for adducting the eye (superior rectus, medial rectus, inferior rectus, and inferior oblique muscles), for elevating the eyelid (levator palpebrae), and for pupil constriction. A left motor neuron (LMN) lesion of one of the oculomotor nerves will result in ipsilateral paralysis, because decussation occurs before this level. As a result of the unopposed activity of the lateral rectus (which rotates the eye out) oculomotor paralysis will result in abduction (outward deviation, or **divergent strabismus**) of the eye and inability to turn the eye in, **ptosis** (drooping of the eyelid), and **mydriasis** (abnormal dilation of the pupil). Control of the III arises predominantly from area 8 of the frontal lobe, with a projection to the superior colliculus, and from there to the contralateral pontine reticular formation and nuclei for the III, IV, and VI nerves. As a result of the extreme coordination of movements of the two eyes for **convergence** (bringing the eyes together) and **conjugate movement** (moving the eyes together to look toward the same side), hemispheric damage affecting ocular movements will result in contralateral involvement. That is, right hemisphere damage results in an inability to turn the eyes to the left side, because the right hemisphere controls movements of the eyes to the left. In other words, the patient with upper motor neuron (UMN) lesion will "look at the lesion."

LMN lesion of the IV trochlear nerve affects the superior oblique muscle. When an eye rotates medially, the superior oblique is able to pull the eye down, and paralysis will result in loss of this ability. The VI abducens nerve controls the lateral rectus, which rotates the eye out. A LMN lesion to this nerve results in **internal strabismus** (eye is rotated in). The concomitant inability to fuse the visual images from both eyes is called **diplopia**, or double vision.

Traumatic injury to the IV trochlear and VI abducens is more frequent than damage to the III oculomotor nerve. Surgical intervention to remedy the diplopia is typically attempted after nine months, giving the nerves an opportunity to recover function and stabilize. Surgery is performed to eliminate double vision in the reading position (see Mackay, Chapman, & Morgan, 1997).

V Trigeminal Nerve (GSA, SVE)

The V trigeminal nerve is an extremely important mixed nerve for speech production, as it provides motor supply to the muscles of mastication and transmits sensory information from the face. As Figure 12-37 indicates, the nerve arises from the motor trigeminal nucleus and sensory nucleus of the trigeminal within the upper pons, emerging from the pons at the level of the superior margin of the temporal bone. An enlargement in the nerve indicates the trigeminal ganglion containing pseudounipolar cells, and there the nerve divides into three components: the ophthalmic, maxillary, and mandibular nerves.

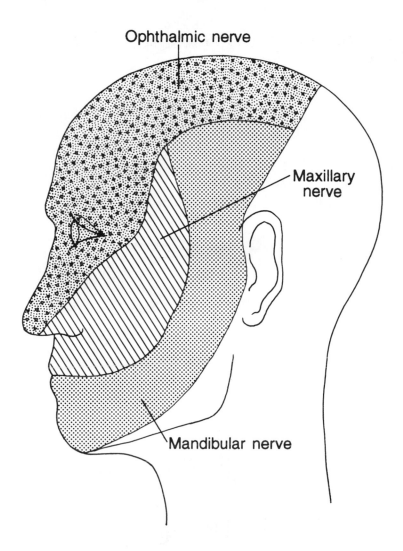

Figure 12-37. Areas served by the nerves arising from the V trigeminal nerve.

The **ophthalmic** is the small, superior nerve of the trigeminal, and is entirely sensory. The *general somatic afferent* component of the ophthalmic branch transmits general sensory information from the skin of the upper face, forehead, scalp, cornea, iris, upper eyelid, conjunctiva, nasal cavity mucous membrane, and lacrimal gland.

The **maxillary nerve** is only sensory, being *general somatic afferent* in nature (see Figure 12-38). It transmits information from the lower eyelid, skin on the sides of the nose, upper jaw, teeth, lip, mucosal lining of buccal and nasal cavities, maxillary sinuses, and nasopharynx.

The **mandibular branch** is both *general somatic afferent* and *special visceral efferent*. This largest branch of the trigeminal nerve exits the skull via the foramen ovale of the sphenoid and gives rise to a number of branching nerves. The afferent component conducts general somatic afferent information from a region roughly encompassing the mandible,

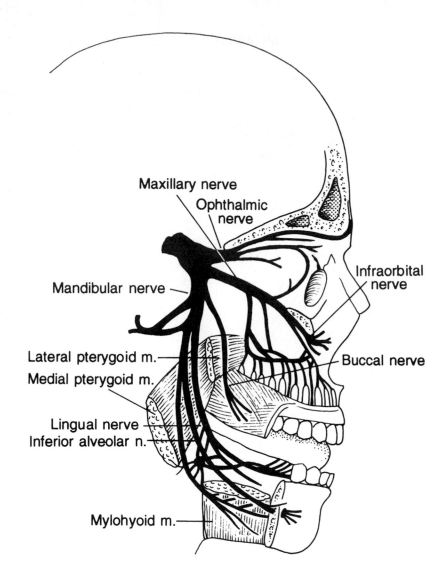

Figure 12-38. Ophthalmic, maxillary, and mandibular branches of the V trigeminal nerve.

including the skin, lower teeth, gums, and lip; a portion of the skin and mucosal lining of the cheek; the external auditory meatus and auricle; the temporomandibular joint; and the region of the temporal bone, as well as kinesthetic and proprioceptive sense of muscles of mastication. The **lingual nerve** conducts somatic sensation from the anterior two-thirds of the mucous membrane of the tongue and floor of the mouth.

The *special visceral efferent* component arises from the trigeminal motor nucleus of the pons, innervates the muscles of mastication (masseter, medial and lateral pterygoids, temporalis), the tensor tympani, the mylohyoid, the anterior digastricus, and the tensor veli palatini muscles. Note that taste is *not* mediated by the trigeminal, but the pain from biting the tip of your tongue is.

Lesions of the V Trigeminal Nerve

The V trigeminal nerve has both motor and sensory components, and all have the potential to be affected by lesions. UMN damage to the V trigeminal will result in minimal motor deficit because of strong bilateral innervation by each hemisphere. With UMN lesion you may see increased **jaw jerk reflex** (elicited by pulling down on the passively opened mandible). LMN damage will result in **atrophy** (wasting) and weakness on the affected side. When your patient closes his or her mouth, the jaw will deviate toward the side of the lesion as a result of the action of the intact internal pterygoid muscle. The jaw will hang open with bilateral LMN damage, which has an extreme effect on speech. The tensor veli palatini is also innervated by the trigeminal, and weakness or paralysis may result in hypernasality because of the role of this muscle in maintaining the velopharyngeal sphincter.

Damage to the sensory component of the V cranial nerve will result in loss of tactile sensation for the anterior two-thirds of the tongue, loss of the corneal blink reflex elicited by touching the cornea with cotton, and alteration of sensation at the orifice of the Eustachian tube, external auditory meatus, tympanic membrane, teeth, and gums. Sensation of the forehead, upper face, and nose region will be lost with ophthalmic branch lesion, and the sensation to the skin region roughly lateral to the zygomatic arch and over the maxilla will be lost with maxillary branch lesion. Damage to the mandibular branch will affect sensation from the side of the face down to the mandible. **Trigeminal neuralgia (tic douloureux)** may also arise from damage to the V cranial nerve. The result of this is severe and sharp shooting pain along the course of the nerve, which may be restricted to areas served by only one of the branches.

VI Abducens Nerve (GSE)

As the name implies, the **VI abducens** (or **abducent**) is an abductor, providing *general somatic efferent* innervation to the lateral rectus ocular muscle. It arises from the abducens nucleus of the pons, which is embedded in the wall of the 4th ventricle, and emerges from the brainstem at the junction of the pons and medulla. The abducens enters the orbit via the superior orbital fissure to innervate the lateral rectus.

VII Facial Nerve (SVE, SVA, GVE)

The facial nerve is quite important to any discussion of speech musculature. This nerve supplies efferent innervation to the facial muscles of expression and tear glands, as well as sense of taste for a portion of the tongue. It communicates with the X vagus, V trigeminal, VIII vestibulocochlear, and IX glossopharyngeal nerves.

The *special visceral efferent* component arises from the motor nucleus of the facial nerve within the reticular formation of the inferior pons. As you may see in Figure 12-39, fibers from both hemispheres of the cerebral cortex terminate on this nucleus. The motor nucleus is

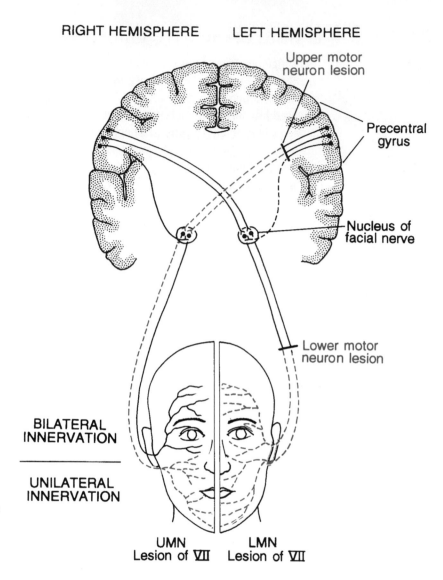

RIGHT HEMISPHERE   LEFT HEMISPHERE

Upper motor
neuron lesion

Precentral
gyrus

Nucleus of
facial nerve

Lower motor
neuron lesion

BILATERAL
INNERVATION

UNILATERAL
INNERVATION

UMN
Lesion of VII

LMN
Lesion of VII

Figure 12-39. Effects of upper and lower motor neuron lesion of the VII facial nerve on facial muscle function. (After view of Gilman & Winans, 1992.)

divided, so that not all muscles are innervated bilaterally. The upper facial muscles receive bilateral cortical input, whereas those of the lower face receive only contralateral innervation. Unilateral damage to the cerebral cortex will produce contralateral deficit in the lower facial muscles, but no noticeable deficit of the upper muscles, because those receive innervation from both cerebral hemispheres. That is, left hemisphere damage could result in right facial paralysis of the oral muscles, but spare the ability to wrinkle the forehead, close the eye, and so forth.

The nerve exits the pons at the cerebellopontine angle to enter the internal auditory meatus (see Figure 12-40), coursing laterally through

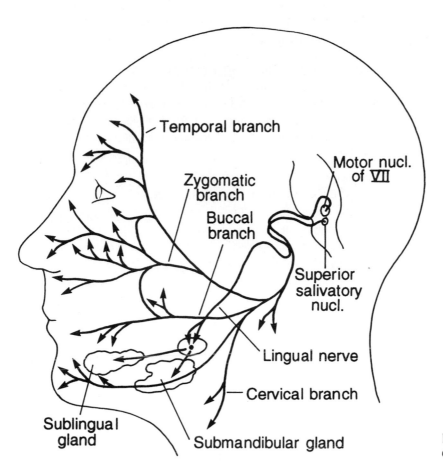

Figure 12-40. General course of the VII facial nerve.

the facial canal of the temporal bone. At the **geniculate ganglion** the nerve turns to continue as a medial prominence in the middle ear cavity. A twig of the facial nerve, the **chorda tympani**, enters the cavity and passes medial to the malleus and tympanic membrane. It ultimately joins the lingual nerve of the V trigeminal.

The facial nerve exits at the stylomastoid foramen of the temporal bone, coursing between and innervating the stylohyoid and posterior digastricus muscles. The nerve branches into **cervicofacial** and **temporofacial** divisions. The cervicofacial division further gives off the buccal, lingual, marginal mandibular, and cervical branches, while the temporofacial division gives rise to the temporal and zygomatic branches.

The *general visceral efferent* component of the facial nerve arises from the **salivatory nucleus** of the pons, forming the **nervus intermedius**. Fibers from the nervus intermedius innervate the **lacrimal gland** (for tearing), the **sublingual gland** beneath the tongue, and the **submandibular gland**.

Lesions of the VII Facial Nerve

Lesions of the facial nerve may significantly affect articulatory function. Because the upper motor neuron supply to the upper face is bilateral, unilateral UMN damage will not result in upper face paralysis. It may, however, paralyze all facial muscles below the eyes. Even then, muscles of facial expression (**mimetic muscles**) may be contracted involuntarily in response to emotional stimuli, because these motor gestures are initiated at regions of the brain that differ from those of speech.

LMN damage will cause upper- and lower-face paralysis on the side of the lesion. This may involve the inability to close the eyelid, and will result in muscle sagging, loss of tone, and reduction in wrinkling around the lip, nose, and forehead. When the individual attempts to smile, the affected corners of the mouth will be drawn toward the unaffected side. Your patient may drool due to loss of the ability to impound saliva with the lips, and the cheeks may puff out during expiration due to a flaccid buccinator.

Bell's palsy (palsy means "paralysis") may result from any compression of the VII nerve, or even from cold weather. It results in paralysis of facial musculature, which remits in most cases within a few months.

Damage to the facial nerve following penetrating facial or cranial trauma is quite common. Damage to the middle ear or skull fractures involving the temporal bone will both result in facial nerve damage. Most fractures of the temporal bone occur along the long axis of the temporal bone, although facial paralysis is much more likely if the fracture is transverse (see Mackay, Chapman, & Morgan, 1997).

The *special visceral afferent* sense of taste (**gustation**) arising from the anterior two-thirds of the tongue is mediated by the facial nerve. Information is transmitted via the chorda tympani to the nervus intermedius, and ultimately to the **solitary tract nucleus**.

VIII Vestibulocochlear Nerve (SSA)

This nerve, also known as the **auditory nerve**, is extremely important for both the speech-language pathologist and the audiologist because it mediates both auditory information and sense of movement in space. The nerve consists of both afferent and efferent components. The *special somatic afferent* portion mediates information concerning hearing and balance, while the efferent component appears to assist in selectively damping the output of hair cells (see Figures 12-41 and 11-12).

Acoustic Branch. Information concerning acoustic stimulation at the **cochlea** is transmitted via short dendrites to the spiral ganglion within the modiolus of the bony labyrinth. The spiral ganglion consists of bodies of bipolar cells whose axons project through the internal auditory meatus, where the nerve joins with the vestibular branch of the VIII

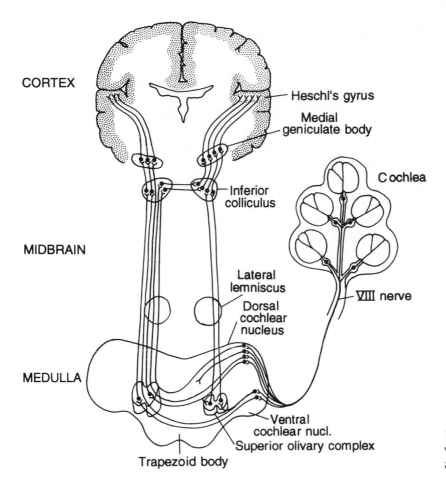

CORTEX

Heschl's gyrus

Medial
geniculate body

Cochlea

Inferior
colliculus

MIDBRAIN

VIII nerve

Lateral
lemniscus

Dorsal
cochlear
nucleus

MEDULLA

Ventral
cochlear nucl.

Superior olivary complex

Trapezoid body

Figure 12-41. Course of the VIII vestibulocochlear nerve and auditory pathway.

nerve. The nerve enters the medulla oblongata at the junction with the pons to synapse with the **dorsal cochlear nucleus (DCN)** and the **ventral cochlear nucleus (VCN)**, lateral to the inferior cerebellar peduncle.

Vestibular Branch. The vestibular branch of the VIII cranial nerve transmits information concerning acceleration and position in space to the bipolar cells of the **vestibular ganglion** within the internal auditory meatus. From within the pons, fibers branch to synapse in nuclei of the pons and medulla, as well as directly to the flocculonodular lobe of the cerebellum. Within the pons and medulla, the vestibular branch communicates with the superior, medial, lateral, and inferior vestibular nuclei. Vestibular nuclei project to the spinal cord, cerebellum, thalamus, and cerebral cortex.

Efferent Component. Although considered to be a sensory device, the cochlea is served by efferent fibers of the **olivocochlear bundle**. Although this pathway has only about 1,600 fibers (compared with the 30,000 fibers

Lesions of the VIII Vestibulocochlear Nerve

Clearly, damage to the VIII nerve will result in ipsilateral hearing loss reflecting the degree of trauma. Damage to the VIII nerve may arise from a number of causes, including physical trauma (skull fracture), tumor growth compressing the nerve (benign but life-threatening tumors of the myelin sheath will result in slow-onset unilateral hearing loss and other symptoms as compression of the brainstem increases), or vascular incident. Damage to the vestibular component of the VIII nerve may result in disturbances of equilibrium arising from loss of information concerning position in space.

Traumatic injury to the VIII vestibulocochlear nerve usually arises from fracture of the temporal bone or penetrating injury, such as that from gunshot wounds. A fracture along the long axis of the temporal bone will often result in sensorineural loss and vertigo without VIII nerve compression or apparent damage to the labyrinth. If the fracture is in the transverse dimension, the VII and VIII nerves may well be sheared or compressed. Vertigo and nystagmus in head injury often occur when the head position is changed (as in turning the head, looking up or down, or turning a corner when walking): In the absence of evidence of physical damage to the labyrinth, it is hypothesized that the vertigo and nystagmus arise from disturbance of calcium particles used within the sensory mechanisms of the vestibular system. Fortunately, most trauma-induced vertigo remits over time (see Mackay, Chapman, & Morgan, 1997).

of the afferent VIII), activation of the bundle has a significant attenuating effect on the output of the hair cells with which they communicate.

The **crossed olivocochlear bundle (COCB)** arises from a region near the **medial superior olive (MSO)** of the olivary complex. Fibers descend, and most of them decussate near the 4th ventricle, and communicate with **outer hair cells**. The **uncrossed olivocochlear bundle (UCOB)** originates near the **lateral superior olive** of the olivary complex, with most of the fibers projecting ipsilaterally to the **inner hair cells** of the cochlea. It is believed that the olivocochlear bundle can be controlled through cortical activity and may be active in signal detection within noise.

Auditory Pathway. The auditory pathway to the cerebral cortex is illustrated in Figure 12-41 (see also Chapter 11, Figure 11-12): Dendrites of VIII nerve fibers synapsing on cochlear hair cells become depolarized following adequate mechanical stimulation via the cochlear traveling wave. Axons of the bipolar cells of the VIII vestibulocochlear nerve project to the cochlear nucleus, which is functionally divided into the dorsal cochlear nucleus (DCN), anteroventral cochlear nucleus (AVCN), and posteroventral cochlear nucleus (PVCN) of the pons. (Some anatomists distinguish only two nuclei, the DCN and the ventral cochlear nucleus.) Projections from the VIII nerve are arrayed **tonotopically** within the cochlear nucleus, reflecting the organization of the cochlear partition. That is, there is an orderly array of fibers representing the information processed within the cochlea, from low to high frequency. This order is maintained throughout the auditory nervous system.

Projections from the cochlear nucleus take the form of **acoustic striae**. The **dorsal acoustic stria** arises from the DCN, coursing around the inferior cerebellar peduncle. It decussates, bypasses the superior olivary complex (SOC) and lateral lemniscus, and makes synapse at the inferior colliculus (IC). Fibers of the **ventral acoustic stria** course anterior to the inferior cerebellar peduncle and terminate in the contralateral superior olivary nuclei. The **intermediate acoustic stria** arises from the PVCN and terminates at the ipsilateral superior olivary complex.

The **medial superior olive (MSO)** and **lateral superior olive** (**LSO**, also known as the **s-segment**) are major auditory nuclei of the superior olivary complex within the pons. Localization of sound in the environment is processed primarily at this level. High-frequency information at the LSO provides the binaural intensity cue for location of sound in space, while low-frequency information projected to the MSO provides the interaural phase (frequency) cue for localization. In addition, the crossed and uncrossed olivocochlear bundles arise from cells peripheral to the MSO and LSO nuclei.

As you can see from the schematic of the auditory pathway, fibers from the SOC ascend to the lateral lemniscus and inferior colliculus, structures apparently involved in localization of sound. You may also notice that there are ample decussations throughout the pathway, following cochlear nucleus synapse. Indeed, the auditory pathway is primarily crossed, although a small ipsilateral component is retained. Unilateral deafness will result from cochlea or VIII nerve damage, but not from unilateral damage to the auditory pathway above the level of the auditory nerve. Although much hearing function will be retained as a result of the redundant pathway, interaction of the two ears is essential for localization of sound in space, and damage to the brainstem nuclei will result in loss of discrimination function. Of course, complete bilateral sectioning of the pathway would result in complete loss of auditory function.

The **medial geniculate body (MGB)**, a thalamic nucleus, is the final auditory relay. The **auditory radiation** (also known as the **geniculotemporal radiation**) projects from the MGB to **Heschl's gyrus** (area 41) of the temporal lobe. This segment of the dorsal surface of the superior temporal convolution is partially hidden in the Sylvian fissure, and projections to the auditory cortex retain tonotopic organization. The adjacent area 42 is an auditory association area, which projects to other areas of the brain, as well as to the contralateral auditory cortex via the corpus callosum.

IX Glossopharyngeal Nerve (GSA, GVA, SVA, GVE, SVE)

The IX glossopharyngeal nerve serves both sensory and motor functions (see Figure 12-42). The motor component arises from the nucleus ambiguus and inferior salivatory nucleus of the medulla, while axons of

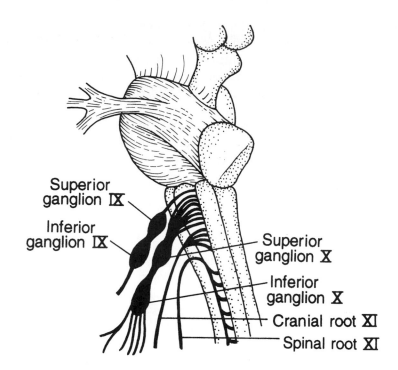

Figure 12-42. Relation of glossopharyngeal nerve to vagus and accessory nerves.

the sensory component terminate in the medulla at the **solitary tract nucleus** and **spinal tract nucleus** of the V trigeminal. The rootlets emerge in the ventrolateral aspect of the medulla, converge, and exit the skull through the jugular foramen of the temporal bone. The nerve courses deep to the styloid process of the temporal bone and beside the stylopharyngeus muscle. It enters the base of the tongue after penetrating the superior constrictor muscle. The nerve has **superior** and **inferior (petrosal) ganglia**.

The *special visceral afferent* function of the nerve mediates sensation from taste receptors of the posterior one-third of the tongue and a portion of the soft palate, with this information delivered to the solitary tract nucleus. Impulses from **baroreceptors** within the carotid sinus convey information concerning arterial pressure within the common carotid artery to the same nucleus. The *general visceral afferent* component provides sensation of touch, pain, and temperature from the posterior one-third of the tongue, as well as from the faucial pillars, upper pharynx, and Eustachian tube to the inferior ganglion.

General somatic afferent information from the region behind the auricle and external auditory meatus is transmitted by the superior branch of the IX glossopharyngeal to the nucleus of the spinal trigeminal via the superior ganglion.

Efferent innervation by the IX glossopharyngeal includes *special visceral efferent* activation of the stylopharyngeus and superior constrictor muscles by means of the nucleus ambiguus. *General visceral efferent*

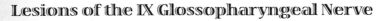

Lesions of the IX Glossopharyngeal Nerve

The IX glossopharyngeal nerve works in concert with the X vagus, making its independent function difficult to determine. Damage to the IX nerve will result in paralysis of the stylopharyngeus muscle, and may result in loss of general sensation (**anesthesia**) for the posterior one-third of the tongue and pharynx, although the vagus may support these functions as well. The cooperative innervation with the vagus results in little effect on the pharyngeal constrictors, although reduced sensation of the auricle and middle ear may indicate IX damage. IX damage may also cause reduced or absent gag reflex, although absence of the reflex does not guarantee that a lesion exists.

innervation of the parotid gland for salivation arises from the inferior salivatory nucleus via the otic ganglion.

X Vagus Nerve (GSA, GVA, SVA, GVE, SVE)

The vagus nerve is both complex and important. Let us examine both motor and sensory components of this nerve. The vagus arises from the lateral medulla oblongata and exits from the skull through the jugular foramen along with the IX glossopharyngeal and XI accessory nerves (see Figure 12-43).

The vagus is served by several nuclei and ganglia. The dorsal vagal nucleus (dorsal motor nucleus) gives rise to visceral efferent fibers for parasympathetic innervation and receives information from the inferior vagal ganglion. The solitarius tract and nucleus serve taste, whereas the nucleus ambiguus provides motor innervation to laryngeal musculature and mucosa. As with the glossopharyngeal nerve, the vagus has inferior (nodose) and superior ganglia.

The *general visceral efferent* component of the vagus arises from the dorsal motor nucleus of the X vagus, providing parasympathetic motor innervation of intestines, pancreas, stomach, esophagus, trachea and bronchial smooth muscle and mucosal glands, kidneys, liver, and the heart. This branch is responsible for inhibiting heart rate. The striated muscles of the larynx, as well as most pharyngeal and palatal muscles, are innervated by the *special visceral efferent* portion of the vagus, served by the nucleus ambiguus.

The *general somatic afferent* component of the vagus delivers pain, touch, and temperature sense from the skin covering the ear drum, posterior auricle, and external auditory meatus to the superior vagal ganglion, and subsequently to the spinal nucleus of the V trigeminal. It is this innervation that triggers nausea or vomiting when the ear drum is touched by external stimuli.

Pain sense from the mucosal lining of the lower pharynx, larynx, thoracic and abdominal viscera, esophagus, and bronchi is conveyed by means of the *general visceral afferent* component, with soma in the

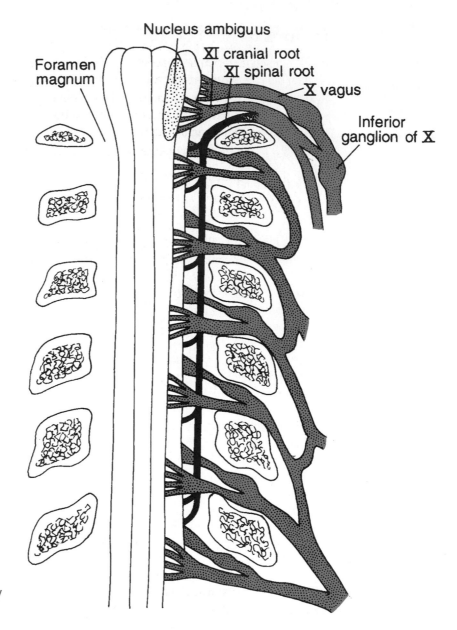

Figure 12-43. Spinal accessory nerve origins.

inferior ganglion, and with axons terminating in the caudal nucleus solitarius and dorsal vagal nucleus. Sensations of nausea and hunger are mediated by the vagus. This GVA component supports maintenance of heartbeat, blood pressure (via baroreceptors), respiration (stretch receptors in the lung signal fully distended tissue to terminate inspiration), and digestion.

Taste sense from the epiglottis and valleculae is mediated by the *special visceral afferent* component of the vagus, with soma of these afferent fibers residing in the inferior ganglion (Gilman & Winans, 1992). Axons from this component terminate in the caudal nucleus solitarius.

These functions are served through four important branches of the vagus. The auricular branch arises from the superior ganglion, while the pharyngeal, recurrent laryngeal, and superior laryngeal branches arise from the inferior ganglion.

The right **recurrent laryngeal nerve** courses under and behind the subclavian artery and ascends between the trachea and the esophagus. The left recurrent laryngeal nerve loops under the aortic arch to ascend between the trachea and esophagus. After entering the larynx between the cricoid and thyroid cartilages, tracheal and esophageal branches provide GVA innervation to the laryngeal mucosa beneath the vocal folds, and SVE innervation serves the intrinsic muscles of the larynx and the inferior pharyngeal constrictor. The auricular branch conveys sensory information from the tympanic membrane and external auditory meatus.

The **pharyngeal branch** of the vagus mediates the SVA taste sense and GVA sensation from the base of the tongue and upper pharynx. It also mediates SVE innervation of the upper and middle pharyngeal

Lesions of the X Vagus Nerve

The X vagus is the most extensive of the cranial nerves, presenting an important constellation of clinical manifestations. Damage to the pharyngeal branch will result in deficit in swallowing, potential loss of gag through interaction with the IX glossopharyngeal nerve, and hypernasality due to weakness of the velopharyngeal sphincter (all velopharyngeal muscles are innervated by the vagus, with the exception of the tensor veli palatini, which is innervated by the trigeminal). Unilateral pharyngeal branch damage will result in failure to elevate the soft palate on the involved side (asymmetrical elevation), producing hypernasality. Bilateral lesion will produce absent or reduced (but symmetrical) movement of the soft palate, causing hypernasality, **nasal regurgitation** (loss of food and liquid through the nose), dysphagia, and paralysis of the pharyngeal musculature.

Lesions of the superior laryngeal nerve may result in loss of sensation of the upper larynx mucous membrane and stretch receptors, as well as paralysis of the cricothyroid muscle. Recurrent laryngeal nerve damage will alter sensation below the level of the vocal folds and stretch receptor information from the intrinsic muscles. Unilateral recurrent laryngeal nerve lesion typically results in a flaccid vocal fold on the side of the lesion, accompanied by hoarse and breathy voice. In bilateral lesion, the vocal folds may rarely be paralyzed in the adducted position, which is life-threatening because of airway occlusion. More commonly, the vocal folds are paralyzed in the paramedian position, compromising the airway by risk of aspiration. Paralysis in the adducted position will result in **laryngeal stridor** (harsh, distressing phonation upon inspiration and expiration). Paralysis in the paramedian position may permit limited breathy and hoarse phonation with limited pitch range due to loss of tensing ability of the vocalis. Vocal intensity range will be extremely limited by the loss of adductory ability.

constrictors, palatopharyngeus, palatoglossus, salpingopharyngeus, levator veli palatini, and musculus uvulae. The only soft-palate muscle not innervated by the vagus is the tensor veli palatini.

The **superior laryngeal nerve** has both internal and external branches. The internal branch enters the larynx through the thyrohyoid membrane, receiving GVA information from the laryngeal region above the vocal folds. The external branch provides SVE innervation of the cricothyroid muscle.

XI Accessory Nerve (SVE)

The XI accessory nerve consists of both cranial and spinal components. It provides *special visceral efferent* innervation directly to the sternocleidomastoid and trapezius muscles and works in conjunction with the vagus to innervate the intrinsic muscles of the larynx, pharynx, and soft palate. The exceptions to this are the tensor veli palatini, which is innervated by the V trigeminal; and the cricothyroid muscles, which are innervated by the superior laryngeal nerve of the vagus (Figure 12-42).

The cranial root arises from the caudal portion of the nucleus ambiguus, where it is joined by the spinal root, to exit through the jugular foramen with the vagus. On exiting the skull, the internal branch of the accessory nerve joins the inferior ganglion of the vagus. The accessory nerve serves both recurrent laryngeal and pharyngeal nerves of the vagus.

The spinal root emerges from the first five spinal segments between the dorsal and ventral rootlets, ascends to enter the skull through the foramen magnum, and joins the cranial accessory nerve prior to exiting the skull (see Figure 12-42). The spinal root makes up the external root of the accessory nerve, and innervates the sternocleidomastoid and trapezius muscles.

XII Hypoglossal Nerve (GSE)

As the name implies, this nerve provides the innervation to motor function of the tongue. This *general somatic efferent* nerve arises from the hypoglossal nucleus of the medulla, exits the skull through the hypoglossal canal, and courses with the vagus. The hypoglossal nerve descends

Lesions of the XI Accessory Nerve

Lesion to the XI accessory nerve may have an effect on the trapezius and sternocleidomastoid muscles. Unilateral lesion affecting the sternocleidomastoid will result in the patient being unable to turn his or her head away from the side of the lesion. (The left sternocleidomastoid rotates the head toward the right side when contracted.) Lesions resulting in paralysis of the trapezius will result in restricted ability to elevate the arm and a drooping shoulder on the side of the lesion.

Lesions of the XII Hypoglossal Nerve

Lesions affecting the XII hypoglossal will have a profound impact on articulation function and speech intelligibility. This nerve provides efferent innervation of intrinsic and extrinsic muscles of the tongue, as well as afferent proprioceptive supply. Unilateral LMN lesion will result in loss of movement on the side of the lesion. Muscular weakness and atrophy on the affected side will result in deviation of the tongue toward the side of the lesion (function of the normal contralateral genioglossus will cause this). **Fasciculations**, or abnormal involuntary twitching or movement of muscle fibers, may occur prior to atrophy, arising from damage to the cell body. At rest the tongue may deviate toward the unaffected side as a result of the tonic pull of the normal styloglossus muscle. Upper motor lesion may result in muscle weakness and impaired volitional movements with accompanying spasticity.

and branches to innervate all intrinsic muscles of the tongue, and all of the extrinsic muscles of the tongue except the palatoglossus, which is innervated via the XI accessory nerve through the pharyngeal plexus.

Each hypoglossal nucleus is served primarily by the contralateral corticobulbar tract, which means that *left* upper motor neuron (UMN) damage will result in *right* tongue weakness. Damage to the lower motor neurons (LMNs) will result in ipsilateral deficit, because the fibers of the corticobulbar tract decussate prior to reaching the hypoglossal nucleus. Thus, left UMN damage or right LMN damage will affect muscles of the right side of the tongue. When the tongue is protruded, it will point to the side of the paralyzed muscles, because contraction of the posterior genioglossus is bilaterally unequal.

In summary, **cranial nerves** are extremely important to the speech-language pathologist.

- Cranial nerves may be **sensory**, **motor**, or **mixed sensory-motor**, and are categorized based on their function as being **general** or **specialized** and as serving **visceral** or **somatic** organs or structures.
- The **I olfactory nerve** serves the sense of smell, and the **II optic nerve** communicates visual information to the brain.
- The **III oculomotor**, **IV trochlear**, and **VI abducens nerves** provide innervation for eye movements.
- The **V trigeminal nerve** innervates muscles of **mastication** and the **tensor veli palatini**, and communicates sensation from the face, mouth, teeth, mucosal lining, and tongue.
- The **VII facial nerve** innervates muscles of **facial expression**, and the sensory component serves taste of the anterior two-thirds of the tongue.
- The **VIII vestibulocochlear nerve** mediates auditory and vestibular sensation.

- The **IX glossopharyngeal nerve** serves the **posterior tongue taste** receptors, as well as somatic sense from the tongue, fauces, pharynx, and Eustachian tube.
- The **stylopharyngeus** and **superior pharyngeal constrictor** muscles receive motor innervation via this nerve.
- The **X vagus nerve** is extremely important for autonomic function as well as somatic motor innervation.
- Somatic sensation of **pain**, **touch**, and **temperature** from the region of the **ear drum** is mediated by the vagus, as well as pain sense from **pharynx**, **larynx**, **esophagus**, and many other regions.
- The **recurrent laryngeal nerve** and **superior laryngeal nerves** supply motor innervation for the intrinsic muscles of the larynx.
- The **XI accessory nerve** innervates the **sternocleidomastoid** and **trapezius** muscles, and collaborates with the vagus in activation of palatal, laryngeal, and pharyngeal muscles.
- The **XII hypoglossal nerve** innervates the **muscles of the tongue** with the exception of the **palatoglossus**.

Anatomy of the Spinal Cord

The spinal cord is the information lifeline to and from the periphery of the body. Movement of axial skeletal muscles occurs by means of information passed through this structure, and sensory information from the periphery must pass through it as well. The spinal cord is a long mass of neurons, with both cell bodies and projections from (and to) those neurons. If you can imagine taking many long lengths of rope, stretching them out and banding them together so it made a long cable, you will have the basic concept of the spinal cord. The spinal cord is the aggregation of many single-nerve fibers into bundles (called **tracts**) of fibers. These bundles provide communication between the peripheral body and the brain, and each bundle has unique properties. Because of this, the spinal cord can be viewed in its length (vertical anatomy) and in cross-section (transverse anatomy). Both of these views are important, because discussion of the spinal cord provides an understanding of how the brain communicates with the rest of the body. Without that communication there would be no reason to have a brain!

Vertical Anatomy

The spinal cord is a longitudinal mass of columns. The columns consist of neurons: Gray portions are neuron cell bodies within the spinal cord, while white portions are the myelinated fibers of tracts that communicate information to and from the brain. The spinal cord is wrapped in **meningeal linings** (meninges), which are thin coverings that were discussed earlier in this chapter (see Figure 12-8).

The spinal cord begins at the foramen magnum of the skull (the superior margin of the atlas or C1), and courses about 46 cm through the vertebral canal produced by the vertebral column (you may want to refresh your memory of the vertebral column by reviewing Figure 3-4). You can think of the spinal cord as being safely contained within a long tube made up of connective tissue (the meningeal linings). The spinal cord is suspended within the tube by means of **denticulate ligaments** that pass through the meningeal linings and attach the spinal cord to the vertebral column. The lower portion of the spinal cord ends in a cone-shaped projection known as the **conus medullaris**, so that the spinal cord is present down to the level of the first lumbar vertebra. There is a fibrous projection from the conus medullaris called the **filum terminale** ("end filament"), and this joins with the toughest part of the tube surrounding the spinal cord (the **dural tube**) and then becomes the **coccygeal ligament** (see Figure 12-8). The coccygeal ligament attaches to the posterior coccyx. Thus, the spinal cord is wrapped in meningeal linings, and is attached to the vertebral column laterally by denticulate ligaments, and is firmly attached to the coccyx by means of the coccygeal ligament.

What you can also see from Figure 12-8 is that there are nerves arising at regular intervals along the cord. The 31 pairs of **spinal nerves** arise from regions related to each vertebra, with the first (spinal nerve C1) arising from the spinal cord on the superior surface of the atlas (C1 vertebra). Thus, there are 8 pairs of cervical spinal nerves instead of 7 (the number of cervical vertebrae), 12 pairs of thoracic nerves, 5 pairs of lumbar and sacral nerves, and 1 pair of coccygeal nerves. The spinal nerves are referred to in the abbreviated manner of vertebrae, with the first thoracic spinal nerve being T1, and so forth.

During embryonic development, the spinal cord is the same length as the vertebral column, but as the brain and body develop, the spinal cord moves up in the canal so that the adult spinal nerves course downward before exiting the vertebral column. (We have seen this same developmental configuration in the relationship between the thorax and the lungs, as you will recall.) When a child is born, the conus medullaris is at the L3 vertebral level, but it will be at the L1 level by adulthood. This changing size relationship is reflected in the relationship between the location of **spinal cord segment** (the functional unit representing the spinal nerve) and vertebra as well. The vertebrae will have a higher number than the cord segment at that vertebral level, as you can see in Figure 12-44. This becomes most marked in the caudal end, where the segment from which the L5 nerve arises corresponds to the L1 vertebra. This relationship gives rise also to a rather descriptive term for the lowermost nerves. The **cauda equina** ("horse's tail") is the tail-like region beneath the filum terminale in which no spinal cord segments will be found. This is, by the way, the region chosen for a lumbar puncture to sample cerebrospinal fluid for medical testing.

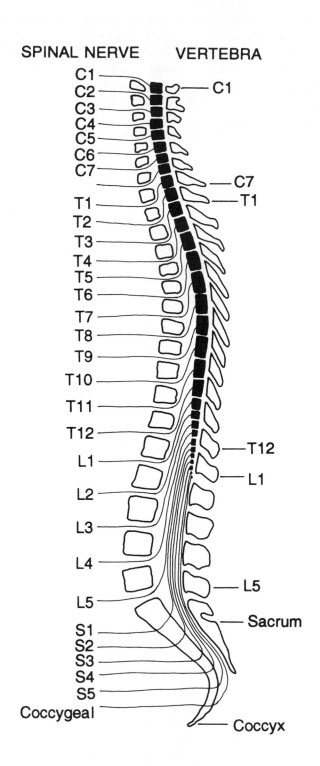

SPINAL NERVE

C1
C2
C3
C4
C5
C6
C7
T1
T2
T3
T4
T5
T6
T7
T8
T9
T10
T11
T12
L1
L2
L3
L4
L5
S1
S2
S3
S4
S5
Coccygeal

VERTEBRA

C1
C7
T1
T12
L1
L5
Sacrum
Coccyx

Figure 12-44. Arrangement of spinal nerves relative to vertebral segment.

Spinal nerves have both sensory (**afferent**) and motor (**efferent**) components. The distribution of sensory function is generally related to segment level, such that upper nerves serve upper body regions, and so forth. A mapping of regions served by spinal nerve afferents reveals a fairly consistent pattern of innervation, with each region served by a nerve being functionally referred to as a **dermatome**. There is overlap of innervation, one of the safeguards of nature against complete loss of sensation. This relationship, shown in Figure 12-45, is not as clear-cut for

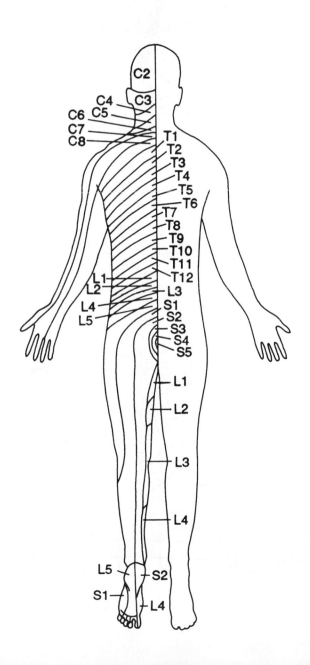

Figure 12-45. Dermatomes reflecting sensory innervation by spinal afferents.

motor function, which is mediated by cooperatives of nerves, referred to as plexuses. A **plexus** is a network of nerves that physically communicate with other nerves.

If you think again of the spinal cord as a series of ropes lashed together, then each of these ropes is a columnar tract, which is a collection of nerve fibers with functional unity (see Figure 12-46). If you were to cut the spinal cord transversely, you might see a segment that looked

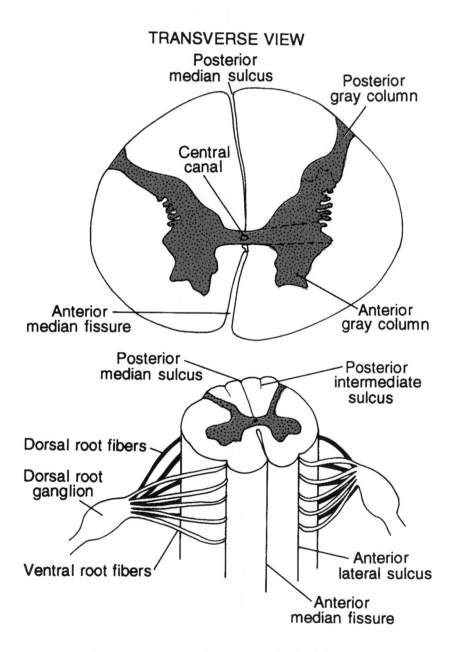

Figure 12-46. Transverse section through spinal cord, with landmarks.

like that in Figure 12-46. In the center of the transverse section you would see a gray "H" shape, with white matter surrounding the gray. The peripheral white segment is made up of myelinated ascending and descending pathways. The central matter is gray due to the concentration of neuron bodies there. Thus, the tracts that we referred to are within the white matter, while the gray matter consists of neuron cell bodies that provide input to the afferent tracts or receive input from efferent tracts.

Transverse Anatomy

Several important landmarks of the sectioned spinal cord are shown in Figure 12-46. At the center of the cell mass is the **central canal**. This central canal is continuous with the 4th ventricle, a space we discussed when we talked about the cerebrum. The anterior surface of the spinal cord has a deep longitudinal **anterior median fissure** that continues through the medulla. Lateral to that is the **anterior lateral sulcus**. In the dorsal aspect you can see the **posterior median sulcus**. Lateral to the posterior median sulcus at the cervical and upper thoracic levels is the **posterior intermediate sulcus**.

The internal spinal cord itself also can be divided into gross regions. The **posterior gray column** (or **horn**) is a mass of nuclei directed posteriorly. The **anterior gray column** makes up the anterior portion of the gray matter. The white matter is divided into funiculi, which are further divided into fasciculi, as will be discussed.

Sensory information enters the spinal cord by means of the afferent neurons, the **dorsal root fibers**. The cell bodies of these sensory neurons combine into the **dorsal root ganglia**, which lie outside the spinal cord (Figures 12-46 and 12-47). Motor information leaves the spinal cord through the ventral root, but there are no "ventral root ganglia" because the cell bodies of motor neurons are housed within the spinal cord instead of outside the cord. The dorsal and ventral roots combine to form the spinal nerve, so that each spinal nerve has both a sensory and a motor component. The spinal nerves divide into posterior and anterior parts (**dorsal** and **ventral rami**) to serve posterior and anterior portions of the body, respectively. Branches of the ventral rami course anteriorly to communicate with the sympathetic ganglia, nuclei of the autonomic nervous system. Efferent neurons of the dorsal and ventral rami communicate with muscle by means of a **motor endplate**. The motor endplate is analogous to the synapse seen as the communication between two neurons. Afferent fibers that enter the spinal cord receive their stimulation from sensors that are peripheral to the spinal cord. We now have all the elements in place for the most basic unit of interaction with the environment, the single-segment reflex arc.

The Reflex Arc. The **segmental spinal reflex arc** is the simplest stimulus-response system of the nervous system, and is the most basic means

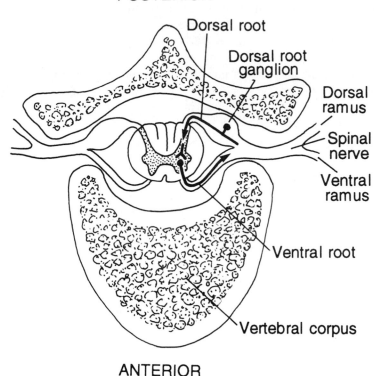

POSTERIOR

Dorsal root

Dorsal root ganglion

Dorsal ramus

Spinal nerve

Ventral ramus

Ventral root

Vertebral corpus

ANTERIOR

Figure 12-47. Transverse section through spinal cord and vertebral segment. Note the dorsal root ganglion and ventral root.

that the nervous system has of responding to its environment (see Figure 12-48). Although we use the term *basic* to imply simplicity, it is not too early to let you know that many speech-language pathologists involved in oral motor therapy recognize that this "basic" response is an essential element of their therapy, because it is a critical component of adequate muscle tone.

Muscle length and tension must be continually monitored by the nervous system. Your brain needs to know where its muscles are in space, and what degree of tone the muscle has. As importantly, a muscle that is supposed to hold a static or stable posture for long periods of time needs to have a system that keeps its length constant. The nervous system has a means of monitoring length and tension that fulfills both of these important functions. The muscle spindle unit senses muscle length and that information is transmitted to the brain for the purposes of programming movement. The muscle spindle also provides a way to monitor muscle length without having to bother the brain with that piece of detail.

Look at Figure 12-48. Sensory information concerning the length of the muscle is transmitted by means of dorsal root fibers to the spinal cord. The dorsal root fibers synapse with the motor neuron in the ven-

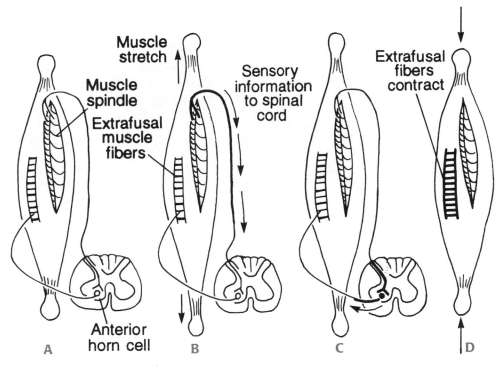

Figure 12-48. Schematic of segmental spinal reflex arc. **A.** The muscle is in a stable state. **B.** The muscle has been passively stretched. Information from the muscle spindle concerning muscle length is transmitted to the spinal cord via the dorsal root ganglion. **C.** Synapse with motor neuron causes efferent activation of muscle fiber. **D.** Extrafusal muscle contracts, shortening the muscle to its original length. *(continues)*

tral cord, and the motor fiber exits the cord to innervate muscle fibers that are being sensed by the muscle spindle. Therefore, if the muscle spindle senses that a muscle has been passively stretched, that information causes the muscle that became longer passively to contract to its original length. The purpose of this reflex is to maintain the length of a muscle fiber that is not being actively contracted, typically for maintenance of posture. If, for instance, you are standing and lean forward slightly, the muscles that are stretched by your leaning will be reflexively contracted until they return to their original length. In this way you can maintain tonic posture automatically without voluntary effort. This is not a trivial or academic detail, because we have muscle spindles in some of the speech musculature, and that makes a very big difference in neuropathology. Let us examine the sequence of the reflex arc in detail.

As you can see in the first panel of Figure 12-48, at rest the muscle is not being stretched and the reflex arc is quiet. In the next panel, the muscle is being stretched and a highly specialized sensor, the muscle spindle, senses that stretching process. This information is passed along the neuron to the cell body in the dorsal root ganglion. The information is then passed to a synapse within the anterior horn cells of the spinal

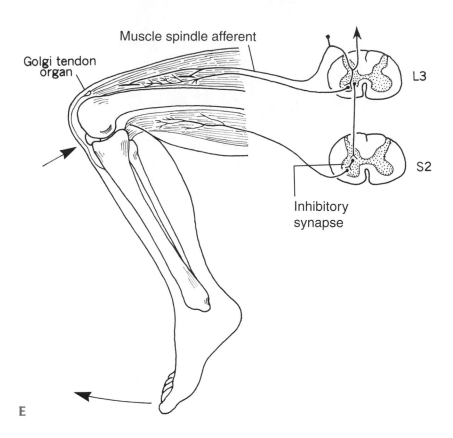

Golgi tendon
organ

Muscle spindle afferent

L3

S2

Inhibitory
synapse

Figure 12-48. *(continued)*
E. Patellar tendon reflex.

E

cord. The axon synapses with the cell body of a motor neuron in the dorsal gray area of the spinal cord, and that causes the muscle it innervates to contract. Thus, when a muscle is passively stretched, it contracts to return to its original length.

To make this muscle contract, an efferent neuron had to be excited. This neuron within the gray matter of the ventral gray matter is known as the **final common pathway** or **lower motor neuron (LMN)**, a very functional unit to remember (see Figure 12-49). The lower motor neuron consists of the dendrites and soma within the spinal cord, as well as the axon and components that communicate with the muscle fiber. In contrast, **upper motor neurons (UMNs)** are efferent fibers descending from upper brain levels. Upper motor neurons bring commands from the upper brain levels that activate or inhibit muscle function by synapsing with lower motor neurons.

Damage to LMNs results in muscle weakness or complete paralysis, just as if you cut the power line leading to your radio. Damage to the UMNs will cause muscle weakness or paralysis because the information from the brain to the lower motor neuron is lost, but this UMN damage will leave reflexes intact because the spinal arc reflex is a lower motor neuron process. This has great clinical significance, which will become clearer in Chapter 13 when we examine function.

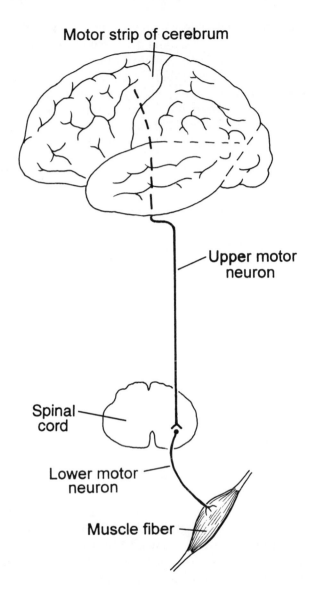

Motor strip of cerebrum

Upper motor neuron

Spinal cord

Lower motor neuron

Muscle fiber

Figure 12-49. Schematic representation of UMN arising from precentral gyrus of cerebral cortex and projecting through corticospinal tract.

These reflexive responses are certainly important, and provide a basic response to the environment. For instance, you reflexively withdraw your hand upon touching the hot burner on a stove. However, for you to make *decisions* about the information, it must reach the cerebral cortex, the seat of conscious thought. You might recall that, when you touched the burner on that stove, you retracted your hand well before you felt the heat and pain. This is the hallmark of interaction between the cerebrum and the reflex. Reflexes "put out the brush fire," but neural circuitry also lets the cerebrum know that something has happened so that other action may be taken (such as putting ice on the burn). The time lag between retracting your hand and feeling the burn is an important reminder that reflexes provide nearly instant, automated response well before the cortex could ever respond. On the other hand, the simple reflex is never going to win you the Nobel Prize. These neurons will not produce conscious thought or mediate cognitive processes.

There must be a system of pathways for information to reach the higher centers or to come from those centers. Within the central nervous system, such pathways are referred to as **tracts**. Tracts are groups of axons with a functional and anatomical unity (that is, they transmit generally the same information to generally the same locations).

Pathways of the Spinal Cord

The spinal cord is a conduit of information, and the channels are built along the longitudinal axis. The spinal cord is compartmentalized, so that it is actually subdivided into functionally and anatomically distinct areas. The gray matter of the spinal cord is divided into nine **laminae** or regions, based on cell type differences. These laminar regions correspond well with the nuclei and regions identified anatomically within the spinal gray.

As you can see from Figure 12-50, a transverse section of the spinal cord is divided into **dorsal**, **lateral**, and **ventral funiculi** (a *funiculus* is

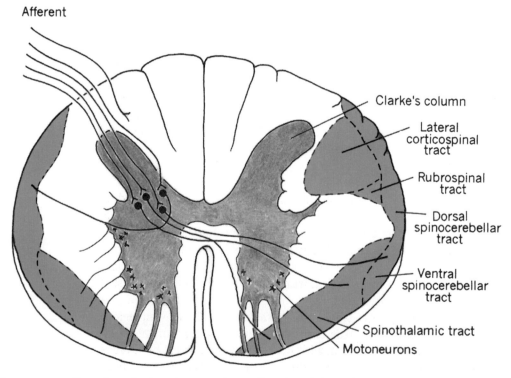

Figure 12-50. Transverse section of a spinal cord segment revealing dorsal, lateral, and anterior funiculi and major ascending tracts.

a large column), which are subdivided into **fasciculi** or tracts of white matter. The size and presence of a tract depend on the level of the spinal cord. Tracts that must serve the muscles of the entire body, for instance, will certainly be larger in the upper spinal cord than in the lower cord. Similarly, the gray matter of the cord will be wider in regions serving more muscles, specifically in the cervical (segments C3 to T2) and thoracic segments (segments T9 to T12). Those regions have more cell bodies to serve the extremities. Tracts of white matter are widest in the cervical region because all descending and ascending fibers must pass through those segments. Sensory pathways tend to be in the posterior portion of the spinal cord, and motor pathways tend toward the anterior aspect, reflecting the dorsal and ventral orientation of the spinal roots (see Table 12-8).

Ascending Pathways. The major ascending sensory pathways include the fasciculus gracilis, fasciculus cuneatus, anterior and lateral spinothalamic tracts, and the anterior and posterior spinocerebellar tracts (see Figure 12-51). Neurons are referred to as first-order, second-order, and so on to indicate the number of neurons in a chain. Thus, the afferent neuron transmitting information from the sensor will be the first-order neuron, the next neuron in the chain following synapse will be the second-order neuron, and so forth up to the terminal point in the neural chain.

Posterior Funiculus. The **fasciculus gracilis** and **fasciculus cuneatus** are separated by the posterior intermediate septum of the posterior funiculus. These tracts convey information concerning touch-pressure and **kinesthetic sense** (sense of movement), as well as vibration sense, which is actually a temporal form of touch-pressure. These columns convey information from group Ia muscle spindle sensors and Golgi tendon organs as well. The Ia spindle fibers convey information about rate of muscle stretch, whereas the Golgi organs appear to respond to stretch of the tendon.

Information concerning sensation in the periphery is conducted by the unipolar first-order neuron of the dorsal root ganglion to the spinal cord. The axons of those neurons ascend on the same side of entry, so that the information is conveyed toward the brain. (The same information remains at the level of entry to form the spinal reflex.) The fasciculus gracilis serves the lower extremities, whereas the fasciculus cuneatus arises from the cervical regions.

The fibers of these tracts ascend **ipsilaterally** (on the same side they entered the cord) until they reach the level of the medulla oblongata of the brainstem to synapse with the **nucleus gracilis** and **nucleus cuneatus**. The axons of the second-order neuron arising from those nuclei combine and **decussate** (cross the midline) to ascend **contralaterally** (on the other side) as the **medial lemniscus** to the **thalamus**, and

Table 12-8. Major ascending and descending pathways.

AFFERENT PATHWAYS			
TRACT	**ORIGIN**	**TERMINATION**	**FUNCTION**
Fasciculus gracilis (lemniscal pathway)	Posterior funiculus	Nuc. gracilis	Touch-pressure, vibration, kinesthetic sense, muscle stretch (spindles), muscle tension (Golgi tendon organs), proprioception for lower extremities
Fasciculus cuneatus (lemniscal pathway)	Posterior funiculus	Nuc. cuneatus	Touch-pressure, vibration, kinesthetic sense, muscle stretch (spindles), muscle tension (Golgi tendon organs), proprioception for upper extremities
Anterior spinothalamic (anterior white commissure and medial lemniscus)	Anterior funiculus	Ventral posterolateral nucleus of thalamus	Light touch
Lateral spinothalamic	Anterior funiculus	Ventral posterolateral nucleus of thalamus	Pain, thermal sense
Anterior spinocerebellar	Lateral funiculus	Vermis of cerebellum	Muscle tension from Golgi tendon organ
Posterior spinocerebellar	Lateral funiculus	Vermis of cerebellum	Muscle tension from Golgi tendon organ

EFFERENT PATHWAYS			
TRACT	**ORIGIN**	**TERMINATION**	**FUNCTION**
Corticospinal	Frontal lobe, cerebrum	Spinal cord	Activation of skeletal muscle of extremities
Corticobulbar	Frontal lobe, cerebrum	Brainstem	Activation of muscles served by cranial nerves
Tectospinal	Superior colliculus, midbrain	C1–C4 spinal cord	Orienting reflex to visual input
Rubrospinal	Red nucleus, midbrain	Spinal cord	Flexor tone
Vestibulospinal	Lateral vestibular nuclei, pons, and medulla	Spinal cord	Extensor tone, spinal reflexes
Pontine reticulospinal	Medial tegmentum, pons	Spinal cord	Voluntary movement
Medullary reticulospinal	Medulla oblongata	Spinal cord	Voluntary movement

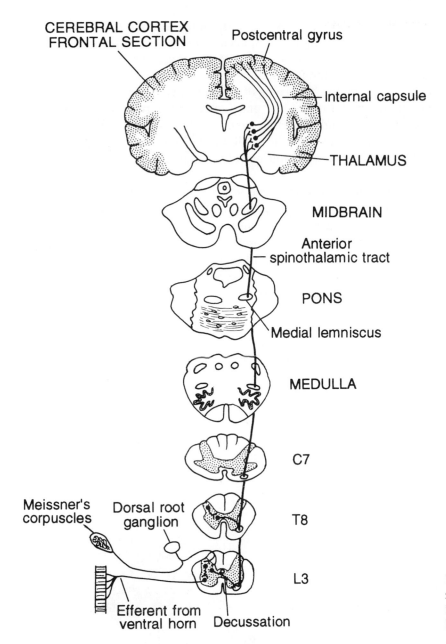

CEREBRAL CORTEX
FRONTAL SECTION

Postcentral gyrus

Internal capsule

THALAMUS

MIDBRAIN

Anterior
spinothalamic tract

PONS

Medial lemniscus

MEDULLA

C7

Meissner's
corpuscles

Dorsal root
ganglion

T8

L3

Efferent from
ventral horn

Decussation

Figure 12-51. Anterior
spinothalamic tract, transmitting
information concerning sense of
light touch.

from the thalamus to the precentral gyrus, which is the major sensory
relay of the brain (for this reason, the pathway is also referred to as the
lemniscal pathway). **Spatiotopic** information (information about the specific region of the body stimulated) is maintained throughout the process.

Damage to these pathways will cause problems in touch discrimination, especially in the hands and feet. Patients may lose **proprioceptive sense** (sense of body position in space), which can greatly impair gait.

Anterior Funiculus. The **anterior spinothalamic tract** conveys information concerning light touch, such as the sense of being stroked by a feather, conveyed from the *spine* to the *thalamus* (see Figure 12-52). Afferent axons of the first-order neuron synapse with anterior spinothalamic tract neurons, the axons of which decussate in the **anterior white commissure** at the level of entry, or perhaps two or three segments higher. The second-order tract neurons ascend to the pons of the brainstem, where fibers enter the **medial lemniscus** to terminate at the ventral posterolateral (VPL) nucleus of the thalamus.

Lateral Funiculus. The last time you stubbed your toe, the information concerning that pain traveled through the **lateral spinothalamic tract**. This important tract transmits information concerning pain and thermal sense. Dorsal root fibers synapse with second-order interneurons which subsequently synapse with third-order tract neurons. These decussate in the anterior white commissure to ascend to the VPL of the thalamus and **reticular formation**. If the spinal cord is cut unilaterally, the result will be *contralateral* loss of pain and thermal sense beginning one segment below the level of the trauma.

Anterior and Posterior Spinocerebellar Tracts. These important tracts convey information concerning muscle tension to the cerebellum. The **posterior spinocerebellar tract** is an uncrossed tract, meaning that information from one side of the body remains on that side during its ascent through

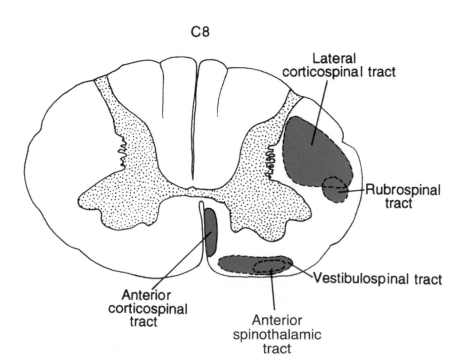

Figure 12-52. Major efferent tracts of the spinal cord as seen in a transverse segment of the cervical spinal cord.

the pathway. Afferent information from Golgi tendon organs and muscle spindle stretch receptors enters the spinal cord via the dorsal root ganglion where axons of these neurons synapse with the second-order tract fibers. Branches of these first-order neurons ascend and descend, so that synapse occurs at points above and below the site of entry as well. The second-order neurons arise from the dorsal nucleus of Clarke, located in the posterior gray of the cord. Upon reaching the medulla oblongata, the second-order neurons enter the **inferior cerebellar peduncle**, the lower pathway to the cerebellum. These axons terminate in the rostral and caudal **vermis** of the cerebellum.

None of the information transmitted by this tract reaches consciousness, although the result of damage to the pathway would. Information from muscles concerning length, rate of stretch, degree of muscle and tendon stretch, and some pressure and touch sense would all be impaired, causing deficit in movement and posture.

The **anterior spinocerebellar tract** is a crossed pathway. Information from Ib afferent fibers serving the Golgi apparatus enters the spinal cord via the dorsal root, where it synapses with the second-order tract neurons. Tract fibers decussate at the same level and ascend through the anterolateral portion of the spinal cord. The tract enters the **superior cerebellar peduncle**, the superior pathway to the cerebellum from the brainstem. Most of the fibers cross to enter the cerebellum on the opposite side of the tract (but the same side as initial stimulation), with the information presumably serving the same function as that of the posterior spinocerebellar tract.

Descending Pathways. Descending motor pathways are the conduits for information commanding muscle contraction that will result in voluntary movement, modification of reflexes, and visceral activation. The most important of these arise from the cerebral cortex, although there are tracts originating in the brainstem as well. The major pathways include the **pyramidal pathways** (the corticospinal and corticobulbar tracts), and the tectospinal, **rubrospinal**, vestibulospinal, pontine reticulospinal, and medullary reticulospinal tracts (see Figure 12-53).

> **rubrospinal:** *L., ruber spina, red thorn*

Corticospinal Tract. As the name implies, this extraordinarily important tract runs from the *cortex* to the *spine*, providing innervation of skeletal muscle (see Figure 12-54). Myelination of the axons of these fibers occurs after birth, and is normally complete by a child's second birthday. The corticospinal tract is made up of more than 1 million fibers, about half of which arise from cells in each frontal lobe of the cerebral cortex (Brodmann areas 4 and 6, areas known as the motor strip and premotor region, to be discussed). The remainder of the neurons supplying the corticospinal tract arise from the region anterior to the motor strip, the premotor region, and from the supplementary motor area on the superior and medial surface of the cerebrum. In addition, some fibers from

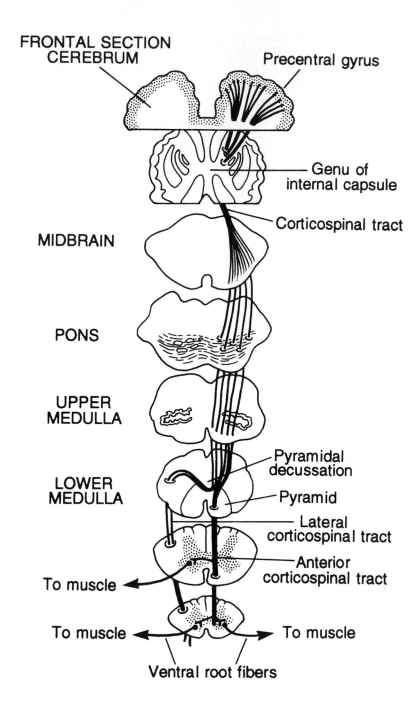

Figure 12-53. Corticospinal pathway as traced from cerebral cortex to spinal cord.

the parietal sensory cortex (areas 1, 2, and 3) project through the corticospinal tract, generally terminating on the dorsal horn cells of the spinal cord. The fibers from the cortex descend as the **corona radiata**, through the **internal capsule** and **crus cerebri** at the level of the midbrain.

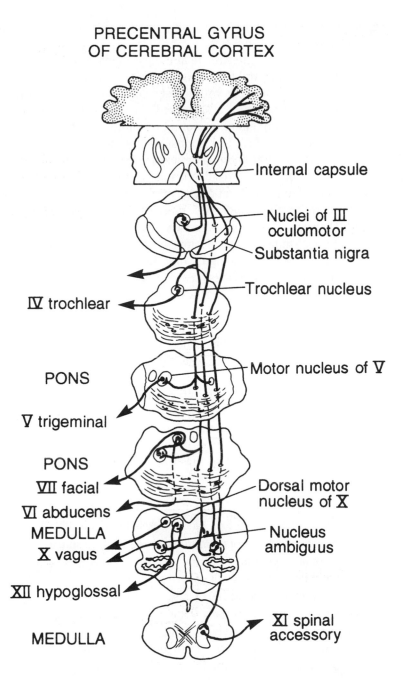

PRECENTRAL GYRUS
OF CEREBRAL CORTEX

Internal capsule

Nuclei of III
oculomotor

Substantia nigra

Trochlear nucleus

IV trochlear

Motor nucleus of V

PONS

V trigeminal

PONS

VII facial

VI abducens

Dorsal motor
nucleus of X

MEDULLA

X vagus

Nucleus
ambiguus

XII hypoglossal

XI spinal
accessory

MEDULLA

Figure 12-54. Corticobulbar tract as traced from cerebral cortex to cranial nerve nuclei.

At the medulla oblongata, the fibers enter the **pyramids** (so called because of the pyramidal column shape), where they undergo the important **pyramidal decussation**. Seventy-five to 90% of corticospinal tract fibers cross to descend as the lateral corticospinal tract in the lateral funiculus. This tract becomes increasingly smaller as it descends through the cord to serve skeletal muscles.

The fibers that do not decussate at the pyramids descend uncrossed as the **anterior corticospinal tract**. On reaching the point of innervation, the axons decussate to synapse with lower motor neurons. This arrangement of partial decussation is a safeguard. Incomplete damage to this pathway may result in retention of voluntary motor function.

The corticospinal tract is responsible not only for activation of muscles but also for inhibition of reflexes. Corticospinal tract lesions (upper motor neuron lesion) result in muscle weakness, loss of voluntary use of musculature, and initial loss of muscle tone. Reduced muscle tone will return to the antigravity muscles and hyperactive tendon reflexes will be seen. The **Babinski reflex** will be elicitable in many individuals with upper motor neuron lesion. When the sole of a relaxed foot is stroked, a positive Babinski sign would be extension of the great toe and spreading of the outer toes. This reflex is normally present in infants, but diminishes through cortical control arising from progressive myelination of the corticospinal tract.

Corticobulbar Tract.   Although the corticobulbar tract is not a tract of the spinal cord, it is included here because it is extraordinarily important for speech production, paralleling the importance of the corticospinal tract for muscles of the trunk and extremities (see Figure 12-54). The corticobulbar tract acts also on sensory information, both facilitating and inhibiting its transmission to the thalamus.

The corticobulbar tract arises from cortical cells in the lateral aspects of the precentral gyrus of the frontal lobe, in the region of the

Terms of Paralysis

Paralysis refers to temporary or permanent loss of motor function. Paralysis is **spastic** in nature if the lesion causing it is of an upper motor neuron. In this type of paralysis, voluntary control is lost through the lesion, but hyperactive reflexes will remain, producing seemingly paradoxical **hyperreflexia** (brisk and overly active reflex responses) and **hypertonia** (muscle tone greater than appropriate) coupled with muscular weakness. **Flaccid** paralysis arises from lesion to the lower motor neuron, and results in **hypotonia** (reduced muscle tone), and **hyporeflexia** (reduced or absent reflex response), with co-occurring muscle weakness.

Paralysis of the lower portion of the body, including legs, is termed **paraplegia**. **Quadriplegia** refers to paralysis of all four limbs, usually arising from damage to the spinal cord above C5 or C6. Spinal cord cut above C3 causes death. If lesions produce paralysis of the same part on both sides of the body, it is referred to as **diplegia**, while **triplegia** involves three limbs. **Monoplegia** refers to paralysis of only one limb or group of muscles. **Hemiplegia** arises from upper motor neuron damage, resulting in loss of function in one side of the body.

motor strip serving the head, face, neck, and larynx. It arises also from the premotor and **somesthetic** (body sense) regions of the parietal lobe of the cortex. Fibers from these areas follow a descent pattern similar to those of the corticospinal tract, passing through the corona radiata and genu of the internal capsule, and entering the brainstem.

These axons branch and decussate at various levels of the brainstem, synapsing with nuclei of cranial nerves to provide bilateral innervation to many muscles of the face, neck, pharynx, and larynx.

Other Descending Pathways. The **tectospinal tract** arises in the superior colliculus ("little hill") of the midbrain, crosses midline in the dorsal tegmental decussation, and descends to the first four cervical spinal cord segments. Because the superior colliculus is a visual relay, it is assumed that this efferent pathway is associated with reflexive postural control arising from visual stimulation, perhaps orienting to the source of visual stimulation.

The **rubrospinal tract** arises from the red nucleus of the midbrain tegmentum. Fibers of this tract cross in the ventral tegmental decussation of the midbrain, and descend with the **medial longitudinal fasciculus (MLF)** of the spinal cord (see Figures 12-49 and 12-52). Most fibers from this tract serve the cervical region, although they descend the length of the spinal cord. The red nucleus receives input from the cerebral cortex and the cerebellum, and appears to be responsible for maintenance of tone in flexor muscles.

The **vestibulospinal tract** arises from the lateral vestibular nucleus of the pons and medulla and descends ipsilaterally the length of the spinal cord. Fibers of this tract facilitate spinal reflexes and promote muscle tone in extensor musculature.

The **pontine reticulospinal tract** arises from nuclei in the medial tegmentum of the pons and descends, primarily ipsilaterally, near the MLF in the spinal cord. The **medullary reticulospinal tract** is formed in the medulla oblongata near the inferior olivary complex and descends in the lateral funiculus. Activity of these neurons have both facilitating and inhibiting effects on motor neurons and hence on voluntary movement.

In summary, the **spinal cord** is comprised of tracts and nuclei.

- The 31 pairs of **spinal nerves** arise from spinal segments, serving sensory and voluntary motor function for the limbs and trunk.
- **Sensory nerves** have their cell bodies within the dorsal root ganglia, whereas **motor neuron** bodies lie within the gray matter of the spinal cord.
- The **spinal reflex arc** is the simplest motor function, providing an efferent response to a basic change in muscle length.
- Several landmarks of the transverse cord assist in identifying the **funiculi** and **fasciculi** of the spinal cord.

- **Upper motor neurons** have their cell bodies rostral to the segment at which the spinal nerve originates, whereas **lower motor neurons** are the final neurons in the efferent chain.
- **Efferent tracts**, such as the corticospinal tract, transmit information from the brain to the spinal nerves.
- **Afferent tracts**, such as the spinothalamic tract, transmit information concerning the physical state of the limbs and trunk to higher brain centers.
- The **corticobulbar tract** is of particular interest to speech-language pathologists because it serves the motor **cranial nerves** for speech.

 CHAPTER SUMMARY

The **nervous system** is a complex, hierarchical structure. Voluntary movement, sensory awareness, and cognitive function are the domain of the **cerebral cortex**. The communication links of the nervous system are **spinal nerves**, **cranial nerves**, and **tracts** of the brainstem and spinal cord. Several organizational schemes characterize the nervous system. The **autonomic** and **somatic nervous systems** control involuntary and voluntary functions. One may divide the nervous system into **central** and **peripheral** nervous systems. **Developmental** characterization separates the brain into **prosencephalon** (**telencephalon** and **diencephalon**), the **mesencephalon** (**midbrain**), and the **rhombencephalon** (**metencephalon** and **myelencephalon**). Monopolar, bipolar, or multipolar **neurons** communicate through synapse by means of **neurotransmitter substance**. Responses may be **excitatory** or **inhibitory**. **Glial cells** provide the fatty sheath for **myelinated** axons, as well as support structure for neurons.

The **cerebral cortex** is protected from physical insult by **cerebrospinal fluid** and the **meningeal linings**, the **dura**, **pia**, and **arachnoid mater**. Cerebrospinal fluid originating within the **ventricles** of the brain and circulating around the spinal cord cushions these structures from trauma associated with rapid acceleration. The **cerebrum** is divided into two **hemispheres** connected by the **corpus callosum**. The **gyri** and **sulci** of the hemisphere provide important landmarks for lobes and other regions of the cerebrum. The **temporal lobe** is the site of auditory reception; the **frontal lobe** is responsible for most voluntary motor activation and use of the important speech region known as **Broca's area**. The **parietal lobe** is the region of somatic sensory reception. The **occipital lobe** is the site of visual input to the cerebrum. The **insular lobe** is revealed by deflecting the temporal lobe, and lies deep in the lateral sulcus. The **operculum** overlies the insula. The functionally defined **limbic lobe** includes the cingulate gyrus, uncus, parahippocampal gyrus, and other deep structures.

The **basal ganglia** are subcortical structures involved in control of movement, and the hippocampal formation of the inferior temporal lobe is deeply implicated in memory function. The **thalamus** of the diencephalon is the final relay for somatic sensation directed toward the cerebrum and other diencephalic structures. The **subthalamus** interacts with the globus pallidus to control movement, and the **hypothalamus** controls many bodily functions and desires. The regions of the cerebral cortex are interconnected by means of a complex network of **projection fibers** that link the cortex with other structures; **association fibers**, which connect regions of the same hemisphere; and **commissural fibers**, which provide communication between corresponding regions of the two hemispheres.

The **anterior cerebral arteries** serve the medial surfaces of the brain, and the **middle cerebral artery** serves the lateral cortex, including the temporal lobe, motor strip, Wernicke's area, and much of the parietal lobe. The **vertebral arteries** branch to form the anterior and posterior spinal arteries, with ascending components serving the ventral brainstem. The **basilar artery** gives rise to the superior and anterior inferior cerebellar arteries to serve the cerebellum, while the **posterior inferior cerebellar artery** arises from the vertebral artery. The basilar artery divides to become the **posterior cerebral arteries**, serving the inferior temporal and occipital lobes, upper midbrain, and diencephalon. The **circle of Willis** is a series of communicating arteries that provide redundant pathways for blood flow to regions of the cerebral cortex, equalizing pressure and flow of blood.

The **cerebellum** coordinates motor and sensory information, communicating with the brainstem, cerebrum, and spinal cord. It is divided into **anterior, middle**, and **flocculonodular** lobes and communicates with the rest of the nervous system via the superior, middle, and inferior **cerebral peduncles**. Position in space is coordinated via the flocculonodular lobe, and adjustment against gravity is mediated by the anterior lobe. The posterior lobe mediates fine motor adjustments. The superior cerebellar peduncle enters the pons and serves the **dentate nucleus, red nucleus**, and **thalamus**. The middle cerebellar peduncle communicates with the pontine nuclei, while the inferior cerebellar peduncle receives input from the spinocerebellar tracts.

The **brainstem** is divided into **medulla, pons**, and **midbrain**. It is more highly organized than the spinal cord and mediates higher-level body functions such as vestibular responses. The **pyramidal decussation** of the medulla is the point at which the motor commands originating in one hemisphere of the cerebral cortex cross to serve the opposite side of the body. The IX, X, XI, and XII cranial nerves emerge at the level of the **medulla**. The **pons** contains four cranial nerve nuclei, the V, VI, VII, and VIII nerves. The **midbrain** contains the important cerebral peduncles, and gives rise to the III and IV cranial nerves. The **reticular formation** is a phylogenetically old set of nuclei essential for life function. The pons and midbrain set the stage for communication with the higher levels of the brain, including the cerebellum and cerebrum. This communication link permits not only **complex motor** acts, but **consciousness, awareness**, and **volitional** acts.

Cranial nerves are extremely important to the speech-language pathologist. Cranial nerves may be **sensory, motor**, or **mixed** sensory-motor, and are categorized based on their function as being **general** or **specialized**, and as serving **visceral** or **somatic** organs or structures. The **V trigeminal** innervates muscles of mastication and the tensor veli palatini, and communicates sensation from the face, mouth, teeth, mucosal lining, and tongue. The **VII facial** nerve innervates muscles of facial expression, and the sensory component serves taste of the anterior two-thirds of the tongue. The **VIII vestibulocochlear** nerve mediates auditory and vestibular sensation. The **IX glossopharyngeal** nerve serves the posterior tongue taste receptors, as well as somatic sense from the tongue, fauces, pharynx, and Eustachian tube. The stylopharyngeus and superior pharyngeal constrictor muscles receive motor innervation via this nerve. The **X vagus** serves autonomic and somatic functions, mediating pain, touch, and temperature from the ear drum and pain sense from the pharynx, larynx, and esophagus. The **recurrent laryngeal** nerve and **superior laryngeal** nerves supply motor innervation for the intrinsic muscles of the larynx. The **XI accessory** nerve innervates the sternocleidomastoid and trapezius muscles, and collaborates with the vagus in activation of palatal, laryngeal, and pharyngeal muscles. The **XII hypoglossal** nerve innervates the muscles of the tongue with the exception of the palatoglossus.

The **spinal cord** is comprised of **tracts** and **nuclei**. The 31 pairs of **spinal nerves** serve the limbs and trunk. **Sensory nerves** have cell bodies in **dorsal root ganglia** and **motor neuron** bodies lie within the spinal cord. **Upper motor neurons** have their cell bodies above the segment at which the spinal nerve originates. **Lower motor neurons** are the final neurons in the efferent chain. **Efferent tracts**, such as the corticospinal tract, transmit information from the brain to the spinal nerves. Afferent tracts, such as the **spinothalamic tract**, transmit information concerning the physical state of the limbs and trunk to higher brain centers. The **corticobulbar tract** is of particular interest to speech-language pathologists because it serves **motor cranial nerves** for speech.

This overview of neuroanatomy should give you some feel for the complexity of this system. The interaction of all these systems provides us with the smooth motor function required for speech, as well as the cognitive and linguistic processes required for comprehension of the spoken word and formulation of a response. Chapter 13 examines some of those processes.

STUDY QUESTIONS

1. The _____ governs voluntary actions.

2. The _____ is responsible for coordinating movement.

3. _____ is the sense of muscle and joint position.

4. _____ are groups of cell bodies in the PNS with functional unity.

5. _____ sense is the sense of the body in motion.

6. Special senses include _____, _____, _____, and _____.

7. The _____ system includes the cerebrum, cerebellum, subcortical structures, brainstem, and spinal cord.

8. The _____ consists of the 12 pairs of cranial nerves and 31 pairs of spinal nerves, as well as the sensory receptors.

9. The _____ governs involuntary activities of involuntary muscles.

10. The _____ governs voluntary activities.

11. Information directed toward the brain is termed _____ while information directed from the brain is termed _____.

12. Developmental divisions: Identify the division referred to by each statement.

    a. _____ refers to the "extended" or "telescoped" brain, and includes the cerebral hemispheres, the white matter immediately beneath it, the basal ganglia, and the olfactory tract.

    b. _____ refers to the olfactory bulb, tract, and striae; pyriform area; intermediate olfactory area; hippocampal formation; and fornix.

    c. _____ includes the thalamus, hypothalamus, pituitary gland (hypophysis), and optic tract.

    d. _____ refers to the midbrain.

    e. _____ includes the pons and cerebellum.

    f. _____ refers to the medulla.

13. On the figure below, identify the parts of the neuron indicated.

a. _____

b. _____

c. _____

d. _____

e. _____

f. _____

g. _____

h. _____

i. _____

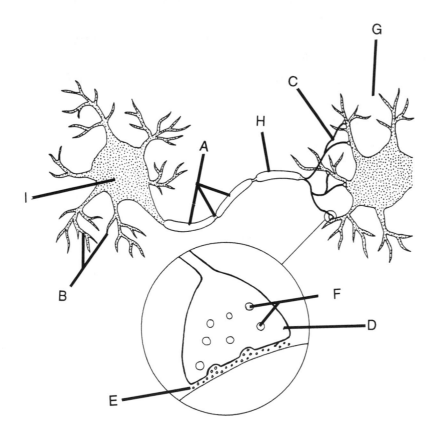

14. On the figure below, identify the parts of the cerebrum indicated.

   a. _____ lobe

   b. _____ lobe

   c. _____ lobe

   d. _____ lobe

   e. _____ gyrus

   f. _____ gyrus

   g. _____ sulcus

   h. _____ sulcus

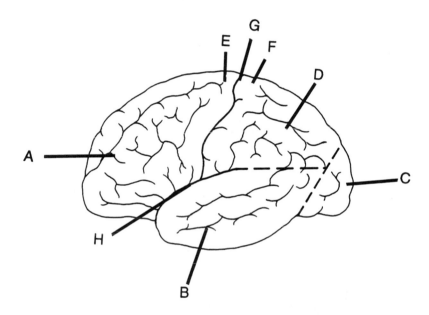

15. On the figure below, identify the parts of the surface of the cerebrum.

a. _____ gyrus

b. _____

c. _____ gyrus

d. _____ area

e. _____ area

f. _____ area

g. _____ gyrus

h. _____ gyrus

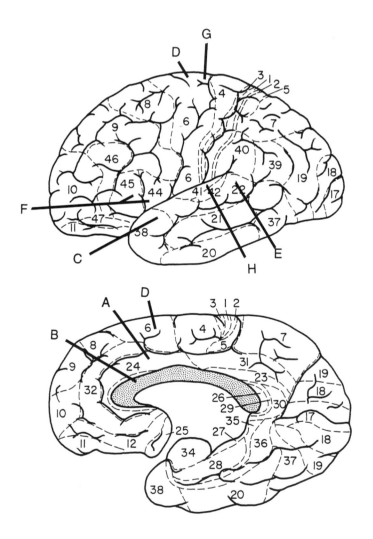

16. On the figure below, identify the components of the ventricle system indicated.

a. _____

b. _____

c. _____

d. _____

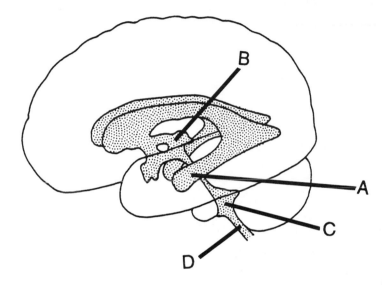

17. On the figure below, identify the arteries and structures indicated.

   a. _____ artery
   b. _____ artery
   c. _____ artery
   d. _____ artery
   e. _____ artery
   f. _____ artery
   g. _____ artery
   h. _____ artery
   i. _____

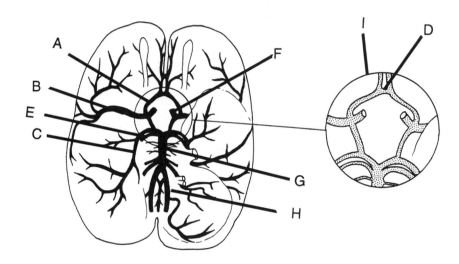

18. Redundancy is nature's safety net. Identify as many redundant systems as you can within the nervous system.

STUDY QUESTION ANSWERS

1. The CEREBRUM governs voluntary actions.
2. The CEREBELLUM is responsible for coordinating movement.
3. PROPRIOCEPTION is the sense of muscle and joint position.
4. GANGLIA are groups of cell bodies in the PNS with functional unity.
5. KINESTHETIC sense is the sense of the body in motion.
6. Special senses include OLFACTION, VISION, GUSTATION, and AUDITION.
7. The CENTRAL NERVOUS SYSTEM includes the cerebrum, cerebellum, subcortical structures, brainstem, and spinal cord.
8. The PERIPHERAL NERVOUS SYSTEM consists of the 12 pairs of cranial nerves and 31 pairs of spinal nerves, as well as the sensory receptors.
9. The AUTONOMIC NERVOUS SYSTEM governs involuntary activities of involuntary muscles.
10. The SOMATIC NERVOUS SYSTEM governs voluntary activities.
11. Information directed toward the brain is termed AFFERENT while information directed from the brain is termed EFFERENT.
12. Developmental divisions: Identify the division referred to by each statement.
    a. TELENCEPHALON refers to the "extended" or "telescoped" brain, and includes the cerebral hemispheres, the white matter immediately beneath it, the basal ganglia, and the olfactory tract.
    b. RHINENCEPHALON refers to the olfactory bulb, tract, and striae; pyriform area; intermediate olfactory area; hippocampal formation; and fornix.
    c. DIENCEPHALON includes the thalamus, hypothalamus, pituitary gland (hypophysis), and optic tract.
    d. MESENCEPHALON refers to the midbrain.
    e. METENCEPHALON includes the pons and cerebellum.
    f. MYELENCEPHALON refers to the medulla.
13. On the figure below, identify the parts of the neuron indicated.
    a. AXON
    b. DENDRITE
    c. TELODENDRIA
    d. TERMINAL END BOUTON
    e. SYNAPTIC CLEFT
    f. SYNAPTIC VESICLES
    g. POSTSYNAPTIC NEURON
    h. MYELIN SHEATH
    i. SOMA
14. On the figure below, identify the parts of the cerebrum indicated.
    a. FRONTAL lobe
    b. TEMPORAL lobe
    c. OCCIPITAL lobe
    d. PARIETAL lobe
    e. PRECENTRAL gyrus
    f. POSTCENTRAL gyrus

g. <u>CENTRAL</u> sulcus

h. <u>LATERAL</u> sulcus

15. On the figure below, identify the parts of the surface of the cerebrum.

    a. <u>CINGULATE</u> gyrus

    b. <u>CORPUS CALLOSUM</u>

    c. <u>SUPERIOR TEMPORAL</u> gyrus

    d. <u>SUPPLEMENTARY MOTOR</u> area

    e. <u>WERNICKE'S</u> area

    f. <u>BROCA'S</u> area

    g. <u>PRECENTRAL</u> gyrus

    h. <u>HESCHL'S</u> gyrus

16. On the figure below, identify the components of the ventricle system indicated.

    a. <u>LATERAL VENTRICLE</u>

    b. <u>THIRD VENTRICLE</u>

    c. <u>FOURTH VENTRICLE</u>

    d. <u>CEREBRAL AQUEDUCT</u>

17. On the figure below, identify the arteries and structures indicated.

    a. <u>ANTERIOR CEREBRAL</u> artery

    b. <u>MIDDLE CEREBRAL</u> artery

    c. <u>POSTERIOR CEREBRAL</u> artery

    d. <u>ANTERIOR COMMUNICATING</u> artery

    e. <u>SUPERIOR CEREBELLAR</u> artery

    f. <u>INTERNAL CAROTID</u> artery

    g. <u>BASILAR</u> artery

    h. <u>VERTEBRAL</u> artery

    i. <u>CIRCLE OF WILLIS</u>

18. Redundancy takes many forms within the nervous system. One of the most obvious is the presence of two cerebral hemispheres, although they are not functionally equal, as we will see in Chapter 13. The fact that the corticospinal tract divides into anterior and lateral corticospinal tracts indicates some safety in spreading the "risk" around. Likewise, the circle of Willis within the cerebrovascular system is an important safety valve. What about the fact there are identical nuclei within each half of the brainstem? How about the fact that the upper face is bilaterally innervated? Can you think of any other redundancies?

REFERENCES

Adams, R. D., Victor, M., & Ropper, A. H. (1997). *Principles of neurology* (6th ed.). New York: McGraw-Hill.

Albom, M. (1997). *Tuesdays with Morrie.* New York: Broadway Books.

Aronson, A. E. (2000). *Aronson's neurosciences pocket lectures.* San Diego, CA: Singular Publishing Group.

Bateman, H. E., & Mason, R. M. (1984). *Applied anatomy and physiology of the speech and hearing mechanism.* Springfield, IL: Charles C. Thomas.

Bear, M. F., Connors, B. W., & Paradiso, M. A. (1996). *Neuroscience: Exploring the brain.* Baltimore: Williams & Wilkins.

Berkovitz, B. K. B., & Moxham, B. J. (2002). *Head and neck anatomy*. United Kingdom: Martin Dunitz Ltd.

Bhatnagar, S. C., & Andy, O. J. (2002). *Neuroscience for the study of communicative disorders* (2nd ed.). Baltimore: Williams & Wilkins.

Bly, L. (1994). *Motor skills acquisition in the first year*. Tucson, AZ: Therapy Skill Builders.

Bowman, J. P. (1971). *The muscle spindle and neural control of the tongue*. Springfield, IL: Charles C. Thomas.

Carpenter, M. B. (1991). *Core text of neuroanatomy* (4th ed.). Baltimore: Williams & Wilkins.

Chusid, J. G. (1985). Correlative neuroanatomy and functional neurology (17th ed.). Los Altos, CA: Lange Medical Publications.

Cotman, C. W., & McGaugh, J. L. (1980). *Behavioral neuroscience*. New York: Academic Press.

Darley, F. L., Aronson, A. E., & Brown, J. R. (1975). *Motor speech disorders*. Philadelphia: W. B. Saunders.

Edvinsson, L., & Krause, D. N. (2002). *Cerebral blood flow and metabolism*. Philadelphia: Lippincott/Williams & Wilkins.

Fields, D. (2004, April). The other half of the brain. *Scientific American*, 53–61.

Filskov, S. B., & Boll, T. J. (1981). *Handbook of clinical neuropsychology*. New York: John Wiley & Sons.

Fiorentino, M. R. (1973). *Reflex testing methods for evaluating CNS development*. Springfield, IL: Charles C. Thomas.

Ganong, W. F. (1981). *Review of medical physiology*. Los Altos, CA: Lange Medical Publications.

Gelfand, S. A. (1990). *Hearing*. New York: Marcel Dekker.

Gelfand, S. A. (2001). *Essentials of audiology* (2nd ed.). New York: Thieme Medical Publishers.

Gilman, S., & Winans, S. S. (1992). *Manter and Gatz's essentials of clinical neuroanatomy and neurophysiology*. Philadelphia: F. A. Davis.

Gilroy, J. (2000). *Basic neurology* (3rd ed.). New York: McGraw-Hill.

Gray, H., Bannister, L. H., Berry, M. M., & Williams, P. L. (Eds.). (1995). *Gray's anatomy*. London: Churchill Livingstone.

Kandel, E. R. (1991). Brain and behavior. In E. R. Kandell, J. R. Schwartz, & T. M. Jessell (Eds.), *Principles of neural science* (3rd ed., pp. 9–48). Norwalk, CT: Appleton & Lange.

Kandel, E. R., Schwartz, J. H., & Jessell, T. M. (1991). *Principles of neural science*. Norwalk, CT: Appleton & Lange.

Kandel, E. R., Schwartz, J. H., & Jessell, T. M. (2000). *Principles of neural science* (4th ed.). New York: McGraw Hill.

Kaufman, D. M. (2000). *Clinical neurology for psychiatrists* (5th ed.). Philadelphia: W. B. Saunders.

Kuehn, D. P., Lemme, M. L., & Baumgartner, J. M. (1989). *Neural bases of speech, hearing, and language*. Boston: College-Hill Press.

Mackay, L. E., Chapman, P. E., & Morgan, A. S. (1997). *Maximizing brain injury recovery*. Gaithersburg, MD: Aspen Publishers.

McMinn, R. M. H., Hutchings, R. T., & Logan, B. M. (1994). *Color atlas of head and neck anatomy*. London: Mosby-Wolfe.

Møller, A. R. (2003). *Sensory systems: Anatomy and physiology*. New York: Academic Press.

Moore, K. L. (1988). *The developing human*. Philadelphia: W. B. Saunders.

Netsell, R. (1986). *A neurobiologic view of speech production and the dysarthrias*. San Diego, CA: College-Hill Press.

Netter, F. H. (1983a). *The CIBA collection of medical illustrations. Vol. 1. Nervous system. Part I. Anatomy and physiology*. West Caldwell, NJ: CIBA Pharmaceutical.

Netter, F. H. (1983b). *The CIBA collection of medical illustrations. Vol. 1. Nervous system. Part II. Neurologic and neuromuscular disorders.* West Caldwell, NJ: CIBA Pharmaceutical.

Netter, F. H. (1997). *Atlas of human anatomy.* Los Angeles: Icon Learning Systems.

Noback, C. R., Demarest, R. J., & Strominger, N. L. (1991). *The nervous system: Introduction and review.* Philadelphia: Williams & Wilkins.

Nolte, J. (2002). *The human brain* (5th ed.). St. Louis, MO: Mosby Year Book.

Poritsky, R. (1992). *Neuroanatomy: A functional atlas of parts and pathways.* St. Louis, MO: Mosby Year Book.

Rohen, J. W., & Yokochi, C. (1993). *Color atlas of anatomy.* New York: Igaku-Shoin.

Twietmayer, A., & McCracken, T. (1992). *Coloring guide to regional human anatomy.* Philadelphia: Lea & Febiger.

Webster, D. B. (1999). *Neuroscience of Communication* (2nd ed.) San Diego, CA: Singular Publishing Group.

Williams, P., & Warrick, R. (1980). *Gray's anatomy* (36th Brit. ed.). Philadelphia: W. B. Saunders.

Winans, S. S., Gilman, S., Manter, J. T., & Gatz, A. J. (2002). *Manter and Gatz's essentials of clinical neuroanatomy and neurophysiology* (10th ed.). Philadelphia: F. A. Davis.

Wood, P. J., & Criss, W. R. (1975). *Normal and abnormal development of the human nervous system.* Hagerstown, MD: Harper & Row.

Yost, W. A. (2000). *Fundamentals of hearing: An introduction* (4th ed.). New York: Academic Press.

Zemlin, W. R. (1998). *Speech and hearing science: Anatomy and physiology* (4th ed.). Needham Heights, MA: Allyn & Bacon.

CHAPTER 13
Neurophysiology

lthough extraordinary advances over the past 30 years have vastly
expanded our understanding of the workings of the brain, we still
have a great deal to learn. We will set out in this chapter to provide at
least some of the pieces to a puzzle. Knowledge of how the nervous system functions is the key to successful treatment by speech-language
pathologists. All therapy works within the limits of the client's nervous
system, because behavior, motivation, learning, and especially speech
and language function depend on the ability to process information and
respond to it. We hope that this introduction to nervous system physiology will tempt you to spend your life examining it.

We will approach our discussion of nervous system function from
the "bottom up," looking first at the simplest responses of the system
(communication between neurons) and working our way up to the all-
important functions of the cerebral cortex (see Table 13-1). The **single
neuron response** and **reflex arc** associated with the spinal cord represent the basic level of information processing, and the brainstem structures provide control of **balance** and other **high-level reflexes**. The
diencephalon supports attention to **stimulation** and **basic** (but highly
organized) **responses to danger.** The cerebellum provides exquisite **integration of sensory information** and **motor planning**, but the cerebrum

Table 13-1. Structures of nervous system and general functions.

STRUCTURE	GENERAL FUNCTION
Spinal arc reflexes	Subconscious response to environmental stimuli
Tracts	Transmit information to cerebrum or periphery
Brainstem	Mediation of high-level reflexes and maintenance of life function; activation of cranial nerves
Diencephalon	Mediates sensory information arriving at cerebrum and provides basic autonomic responses for body maintenance
Cerebellum	Integrates somatic and special sensory information with motor planning and command for coordinated movement
Cerebrum	Processes conscious sensory information, plans and executes voluntary motor act, analyzes stimuli, performs cognitive functions, decodes and encodes linguistic information

is the site of **consciousness, planning, ideation**, and **cognition**. When you are caught off guard by a loud noise, your lower neural processes will register the noise, cause you to orient to it, cause you to flinch, and even possibly to move away from it. Only your cerebrum evaluates the input to determine the nature and meaning of the noise. Your eyes can receive light reflected off of the Mona Lisa; your brainstem visual pathways can process information concerning shapes, forms, textures, and colors—but it takes your cerebrum to wonder why she is smiling.

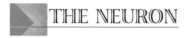

THE NEURON

Neuron Function

The nervous system is composed of billions of neurons whose singular function is to communicate. The communication between neurons occurs at the **synapse**, the union of two neurons. The synapse consists of the end bouton and the synaptic vesicles, the synaptic cleft, and the region of the postsynaptic neuron that contains the ion channels. You will recall from the last chapter that when neurotransmitter is released into the synaptic cleft, the postsynaptic neuron (the neuron after the synapse) will either be inhibited from acting or excited to act. Let's examine transmission of information at the neuronal level. To do that, we must address energy gradients, electrical charge, and membrane permeability.

Gradients

The analogy of a water tower will help explain gradients. Engineers build water towers to hold water so that you can turn on your tap for a drink or a shower. Water is pumped up into the tower using electrical energy, and the energy expended to do that is stored in the elevated water. Because the energy has the **potential** of being expended, it is referred to as *potential energy*. There is a **gradient** of pressure between the tank and your faucet, and the water will flow from the point of higher pressure to the point of lower pressure. You know that water will not naturally flow up the pipe to the tower, but it will flow quite freely if you break a pipe in your house. That sets the stage for discussing the passage of ions through the membranous wall of a neuron. Gradients are established between inside and outside of the cell, and ions have a tendency to flow to equalize that "pressure." We have pumps that move ions to increase that gradient, and we have faucets that we turn on to let those ions flood in. There are two basic forms of gradient that drive ion transport: electrochemical and concentration gradients.

Electrochemical Gradient. In neurons, a gradient is established using electrical charge and molecule density rather than gravity pulling on water, but the analogy with the water tower holds. You may remember from playing with magnets that the positive poles of two magnets repel each other, but opposite poles attract. **Ions** are atoms that have either lost or gained an **electron** (negative particle), causing them to acquire either a positive or negative charge, much like your magnet. Just as with your magnets, positive ions will be repelled by other positive ions but will be attracted to negative ions.

Concentration Gradient. A second type of gradient is derived from concentration of ions. If there is a high concentration of molecules on one side of a membrane (a high **concentration gradient**), the molecules will tend to migrate until there are equal numbers of molecules on either side of the membrane. When charged particles move, the movement produces an electrical current. That is to say, if ions move across a membrane to enter or leave a cell, the very act of moving creates an electrical current. This is important for several reasons. First, current is a prime mover in activating the cell membrane, in that it activates ion channels to open to promote more movement, as will be discussed. Secondly, this is the electrical activity that physicians record when they perform electroencephalography: Electroencephalographic (EEG) traces are the sum of much neural activity within the brain, produced by "generators." More importantly for our field, the electrical activity of neurons is recorded by the audiologist when he or she performs **auditory brainstem response (ABR)** testing. This permits the audiologist to determine whether the auditory pathway is intact by measuring electroencephalographic emanations that have been time-locked to a stimulus such as a pure-tone source or a click. While you will learn more of this in your study of audiologic procedures, the ABR and similar measures of brain function are extremely important tools used by audiologists.

Ions cannot pass through membranous walls unless those walls are **permeable**. **Permeability** is the ease with which ions may pass through a membrane. The wall of a neuron is considered to be semipermeable, meaning that *some* ions may pass through it, given appropriate circumstances. Ions may pass into or out of a healthy neuron wall through two mechanisms: passive and active transport.

Passive Transport. Ions in higher concentration are held back from crossing the neural membrane by special proteins that serve as gatekeepers. **Voltage-sensitive proteins** are those that open when they receive adequate electrical stimulation. There also are **channel proteins** that allow specific ions to pass through the membrane. Essentially, these proteins prohibit ions from passing across the membrane until specific circumstances occur. When the circumstances of transport are met, these proteins will then only let specific ions pass through the membrane wall. The movement is considered to be passive transport because no energy is expended to move the ions across the barrier; rather, the gradient established by inequalities between the two sides of the membrane causes ion movement.

Active Transport. The second mechanism for moving ions (**ion transport**) is active pumping. You will recall that in the water tank analogy, something had to pump water up into the tank. To do so required an *active* process that used energy. There are ion pumps whose role is to move sodium (Na) and potassium (K) ions against the gradient (i.e., pump them "uphill"). The energy used by these **sodium-potassium pump** proteins is in the form of adenosine triphosphate, or ATP, a product of the mitochondria of the cell. The pumps operate continually, moving three sodium ions out for every two potassium ions moved in. Active transport is required to readjust the balance of ions across the membrane so that there is a gradient between the outside and inside of a neuron. Ions move passively across a membrane as a result of a gradient, but when that gradient is eliminated active transport is responsible for reestablishing it. We now have the pieces we need to "fire" a neuron.

Figure 13-1 shows a neuron at rest. The minus signs inside the neuron indicate a negative charge, arising from the relatively smaller number of positive ions within the **intracellular space** (the space within individual cells) than outside in the **interstitial space** (the space between cells). At rest, there is a potential difference of 270 millivolts, a gradient that will promote ion movement if a channel opens to permit that movement. This charge is referred to as the **resting membrane potential (RMP)**. At rest, there are 30 times as many K^+ ions inside as

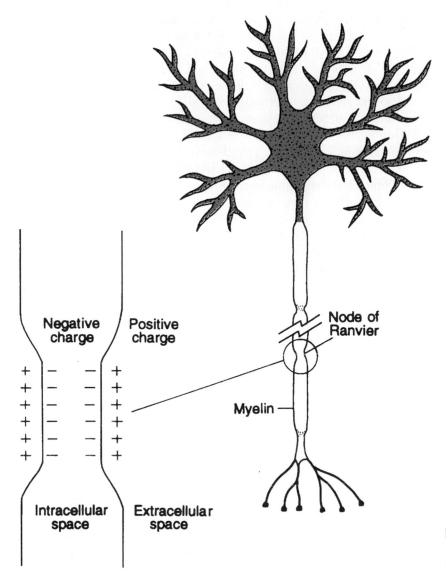

Figure 13-1. A quiescent neuron, showing equilibrium of membrane potential.

outside, and 10 times as many Na^+ ions outside as inside. K^+ is continually leaking out of the cell and is continually being pumped back in by the sodium-potassium pumps. If the membrane were to permit free ion flow, the chemical gradient would drive Na^+ into the cell and K^+ out of the cell. The smaller number of charged particles within the cell drives the potential difference to -70 mV.

An **action potential (AP)** is a change in electrical potential that occurs when the cell membrane is stimulated adequately to permit ion exchange between intra- and extracellular spaces. When a critical threshold of stimulation is reached, the Na^+ ion gates open up, causing the large number of ions to flood the intracellular space and thus raising the intracellular potential to +50 mV over the course of about 1 millisecond (this is a net change of about 120 mV). This equalization of the ion gradient is called **depolarization**. For about 0.5 ms, no amount of stimulation of that region of the membrane will cause it to depolarize again. This phase of depolarization is termed the **absolutely refractory period** (or **absolute refractory period**). The absolutely refractory period is the time during which the cell membrane cannot be stimulated to depolarize. During the absolutely refractory period, the K^+ channels open up and K^+ ions flow out of the intracellular space. The sodium gates will spontaneously close and become inactivated (**sodium inactivation**), and the sodium-potassium pump removes most of the Na^+ ions while increasing the intracellular concentration of K^+ ions. Potassium channels are slower than sodium channels, and the outflow of K^+ ions actually promotes restoration of the RMP, because it increases the relative positivity of the extracellular fluid and, thus, the negativity of the intracellular fluid.

There is a period after the absolutely refractory period during which the membrane may be stimulated, but stimulation will have to be much greater than that required to depolarize it initially. The **relatively refractory period** is a period during which the membrane may be stimulated to excitation again, but only with greater than typical stimulation. This period follows the absolutely refractory period. The relatively refractory period lasts from 5 to 10 ms.

For action potentials to be generated, the membrane channels have to break down. Portions of the cell membrane may be depolarized, but other parts of the membrane will not be depolarized until a critical threshold has been reached. The **critical limit** at which the membrane channels break down is approximately –50 mV. That is, portions of cell membrane may be depolarized, but an action potential is not generated until ion movement is sufficient to elevate the membrane potential from –70 to –50 mV. If the membrane receives sufficient stimulation to cause the potential difference to drop to –50 mV, an action potential will be generated, causing a cascade of ion movement and total depolarization of the neuron. If stimulation does not result in sufficient ion transfer to reach this level, an action potential will not be triggered and the RMP will be restored by the ongoing action of the ion pump. This is an important modulating function of neurons, as we will see: It keeps neurons from firing until there is an adequate stimulus.

This whole cycle from RMP to AP and back to RMP takes about 1 ms in most neurons, and this is a defining time period. This means that a neuron may respond every 1/1,000 of a second, or 1,000 times per second. Even if it is stimulated 2,000 times per second, it will not be able to respond more often.

Propagation. An action potential would do no good at all if it did not propagate, because no information would be passed to the next neuron or to a muscle fiber. **Propagation** refers to the spreading effect of wave action, much as the wave generated by throwing a rock in a pond spreads out from the stone's point of contact with the water. The action potential is propagated in a wave of depolarization. When the membrane undergoing the local polarization reaches the critical limit, ions flow rapidly across the membrane, as we discussed. Because the adjacent membrane contains voltage-sensitive protein channels, the current flow stimulates those regions to depolarize as well. In this manner the depolarization spreads along the membrane, ultimately reaching the terminal of the axon. This regeneration of the action potential along the entire length of the axon will produce precisely the same voltage difference.

The neuron responds in an **all-or-nothing manner**. That is, it either depolarizes or it does not. If it fails to depolarize, no action potential is generated and no information is conveyed. If the critical threshold for depolarization is reached, an action potential will be produced and information will be transmitted. The neuron acts like a light switch in this sense, and the only variation in information is in the frequency with which the neuron is "turned on," referred to as **spike rate** or **rate of discharge**.

Propagation of the action potential is facilitated by axon diameter and myelin. Fibers with larger diameters propagate at a much higher rate than smaller fibers, and myelin further speeds up propagation. Figure 13-2 shows that myelin is laid down on the axon in "donuts" with

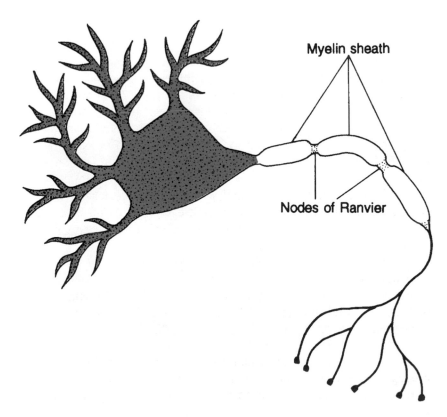

Myelin sheath

Nodes of Ranvier

Figure 13-2. Myelin sheath and nodes of Ranvier.

The node of Ranvier is described in Chapter 12.

nodes of exposed membrane between them. Voltage-sensitive channels are found within the membrane of the **nodes of Ranvier**, but generally are absent in the myelinated regions. The myelin insulates the fiber so that even if there were channels they would serve no function, because ions could not pass through them.

Thus, the membrane becomes depolarized at one node, and the effect of that depolarization is felt at the next node where the membrane depolarizes as well. The propagating action potential is "passed" from node to node, and this jumping is referred to as **saltatory conduction**. Clearly, in long fibers, many precious milliseconds can be saved by skipping from node to node.

When the impulse reaches the terminal point on the axon, a highly specialized process begins. The synaptic vesicles within the terminal end boutons contain a neurotransmitter substance that will permit communication between the two neurons. A **neurotransmitter** is a substance that is released from the terminal end bouton of an axon and causes either excitation or inhibition of another neuron or excitation of a muscle fiber. When the action potential reaches the terminal point, the vesicles are stimulated to migrate to the membrane wall, where they will dump their neurotransmitter through the membrane into the synaptic cleft (see Figure 13-3 and Table 13-2).

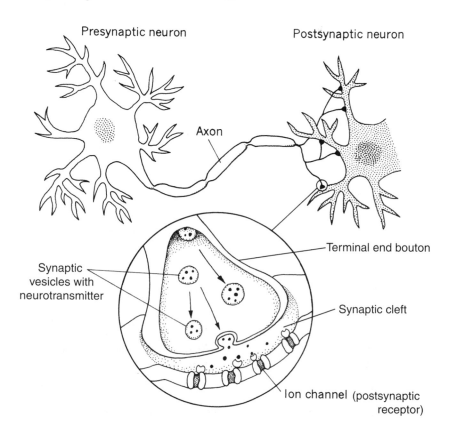

Figure 13-3. A. Expanded view of synapse between two neurons. *(continues)*

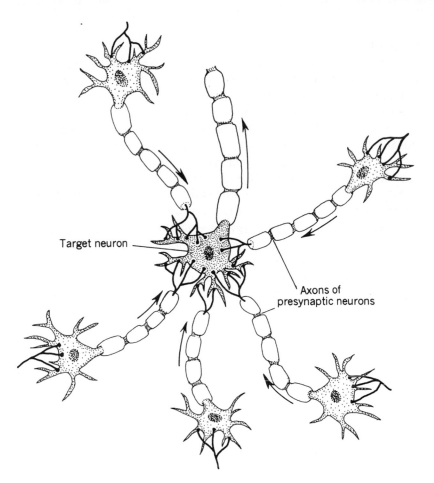

Labels in figure:
Target neuron

Axons of presynaptic neurons

Figure 13-3. *(continued)* **B.** Convergence of multiple neurons upon a single postsynaptic neuron.

Table 13-2. Some neurotransmitters of the peripheral and central nervous system.

NEUROTRANSMITTER	SITE	SPECIFIC REGION (FUNCTION)
Acetylcholine	PNS	Myoneural junction (excitatory)
	CNS	Forebrain, brainstem (modulatory), basal ganglia (inhibitory)
Dopamine	CNS	Limbic system (modulatory), basal ganglia (excitatory)
Norepinephrine	CNS	Brainstem reticular formation (regulatory)
Serotonin	CNS	Brainstem, limbic system (regulatory)
Gamma-aminobutyric acid (GABA)	CNS	Basal ganglia (inhibitory), other CNS structures
Endorphins	CNS	Throughout CNS (pain regulation)

See Bhatnagar & Andy, 1995, and Cotman & McGaugh, 1980, for further discussion.

The neurotransmitter travels across the cleft very quickly (100 microseconds [μs]) and is dumped into the cleft to activate receptor proteins on the **postsynaptic neuron**. Presence of neurotransmitter in the cleft triggers ion channels to open. Neurotransmitters fit specific ion channels, and if a given neurotransmitter does not match a receptor channel protein, the postsynaptic neuron will not fire. That is, the neurotransmitter is a "key" and the receptor is a "lock": If the key does not fit, the gate will not open.

The neurotransmitter may have either an excitatory or an inhibitory effect on the neuron. **Excitatory effects** increase the probability that a neuron will depolarize, whereas **inhibition** decreases that probability. Excitatory stimulation generates an **excitatory postsynaptic potential (EPSP)**, whereas inhibitory synapses produce **inhibitory postsynaptic potentials (IPSPs)**. Excitation causes depolarization, whereas inhibition causes **hyperpolarization**, greatly elevating the threshold of firing. Generally, inhibitory synapses are found on the soma. Synapses on the dendrite are usually excitatory. Synapses on the axon tend to reduce the amount of neurotransmitter substance released into the synaptic cleft, thereby modulating neurotransmitter flow.

The EPSP actually begins as a **micropotential**, depolarizing the membrane by only about 3 mV. If there is a sufficient number of miniature EPSP depolarizations, the sum of their depolarization will reach the critical threshold and an action potential will be generated, as before. You may think of this as voting by neurons. Hundreds or even thousands of neurons make synapse on a given neuron, and that means that the output of that single neuron reflects the "conventional wisdom" of all those neurons. If sufficient numbers of those synapses are activated, the majority wins in an election that you cannot see: Each neuron casts its "votes" in favor of (or against) activation, in the form of activation of a small portion of the receptive membrane. If there are sufficient numbers of depolarizations, there will be an action potential. This is called spatial summation. **Spatial summation** refers to the quality of some neurons that require many near-simultaneous synaptic activations, representing many points of contact arrayed over the surface of the neuron. Likewise, there can be **temporal summation**, in which a smaller number of regions depolarize virtually simultaneously. To stretch our voting analogy to fit temporal summation, votes would have to be cast at approximately the same time to be counted (late-arriving mail-in ballots wouldn't help make the decision).

Single neurons may take input from thousands of other neurons to produce a single response, a process called **convergence**. In this configuration, a mass of information is distilled into a single response. In contrast, **divergence** occurs when the axon of one neuron makes synapse with many thousands of other neurons. Its single piece of information is transmitted to a vast array of other neurons.

Myasthenia Gravis

Myasthenia gravis is a neuromuscular disease; its primary effect is on the neuromuscular junction. It appears that an individual's autoimmune system develops an immune response to the neurotransmitter receptor of the neuromuscular junction, building antibodies that block the receptor. Blocked receptors are unable to respond to neurotransmitter substance, so that, as the disease progresses, greater numbers of receptors become blocked and increasingly fewer ion channels can be activated to depolarize a neuron.

The individual with myasthenia gravis will complain of extreme fatigue as the day progresses: He or she may feel reasonably well in the morning, but become exhausted by noon. The speech-language pathologist is quite often the first person to suspect myasthenia gravis because the individual notices that speech has become more difficult and people are having difficulty understanding what he or she says. Reduced velar function is often an early sign, producing hypernasal speech with reduced intelligibility.

The neurotransmitter substance released into the synaptic cleft does not go to waste. As soon as it is released, enzymes specific to it break it down for resynthesis of the neurotransmitter within the neuron.

In summary:

- Communication between neurons of the nervous system occurs at the **synapse**.
- **Neurotransmitter** passing through the **synaptic cleft** will either **excite** or **inhibit** the postsynaptic neuron.
- If a neuron is excited sufficiently, an **action potential** will be generated.
- Stimulation of a neuron membrane to **depolarize** causes exchange of ions between the extracellular and intracellular spaces, and the ion movement results in a large and predictable change in voltage across the membrane.
- The **resting membrane potential** is the electrical potential measurable prior to excitation.
- The **absolutely refractory period** after excitation is an interval during which the neuron cannot be excited to fire, whereas it may fire during the **relatively refractory period**, given adequate stimulation.
- Because an **action potential** always results in the same neural response, the neuron is capable of representing differences in input only through rate of response.
- Myelinated fibers conduct the wave of depolarization more rapidly than demyelinated fibers, primarily because of **saltatory conduction**.

Muscle Function

A similar process occurs at the **neuromuscular junction**, the point where nerve and muscle communicate. In this case the product of the communication will be a muscle twitch rather than an action potential. The basic unit of skeletal muscle control is the **motor unit**, consisting of the motor neuron, its axon, and the muscle fibers it innervates.

Figure 13-4 shows a neuromuscular junction, which looks very much like a synapse. In this case, however, there is a **terminal endplate** on the axon, with a synaptic cleft as before. The neurotransmitter **acetylcholine** is dumped into the active zone, and a **miniature end plate potential (MEPP)** will be generated. If there are sufficient numbers of MEPPs, a muscle action potential will be generated. This is directly analogous to synapse, in that it takes many activated regions to excite a muscle fiber. In addition, we will see that we have to activate many muscle fibers to actually move a muscle and do work.

You know that movement requires muscular effort, and that muscle can only contract, shortening the distance between two points. This is a good opportunity to examine that function at the microscopic level.

If you were to look at a cotton rope, you would see that the rope is actually made up of smaller ropes, wrapped in a spiral. If you were to look closer you could see that those smaller spiral ropes are made up of

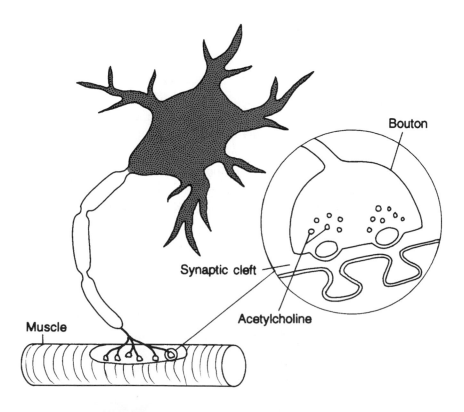

Figure 13-4. Neuromuscular junction between neuron and muscle fiber.

individual strings, and your microscope would show you that those strings were made of cotton fibers that had been spun into thread. *There are successively smaller elements from which the rope is made, and they all have similar orientation and structure.* The same is true for muscle.

As you can see from Figure 13-5, skeletal (striated) muscle is a long ropelike structure made up of strands of muscle fiber, each running the length of the muscle and having many nuclei. Each muscle fiber is made up of long **myofibrils**, and myofibrils are composed of either **thin** or **thick myofilaments**.

Thin myofilaments are composed of a pair of **actin** protein strands coiled around each other to form a spiral or helix. Double strands of **tropomyosin** that are laced with molecules of **troponin** wrap around this helix. **Thick filaments** are composed of myosin molecules arranged in staggered formation. These two components (actin and myosin) are key players in movement: The actin and myosin filaments slide past each

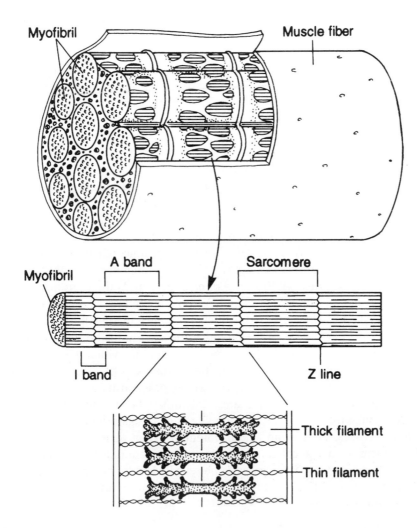

Figure 13-5. Exploded view of muscle fiber components. Each muscle fiber is made up of thin and thick filaments. (After view of Campbell, 1987.)

other during muscle contraction, with **bridging arms** reaching from the myosin to the actin. The tropomyosin and troponin facilitate the bridging arms, as you shall see.

When the myofilaments group together to form muscle myofibrils, a characteristic striated appearance is seen. This is the product of alternating dark and light myofilaments. Each of these combined units is known as a **sarcomere**. The sarcomere is the building block of striated muscle. An area known as the **Z line** marks the margin of the sarcomere, and the thin filaments are bound at this point. The thick filaments are centered within the sarcomere, much like overlapping bricks in a wall. The **A band** is the region of overlap between thin and thick fibers at rest, and the **H zone** in the center of the sarcomere is a region with only thick filaments. The two myofilaments slide across each other as the muscle shortens, bringing the centers of the thin and thick filaments closer together. Here is how that happens.

When the muscle is at rest, the regulatory proteins of tropomyosin on the thin filaments block the binding sites, prohibiting formation of cross-bridges. The regulatory proteins are guards that prohibit the myosin and actin from interacting. For a cross-bridge to form, the tropomyosin must be moved out of the way to free up the binding sites, and that function is performed by calcium. When calcium is present in the environment, it changes the configuration of the proteins, revealing the binding site on the thin filaments and facilitating development of cross-bridges. Calcium has the "password" that causes the tropomyosin "guards" to move away from the binding sites and to permit cross-bridges to form. What causes the calcium to enter the environment, though?

Calcium is found within the **sarcoplasmic reticulum** of the muscle cytoplasm. (Sarcoplasmic reticulum is a form of the cellular endoplasmic reticulum.) An action potential generated at the neuromuscular junction is conveyed deep into the muscle cell by a series of transverse tubules that are in contact with the sarcoplasmic reticulum. The AP depolarizes the membrane of the sarcoplasmic reticulum, permitting calcium ions to be released. Presence of calcium causes the morphology of tropomyosin and troponin to change, exposing binding sites and permitting myosin to bridge from the thick filaments to the thin filaments. Adenosine triphosphate (ATP) provides the energy to the bridging arm (that's the same "energy" that you "run out of" when you become fatigued from overwork), which reaches across to a binding site on the thin filaments, pulls, and releases even as other arms are pulling and releasing. When the AP terminates, calcium is taken back up into the sarcoplasmic reticulum, the binding site is once again hidden, and contraction ceases. That is, an action potential at the neuromuscular junction causes release of calcium into the environment of actin and myosin. Calcium causes the binding sites to be revealed so that cross-bridges can be formed between the two molecules—at that point, muscle contraction has begun.

This seems like a lot of work to contract a muscle, and it is. Work requires energy, and ATP supplies it. The actual contraction is much like pulling yourself up a mountainside using a rope. You grab the rope (cross-bridge) and pull, hand-over-hand, drawing yourself upward. Your arms are like the myosin arms, the rope is like the thin filament of actin, and you are the thick filament. This is the **sliding filament model** of muscle contraction.

In this process, the center of the sarcomere (the H zone) will disappear as the sarcomere shortens. There are about 350 heads on each thick filament that can bridge across to the thin filaments, and each bridge can perform its hand-over-hand act five times per second. If you remember that it takes many myofilaments to make up one muscle fiber, and that a muscle bundle is made up of many muscle fibers, you will begin to realize the magnitude of activity involved in moving your little finger!

Muscle Control

This still does not tell us how a muscle does its job. When the AP is generated and the sarcoplasmic reticulum releases calcium, there is an all-or-none response, and the muscle twitches. From your study, you already know that muscles come in all sizes, from the massive to the minute. In addition, muscles must perform vastly different functions, ranging from gross, slow movement to quick, precise action. How do we manage this?

The answer to this question lies largely in allocation of resources. For fine movement, only a limited number of muscle fibers need be recruited for movement, because you are not trying to move as much mass. In contrast, heavy lifting requires recruitment of many muscle fibers. This makes sense if you consider the effort involved in moving objects. It only takes one person to move a chair, but it might take four or five individuals to lift a piano.

Neuromotor innervation accounts for much of the allocation of resources: Each muscle fiber is innervated by one motor neuron, but each motor neuron may innervate a large number of muscle fibers. The more motor neurons that are activated, the greater the number of fibers that will contract. Use of many motor nerves to activate a muscle is called **multiple motor unit summation**.

Another mechanism of control comes from a functional difference between how various muscles act. There are two basic types of muscle fibers: slow twitch and fast twitch fibers. As their name implies, **slow twitch fibers** take a longer time to move, whereas fast twitch fibers are capable of much more rapid movement. Slow twitch muscle fibers remain contracted five times longer than fast twitch fibers, perhaps because calcium remains in the cytoplasm for longer periods. Slow twitch fibers are typically found in muscles that must contract for long periods of time, such as those used to support your body against gravity. Fast twitch muscles, in contrast, are used to meet rapid contraction requirements. Now remember our discussion of the tongue anatomy and physiology: Recall that the tongue tip moves much more rapidly than the massive dorsum, but it is not *only* mass of the musculature that determines speed of response. The rapidly moving tongue tip is supplied with *fast twitch fibers*, but slow-moving deep tongue muscles have *slow twitch fibers*.

There is another significant difference between slow and fast twitch fibers. One neuron may innervate thousands of slow twitch fibers, but neurons serving fast twitch fibers may innervate only 10 or 20 muscle fibers. With this difference in innervation ratio you can get extremely fine control: If you need to tense the vocal folds quickly for pitch change, you want to be able to control precisely the fraction of a millimeter required to keep your voice from going sharp while singing. This control comes from being able to activate progressively more motor units in fine steps. In contrast, maintaining an erect posture requires less precision and more stamina.

To summarize:

- Activation of a muscle fiber causes release of calcium into the environment of **thick myofilaments**, revealing the binding sites on the **thin filaments** that permit **cross-bridging** from the thick filaments.

- The action of the bridging causes the myofilaments to slide past each other, thereby shortening the muscle.

- **Slow twitch** muscle fibers remain contracted longer than **fast twitch** fibers, with the former being involved in maintenance of posture and the latter in fine and rapid motor function.

Muscle Spindle Function

We touched on the activities of the muscle spindle in Chapter 12, but let us discuss its function more thoroughly. If you examine Figure 13-6, you will see the major players in posture and motor control in general. It is sobering to realize that the lowest level of motor response (the stretch reflex) is intimately related to the highest levels of motor response requiring extraordinary skill and dexterity, such as fine motor control of the fingers. Discussion of the muscle spindle will provide the background necessary to talk about higher-level motor control.

The role of the muscle spindle is to provide feedback to the neuromotor system about muscle length and thus information about motion and position. Before we explain that function, let us examine the structure of this important sensory element.

There are two basic types of striated muscle fibers with which we must be concerned. **Extrafusal muscle** fibers make up the bulk of the muscles discussed over the past several chapters. Deep within the struc-

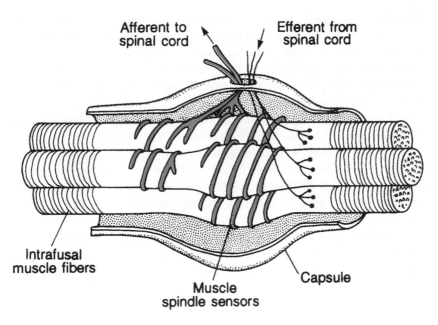

Afferent to spinal cord

Efferent from spinal cord

Intrafusal muscle fibers

Muscle spindle sensors

Capsule

Figure 13-6. Schematic representation of a muscle spindle.

ture of the muscle is another set of muscle fibers, referred to as **intra-fusal muscle** fibers. These fibers have a parallel course to the extrafusal fibers and would not really be obvious on gross examination of a muscle. Close examination would reveal short **intrafusal fibers** that attach to the muscle and are capable of sensing changes in the length of the muscle. At or near the **equatorial region** of the intrafusal muscle fiber are the stretch sensors themselves, with the combination of muscle and sensor known as the **muscle spindle**, so named because of its spindle shape.

The intrafusal fibers may be classified as being either **thin** or **thick**. Thick muscle fibers typically are outfitted with a capsule that contains nuclear bag fibers, and thin muscle fibers house nuclear chain fibers. **Nuclear bag fibers** are groups of stretch receptors collected in a cluster at the equatorial region of the intrafusal muscle fiber. **Nuclear chain fibers,** in contrast, are a row of stretch sensors in the equatorial region. These two configurations serve different functions, as we shall see. The placement of the capsules in the equatorial region is important, because that portion of these fibers is noncontractile.

The muscle spindle has both afferent and efferent innervation. The afferent component conveys the sensation of muscle length change to the central nervous system, while the efferent system sends nerve impulses that cause the intrafusal fibers to contract. The innervation pattern is important. Nuclear bag fibers send information to the CNS by means of **Group Ia primary** afferent fibers, which wrap around the capsule in a spiral formation. Group Ia fibers are large, and when the muscle is stretched, the nuclear bag changes shape. That distortion causes the nerve to fire, sending information to the spinal cord. Bags surrounding

The term nuclear bag fiber *refers to the portion of the muscle spindle that is formed by a cluster of stretch sensors situated on the equatorial region of the muscle fiber.*

nuclear chain fibers may have primary Ia afferents as well, but may instead have **Group II secondary** afferent fibers. These are smaller fibers conveying a functionally different response, although they also respond to stretching of the muscle.

Extrafusal (general skeletal muscle) and intrafusal (muscle spindle) muscle fibers have distinctly different innervation. Extrafusal muscle is innervated through **alpha** motor fibers, which are larger in diameter than the **gamma** (or **fusimotor**) efferent fibers of the intrafusal muscle.

As you can see, there is a great deal of physical differentiation going on with this sensorimotor system. There are two types of sensors, two types of afferent fibers delivering information to the CNS, and a specialized efferent system (gamma efferents) that can cause the intrafusal muscle to contract.

The muscle spindle responds to both phasic and tonic muscle lengthening. **Phasic lengthening** refers to the period during which a muscle is undergoing a *change* in length. This information is transduced by the nuclear bag fibers and conveyed via Group Ia afferents to the CNS. **Tonic lengthening** refers to a muscle that is *maintained* in a lengthened condition, and this information is conveyed via the nuclear chain fibers by means of either type of afferent. It turns out that both pieces of information are essential for motor control.

Figure 13-7 will help us discuss how this system helps you control your muscles. A useful way to describe how the spindle works is to think of posture control. If you were to pay close attention to your body as you

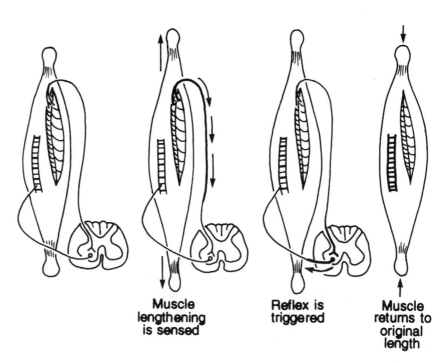

Figure 13-7. Schematic representation of muscle spindle function to control muscle length.

Muscle
lengthening
is sensed

Reflex is
triggered

Muscle
returns to
original
length

stand in line at the post office, you would notice that you sway ever so slightly. That slight movement you feel is a trigger for the intrafusal system.

When you lean a little, some of your leg muscles stretch. When they do so, the spindle sends notice to the motor neuron within the spinal column that the muscle has changed position. The motor neuron with which it synapses immediately activates the extrafusal muscle mass to contract, thereby counteracting that "accidental" stretching that occurred in response to gravity. Notice that you passively stretched the muscle spindle fibers and then the muscles of your leg with which those spindles are associated contracted to return the muscle to its original length.

One more thing to note in Figure 13-7 is that this afferent synapses with another neuron. In the drawing, the spindle within the flexor is sending its information centrally. The afferent makes **inhibitory** synapse with extensors associated with the same joint, so that you are not only actively contracting flexors but also actively inhibiting contraction of extensors.

There are hosts of reflexive responses, mediated by the spinal cord, brainstem, and even through cortical response. While it is clearly beyond the scope of this review to discuss those, you may wish to examine Table 13-3 for a sampling of some of those reflexes.

Lesions and the Gamma Efferent System

To appreciate the effects of lesions to the extrapyramidal system, it might help to do a quick exercise. Do this: Reach across the desk top to pick up a pencil. As you do this, pay attention to what your muscles are doing. Even as you reach for the pencil, your elbow rotates to accommodate the needs of your arm and hand to make contact with the object. As you get close to the target, your fingers start to close and the rate of movement of your arm slows down. For all of this to happen, your brain must know how fast your muscles are changing length, as well as where the target is located in space relative to your hand and body. Contraction of extensors obviously is important, but your brain must also contract flexors to help control extensor contraction, lest the movement be ballistic.

Damage to the cerebellum will reduce activation of the fusimotor system. Because this system maintains muscle tone through mild, constant muscle contraction, muscles in a patient with lesions to the cerebellum will lose tone and become flaccid. In contrast, loss of the moderating control by the cerebrum through lesion will cause hypertonia in antigravity musculature and extensors, because the stretch reflexes are unrestrained. In this condition, the alpha system is either disabled or not well coordinated with the gamma system due to the lesion, and spasticity results.

Lesions and conditions of the basal ganglia will have various effects, among them the rigidity of Parkinson's disease. In this condition, intrafusal systems for both extensors and flexors are unrestrained, resulting in simultaneous contraction of antagonists and rigidity. Other basal ganglia lesions will result in general hypertonicity.

Table 13-3. A sample of reflexes mediated by spinal cord and brainstem. Note that several variations have been eliminated for brevity, as have specific stimulus conditions.

SPINAL REFLEXES	
Palmar grasp reflex	Placing object on ventral surface of fingers causes fingers to flex (up to 3 to 4 months).
Sucking reflex	Stroking lips laterally causes sucking action (ends at 6 months to 1 year).
Knee-jerk tendon	Rapid stretching of patellar tendon by tapping on knee at tendon causes extension of leg (present after 6 months).
Flexor withdrawal	In supine, head in mid position; leg flexes when sole of foot stimulated (ends at 2 months).
Extensor thrust	In supine, head in mid position, one leg extended, one flexed; leg remains flexed when sole stimulated (ends at 2 months).
Crossed extension	In supine, head in mid position, one leg extended, one flexed; when extended leg is flexed, the opposite leg will extend (before 2 months) or remain flexed (after 2 months).
Crossed extension	In supine, head in mid position, legs extended; stimulation of medial leg surface causes adduction (ends at 2 months).

BRAINSTEM REFLEXES	
Asymmetrical tonic neck reflex (ATNR)	In supine, arms and legs extended, head in mid position; if head turned, arm on face side extends, arm on opposite side flexes (ends 4–6 months).
Symmetrical tonic neck reflex	In quadruped, on tester's knee; ventroflex (toward belly), no change in arm/leg tone (before 6 months) or arms flex or increase tone and legs extend or increase tone (after 6 months).
Tonic labyrinthine supine reflex	In supine, arms and legs extended; passive flexing of arms and legs does not increase tone (before 6 months) or does increase tone (after 6 months).
Tonic labyrinthine prone reflex	In prone, head mid position, no increase in flexor tone (before 4 months) or cannot dorsiflex head, retract shoulders, or extend arms and legs (after 4 months).
Associated	In supine, have individual squeeze object; increases tone in opposite arm and hand (before 6 months) or no change in opposite-side tone (after 6 months).
Positive supporting reactions	In standing position, bounce individual on soles of feet; no increase in leg tone (up to 8 months) or increase in extensor tone (after 8 months).
Neck righting reflex	In supine, head in mid position, arms and legs extended; rotate head and body will rotate (before 6 months) or not rotate (after 6 months).
Body righting; acting on the body	In supine, head in mid position, arms and legs extended; rotate head to one side and body rotates as a whole (before 6 months) or head turns, then shoulders, and finally pelvis (after 6 months).
Labyrinthine righting; acting on the head	Blindfolded and suspended in prone; head does not raise (before 2 months) or raises with face vertical and mouth horizontal (after 1 month).
Optical righting	Held in space in prone, head does not raise (before 2 months) or raises to face vertical and mouth horizontal (after 2 months).

(continues)

Table 13-3. *(continued)*

BRAINSTEM REFLEXES *(continued)*	
Moro reflex	In semireclined, drop head backward; arms extend, arms rotate, fingers extend and abduct (under 4 months).
Landau reflex	Held in space supported at thorax in prone; raise head and spine and legs extend and remain in flexed position (from 6 months).
Positive extensor thrust (parachute reaction)	In prone, arms extended overhead, suspended in space by pelvis; move suddenly downward; arms extend, fingers abduct and extend to protect head (after 6 months).
Rooting reflex and sucking reflex	Stroke the side of the mouth at the corner of the lips laterally; the infant will orient toward the fingers with a sucking motion of the lips (before 6 months).
Jaw reflex	Pull down on the mandible briskly, or draw down on the masseter with deep pressure and the mandible will snap to close (before 6 months).

For a thorough review of reflexes, elicitation procedures, and normal and pathological responses, see Bly (1994) and Fiorentino (1973).

What if you move your legs purposefully? How do the muscle spindles oppose *that* movement? When a new posture is reached, the intrafusal muscle contracts to adjust the tension on the spindle, accommodating the new posture. Likewise, the muscle spindle afferent information is delivered to the cerebral cortex and to the cerebellum. When voluntary movement is initiated, both alpha and gamma systems are activated. There is speculation that the gamma system receives information from the cortex concerning the desired or *target* muscle length, and thus the gamma system provides feedback to the cortex when this length has been achieved. Thus, the gamma system may be a regulatory mechanism for voluntary movement: Damage to this system has devastating effects.

Golgi Tendon Organs

Another type of sensor, which is less well understood, is the Golgi tendon organ (GTO), a sensor located at the tendon and sensitive to the degree of tension on the muscle. If the muscle is passively stretched, it takes a great deal to excite a GTO. However, if a muscle is contracted, the GTO is quite sensitive to the tension placed on it.

The GTO probably works in close conjunction with the muscle spindle. The muscle spindle is active any time a muscle is *lengthened,* while the GTO is sensitive to the *tension* placed on the muscle. If a muscle is tensed isometrically, lengthening will be minimal but the GTO will react to the tension placed on it by contraction. Likewise, if a muscle is passively stretched, the muscle spindle will respond but the tendon organ will not.

Other Sensation and Sensors

There are a host of other receptors, as we discussed in Chapters 9 and 12. Sensory receptors are nerve endings that have become specialized to **transduce** (change) energy from one form to another.

When one of these sensors is stimulated, it sends information concerning that stimulation to the CNS for processing. You will not be aware of stimulation unless a threshold of stimulation is reached. This **threshold** varies from sensor to sensor, and even from individual to individual. A stimulus capable of eliciting a response from a given receptor is termed the **adequate stimulus**. The receptor converts the energy exciting it into electrochemical energy, producing what is referred to as a **receptor potential** or **generator potential**, depending on how far the information is being transferred. The magnitude of the potential is related to that of the stimulus, and it typically will be constant until the stimulus is removed.

Sensors vary in morphology and function, but fall into the general classes of encapsulated and nonencapsulated. Encapsulated sensors tend to be pressure sensitive, transducing pressure applied to the skin into electrochemical energy sensed by the nervous system. Some sensors are **rapidly adapting**, in that they respond only to *change* in stimulation. These sensors are particularly well suited for transduction of vibration, whereas **slowly adapting** sensors respond better to long-duration stimulation. Pain, temperature, and some mechanoreceptors are simply unshielded nerve endings that respond when stimulated by one or several different stimuli. The sensation of joint position in space apparently is the product of many of these encapsulated and nonencapsulated sensors.

To summarize:

- **Muscle spindles** provide feedback to the neuromotor system about muscle length, tension, motion, and position.
- Muscle spindles running parallel to intrafusal muscle fibers sense lengthening of muscle, whereas **Golgi tendon organs** sense muscle tension.
- **Nuclear bag fibers** convey information concerning acceleration, whereas the **nuclear chain fibers** are responsive to sustained lengthening.
- When a muscle is passively stretched, a **segmental reflex** is triggered; this in turn activates the **extrafusal muscles** paralleling the muscle spindles, thereby shortening the muscle.
- **Golgi tendon organs** apparently respond to the tension of musculature during active contraction.
- There are many other receptor types, but the common thread is that they all transduce internal or external environment information into electrochemical impulses.
- When a sensor is stimulated beyond its threshold for response, it sends information concerning that stimulation to the CNS for processing.

HIGHER FUNCTIONING

We have been discussing responses that occur at the lowest levels of the nervous system and often do not even reach consciousness. Although it is essential for your brain to know what your tongue muscles are doing, it is obvious that there is more to speech than movement of muscles.

A lively debate concerning localization of function within the brain has been going on for well over 100 years. On the one hand, **localizationists** (or "materialists" as they were called in the 1860s) held that, given sufficiently sensitive tools, specific functions could be localized to specific brain regions. The opposing view, held by "**spiritualists**," was that it was degrading to think that the human body (much less the brain) could be so mechanically dissected, and that functions such as language or mathematics could not be isolated to a single brain region. Perhaps the first localizationist was Joseph Gall, who also proposed that a properly knowledgeable individual could identify specific cognitive traits of an individual by reading the bumps on that person's head (**phrenology**) (Kandel, 1991).

While phrenology did not retain many followers, one admirer of Gall, Paul Broca, was the first to identify the region for expressive language within the dominant hemisphere of the brain (Kandel, 1991; Schuell, Jenkins, & Jimenez-Pabon, 1964). Others provided counterevidence, including patients whose acquired language deficit clearly arose from another region distal from the area identified by Broca. Such notables as Sigmund Freud refuted the notion of localization of function, saying that although some specific locations for basic processes might be found, that still did not explain complex cognitive function (Schuell, Jenkins, & Jimenez-Pabon, 1964).

Carl Wernicke entered the battle, clearly identifying a language center within the temporal lobe distinct from that identified by Broca. Indeed, as the twentieth century dawned, localization of function was demonstrated through ablation studies of the occipital and temporal lobes of dogs, eliminating visual and auditory recognition, respectively. Researchers found that they could stimulate specific locales of a dog's cerebrum and cause single, replicable movements of the limbs (Schuell, Jenkins, & Jimenez-Pabon, 1964).

Although such notable researchers as Karl Lashley countered the growing body of evidence, research that examined brain-damaged soldiers during the First and Second World Wars revealed a great deal of "regional" consistency of symptoms, and these findings led us into the study and treatment of acquired language disorders (Kandel, 1991).

Parallel work by microbiologists such as Nobel laureates David Hubel and Torsten Wiesel, in their work with monkeys (Hubel, 1979) and Colin Blakemore and Grahame Cooper (1970), working with cats, revealed a degree of specificity in the nervous system that must have surpassed even Broca's dreams. Researchers have found neurons within the nervous system that respond to exactly one form of stimulation (for example, vertical lines presented to the visual system) and no other stimulation. These findings revealed extremes of localization of function.

That having been said, there appears no end to the complexity of the nervous system. Despite precise localization of function within the brain, no one is willing to say that any single region is solely responsible for complex cognitive function. Rather, it is the interaction of diverse regions that gives us the ability to think, learn, speak, and communicate.

We will take a regional approach to review of the function of the cerebral cortex. Although it is clear that regions of the cerebral cortex, such as the motor strip, are highly specialized for specific functions, other regions of the cortex are less well defined. To further confound things, the developing brain is **plastic**. The brains of infants who receive trauma are more likely to overcome damage to function than adults receiving the same trauma. This and other evidence has led to theories of **equipotentiality**, which state that the brain functions as a whole. One could strike a balance with the notion of **regional equipotentiality**. There seems to be a functional unity by regions, but the degree of functional loss to an individual receiving trauma also is related to the total volume of damaged tissue. Our discussion will focus on the functional regions and association pathways of the brain, and on the interconnections among regions.

The cortex appears to be organized around regions of **primary** activity for a given area, including the primary receptive area for somatic sense, primary motor area, primary auditory cortex, and primary region of visual reception (see Figure 13-8). Adjacent to these are **higher-order areas of processing**. That is, there are secondary, tertiary, and even quaternary areas of higher-order processing adjacent to the primary receptive areas for sensation. There also are higher-order areas of processing for motor function, as we shall see. Beyond the higher-order areas of processing are **association areas** in which the highest form of human thought occurs. That is, we receive information from our senses at primary reception areas and we extract the information received and put it together with other information associated with the modality at higher-order areas of processing. This information is passed to association areas for the highest level of cognitive processing.

The **primary reception area for vision (VI)** is located within the calcarine fissure of the occipital lobe (area 17). At that location, precise maps of information received at the retinae are projected. The **secondary visual processing region** is considered to be area 18 of the occipital lobe, with even higher-level processing regions found in the temporal lobe (areas 20, 21) and occipital lobe (area 19 and the region anterior to it). Area 7 of the parietal lobe performs higher-level processing of visual information as well. Because higher-level processing sites seem to be concerned with feature extraction, the precise visual field map projected

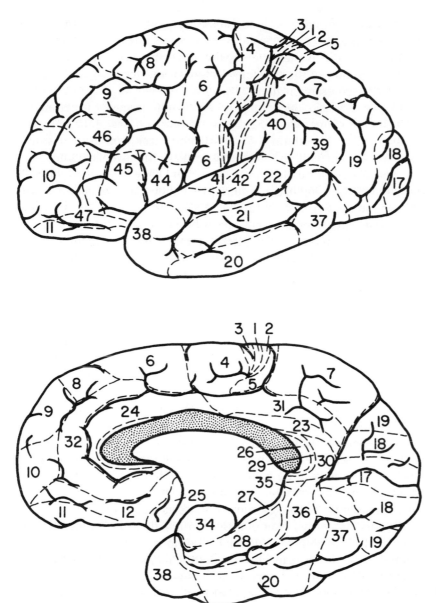

Figure 13-8. Brodmann's area map of lateral and medial cerebrum.

onto the primary cortex is generally not found at those higher-level processing sites.

Somatic sense is received by the parietal lobe, with the primary reception area (SI) being the postcentral gyrus (areas 1, 2, and 3). Again, studies have repeatedly demonstrated that body sense is projected somatotopically along this strip, but this projection is much less apparent at the secondary sites. The opercular portion of the parietal lobe is considered to be the higher-order processing region, as is area 5 of the parietal lobe (Kupfermann, 1991).

The cochlea and the brainstem nuclei serving it have a tonotopic array, which is the correlate of the spatiotopic array seen in the motor strip. High-frequency sounds are resolved at the basal end of the cochlea, whereas low-frequency sounds are resolved at the cochlea apex. Frequency is spread out in an orderly, sequential array along the basilar membrane of the cochlea, and this tonotopic arrangement is seen in the projections at nearly all levels of the auditory pathway.

Auditory information is tonotopically projected at Heschl's gyrus (area 41) of the temporal lobe (AI), whereas the superior temporal gyrus (area 22) performs higher-level processing of the auditory input. There is some retention of the tonotopic nature of the received signal at the higher-level processing region.

Three regions of the brain play central roles in **motor function**, but to discuss these areas we must clarify the three phases of the voluntary motor act. First, to perform a voluntary motor task, you must identify a target, such as making the tongue tip contact the alveolar ridge. Next, you must develop a plan to achieve the target behavior. Finally, you must execute the plan, a process requiring the movement of muscles with accurate timing, force, and rate.

These three functions appear to be governed by three different regions of the cerebral cortex. First, the target must be identified, and this is a function of the posterior parietal lobe. The posterior parietal lobe (areas 5, 7, 39, and 40) processes information about somatic sensation related to **spatial orientation**, including integration of information about position of body parts in space and visual information. Inputs to these parietal regions arise from the thalamus: The venteroposterolateral thalamic nucleus (VPLo) projects body sense information from distant receptors; the caudal ventrolateral thalamic nucleus (VLc) and VPLo project cerebellar information to the posterior parietal regions; and the VLc and ventral anterior nucleus (VA) project information from the basal ganglia to the posterior parietal lobe. In this way, the posterior parietal lobe receives a complete "body map" of the location and condition of all body parts, including the speech articulators.

The second area, the **premotor region** (area 6), anterior to the motor strip, appears to be involved in planning the action. The premotor region takes information from the parietal lobe (areas 1, 2, and 3) concerning the immediate location of muscles and joints and integrates that information with a plan of action. In addition, the **supplementary motor area** (**SMA**; superior and medial portions of area 6) is involved in even more complex acts, including speech initiation. The SMA is strongly involved in the preparatory speech act, as well as in the decision to initiate the act. If an individual is only told to mentally rehearse, the SMA will be activated without the premotor region becoming involved.

Finally, the precentral gyrus or **motor strip** (MI) found in area 4 is responsible for execution of voluntary movement. The motor strip neurons make up half of the pyramidal tract, the major motor pathway. Commands to muscles from the motor strip include information concerning the degree of force and timing of contraction.

Motor System Lesions

Damage to specific regions of the brain have been used repeatedly to infer the function of those regions. Clearly, if a portion of the brain is damaged and specific dysfunction can be consistently identified, that portion of the brain can be assumed to be intimately involved in the lost function. That having been said, specific regions of function for higher cognitive processes are difficult to specify, precisely because the processes involved are so complex and require multiple subsystems to function. In the same vein, removing the knob of a radio may make it impossible to receive a radio signal, but that doesn't mean that the knob was the *only* component involved in receiving a signal. It is important to realize that speech, language, and cognitive processes are exceedingly complex, and our understanding of localized function is revised continuously. Nonetheless, it is fruitful to examine the information we have gleaned from years of observing the results of brain damage.

A lesion to the motor strip will result in muscular weakness and loss of motor function on the side of the body opposite the lesion. **Dysarthria** is a speech disorder arising from paralysis, muscular weakness, and dyscoordination of speech musculature. The type of dysarthria is broadly defined by the site of the lesion.

Flaccid dysarthria arises from damage to lower motor neurons (LMNs) or their cell bodies. Thus, flaccid dysarthria generally reflects damage to the cranial nerves serving speech muscles. As we discussed in Chapter 12, focal lesions to cranial nerves have focal effects on the musculature they serve, and this is manifested in the various subtypes of flaccid dysarthria that one sees clinically. For instance, damage to the VII facial nerve will result in facial paralysis, whereas damage to the V trigeminal will produce paralysis of the muscles of mastication. Damage to the recurrent laryngeal nerve of the X vagus will result in flaccid dysphonia. In all cases, the result will be a flaccid paralysis, manifested as a muscular weakness and **hypotonia** (low muscle tone). If the cell body is involved in the lesion, there may also be **fasciculations** or twitching movements of the affected articulator. In addition, because the damage occurs distal to the interneurons serving the reflex arc (which is a central phenomenon within the brainstem or spinal cord), reflexive responses mediated by the nerve are either reduced or absent. You can normally elicit a jaw jerk reflex by pulling down on a slack jaw, but this reflex may be reduced or absent in flaccid dysarthria if the V trigeminal is involved.

Specific cranial nerve functions and disorders are discussed in Chapter 12.

Spastic dysarthria arises from bilateral damage to upper motor neurons (UMNs) of the pyramidal (direct) and extrapyramidal (indirect) motor pathways. The direct pathway generally is excitatory, being involved with execution of skilled motor acts. The indirect pathway generally is inhibitory, controlling background activities such as maintenance of muscle tone, posture, and agonist contraction to control the trajectory for movement.

Bilateral UMN damage results in an inability to execute skilled movements (paralysis) and muscle weakness. Damage to the extrapyramidal system results in *loss of inhibition* of reflexes, or **hyperreflexia**, as well as increased muscle tone, or **hypertonia**. Thus, the jaw jerk reflex mentioned in the discussion of flaccid dysarthria would now be very easily triggered, to the point that the individual could not control the response.

The person with spastic dysarthria demonstrates reduced force of contraction of muscles from the pyramidal lesion, and this is further confounded by easily elicited reflexive contractions arising from attempting to use the articulators. That is, attempts by the affected individual to lower his or her jaw will result in reflexive contraction of the muscles that elevate the jaw, thereby foiling the attempt. Therapy obviously will be directed toward regaining control over those reflexes!

When a unilateral lesion occurs in the region of facial muscle control, the result is **unilateral upper motor neuron dysarthria** (UUMN) (Duffy, 1995). The effects of UUMN dysarthria are less devastating than those of a bilateral lesion. UUMN results in spastic signs on the side contralateral to the lesion for the tongue and lower facial muscles, because they have unilateral (contralateral) innervation, whereas other articulatory muscles are bilaterally innervated.

Ataxic dysarthria arises from damage to the cerebellum or to the brainstem vestibular nuclei, or both. Because the cerebellum is responsible for coordination of motor activity, ataxic dysarthria is characterized by loss of coordination, deficits in achieving an articulatory target, and problems in coordinating rate, range, and force of movement. Speech in ataxic dysarthria will be distorted because irregular articulation results from **overshoot** (moving an articulator beyond its target) and **undershoot** (moving an articulator an insufficient distance to reach the target). **Dysdiadochokinesia**, a deficit in the ability to make repetitive movements, is a dominant characteristic, as is **dysprosody**, or deficit in maintenance of the intonation and linguistic stress of speech.

Hyperkinetic and hypokinetic dysarthria are the result of damage to different regions of the extrapyramidal system. **Hyperkinetic dysarthria** is characterized by extraneous, involuntary movement of speech musculature *in addition to* movement produced voluntarily. That is, in hyperkinetic dysarthria, articulators move without voluntary muscular contraction, and this is overlaid on the speech act. Hyperkinesias are seen primarily in damage to the basal ganglia circuitry, especially that responsible for inhibiting movement.

Damage to the subthalamic nucleus, which inhibits the globus pallidus, results in uncontrolled flailing known as **ballism**. If damage to the basal ganglia results in a decrease in the neurotransmitter acetylcholine (ACh) or an increase in dopamine (DA), extraneous **choreiform** movements (involuntary twitching and movement of muscles) will result, such as those seen in Huntington's disease. Hyperkinesias take a number of forms, ranging from **tics** (rapid movement of small groups of muscle fibers) and **tremors** (rhythmic contractions) to **athetosis** (slow, writhing movements) and **dystonia** (involuntary movement to a posture, with the posture being held briefly).

Hypokinetic dysarthria is characterized by paucity of movement, most often caused by Parkinson's disease. The disease arises from damage to the substantia nigra, the cell mass responsible for production of dopamine (DA). Dopamine is used by the basal ganglia to balance ACh, and a shortage of DA results in inhibited initiation of motor function, reduction of range of movement, co-contraction of agonists and antagonists (resulting in **rigidity**), and a characteristic pill-rolling tremor of the hands. Speech in Parkinson's disease will be rushed, with reduced duration of speech sounds, reduced vocal intensity, and reduced fluctuation in fundamental frequency.

Mixed dysarthrias arise from damage to more than one of the controlling systems. **Mixed spastic-flaccid dysarthria** is found in amyotrophic lateral sclerosis, a disease that attacks the myelin of UMN and LMN fibers. **Mixed spastic-ataxic dysarthria** results from damage to the UMN and cerebellar control circuitry, as often seen in multiple sclerosis. **Mixed hypokinetic-ataxic-spastic dysarthria** occurs with the degeneration of Wilson's disease (hepatolenticular degeneration). Generally, one may see any combination of dysarthrias, based on the systems involved in the disease process (Duffy, 1995).

The dysarthrias are all characterized by some degree of loss of motor function accompanied by muscular weakness and dyscontrol. In contrast, **dyspraxia** is a dysfunction of motor planning *in the absence of muscular weakness* or muscular dysfunction.

Damage to the premotor region results in gross dyspraxia for the motor function mediated by the area broadly served by the adjacent motor strip neurons. With damage to the SMA, an individual will have difficulty initiating speech, and the effect is bilateral. Verbal dyspraxia appears to be directly related to damage of the precentral region of the dominant insular cortex. This region is deep to **Broca's area**, an area intimately involved in expressive language function. Verbal dyspraxia is characterized by significant loss of fluency and groping behavior associated with even the simplest articulations. Dyspraxia occurs in the absence of the muscular weakness typical of an individual with motor strip damage, but the ability to contract the musculature voluntarily is impaired. One may also experience **oral apraxia**, which is a deficit in the ability to perform nonspeech oral gestures, such as imitatively puffing up the cheeks or blowing out a candle. A word of caution is due, however: Lesions are rarely so focal; it is much more often the case that frontal lobe damage that causes dyspraxia will be of a magnitude to also include regions of the motor strip. That is, dyspraxia and dysarthria very often co-occur.

If an individual has damage to the posterior parietal cortex, the result will be difficulty focusing on the target of action. This individual will have difficulty locating objects in space and may even ignore or neglect the side of the body served by the damaged parietal lobe tissue, because he or she cannot use that information. In addition, damage to the region of the supramarginal gyrus will result in verbal apraxia affecting long and complex sequences, as compared with damage to the speech premotor region, which results in deficits of simple articulatory gestures.

Afferent Inputs

The motor strip is populated by giant Betz cells, and this area receives input from the thalamus, sensory cortex, and premotor area. Regions involved in fine motor control (such as those activating facial regions or the fingers) are very richly represented. There is heavy sensory input to this motor region, underscoring the notion that control of movement is strongly influenced by information about the ongoing state and position of the musculature. Some muscle spindle afferents terminate in the motor strip, and spinal reflexes are modified and controlled, at least in part, by activity from this region. The portion of the motor strip serving a particular part of the body will receive tactile and proprioceptive information from the same body region, providing an effective path for modification of the motor plan even as it is being executed.

The premotor region appears to be involved in preparation for movement, anticipation of movement, and organization of skilled movement. It receives somatic sensory information from the parietal lobe, as well as sensory information from the thalamus, and projects its output to the motor strip. Afferent parietal information to the supplementary motor area also supports its involvement in active planning and rehearsal of the motor act, as well as decision-making about movement. Broca's area (regions 44 and 45 of the frontal lobe) uses parietal lobe information to perform a high-level planning function for movement of the speech articulators for speech function, as will be discussed.

Association Regions

Association areas are considered to provide the highest order of information processing of the cerebral cortex. It appears that higher-order integration areas extract detailed information from the signal input to the primary areas, whereas association areas permit that information to flow among the various processing sites, effectively connecting modalities. These regions are involved in intellect, cognitive functions, memory, and language.

There are three major association areas of interest: the temporal-occipital-parietal association cortex (TOP), the limbic association cortex, and the prefrontal association cortex.

The **temporal-occipital-parietal region** is of the utmost importance to speech-language pathologists, because it includes the areas associated with language in humans. This region includes portions of the temporal, parietal, and occipital lobes (areas 39, 40, and portions of 19,

21, 22, and 37). It receives input from auditory, visual, and somatosensory regions, permitting the integration of this information into language function.

The **limbic association area** (regions 23, 24, 38, 28, and 11) includes regions of the parahippocampal gyrus and temporal pole (temporal lobe), cingulate gyri (parietal and frontal lobes), and orbital surfaces (inferior frontal lobe). The limbic system is involved with motivation, emotion, and memory, making it an ideal association area. Clearly, memory function is served by reception of information from diverse sensory inputs.

The **prefrontal association area** (anterior to area 6) is involved with integration of information in preparation for the motor act, as well as higher-level cognitive processes. The premotor regions, consisting of the premotor gyrus and supplemental motor area, appear to be vital to initiation of motor activity, whereas the prefrontal region anterior to these regions is involved in the motor plan. According to Kupferman (1991), the premotor region receives input from the primary sensory reception areas or low-order processing regions, while the prefrontal regions derive their input from the higher-order regions. Both premotor and prefrontal regions project to the motor strip, permitting both low-order and abstract sensory perceptions to influence the motor act. Broca's area (regions 44 and 45), the frontal operculum, and the insula also are involved in motor programming. These regions share qualities of both the prefrontal association region and the premotor gyrus, because damage to them results in both motor-planning and higher-level language deficits, including word retrieval problems.

In addition to this, the orbitofrontal region (the region on the underbelly of the cerebrum that overlies the orbit region) is involved in limbic system function, as well as motor planning memory associated with delayed execution.

To summarize, the complexity of higher functions of the brain is reflected in the inability to assign precise locations for specific functions.

- General regions, such as **Wernicke's area**, can be ascribed broad function, and this view facilitates examination of brain function and dysfunction.

- A broad view of brain function classifies regions of the cerebrum as primary, higher-order, and association regions.

- **Primary** sensory and motor regions include the **primary reception area** for somatic sense, **primary motor area, primary auditory cortex**, and **primary** region of **visual reception**.

- Adjacent to these are higher-order areas of processing, apparently responsible for extracting features of the stimulus.

- **Association areas** are the regions of highest cognitive processing, where sensory information is integrated with memory.

- The **prefrontal area** appears to be involved in higher function related to motor output (such as inhibition of motor function and the ability to change motor responses), whereas the **temporal-occipital-parietal association area** is involved in language function.
- The limbic association area integrates information relating to affect, motivation, and emotion.
- **Flaccid dysarthria** results from damage to LMNs, whereas UMN lesions result in **spastic dysarthria**.
- **Ataxic dysarthria** arises from cerebellar damage.
- **Hyperkinetic dysarthria** is the result of damage to inhibitory processes of the extrapyramidal system, whereas **hypokinetic dysarthria** results from lesion to excitatory mechanisms.
- **Apraxia** arises from lesion to the regions associated with preparation and planning for the motor act: specifically the supramarginal gyrus of the parietal lobe, Broca's area, insula, and the SMA.

Hemispheric Specialization

Despite the gross similarities between the two cerebral hemispheres, the brain is essentially asymmetrical, and the functional and anatomic asymmetries underlie basic processing differences of extreme importance to speech-language pathologists. When researchers have examined large numbers of brains, they have found that the lateral fissure is slightly longer on the left hemisphere than on the right. The area of primary auditory reception (the planum temporale, or Heschl's gyrus) is larger on this side as well. This anatomical asymmetry supports an extremely rich body of functional asymmetry between the two hemispheres.

If you write with your right hand, you may count yourself among the broad majority of individuals who exhibit functional dominance for language and speech in the left hemisphere. Motor pathways decussate as they descend, and auditory pathways decussate in ascension, with the result being that your right hand (and right ear) are dominated by activities of the left hemisphere.

The two hemispheres continually work in concert with each other, being anatomically connected via the corpus callosum. Virtually all right-handed individuals will show language function in the left hemisphere, whereas 30% of left-handers will either have their language function within the right hemisphere or have it shared between the two hemispheres. Thus, one will speak of the "dominant hemisphere" for language as being, typically, the left hemisphere, knowing full well that there is a group for whom the reverse is true. With that in mind, let us examine some of the hemispheric differences that have been found.

decussate: *L., decussare, to make an X; to decussate means to cross over*

A great deal of the information we have gained concerning hemispheric specialization has come from treatment of seizure disorders. These disorders often involve the temporal lobe, which, as you shall soon see, is intimately involved with language function. When surgical procedures are planned to alleviate seizures, the neurosurgeon does everything possible to spare the speech and language regions. To learn where these regions are, he or she may electrically stimulate regions of the brain to determine their location prior to removing a portion of the cortex, in a procedure known as **brain mapping**. The physician also may inject the carotid artery of one or the other of the hemispheres with amytal sodium, a barbiturate, thereby incapacitating the hemisphere. In this way the surgeon can determine which hemisphere is dominant for language function. Among the surgical procedures used to terminate seizures is severing of the communication link between the two cortices, the corpus callosum.

Individuals in whom the corpus callosum has been severed have provided a great deal of the evidence concerning hemispheric specialization. Auditory information presented to the right ear is processed predominantly by the left hemisphere, and left-ear information is received by the right hemisphere. By careful examination of responses, researchers have found that short-duration acoustic information (such as consonants, transitions, and stop consonant bursts) is processed most efficiently by the left hemisphere in right-handed individuals. The left hemisphere seems to be specialized for the process of analysis, favoring discrete, sequential, rapidly changing information. Spoken and written language perception and production are clearly favored by this hemisphere, whereas the "nondominant" right hemisphere favors more spatial and holistic elements, such as face recognition, speech intonation, melody, and perception of form. This is not to say that the right hemisphere has nothing to say. It has been demonstrated that it has a reasonably large vocabulary (dominated by nouns), but rudimentary grammar. Although expressive abilities are quite limited, the right hemisphere can follow commands and demonstrate knowledge of verbal information through gesture and pointing using the left hand.

Thus, in the majority of individuals, language processing is lateralized to the left hemisphere, and speech production is controlled by the same hemisphere. Interpretation of the speaker's intention, as presented through intonation and facial expression, is processed by the right hemisphere. As you shall soon see, damage to the two hemispheres produces markedly different deficits.

Lesion Studies

Damage to the nervous system can come from many sources. **Cerebrovascular accident (CVA)** refers to lesions that cause cessation of blood flow (**ischemia**) to neural tissue, either through hemorrhage (rupturing of a blood vessel), thrombosis (closure of a blood vessel by means of a foreign object, such as a blood clot), or embolism (closure of a blood vessel by a floating clot). Hemorrhage can occur when an aneurysm (ballooning of a blood vessel due to a weak wall) is subjected to increased blood pressure (hypertension). Aneurysms can be repaired if discovered prior to hemorrhage (see Figure 13-9). Chronic high blood pressure can lead to lacunar (hypertensive) strokes, which are insidious in onset but can lead to aphasia, dysarthria, and dementia.

Damage can also occur from traumatic brain injury (TBI). Injuries depend on the type of trauma (see Figure 13-10). Open injury occurs from trauma that fractures the skull, including gunshot wounds. Closed head injury (CHI) can be translational (front-back or side-side) or angular (rotatory). Translational injuries occur when an object strikes the skull, or more likely, when the skull strikes an object. Being thrown from a car as a result of a motor vehicle accident (MVA) often damages the frontal lobe (Figure 13-10A), while rotational injury causes diffuse axonal damage (Figure 13-10C).

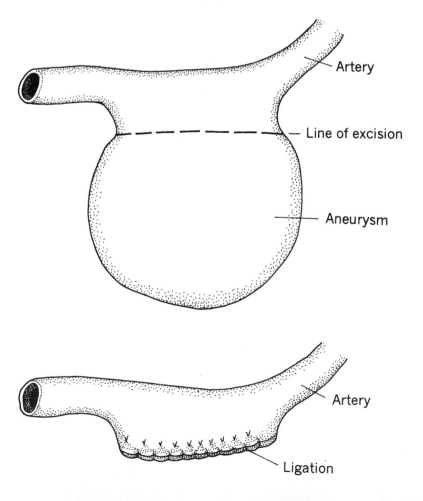

Figure 13-9. Repair of an aneurysm to prevent hemorrhage.

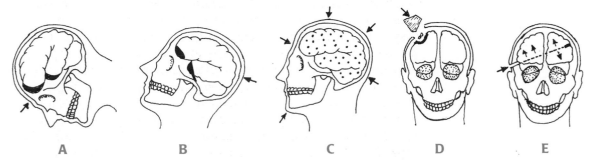

Figure 13-10. Effects of trauma on the cerebrum and related structures. **A.** Closed head injury (CHI) producing direct effect (*coup*) on frontal region. **B.** Trauma to posterior skull causes injury opposite the site of impact (*contra-coup*). **C.** Diffuse trauma arising from rotational injury and resulting in nonlocalized axonal tearing. **D.** Open head injury, resulting from skull fracturing upon impact with a foreign object. **E.** Bullet projectile entering skull, with shock wave causing massive brain damage despite its small diameter.

CVA is the most frequent cause of aphasia and TBI is the most frequent cause of acquired cognitive deficit. That having been said, either class of disorder can cause a wide spectrum of language and cognitive dysfunction.

Aphasia

A primary source of information concerning function of the cerebral cortex in humans is lesion studies. Researchers have examined the behavioral outcome of accidental or surgical lesions in individuals, thus developing our understanding of cortical function.

A Story with a Happy Ending

We promised that we would tell you a story of aneurysm and hemorrhage with a happy ending. While at a public event one Saturday, a dear friend (S) developed a debilitating headache. When her headache didn't improve after an hour of nursing it in the cab of her truck, her husband began the long drive home. Her husband wisely decided that a stop by the local hospital was in order, and the emergency physician suggested magnetic resonance imaging (MRI) to help determine the source of the pain. As the MRI was activated, S became unconscious.

As we later learned, S had a history of aneurysms in her family, and had been examined frequently and repeatedly to ensure that there were no surprises in her future. Despite these precautions, an aneurysm had developed at the base of her brain and hemorrhaged as the MRI was activated. Life-flight took her to a metropolitan center that specialized in management of hemorrhage, and friends and family watched anxiously as S slowly became aware of her surroundings. To everyone's great joy and relief, her recovery was remarkably complete, and she was able to return to her life and work unencumbered. The quick action of the emergency room medical team and the stroke unit at the receiving hospital gave S the chance to be called the "miracle woman" by all who know her.

Of particular interest to our field are the regions associated with speech and language. We have long known that damage to Wernicke's area (posterior area 22) typically results in the disruption of language known as receptive or fluent **aphasia**. Similarly, we have come to recognize that damage to Broca's area (areas 44 and 45) severely disrupts the oral manifestation of language (speech). Through cortical mapping and precise lesion studies, researchers have described these conditions and sites of lesions more precisely, providing us with some insight into how the cerebral cortex functions.

As you know, Heschl's gyrus of the temporal lobe has the primary responsibility for auditory reception; the region adjacent to it in the superior temporal gyrus is a higher-order processing region; and the hippocampus is involved with memory. Portions of the inferior and middle temporal gyri are regions of higher-level integration of visual information. Wernicke's area is posterior to this, technically comprised of the posterior superior gyrus of the temporal lobe, but we know that language function involves a markedly larger area, generally including the temporal-occipital-parietal association areas.

Damage to Heschl's gyrus may result in cortical deafness, the inability to hear information that has passed through the lower auditory nervous system. Lesions of the higher-order processing region adjacent to AI will produce a deficit in processing complex auditory information, and if the lesion involves the inferior temporal lobe (area 28), the individual may experience a memory deficit associated with visual information.

With the notion of the auditory and visual input function of the temporal lobe in mind, let us examine lesions involving Wernicke's area. **Wernicke's aphasia** is referred to as a "fluent aphasia," because individuals with this condition have relatively normal flow of speech. Their expressive language may have relatively normal syntactic structure, but the content of their productions will be markedly reduced. They will often substitute words (**verbal paraphasias**) or create entirely new words (**neologisms**). If you think of the proximity to the auditory reception areas and the discussion of auditory integration, it will not surprise you that the individual with Wernicke's aphasia will have a great deal of difficulty understanding what he or she hears and will not be able to accurately repeat speech of others.

The condition known as **Broca's aphasia** is a stark contrast to Wernicke's aphasia. Broca's aphasia arises not only from lesions to Broca's area (areas 44 and 45), but also from lesions of the operculum of the frontal and parietal regions, the insula, and the supramarginal gyrus of the parietal lobe. That is, Broca's aphasia arises from lesions of areas served by the upper division of the middle cerebral artery. Broca's area is involved with the planning of speech, and the aphasia associated with it is far from fluent. Although the individual with Broca's aphasia generally retains comprehension of auditory or visual input, the patient's expressive abilities may be severely impaired. Length and complexity of utterances will be markedly reduced, and speech may require extreme effort.

Wernicke's and Broca's areas communicate directly with each other by means of the arcuate fasciculus, providing a very strong link between the receptive component of language and its expression. When these fibers or the supramarginal gyrus of the parietal lobe have been damaged, the patient will show signs of **conduction aphasia**. This individual will have good comprehension of speech or written material, and relatively fluent spontaneous speech, but impaired ability to repeat utterances heard. There also will be phoneme substitutions (**literal paraphasias**).

If damage to the brain includes Wernicke's and Broca's areas and areas below the cortex, the result may be **global aphasia**. In this condition, both expressive and receptive abilities are severely impaired. Speech is halting and nonfluent at best, with poverty of grammatical structures and significant comprehension deficit. Gesture and facial expressions may be the primary means of communication for this individual.

You can see how these areas of deficit fit together. Damage to regions of the temporal lobe tends to cause receptive language problems, depending on the location of the lesion, whereas damage to the frontal speech regions may leave receptive abilities intact but cause a deficit in expression of language (speech).

We have been conveniently ignoring the fact that the cerebral cortex is firmly attached to subcortical structures, including the basal ganglia and thalamus. Improvement in brain imaging techniques has

Impact of Aphasia

The life of an individual with aphasia is significantly changed by the cerebrovascular event. With the brain lesion comes an instant change in how the individual can interact with his or her environment, with how readily linguistic information can be used to process information and to communicate, and with how easily cognitive processes can be performed.

The individual with left-hemisphere stroke of the frontal lobe faces difficulty in output that leaves her or him dysfluent and very aware of the jumble of verbal output. If the lesion is in the posterior regions, speech will be more fluent, but may be "empty" of content, and the person may have difficulty with comprehension, not realizing that his or her speech is not doing what was intended.

It is extremely important to enlist the help of your client's spouse or close friend very early in the process. This "significant other" will be most able to extend your therapy into every aspect of her or his life, and will become the individual's most valuable communication partner. Including a partner early on will give you the opportunity to move your client back into the world of communication.

revealed that damage to many of these areas results in language impairment, although these reports emphasize the importance of not assuming a strict localizationist stance. Damage to the thalamus may have a significant impact on attention, but also has resulted in a type of aphasia that includes difficulty in naming objects (**anomia**), generation of novel words (neologisms), and word or sound substitutions. Damage to the basal ganglia has resulted in nonfluent aphasia as well if there is damage to the putamen or caudate nucleus. It is likely that the hierarchical nature of the brain involves using these phylogenetically older structures to integrate information necessary for expression and reception, and that disruption of the pathways always results in some deficit.

Although damage to the posterior language area (TOP) always results in receptive deficit, *any* individual with aphasia will have some degree of receptive impairment. Similarly, word-finding problems are nearly universal in individuals experiencing aphasia. Both of these deficits should remind you that strict localization of function is not always demonstrable.

Dyspraxia

Sometimes lesions can result in **primary oral** or **primary verbal dyspraxia**, a deficit in the ability to program the articulators for nonspeech (oral dysapraxia) or speech production (verbal dyspraxia) in the absence of muscular weakness or paralysis. Dyspraxia often co-occurs with aphasia and is viewed by many to be a component of Broca's aphasia. Errors in dyspraxia tend to be phoneme substitution errors, although they are much less predictable than articulation errors arising from other causes. Because the person with dyspraxia often has good comprehension, he or she may be quite aware of the errors and will struggle to correct them. This struggle will result in loss of speech fluency (and a great deal of frustration for the speaker). As the desired articulatory configuration becomes more complex (as in producing consonant clusters instead of singletons), the client's speech difficulty will increase.

At least two regions are involved in dyspraxia. If damage is restricted to the frontal lobe in the insular cortex (Dronkers, 1996), the individual will have difficulty producing even the simplest gestures with the articulators (referred to as **executive dyspraxia**). Damage to the supramarginal gyrus of the parietal lobe results in difficulty sequencing more complex articulatory gestures (**planning dyspraxia**).

Other Deficits

Not all lesions affect language directly. Left-frontal lobe lesions often result in deficits in cognitive functions. *Cognition* can be defined as the ways in which we perceive and process information: Cognitive processes include such diverse functions as memory, attention, and perception. The frontal lobe appears to be the primary site for cognitive functions, as well as the locus of the **executive functions** by which we exercise control over cognitive processes. Executive functions include the ability to set goals, sequence motor behaviors, and self-monitor behavior. Through the interplay of cognitive processes and the control of the executive functions, we are able to perceive information that is projected from myriad areas of the body and cerebrum, compare it with our stored memories or with previous analyses, evaluate those stimuli, and plan an appropriate response. In the same vein, our executive functions help us to control those responses so that we do not impulsively say or do something inappropriate.

Although individuals experiencing CVAs may demonstrate loss of cognitive functions, the fact that these functions appear to be localized predominantly in the prefrontal region explains why clients who have suffered traumatic brain injury (TBI) more often have deficits in these areas. Because most traumatic brain injury arises from vehicle accidents, the most frequently injured region is the frontal lobe. TBI frequently results in impaired decision-making ability and difficulty changing strategies in problem-solving. There is often a loss of response inhibition, and the ability to evaluate the context of communication results in lost social communication ability, also known as a deficit in pragmatics or use of language. Control of emotion may be compromised by frontal lobe lesions, resulting in **emotional lability** (excessive and uncontrollable emotional response not necessarily related to the stimulus) or reduced emotion. Personality characteristics are often altered by frontal lobe lesion.

If the parahippocampal region of the cerebral cortex is involved, the client may have difficulty learning complex tasks and remembering information received through sensory modalities. Penfield and Roberts (1959) found that removal of both hippocampi produced profound long-term memory deficit, whereas much milder problems arose from unilateral lesion. Removal of the left hippocampus results in difficulty remembering verbal information.

Although right-hemisphere lesions generally do not result in aphasia, they do have linguistic and social significance. Lesions to this hemisphere may result in a deficit of the ability to process information contained in intonation of speech, so that nuance is lost. Communication of emotion, intent, and humor may be impaired in this individual. Individuals with right-hemisphere lesions often make linguistically inappropriate responses, most likely arising from the inability to process these pragmatic functions. Because the right hemisphere appears to be responsible for getting the "big picture," individuals who have suffered right-hemisphere damage lose some of their ability to get the gist of information and to recognize that they need to provide background contextual information during conversation ("given-new" violation), and have difficulty interpreting emotional and paralinguistic information. They often have difficulty making inferences from details (such as interpreting the many parts of a picture by inferring the relation of the parts). (For an excellent review of right-hemisphere dysfunction, see Myers [1999].)

To summarize:

- The **hemispheres** of the brain display clear functional differences.
- The **left hemisphere** in most individuals is dominant for language and speech, processes brief-duration stimuli, and performs detailed analysis.
- The **right hemisphere**, in contrast, appears to process information in a more holistic fashion, preferring spatial and tonal information.
- **Face recognition** appears to be a right-hemisphere function.
- Lesion studies have shown that damage to **Wernicke's area** in the dominant hemisphere usually results in a receptive language deficit with relatively intact speech fluency, whereas damage to **Broca's area** results in loss of speech fluency manifested as Broca's aphasia.
- Damage to the **arcuate fasciculus** connecting these two regions will result in **conduction aphasia**, and damage to all of these regions will produce **global deficit**.
- **Verbal dyspraxia** may result from damage to Broca's area, but also has been seen with lesions to the supramarginal gyrus, supplementary motor area, frontal operculum, and insula.
- **Nondominant hemisphere lesions** often result in deficit in **pragmatics**, especially related to monitoring facial responses of communication partners, information carried in the intonation of speech, and communicative nuance.
- **Frontal lobe lesions** may result in deficits in judgment and response inhibition, whereas damage to the **hippocampus** will affect short-term memory, especially as it relates to auditory information.

Motor Control for Speech

The production of speech is an extraordinarily complex process. We tend to view area 4 as the "prime mover," but it would be more accurate to view it as the location where the very complex planning, programming, and preparation reach fruition. Movement is initiated at the motor strip, but only after it has been conceived, and after the steps involved for muscle activity have been prepared. To further confound things, control of speech musculature must be precisely coordinated, a process involving afferent input from the muscles.

Input to the motor strip arises from the premotor regions that are involved in preparation of the motor act. The premotor gyrus and supplemental motor area receive input concerning state of the musculature from the postcentral gyrus, and it appears that knowledge of articulator position in space is established here. In addition, Broca's area (areas 44 and 45) communicates with the TOP by means of the arcuate fasciculus and is intimately involved in articulatory planning. The supramarginal gyrus of the parietal lobe appears to be involved in early, linguistically based planning of the articulatory gesture. The prefrontal association area receives input from diffuse sensory integration regions of the cerebrum, and this information is used to make decisions concerning execution of the motor act (such as inhibiting a response). Prefrontal and premotor regions project to the precentral gyrus, as does Broca's area, so that both immediate planning and cognitive strategies associated with speech influence the output.

The primary motor cortex (MI) receives information concerning the state of muscles, tendons, and tissue through several means. The sensory cortex (SI) receives this information in a well-organized fashion. Area 3 receives muscle afferent information from Group Ia fibers terminating in the thalamus and from mechanoreceptors of the skin that are apparently very important for speech muscles of the face. Area 1 receives mechanoreceptor input as well, and area 2 receives joint sense. This information is all directed to the MI, either directly or via other SI areas, apparently to modulate the motor command based on current status.

This sensory information obviously is not the only information processed by the MI. The premotor region (lateral area 6) is involved in organization of the motor act for skilled, voluntary movement, and its output is directly routed to the MI in both hemispheres. It receives somatic and visual information and apparently integrates this into its motor plan. The SMA (which is located in medial area 6) appears to be involved in the programming of speech and other sequential movements, as well as control of some reflexes. The SMA receives information concerning tactile, auditory, and visual senses. It should be remembered that information from the cerebellum and basal ganglia is exchanged with the MI, SMA, and premotor region as well. Indeed, lesions of the SMA or basal ganglia can result in akinesia (loss of the ability to initiate movement), and lesions of the premotor cortex may result in apraxia (dysfunction in ability to program movement). Loss of regions of the MI will result in paralysis or weakness of involved muscle groups, reduction in fine motor control, and spasticity arising from the unmodulated reflexes.

Thus, the motor impulse that is initiated by the MI is really the end product of planning and programming (Broca's area, SMA, and premotor area 6), with the strategic formulations arising from areas 8, 9, and 10 of the frontal lobe. The motor areas are influenced by the current state of the musculature of the body via somatosensory afferents to the SI, thalamus, and cerebellum. The afferent information concerning the tissues being acted on will help the MI area modify its output to accommodate fine motor control.

In this way, the motor impulse initiated by the motor strip is the end product of planning and programming, with the strategic formulations arising from the prefrontal region. Remember the executive function of the prefrontal region, and you may think twice about blurting an answer out before it is well formed—and inhibit the response. The motor areas are influenced by the current state of the musculature of the body. Likewise, the executor will carefully examine the propriety of the verbal output in terms of the situation, and may be instrumental in revising the content and form to meet specific needs (e.g., your response to your minister's question at church is markedly different from the same question posed by your best friend while at the drive-in).

Clearly, the execution of speech involves extensive interaction of the areas of the brain in a rapidly coordinated fashion. Studies have revealed that we are amazingly versatile in overcoming obstacles to speech production (this is good news for the budding speech-language pathologist). Try this: Say "Sammy is a friend of mine." Now place your pencil between your molars on the side of your mouth, bite down lightly, and say it again a few times. Were you able to produce intelligible speech? Although the pencil interfered with some dental or labial productions, on the whole you were not only intelligible, but accurate. If the program for the individual articulators were "written in stone," you would not have been able to tolerate this aberration (use of a bite block), and your speech would have been unintelligible. Through this sort of examination, we realize that you probably develop an internal standard of what you want your speech to sound like, and then do whatever is necessary to match that standard. Thus, your role as a speech-language pathologist could well include helping your client develop that internal standard. Conditions that alter the internal model will inevitably alter the output.

A bite block is a device used to stabilize the mandible. Often made of hard acrylic or dental impression material, the bite block is used to eliminate the contribution of the mandible to tongue movement for diagnostic and therapeutic purposes. For an excellent discussion on preparation and use of the bite block, see Dworkin (1994).

CHAPTER SUMMARY

Communication between neurons of the nervous system occurs at the **synapse**, and **neurotransmitter** passing through the **synaptic cleft** will either excite or inhibit the postsynaptic neuron. When the neuron is sufficiently stimulated, an **action potential** will be generated, causing membrane depolarization and exchange of ions between the **extracellular** and **intracellular** spaces. **Ion movement** results in a large and predictable change in voltage across the membrane. **Resting membrane potential** is the relatively stable state of the neuron at rest, while the **absolutely refractory period**, after excitation, is an interval during which the neuron cannot be excited to fire. During the **relatively refractory period**, a neuron may be stimulated to fire, given increased stimulation. Neurons are capable of representing differences in input only through **rate** of response. **Myelinated fibers** conduct the wave of depolarization more rapidly than **demyelinated fibers**, primarily because of saltatory conduction.

Muscle is comprised of thick and thin **myofilaments** that slide across each other during contraction. **Activation** of a muscle fiber causes release of calcium into the environment of **thick myofilaments**, revealing the binding sites on the **thin filaments** that permit cross-bridging from the thick filaments. **Muscle shortening** is the product of repeated contraction of the cross-bridges. **Slow twitch** muscle fibers remain contracted longer than **fast twitch fibers**, with the former being involved in maintenance of posture and the latter in fine and rapid motor function.

Muscle spindles provide feedback to the neuromotor system about muscle length, tension, motion, and position. Muscle spindles running parallel to intrafusal muscle fibers are sensors for muscle length, whereas **Golgi tendon organs** sense muscle tension. **Nuclear bag fibers** convey information concerning acceleration and **nuclear chain fibers** respond to sustained lengthening. When a muscle is passively stretched, a **segmental reflex** is triggered. Extrafusal muscles paralleling the muscle spindles are activated and the muscle is shortened. Golgi tendon organs apparently respond to the tension of musculature during active contraction.

Higher function of the brain defies a strict localization approach to functional organization. General regions, such as Wernicke's area, can be ascribed broad function, and this view facilitates examination of brain function and dysfunction. Brain function may be classified into regions of **primary, higher-order**, and **association regions**. **Primary sensory** and **motor regions** include the primary reception area for somatic sense, primary motor area, primary auditory cortex, and primary region of visual reception. **Higher-order** areas of processing are apparently responsible for extracting features of the stimulus. **Association areas** are the regions of highest cognitive processing, integrating sensory information with memory. The **prefrontal area** appears to be involved in higher function related to motor output, while the **temporal-occipital-parietal association area** is involved in spoken and written language function. The **limbic association area** integrates information relating to affect, motivation, and emotion.

Dysarthria is a speech disorder resulting from damage to the motor execution system of the central nervous system; it causes muscular weakness and reduction in motor control. **Flaccid dysarthria** results from damage to LMNs, whereas UMN lesions result in **spastic dysarthria**. **Ataxic dysarthria** arises from cerebellar damage. **Hyperkinetic dysarthria** is the result of damage to inhibitory processes of the extrapyramidal system, whereas **hypokinetic dysarthria** results from lesion to excitatory mechanisms. **Apraxia** arises from lesion to the regions associated with preparation and planning for the motor act, specifically the supramarginal gyrus of the parietal lobe, Broca's area, and the SMA. Apraxia is a deficit in **motor planning**, existing without muscular weakness or paralysis.

The hemispheres of the brain display clear functional differences. Language and speech, brief-duration stimuli, and detailed information are processed in the **left hemisphere** in most individuals. The **right hemisphere** appears to process information in a more holistic fashion, preferring spatial and tonal information. Lesions to **Wernicke's area** in the dominant hemisphere result in receptive language deficit with relatively intact speech fluency, whereas damage to **Broca's area** results in loss of speech fluency. Damage to the **arcuate fasciculus** connecting these two regions will result in **conduction aphasia**, and damage to all of these regions will produce **global deficit**. **Verbal dyspraxia** may result from damage to Broca's area, the supramarginal gyrus, the supplementary motor area, the frontal operculum, and the insula. **Right-hemisphere lesions** often result in deficit in pragmatics, misinterpretation of information carried in the speech intonation, and loss of communicative nuance. **Frontal lobe lesions** often result in impaired judgment and failure to inhibit responses, whereas damage to the **hippocampus** will affect short-term memory.

Movement is initiated at the **motor strip**, but a great deal of planning occurs prior to that point. The **premotor regions**, including Broca's area, are involved in planning for the motor act, and project that plan to the motor strip. The **prefrontal association area** also provides input to the motor strip concerning higher cognitive elements of the speech act, and the lowest levels of information (information about muscle stretch and tension) are also fed to the motor strip.

STUDY QUESTIONS

1. _____ is a change in electrical potential that occurs when a cell membrane is stimulated adequately to permit ion exchange between the intra- and extracellular spaces.

2. The _____ is the time during which the cell membrane cannot be stimulated to depolarize.

3. The _____ is a period during which the membrane may be stimulated to excitation again, but only with greater than typical stimulation.

4. The _____ of the axon myelin promote saltatory conduction.

5. The substance known as _____ is discharged into the synaptic cleft, stimulating the postsynaptic neuron.

6. Activation of a muscle fiber causes release of calcium into the environment of _____ myofilaments.

7. _____ twitch muscle fibers remain contracted longer than _____ twitch fibers.

8. _____ provide feedback to the neuromotor system about muscle length, tension, motion, and position.

9. Higher cognitive processing occurs generally in _____ areas.

10. The _____ area is involved in language function.

11. _____ dysarthria results from damage to LMNs, whereas UMN lesions result in spastic dysarthria.

12. _____ dysarthria is the result of damage to inhibitory processes of the extrapyramidal system.

13. _____ arises from cerebellar damage.

14. _____ arises from lesion to the regions associated with preparation and planning for the motor act, specifically the supramarginal gyrus of the parietal lobe, Broca's area, and the SMA.

15. The _____ area of the cerebrum appears to be involved in higher function related to motor output (such as inhibition of motor function and the ability to change motor responses), whereas the temporal-occipital-parietal association area is involved in language function.

16. The _____ area integrates information relating to affect, motivation, and emotion.

17. The _____ hemisphere in most individuals is dominant for language and speech, processes brief-duration stimuli, and performs detailed analysis.

18. The _____ hemisphere appears to process information in a more holistic fashion, preferring spatial and tonal information.

19. Damage to _____ area in the dominant hemisphere usually results in a receptive language deficit with relatively intact speech fluency.

20. Damage to _____ area in the dominant hemisphere often results in loss of speech fluency manifested as Broca's aphasia.

21. Damage to the _____ fasciculus will result in conduction aphasia.

22. A client of yours had a stroke, and reveals some muscular weakness on the left side of her body. Her speech is precisely articulated but intonation is flat. She complains that, despite her lack of physical problems, she has noticed that her friends don't call any more. Where is the site of lesion, and where should therapy be directed?

STUDY QUESTION ANSWERS

1. ACTION POTENTIAL is a change in electrical potential that occurs when a cell membrane is stimulated adequately to permit ion exchange between the intra- and extracellular spaces.

2. The ABSOLUTELY REFRACTORY PERIOD is the time during which the cell membrane cannot be stimulated to depolarize.

3. The RELATIVELY REFRACTORY PERIOD is a period during which the membrane may be stimulated to excitation again, but only with greater than typical stimulation.

4. The NODES OF RANVIER of the axon myelin promote saltatory conduction.

5. The substance known as NEUROTRANSMITTER is discharged into the synaptic cleft, stimulating the postsynaptic neuron.

6. Activation of a muscle fiber causes release of calcium into the environment of THICK myofilaments.

7. SLOW twitch muscle fibers remain contracted longer than FAST twitch fibers.

8. MUSCLE SPINDLES provide feedback to the neuromotor system about muscle length, tension, motion, and position.

9. Higher cognitive processing occurs generally in ASSOCIATION areas.

10. The TEMPORO-OCCIPITAL-PARIETAL ASSOCIATION area is involved in language function.

11. FLACCID dysarthria results from damage to LMNs, whereas UMN lesions result in spastic dysarthria.

12. HYPERKINETIC dysarthria is the result of damage to inhibitory processes of the extrapyramidal system.

13. ATAXIC DYSARTHRIA arises from cerebellar damage.

14. APRAXIA arises from lesion to the regions associated with preparation and planning for the motor act, specifically the supramarginal gyrus of the parietal lobe, Broca's area, and the SMA.

15. The PREFRONTAL area of the cerebrum appears to be involved in higher function related to motor output (such as inhibition of motor function and the ability to change motor responses), whereas the temporal-occipital-parietal association area is involved in language function.

16. The LIMBIC ASSOCIATION area integrates information relating to affect, motivation, and emotion.

17. The LEFT hemisphere in most individuals is dominant for language and speech, processes brief-duration stimuli, and performs detailed analysis.

18. The RIGHT hemisphere appears to process information in a more holistic fashion, preferring spatial and tonal information.

19. Damage to WERNICKE'S area in the dominant hemisphere usually results in a receptive language deficit with relatively intact speech fluency.

20. Damage to BROCA'S area in the dominant hemisphere often results in loss of speech fluency manifested as Broca's aphasia.

21. Damage to the ARCUATE fasciculus will result in conduction aphasia.

22. This individual suffered frontal lobe damage of the right hemisphere. Speech was unaffected because the left hemisphere dominates speech and many language functions. Nonetheless, she has a reduction in the ability to examine the context of communication (right hemisphere) and may be insensitive to cues that her friends are giving her that would otherwise cause her to change some communication strategy. An important goal of therapy would be to increase her awareness of the pragmatic cues and to develop strategies to increase her sensitivity to context.

REFERENCES

Adams, R. D., Victor, M., & Ropper, A. H. (1997). *Principles of neurology* (6th ed.). New York: McGraw-Hill.

Albom, M. (1997). *Tuesdays with Morrie.* New York: Broadway Books.

Aronson, A. E. (2000). *Aronson's neurosciences pocket lectures.* San Diego, CA: Singular Publishing Group.

Bear, M. F., Connors, B. W., & Paradiso, M. A. (1996). *Neuroscience: Exploring the brain.* Baltimore: Williams & Wilkins.

Bechera, A., Tranel, D., Damasio, H., Adolphs, R., Rockland, C., & Damasio, A. R. (1995). Double dissociation of conditioning and declarative knowledge relative to the amygdala and hippocampus in humans. *Science, 269,* 1115–1118.

Berkovitz, B. K. B., & Moxham, B. J. (2002). *Head and neck anatomy.* United Kingdom: Martin Dunitz Ltd.

Bhatnagar, S. C., & Andy, O. J. (1995). *Neuroscience for the study of communicative disorders.* Baltimore: Williams & Wilkins.

Blakemore, C., & Cooper, G. F. (1970). Development of brain depends on the visual environment. *Nature, 228,* 477–478.

Bly, L. (1994). *Motor skills acquisition in the first year.* Tucson, AZ: Therapy Skill Builders.

Bowman, J. P. (1971). *The muscle spindle and neural control of the tongue.* Springfield, IL: Charles C. Thomas.

Campbell, N. A. (1987). *Biology.* Menlo Park, CA: Cumming.

Carpenter, M. B. (1978). *Core text of neuroanatomy* (2nd ed.). Baltimore: Williams & Wilkins.

Chusid, J. G. (1979). *Correlative neuroanatomy and functional neurology* (17th ed.). Los Altos, CA: Lange Medical Publications.

Collins, M. J. (1989). Differential diagnosis of aphasic syndromes and apraxia of speech. In Square-Storer (Ed.), *Acquired apraxia of speech in aphasic adults* (pp. 87–114). London: Taylor and Francis.

Cotman, C. W., & McGaugh, J. L. (1980). *Behavioral neuroscience.* New York: Academic Press.

Crary, M. A. (1993). *Developmental motor speech disorders.* San Diego, CA: Singular Publishing Group.

Darley, F. L., Aronson, A. E., & Brown, J. R. (1975). *Motor speech disorders.* Philadelphia: W. B. Saunders.

Dronkers, N. F. (1996). A new brain region for coordinating speech articulation. *Nature, 384,* 159–161.

Duffy, J. R. (1995). *Motor speech disorders.* St. Louis, MO: Mosby.

Dworkin, J. P. (1994). *Motor speech disorders: A treatment guide.* St. Louis, MO: C. V. Mosby.

Edvinsson, L., & Krause, D. N. (2002). *Cerebral blood flow and metabolism.* Philadelphia: Lippincott/Williams & Wilkins.

Filskov, S. B., & Boll, T. J. (1981). *Handbook of clinical neuropsychology.* New York: John Wiley & Sons.

Fiorentino, M. R. (1973). *Reflex testing methods for evaluating CNS development.* Springfield, IL; Charles Thomas Publishers.

Ganong, W. F. (1981). *Review of medical physiology.* Los Altos, CA: Lange Medical Publications.

Gelfand, S. A. (1990). *Hearing.* New York: Marcel Dekker.

Gelfand, S. A. (2001). *Essentials of audiology* (2nd ed.). New York: Thieme Medical Publishers.

Ghez, C. (1991). Voluntary movement. In E. R. Kandel, J. H. Schwartz, & T. M. Jessell (Eds.), *Principles of neural science* (3rd ed., pp. 609–625). Norwalk, CT: Appleton & Lange.

Gilman, S., & Winans, S. S. (1982). *Manter and Gatz's essentials of clinical neuroanatomy and neurophysiology*. Philadelphia: F. A. Davis.

Gilroy, J. (2000). *Basic neurology* (3rd ed.). New York: McGraw-Hill.

Gray, H., Bannister, L. H., Berry, M. M., & Williams, P. L. (Eds.). (1995). *Gray's anatomy*. London: Churchill Livingstone.

Hubel, D. H. (1979). The visual cortex of normal and deprived monkeys. *Scientific American, 67*, 532–543.

Kandel, E. R. (1991). Brain and behavior. In E. R. Kandel, J. H. Schwartz, & T. M. Jessell (Eds.), *Principles of neural science* (3rd ed., pp. 5–17). Norfolk, CT: Appleton & Lange.

Kandel, E. R., Schwartz, J. H., & Jessell, T. M. (2000). *Principles of neural science* (4th ed.). New York: McGraw-Hill.

Kandel, E. R., Siegelbaum, S. A., & Schwartz, J. H. (1991). Synaptic transmission. In E. R. Kandel, J. H. Schwartz, & T. M. Jessell (Eds.), *Principles of neural science* (3rd ed., pp. 1–1135). Norwalk, CT: Appleton & Lange.

Kaufman, D. M. (2000). *Clinical neurology for psychiatrists* (5th ed.). Philadelphia: W. B. Saunders.

Kelly, J. P. (1991). The neural basis of perception and movement. In E. R. Kandel, J. H. Schwartz, & T. M. Jessell (Eds.), *Principles of neural science* (3rd ed., pp. 792–803). Norwalk, CT: Appleton & Lange.

Kuehn, D. P., Lemme, M. L., & Baumgartner, J. M. (1989). *Neural bases of speech, hearing, and language*. Boston: College-Hill Press.

Kupferman, I. (1991). Localization of higher cognitive and affective functions: The association cortices. In E. R. Kandel, J. H. Schwartz, & T. M. Jessell (Eds.), *Principles of neural science* (3rd ed., pp. 823–838). Norwalk, CT: Appleton & Lange.

Mackay, L. E., Chapman, P. E., & Morgan, A. S. (1997). *Maximizing brain injury recovery*. Gaithersburg, MD: Aspen Publishers.

Mayeux, R., & Kandel, E. R. (1991). Disorders of language: The aphasias. In E. R. Kandel, J. H. Schwartz, & T. M. Jessell (Eds.), *Principles of neural science* (3rd ed., pp. 839–851). Norwalk, CT: Appleton & Lange.

Møller, A. R. (2003). *Sensory systems: Anatomy and physiology*. New York: Academic Press.

Myers, P. (1999). *Right hemisphere damage*. San Diego, CA: Singular Publishing Group.

Netter, F. H. (1983). *The CIBA collection of medical illustrations. Vol. 1. Nervous system. Part I. Anatomy and physiology*. West Caldwell, NJ: CIBA Pharmaceutical.

Netter, F. H. (1983). *The CIBA collection of medical illustrations. Vol. 1. Nervous system. Part II. Neurologic and neuromuscular disorders*. West Caldwell, NJ: CIBA Pharmaceutical Company.

Noback, C. R., Demarest, R. J., & Strominger, N. L. (1991). *The nervous system: Introduction and review*. Philadelphia: Williams & Wilkins.

Noback, C. R., Strominger, N. L., & Demarest, R. J. (1991). *The human nervous system*. Philadelphia: Lea & Febiger.

Nolte, J. (1993). *The human brain*. St. Louis, MO: Mosby Year Book.

Penfield, W., & Roberts, L. (1959). *Speech and brain-mechanisms*. Princeton, NJ: Princeton University Press.

Poritsky, R. (1992). *Neuroanatomy: A functional atlas of parts and pathways*. St. Louis, MO: Mosby Year Book.

Raymond, J. L., Lisberger, S. G., & Mauk, M. D. (1996). The cerebellum: A neuronal learning machine. *Science. 272*, 1126–1131,

Schuell, H., Jenkins, J., & Jiménes-Pabon, E. (1964). *Aphasia in adults: Diagnosis, prognosis, and therapy*. New York: Hoeber.

Square-Storer, P., & Roy, E. A. (1989). The apraxias: Commonalities and distinctions. In P. Square-Storer (Ed.), *Acquired apraxia of speech in aphasic adults* (pp. 20–63). London: Taylor and Francis.

Twietmeyer, A., & McCracken, T. (1992). *Coloring guide to regional human anatomy*. Philadelphia: Lea & Febiger.

Webster, D. B. (1999). *Neuroscience of communication* (2nd ed.). San Diego, CA: Singular Publishing Group.

Williams, P., & Warrick, R. (1980). *Gray's anatomy* (36th British ed.). Philadelphia: W. B. Saunders.

Winans, S. S., Gilman, S., Manter, J. T., & Gatz, A. J. (2002). *Manter and Gatz's essentials of clinical neuroanatomy and neurophysiology* (10th ed.). Philadelphia: F. A. Davis.

Wood, P. J., & Criss, W. R. (1975). *Normal and abnormal development of the human nervous system*. Hagerstown, MD: Harper & Row.

Yost, W. A., & Nielsen, D. W. (1977). *Fundamentals of hearing*. New York: Holt, Rinehart, and Winston.

Zemlin, W. R. (1998). *Speech and hearing science: Anatomy and physiology* (4th ed.) Needham Heights, MA: Allyn & Bacon.

APPENDIX A
Anatomical Terms

Anatomical position:	Upright, palms forward, eyes directly ahead, feet together
Anterior:	Toward the front of the body or subpart
Asthenia:	Weakness
Bifurcation:	A fork; split into two parts
Caudal:	Toward the tail or coccyx
Central:	Relative to the center of a structure
Cranial:	Toward the head
Deep:	Further from the surface
Distal:	Further from the trunk or thorax; further from the attached end
Dorsal:	Pertaining to the back of the body or posterior surface
Extension:	Straightening or moving out of the flexed position
External:	Toward the exterior of a body
Flexion:	The act of bending
Frontal plane:	Divides the body into anterior and posterior halves
Horizontal plane:	Divides the body or body part into upper and lower halves
Inferior:	The lower point; nearer the feet
Insertion:	Distal attachment of a muscle
Internal:	Enclosed or on the interior
Lateral:	Away from the midline of the body or subpart
Medial/Mesial:	Toward the midline of the body or subpart
Origin:	Proximal attachment of a muscle

Palmar:	Pertaining to the palm of the hand
Peripheral:	Relative to the periphery or away from the center
Plantar:	Pertaining to the sole of the foot
Posterior:	Toward the back of the body or subpart
Prone:	Body in horizontal position with face down
Proximal:	Closer to the trunk or thorax; nearer to the attached end
Radial:	Pertaining to the radius bone
Sagittal plane:	Divides the body or body part into right and left halves
Superficial:	Near to the surface
Superior:	The upper point; nearer the head
Supine:	Body in horizontal position with face up
Ventral:	Pertaining to the belly or anterior surface

APPENDIX B

Useful Combining Forms

-a-	Without; lack of	con-	With or together with
ab-	Away from	contra-	Opposite
ad-	Toward	cor-	Heart
-algia	Pain	corp-	Body
amphi-	On both sides	crus-	Cross; leglike part
an-	Without; lack of	crur-	Cross; leglike part
ana	Up	cryo-	Cold
angio-	Blood vessels	-cule	Implies something very small
ante-	Before	-culus	Diminutive form of a noun
antero-	Before	-culum	Diminutive form of a noun
apo-	Away from	-cyte	Cell
arthr-	A joint	de-	Away from
bi-	Two	dextro-	Right
blast-	Germ	-dynia	Pain
brachy-	Short	dys-	Bad; with difficulty
brady-	Slow	e-	Out from
capit-	Head, or toward the head end	ec-	Out of
-carpal	Wrist	ecto-	On the outer side; toward the surface
-cele	Tumor		
cephalo-	Head, or toward the head end	-ectomy	Excision
circum	Around	-emia	Blood
-cle	Implies something very small	endo-	Toward the interior; within
com-	With or together with	ento-	Toward the interior; within

ep-	Upon or above something else		myo-	Pertaining to muscle
epi-	Upon or above something else		naso-	Nose
etio-	Cause or origin		neo-	New
ex-	Out of, toward the surface		neuro-	Nerve
extero-	Aimed outward or nearer to the surface		oculo-	Eye
extra-	Outside		-oma	Morbid condition of a part, often a tumor
-gen	Producing		oro-	Mouth
-genic	Producing		ortho	Straight
hemi-	Half		-osis	Condition
hyper-	Above; increased, or too much of something		osseo-	A hardened or bony part, but not strictly
hypo-	Below; decreased, or too little of something		osteo-	Bone
idio-	Peculiar		pachy-	Thick
-ilos	Diminutive form of noun		palato-	Palate
infra-	Below		para	Beside; partial
inter-	Between		patho-	Abnormal in some way
intero-	Aimed inward or farther from the surface		-pathy	Disease
intra-	Within		-penia	Poverty
intro-	Into		ped-	Child
ipsi-	Same		ped-	Foot
iso-	Equal		per	Through; passing through; before
-itis	Inflammation or irritation		peri	Around
-ium	Diminutive form of noun		-phage	Eating
latero-	Side		-phagia	Eating
lepto-	Thick		-pher-	Bearing or carrying
leuco-	White		-plasia	Growth
levo-	Left		-plastic	Capable of being molded
macro-	Large		-plasty	Molding, forming
medio-	Middle		-poiesis	Making
megalo-	Large		poly-	Many
meso-	Middle		post-	After; behind
meta-	After; mounted or built upon		postero-	Behind
micro-	Small		pre-	Before; in front of
mono-	Single		pro-	Before; in front of
morph-	Form		proto-	Primitive; simple form
my-	Pertaining to muscle		quadra-	Four
myelo-	Pertaining to spinal cord		quadri-	Four
			-raphy	Suturing or stitching
			re-	Back or again; curved back

retro-	Backward, toward the rear	supra-	Above, upon
-rrhea	A flowing	sym-	With or together
scirrho-	Hard	syn-	With or together
sclero-	Hard	tachy-	Swift; fast
-sclerosis	Hardening	-tarsal	Ankle
scolio-	Curved	telo-	Far from, toward the extreme
semi-	Half	tetra-	Four
sinistro-	Left	-tomy	Cutting
soma-	Pertaining to the body	trans-	Beyond or on the other side
somato-	Pertaining to the body	tri-	Three
steno-	Narrow	-trophic	Related to nourishment
strepto-	Swift	-trophy	Growth, usually by expanding
sub-	Under	-tropy	Implies seeking or heading for something
sup-	Under; moderately		
super-	Above; excessively	uni-	One

Muscles of Respiration

 THORACIC MUSCLES OF INSPIRATION

Primary Inspiratory Muscle

Muscle:	**Diaphragm**
Origin:	Xiphoid process of sternum, inferior margin of the rib cage (ribs 7 through 12), corpus of L1, transverse processes of L1 through L5
Course:	Fibers course up and medially
Insertion:	Central tendon of diaphragm
Innervation:	Phrenic nerve arising from cervical plexus of spinal nerves C3, C4, C5
Function:	Depresses central tendon of diaphragm, enlarges vertical dimension of thorax, distends abdomen

Accessory Thoracic Muscles of Inspiration

Muscle:	**External intercostal**
Origin:	Inferior surface of ribs 1 through 11
Course:	Down
Insertion:	Upper surface of rib immediately below
Innervation:	Intercostal nerves: thoracic intercostal nerves arising from T2 through T6 and thoracoabdominal intercostal nerves from T7 through T11
Function:	Elevates rib

Muscle:	**Levator costarum, longis**
Origin:	Transverse processes of T7 through T11
Course:	Down and obliquely out
Insertion:	Bypasses the rib below the point of origin, inserting rather into the next rib
Innervation:	Dorsal rami (branches) of the intercostal nerves arising from spinal nerves T2 through T12
Function:	Elevates rib cage

Muscle:	**Levator costarum, brevis**
Origin:	Transverse processes of vertebrae C7 through T11
Course:	Obliquely down and out
Insertion:	Tubercle of the rib below
Innervation:	Dorsal rami (branches) of the intercostal nerves arising from spinal nerves T2 through T12
Function:	Elevates rib cage

Muscle:	**Serratus posterior superior**
Origin:	Spinous processes of C7 and T1 through T3
Course:	Down and laterally
Insertion:	Just beyond the angles of ribs 2 through 5
Innervation:	Ventral intercostal portion of spinal nerves T1 through T4 or T5
Function:	Elevates rib cage

Accessory Muscles of Neck

Muscle:	**Sternocleidomastoid**
Origin:	Mastoid process of temporal bone
Course:	Down and in
Insertion:	Superior manubrium sterni; clavicle
Innervation:	XI accessory, spinal branch arising from spinal cord in the regions of C2 through C4 or C5
Function:	Elevates sternum and, by association, rib cage

Muscle:	**Scalenus anterior**
Origin:	Transverse processes of vertebrae C3 through C6
Course:	Down
Insertion:	Superior surface of rib 1
Innervation:	C4 through C6
Function:	Elevates rib 1

Muscle:	**Scalenus medius**
Origin:	Transverse processes of vertebrae C2 through C7
Course:	Down

Insertion:	Superior surface of the first rib
Innervation:	Cervical plexus derived from C3 and C4 and spinal nerves C5 through C8
Function:	Elevates rib 1

Muscle:	**Scalenus posterior**
Origin:	Transverse processes of C5 through C7
Course:	Down
Insertion:	Second rib
Innervation:	Spinal nerves C5 through C8
Function:	Elevates rib 2

Muscle:	**Trapezius**
Origin:	Spinous processes of C2 to T12
Course:	Fans laterally
Insertion:	Acromion of scapula and superior surface of clavicle
Innervation:	XI accessory, spinal branch arising from spinal cord in the regions of C2 through C4 or C5
Function:	Elongates neck, controls head

Muscles of Upper Arm and Shoulder

Muscle:	**Pectoralis major**
Origin:	Sternal head: length of sternum at costal cartilages; clavicular head: anterior clavicle
Course:	Fanlike laterally, converging at humerus
Insertion:	Greater tubercle of humerus
Innervation:	Brachial plexus (spinal nerves C5 through C8 and T1)
Function:	Elevates sternum, and subsequently increases transverse dimension of rib cage

Muscle:	**Pectoralis minor**
Origin:	Anterior surface of ribs 2 through 5 near chondral margin
Course:	Up and laterally
Insertion:	Coracoid process of scapula
Innervation:	Superior branch of the brachial plexus (spinal nerves C4 through C7 and T1)
Function:	Increases transverse dimension of rib cage

Muscle:	**Serratus anterior**
Origin:	Ribs 1 through 9, lateral surface of thorax
Course:	Up and back
Insertion:	Inner vertebral border of scapula
Innervation:	Brachial plexus, long thoracic nerve from C5 through C7
Function:	Elevates ribs 1 through 9

Muscle:	**Subclavius**
Origin:	Inferior surface of clavicle
Course:	Oblique and medial
Insertion:	Superior surface of rib 1 at chondral margin
Innervation:	Brachial plexus, lateral branch, from fifth and sixth spinal nerves
Function:	Elevates rib 1

Muscle:	**Levator scapulae**
Origin:	Transverse processes of C1 through C4
Course:	Down
Insertion:	Medial border of scapula
Innervation:	C3 through C5 of cervical plexus
Function:	Neck support, elevates scapula

Muscle:	**Rhomboideus major**
Origin:	Spinous processes of T2 through T5
Course:	Down and laterally in
Insertion:	Scapula
Innervation:	Spinal C5 from the dorsal scapular nerve of upper root of brachial plexus
Function:	Stabilizes shoulder girdle

Muscle:	**Rhomboideus minor**
Origin:	Spinous processes of C7 and T1
Course:	Down and laterally in
Insertion:	Medial border of scapula
Innervation:	Spinal C5 from the dorsal scapular nerve of upper root of brachial plexus
Function:	Stabilizes shoulder girdle

Thoracic Muscles of Expiration

Muscle:	**Internal intercostal**
Origin:	Superior margin of ribs 1 through 11
Course:	Up and medially
Insertion:	Inferior surface of the rib above
Innervation:	Intercostal nerves: thoracic intercostal nerves arising from T2 through T6 and thoracoabdominal intercostal nerves from T7 through T11
Function:	Depresses ribs 1 through 11

Muscle:	**Innermost intercostal**
Origin:	Superior margin of ribs 1 through 11; sparse or absent in superior thorax

Course:	Up and medially
Insertion:	Inferior surface of the rib above
Innervation:	Intercostal nerves: thoracic intercostal nerves arising from T2 through T6 and thoracoabdominal intercostal nerves from T7 through T11
Function:	Depresses ribs 1 through 11

Muscle:	**Transversus thoracis**
Origin:	Inner thoracic lateral margin of sternum
Course:	Laterally
Insertion:	Inner chondral surface of ribs 2 through 6
Innervation:	Thoracic intercostal nerves and thoracoabdominal intercostal nerves and subcostal nerves derived from T2 through T6 spinal nerves
Function:	Depresses rib cage

Posterior Thoracic Muscles

Muscle:	**Subcostal**
Origin:	Inner posterior thorax; sparse in upper thorax; from inner surface of rib near angle
Course:	Down and lateral
Insertion:	Inner surface of second or third rib below
Innervation:	Intercostal nerves of thorax, arising from the ventral rami of the spinal nerves
Function:	Depresses thorax

Muscle:	**Serratus posterior inferior**
Origin:	Spinous processes of T11, T12, L1 through L3
Course:	Up and laterally
Insertion:	Lower margin of ribs 7 through 12
Innervation:	Intercostal nerves from T9 through T11 and subcostal nerve from T12
Function:	Contraction tends to pull rib cage down, supporting expiratory effort

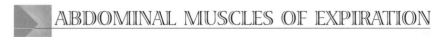

ABDOMINAL MUSCLES OF EXPIRATION

Anterolateral Abdominal Muscles

Muscle:	**Transversus abdominis**
Origin:	Posterior abdominal wall at the vertebral column via the thoracolumbar fascia of the abdominal aponeurosis
Course:	Lateral

Insertion:	Transversus abdominis aponeurosis and inner surface of ribs 6 through 12, interdigitating at that point with the fibers of the diaphragm; inferior-most attachment is at the pubis
Innervation:	Thoracic and lumbar nerves from the lower spinal intercostal nerves (derived from T7 to T12) and first lumbar nerve, iliohypogastric and ilioinguinal branches
Function:	Compresses abdomen

Muscle:	**Internal oblique abdominis**
Origin:	Inguinal ligament and iliac crest
Course:	Fans medially
Insertion:	Cartilaginous portion of lower ribs and the portion of the abdominal aponeurosis lateral to the rectus abdominis
Innervation:	Thoracic and lumbar nerves from the lower spinal intercostal nerves (derived from T7 to T12) and first lumbar nerve, iliohypogastric and ilioinguinal branches
Function:	Rotates trunk, flexes trunk, compresses abdomen

Muscle:	**External oblique abdominis**
Origin:	Osseous portion of the lower seven ribs
Course:	Fans downward
Insertion:	Iliac crest, inguinal ligament, and abdominal aponeurosis lateral to rectus abdominis
Innervation:	Thoracoabdominal nerve arising from T7 through T11 and subcostal nerve from T12
Function:	Bilateral contraction flexes vertebral column and compresses abdomen; unilateral contraction results in trunk rotation

Muscle:	**Rectus abdominis**
Origin:	Originates as four or five segments at pubis inferiorly
Course:	Up to segment border
Insertion:	Xiphoid process of sternum and the cartilage of ribs 7 through 12, lower ribs
Innervation:	T7 through T11 intercostal nerves (thoracoabdominal) subcostal nerve from T12 (T7 supplies upper segment, T8 supplies the second, T9 supplies remainder)
Function:	Flexion of vertebral column

Posterior Abdominal Muscles

Muscle:	**Quadratus lumborum**
Origin:	Iliac crest
Course:	Fans up and in
Insertion:	Transverse processes of the lumbar vertebrae and inferior border of rib 12
Innervation:	Thoracic nerve T12 and L1 through L4 lumbar nerves
Function:	Bilateral contraction fixes the abdominal wall in support of abdominal compression

MUSCLES OF UPPER LIMB

Muscle:	**Latissimus dorsi**
Origin:	Lumbar, sacral, and lower thoracic vertebrae
Course:	Up fanlike
Insertion:	Humerus
Innervation:	Brachial plexus, posterior branch; fibers from the regions C6 through C8 form the long subscapular nerve
Function:	For respiration, stabilizes posterior abdominal wall for expiration

Muscles of Phonation

 ## INTRINSIC LARYNGEAL MUSCLES

Muscle:	**Aryepiglotticus muscle**
Origin:	Continuation of oblique arytenoid muscle from arytenoid apex
Course:	Back and up as muscular component of aryepiglottic fold
Insertion:	Lateral epiglottis
Innervation:	X vagus recurrent laryngeal nerve
Function:	Constricts laryngeal opening

Muscle:	**Lateral cricoarytenoid**
Origin:	Superior-lateral surface of the cricoid cartilage
Course:	Up and back
Insertion:	Muscular process of the arytenoid
Innervation:	X vagus, recurrent laryngeal nerve
Function:	Adducts vocal folds, increases medial compression

Muscle:	**Transverse arytenoid**
Origin:	Lateral margin of posterior arytenoid
Course:	Laterally
Insertion:	Lateral margin of posterior surface, opposite arytenoid
Innervation:	X vagus, recurrent laryngeal nerve
Function:	Adducts vocal folds

Muscle: **Oblique arytenoid**

Origin:	Posterior base of the muscular processes
Course:	Obliquely up
Insertion:	Apex of the opposite arytenoid
Innervation:	X vagus, recurrent laryngeal nerve
Function:	Pulls the apex medially

Muscle: **Posterior cricoarytenoid**

Origin:	Posterior cricoid lamina
Course:	Up and out
Insertion:	Posterior aspect of the muscular process of arytenoid cartilage
Innervation:	X vagus, recurrent laryngeal nerve
Function:	Abducts vocal folds

Muscle: **Cricothyroid**

Origin:	Pars recta: anterior surface of the cricoid cartilage beneath the arch; Pars oblique: cricoid cartilage lateral to the pars recta
Course:	Pars recta: up and out; Pars oblique: obliquely up
Insertion:	Pars recta: lower surface of the thyroid lamina
	Pars oblique: thyroid cartilage between laminae and inferior horns
Innervation:	External branch of superior laryngeal nerve of X vagus
Function:	Depresses thyroid relative to cricoid, tenses vocal folds

Muscle: **Thyrovocalis (medial thyroarytenoid)**

Origin:	Inner surface, thyroid cartilage near notch
Course:	Back
Insertion:	Lateral surface of the arytenoid vocal process
Innervation:	X vagus, recurrent laryngeal nerve
Function:	Tenses vocal folds

Muscle: **Thyromuscularis (lateral thyroarytenoid)**

Origin:	Inner surface of thyroid cartilage near the notch
Course:	Back
Insertion:	Muscular process and base of arytenoid cartilage
Innervation:	X vagus, recurrent laryngeal nerve
Function:	Relaxes vocal folds

Muscle: **Superior thyroarytenoid**

Origin:	Inner surface of thyroid cartilage near the angle
Course:	Back

Insertion: Muscular process of arytenoid
Innervation: X vagus, recurrent laryngeal nerve
Function: Relaxes vocal folds

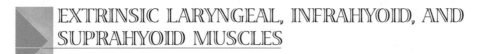

EXTRINSIC LARYNGEAL, INFRAHYOID, AND SUPRAHYOID MUSCLES

Hyoid and Laryngeal Elevators

Muscle: **Digastricus, anterior and posterior**

Origin: Anterior: inner surface of the mandible, near symphysis; Posterior: mastoid process of temporal bone
Course: Medial and down
Insertion: Hyoid, by means of intermediate tendon
Innervation: Anterior: V trigeminal nerve, mandibular branch, via the mylohyoid branch of the inferior alveolar nerve; Posterior: VII, digastric branch
Function: Anterior belly: draws hyoid up and forward; Posterior belly: draws hyoid up and back; together: elevate hyoid

Muscle: **Stylohyoid**

Origin: Styloid process of temporal bone
Course: Medially down
Insertion: Corpus hyoid
Innervation: Motor branch of the VII facial nerve
Function: Elevates and retracts hyoid bone

Muscle: **Mylohyoid**

Origin: Mylohyoid line, inner surface of mandible
Course: Fanlike to median fibrous raphe and hyoid
Insertion: Corpus of hyoid
Innervation: Alveolar nerve, V trigeminal, mandibular branch
Function: Elevates hyoid or depresses mandible

Muscle: **Geniohyoid**

Origin: Mental spines, inner surface of mandible
Course: Back and down
Insertion: Corpus, hyoid bone
Innervation: XII hypoglossal nerve and C1 spinal nerve
Function: Elevates hyoid bone, depresses mandible

Muscle: **Hyoglossus**

Origin:	Greater cornu hyoid
Course:	Up
Insertion:	Side of tongue
Innervation:	Motor branch of the XII hypoglossal
Function:	Elevates hyoid; depresses tongue

Muscle: **Genioglossus**

Origin:	Inner surface of mandible, mental spines
Course:	Up and back
Insertion:	Tongue and corpus hyoid
Innervation:	Motor branch of XII hypoglossal
Function:	Elevates hyoid; depresses, retracts, and protrudes tongue

Muscle: **Thyropharyngeus of inferior pharyngeal constrictor**

Origin:	Posterior pharyngeal raphe
Course:	Down, fanlike laterally
Insertion:	Thyroid lamina and inferior cornu
Innervation:	X vagus, recurrent laryngeal nerve (external laryngeal branch) and X vagus, superior laryngeal nerve (pharyngeal branch) and XI accessory
Function:	Elevates larynx and constricts pharynx

Hyoid and Laryngeal Depressors

Muscle: **Sternohyoid**

Origin:	Manubrium sterni and clavicle
Course:	Superiorly
Insertion:	Inferior margin of hyoid corpus
Innervation:	Ansa cervicalis from spinal C1 through C3
Function:	Depresses hyoid

Muscle: **Omohyoid, superior and inferior heads**

Origin:	Superior: corpus hyoid; Inferior: upper border, scapula
Course:	Superior: down; Inferior: down and laterally
Insertion:	Corpus hyoid
Innervation:	Superior: superior ramus of ansa cervicalis from C1; Inferior: ansa cervicalis, spinal C2 and C3
Function:	Depresses hyoid

Muscle: **Sternothyroid**

Origin:	Manubrium sterni
Course:	Up and out
Insertion:	Oblique line, thyroid cartilage
Innervation:	Spinal nerves C1, C2, and C3
Function:	Depresses thyroid cartilage

Muscle: **Thyrohyoid**

Origin:	Oblique line, thyroid cartilage
Course:	Up
Insertion:	Greater cornu, hyoid
Innervation:	XII hypoglossal nerve and fibers from spinal C1
Function:	Depresses hyoid or elevates thyroid

APPENDIX E

Muscles of Face, Soft Palate, and Pharynx

 FACIAL MUSCLES

Muscle: **Risorius**

Origin:	Posterior region of the face along the fascia of the masseter
Course:	Forward
Insertion:	Orbicularis oris at corners of mouth
Innervation:	Buccal branch of the VII facial nerve
Function:	Retracts lips at the corners

Muscle: **Buccinator**

Origin:	Pterygomandibular ligament
Course:	Forward
Insertion:	Orbicularis oris at corners of mouth
Innervation:	Buccal branch of the VII facial nerve
Function:	Moves food onto the grinding surfaces of the molars; constricts oropharynx

Muscle: **Levator labii superioris**

Origin:	Infraorbital margin of the maxilla
Course:	Down and in to the upper lip
Insertion:	Mid-lateral region of the upper lip
Innervation:	Buccal branches of the VII facial nerve
Function:	Elevates upper lip

Muscle:	**Zygomatic minor**
Origin:	Facial surface of the zygomatic bone
Course:	Downward
Insertion:	Mid-lateral region of upper lip
Innervation:	Buccal branches of the VII facial nerve
Function:	Elevates upper lip

Muscle:	**Levator labii alaeque nasi superioris**
Origin:	Frontal process of maxilla
Course:	Vertically along the lateral margin of the nose
Insertion:	Mid-lateral region of the upper lip
Innervation:	Buccal branches of the VII facial nerve
Function:	Elevates upper lip

Muscle:	**Zygomatic major (zygomaticus)**
Origin:	Lateral to the zygomatic minor on zygomatic bone
Course:	Obliquely down
Insertion:	Corner of the orbicularis oris
Innervation:	Buccal branches of the VII facial nerve
Function:	Elevates and retracts angle of mouth

Muscle:	**Depressor labii inferioris**
Origin:	Mandible at the oblique line
Course:	Up and in
Insertion:	Lower lip
Innervation:	Mandibular marginal branch of facial nerve
Function:	Dilates orifice by pulling lip down and out

Muscle:	**Depressor anguli oris (triangularis)**
Origin:	Lateral margins of mandible on oblique line
Course:	Fanlike up
Insertion:	Orbicularis oris and upper lip at corner
Innervation:	Mandibular marginal branch of the facial nerve
Function:	Depresses corners of mouth and helps to compress upper lip against lower lip

Muscle:	**Mentalis**
Origin:	Region of the incisive fossa of mandible
Course:	Down
Insertion:	Skin of the chin below
Innervation:	Mandibular marginal branch of the facial nerve
Function:	Elevates and wrinkles chin and pulls lower lip out

Muscle: **Orbicularis oris inferior and superior**

Origin: Corner of lips
Course: Laterally within lips
Insertion: Opposite corner of lips
Innervation: VII facial nerve
Function: Constricts oral opening

Muscle: **Platysma**

Origin: Fascia overlaying pectoralis major and deltoid
Course: Up
Insertion: Corner of the mouth, region below symphysis mente, lower margin of the mandible, and skin near the masseter
Innervation: Cervical branch of the VII facial nerve
Function: Depresses mandible

Intrinsic Tongue Muscles

Muscle: **Superior longitudinal**

Origin: Fibrous submucous layer near the epiglottis, the hyoid, and from the median fibrous septum
Course: Fans forward and outward
Insertion: Lateral margins of the tongue and region of apex
Innervation: XII hypoglossal nerve
Function: Elevates, assists in retraction of, or deviates tip of tongue

Muscle: **Inferior longitudinal**

Origin: Root of the tongue and corpus hyoid
Course: Forward
Insertion: Apex of the tongue
Innervation: XII hypoglossal nerve
Function: Pulls tip of the tongue downward, assists in retraction, deviates tongue

Muscle: **Transverse**

Origin: Median fibrous septum
Course: Laterally
Insertion: Side of the tongue in the submucous tissue
Innervation: XII hypoglossal nerve
Function: Narrows tongue

Muscle:	**Vertical**
Origin:	Base of the tongue
Course:	Vertically
Insertion:	Membranous cover
Innervation:	XII hypoglossal nerve
Function:	Pulls tongue down into floor of mouth

Extrinsic Tongue Muscles

Muscle:	**Genioglossus**
Origin:	Inner mandibular surface at symphysis
Course:	Fans up back and forward
Insertion:	Tip and dorsum of tongue and corpus hyoid
Innervation:	XII hypoglossal nerve
Function:	Anterior fibers retract tongue; posterior fibers protrude tongue; together, anterior and posterior fibers depress tongue

Muscle:	**Hyoglossus**
Origin:	Length of greater cornu and lateral body of hyoid
Course:	Upward
Insertion:	Sides of tongue between styloglossus and inferior longitudinal muscles
Innervation:	XII hypoglossal nerve
Function:	Pulls sides of tongue down

Muscle:	**Styloglossus**
Origin:	Anterolateral margin of styloid process
Course:	Forward and down
Insertion:	Inferior sides of the tongue
Innervation:	XII hypoglossal nerve
Function:	Draws tongue back and up

Muscle:	**Chondroglossus**
Origin:	Lesser cornu hyoid and corpus
Course:	Up
Insertion:	Interdigitates with intrinsic muscles of the tongue medial to hyoglossus
Innervation:	XII hypoglossal nerve
Function:	Depresses tongue

Mandibular Elevators and Depressors

Muscle: **Masseter**

Origin: Zygomatic arch

Course: Down

Insertion: Ramus of the mandible and coronoid process

Innervation: Anterior trunk of mandibular nerve arising from the V trigeminal

Function: Elevates mandible

Muscle: **Temporalis**

Origin: Temporal fossa of temporal and parietal bones

Course: Converging downward and forward, through the zygomatic arch

Insertion: Coronoid process and ramus

Innervation: Temporal branches arising from the mandibular nerve of V trigeminal

Function: Elevates mandible and draws it back if protruded

Muscle: **Medial pterygoid (internal pterygoid)**

Origin: Medial pterygoid plate and fossa

Course: Down and back

Insertion: Mandibular ramus

Innervation: Mandibular division of the V trigeminal nerve

Function: Elevates mandible

Muscle: **Lateral pterygoid (external pterygoid)**

Origin: Lateral pterygoid plate and greater wing of sphenoid

Course: Back

Insertion: Pterygoid fovea of the mandible

Innervation: Mandibular branch of the V trigeminal nerve

Function: Protrudes mandible

Muscle: **Digastricus, anterior belly**

Origin: Inner surface of mandible at digastricus fossa, near the symphysis

Course: Medially and down

Insertion: Intermediate tendon to juncture of hyoid corpus and greater cornu

Innervation: Mandibular branch of V trigeminal nerve via the mylohyoid branch of the inferior alveolar nerve

Function: Pulls hyoid forward; depresses mandible if in conjunction with digastricus posterior

Muscle: **Digastricus, posterior belly**

Origin: Mastoid process of temporal bone

Course: Medially and down

Insertion:	Intermediate tendon to juncture of hyoid corpus and greater cornu
Innervation:	Digastric branch of the VII facial nerve
Function:	Pulls hyoid back; depresses mandible if in conjunction with anterior digastricus

Muscle:	**Mylohyoid**
Origin:	Mylohyoid line, inner mandible
Course:	Back and down
Insertion:	Median fibrous raphe and inferiorly to hyoid
Innervation:	Alveolar nerve, arising from the V trigeminal nerve, mandibular branch
Function:	Depresses mandible

Muscle:	**Geniohyoid**
Origin:	Mental spines of the mandible
Course:	Medially
Insertion:	Corpus hyoid
Innervation:	XII hypoglossal nerve and C1 spinal nerve
Function:	Depresses mandible

MUSCLES OF THE VELUM

Muscle:	**Levator veli palatini (levator palati)**
Origin:	Apex of petrous portion of temporal bone and medial wall of the Eustachian tube cartilage
Course:	Down and forward
Insertion:	Palatal aponeurosis of soft palate, lateral to musculus uvulae
Innervation:	Pharyngeal plexus from XI accessory and X vagus nerves
Function:	Elevates and retracts posterior velum

Muscle:	**Musculus uvulae**
Origin:	Posterior nasal spines of the palatine bones and palatal aponeurosis
Course:	Runs the length of soft palate
Insertion:	Mucous membrane cover of the velum
Innervation:	Pharyngeal plexus of XI accessory and X vagus nerves
Function:	Shortens soft palate

Muscle:	**Tensor veli palatini (tensor veli palati)**
Origin:	Scaphoid fossa of sphenoid, sphenoid spine, and lateral Eustachian tube wall
Course:	Down, terminates in tendon which passes around pterygoid hamulus, then is directed medially
Insertion:	Palatal aponeurosis

Innervation:	Mandibular nerve of V trigeminal
Function:	Assists in dilating Eustachian tube

Muscle: **Palatoglossus**

Origin:	Anterolateral palatal aponeurosis
Course:	Down
Insertion:	Sides of posterior tongue
Innervation:	Pharyngeal plexus from XI accessory and X vagus nerves
Function:	Elevates tongue or depresses soft palate

Muscle: **Palatopharyngeus**

Origin:	Anterior hard palate midline of soft palate
Course:	Laterally and down
Insertion:	Posterior margin of thyroid cartilage
Innervation:	Pharyngeal plexus from XI accessory and pharyngeal branch of X vagus nerve
Function:	Narrows pharynx, lowers soft palate

MUSCLES OF PHARYNX

Muscle: **Superior pharyngeal constrictor**

Origin:	Pterygomandibular raphe
Course:	Posteriorly
Insertion:	Median raphe of pharyngeal aponeurosis
Innervation:	XI accessory nerve and X vagus via pharyngeal plexus
Function:	Pulls pharyngeal wall forward and constricts pharyngeal diameter

Muscle: **Middle pharyngeal constrictor**

Origin:	Horns of the hyoid and stylohyoid ligament
Course:	Up and back
Insertion:	Median pharyngeal raphe
Innervation:	XI accessory nerve and X vagus via pharyngeal plexus
Function:	Narrows diameter of pharynx

Muscle: **Inferior pharyngeal constrictor: cricopharyngeus**

Origin:	Cricoid cartilage
Course:	Back
Insertion:	Orifice of esophagus
Innervation:	XI accessory nerve and X vagus via pharyngeal plexus
Function:	Constricts superior orifice of esophagus

Muscle:	**Inferior pharyngeal constrictor: thyropharyngeus muscle**
Origin:	Oblique line of thyroid lamina
Course:	Up and back
Insertion:	Median pharyngeal raphe
Innervation:	XI accessory nerve and X vagus via pharyngeal plexus
Function:	Reduces diameter of lower pharynx

Muscle:	**Salpingopharyngeus**
Origin:	Lower margin of Eustachian tube
Course:	Down
Insertion:	Converges with palatopharyngeus
Innervation:	X vagus and spinal accessory nerve via the pharyngeal plexus
Function:	Elevates lateral pharyngeal wall

Muscle:	**Stylopharyngeus**
Origin:	Styloid process
Course:	Down
Insertion:	Into pharyngeal constrictors and posterior thyroid cartilage
Innervation:	Muscular branch of IX glossophyarngeal nerve
Function:	Elevates and opens pharynx

APPENDIX F
Sensors

GENERAL CLASSES

Interoceptors: Monitor events within the body (e.g., distention of stomach, blood pH)

Exteroceptors: Respond to stimuli outside of body (touch, hearing, vision)

Proprioceptors: Monitor change in body position or position of its parts (body position sense) (e.g., muscle and joint sensors, vestibular sensation)

SPECIFIC TYPES

Teloreceptors: Respond to stimuli separate from body (hearing, vision)

Contact receptors: Respond to stimuli that touch body (e.g., tactile, pain, deep and light pressure, temperature)

Chemoreceptors: Respond to chemical change (smell, taste, pH, etc.)

Photoreceptors: Respond to light changes (vision)

Thermoreceptors: Respond to heat

Mechanoreceptors: Respond to mechanical force (touch, muscle length and tension, auditory, vestibular receptors, etc.)

Nociceptors: Pain sensors

CLASSES OF SENSATION

Somatic sense: Related to pain, temperature, mechanical stimulation of somatic structures (skin, muscle, joints)

Kinesthesia: Sense of motion

Special senses: Senses mediating specific exteroceptive information such as vision, audition, olfaction

APPENDIX G
Cranial Nerves

 ## CLASSES OF CRANIAL NERVES

GSA	**General Somatic Afferent:**	Related to pain, temperature, mechanical stimulation of somatic structures (skin, muscle, joints)
GVA	**General Visceral Afferent:**	From receptors in visceral structures (e.g., digestive tract)
GVE	**General Visceral Efferent:**	Autonomic efferent fibers
GSE	**General Somatic Efferent:**	Innervates skeletal (striated) muscle
SSA	**Special Somatic Afferent:**	Special senses—sight, hearing, equilibrium
SVA	**Special Visceral Afferent:**	Special senses of smell, taste
SVE	**Special Visceral Efferent:**	Innervation of muscle of branchial arch origin: larynx, pharynx, face

 ## CRANIAL NERVES, SOURCES, AND FUNCTIONS

I. Olfactory

SVA: Sense of smell

Source: Mitral cells of olfactory bulb

II. Optic

SSA: Vision

Source: Rod and cone receptor cells synapse with bipolar interneurons which synapse with multipolar ganglionic neuron; optic nerve is axon of multipolar ganglionic neurons; nerve becomes myelinated after exiting eye socket and entering cranium; left and right nerves decussate at chiasm and project as optic tract to lateral geniculate body; projects to occipital cortex via optic radiations; left nasal nerve portion and right temporal nerve portion join after chiasm; left temporal nerve portion and right nasal aspect of nerve join after chiasm; visual field result is that left nasal and right temporal visual fields (right portion of image) project to left cerebral cortex; left temporal and right nasal visual fields (left portion of image) project to right cerebral cortex

III. Oculomotor

GSE: All extrinsic ocular muscles except superior oblique and lateral rectus

Source: Oculomotor nucleus

GVE: Light and accommodation reflexes

Source: Edinger-Westphal nucleus

IV. Trochlear

GSE: Superior oblique muscle of eye (turns eye down when eye is adducted)

Source: Trochlear nuclei

V. Trigeminal

GSA: Exteroceptive afferent for pain, thermal, tactile from face, forehead, mucous membrane of mouth and nose, teeth cranial dura; proprioceptive (deep pressure, kinesthesis) from teeth, gums, temporomandibular joint, stretch receptors of mastication

Source: Sensory nucleus of trigeminal

SVE: To muscles of mastication, tensor tympani, tensor veli palatini

Source: Motor nucleus of trigeminal

Components of V Trigeminal:

Ophthalmic branch: Sensory only

  GSA: From cornea, iris, upper eyelid, front of scalp

Maxillary branch: Sensory only

  GSA: From lower eyelid, nose, palate, upper jaw

Mandibular branch: Sensory and motor

  GSA: From lower jaw and teeth, mucosa, cheeks, temporomandibular joint, anterior two-thirds of tongue

  SVE: To muscles of mastication (internal and external pterygoid, temporalis, masseter), tensor tympani

VI. Abducens

GSE: Lateral rectus muscle for ocular abduction

Source: Abducens nucleus

VII. Facial

SVE: To facial muscles of expression, platysma, buccinator

Source: Motor nucleus of VII

SVA: Taste, anterior two-thirds of tongue

Source: Solitary nucleus

GSA: Cutaneous sense of EAM and skin of ear

Source: Trigeminal nuclei

GVE: Lacrimal gland (tears); mucous membrane of mouth and nose

Source: Superior salivatory and lacrimal nuclei

VIII. Vestibulocochlear

SSA: Vestibular and cochlear sensation

Cochlear (auditory) portion: Sensors are hair cells; cell bodies in spiral ganglion; axons are VIII nerve, auditory portion; low-frequency (apical) fibers terminate at ventral cochlear nucleus (VCN) and high-frequency fibers (basal) terminate at dorsal cochlear nucleus (DCN); transfer of auditory sensation to central nervous system

Source: Spiral ganglion

Vestibular portion: From semicircular canals, utricle, saccule; project to vestibular nuclei of medulla and subsequently to all levels of brainstem, spinal cord, cerebellum, thalamus, and cerebral cortex; maintenance of extensor tone, anti-gravity responses, balance, sense of position in space; coordinated eye/head movement through projection to III oculomotor, IV trochlear, VI abducens cranial nerves

Source: Vestibular ganglion

IX. Glossopharyngeal

GVA: Somatic (tactile, thermal, pain sense) from posterior one-third of tongue, tonsils, upper pharynx, Eustachian tube, mastoid cells

Source: Solitary nucleus

SVA: Taste, posterior one-third of tongue

Source: Inferior salivatory nucleus

GSA: Somatic sense of EAM and skin of ear

Source: Trigeminal nuclei

SVE: Innervation of stylopharyngeus, superior pharyngeal constrictor

Source: Inferior salivatory nucleus

GVE: Parotid gland

Source: Inferior salivatory nucleus

X. Vagus

GSA: Cutaneous sense from external auditory meatus

Source: Trigeminal nuclei

GVA: Sensory from pharynx, larynx, trachea, esophagus, viscera of thorax, abdomen

Source: Solitary nucleus

SVA: Taste buds near epiglottis and valleculae

Source: Solitary nucleus

GVE: To parasympathetic ganglia, thorax, and abdomen

Source: Dorsal motor nucleus of X

SVE: Striated muscle of larynx and pharynx

Source: Nucleus ambiguus

XI. Accessory

SVE, cranial portion: Joins with X vagus to form recurrent laryngeal nerve to innervate intrinsic muscles of larynx

SVE, spinal portion: Innervates sternocleidomastoid and trapezius

Source: Cranial portion: nucleus ambiguus of medulla; Spinal portion: Anterior horn of C1 through C5 spinal nerves; unite and ascend; enter skull via foramen magnum; exit with vagus at jugular foramen

XII. Hypoglossal

GSE: Muscles of tongue

Source: Nucleus of hypoglossal nerve

Clinical Note: Lesion of LMN produces ipsilateral damage (tongue deviates toward side of damage)

APPENDIX H

Pathologies That Affect Speech Production

The following list is far from exhaustive, but is rather a sampler of the many speech, language, and hearing problems that can arise from physical sources.

Respiration Subsystem	Impact
Emphysema:	Reduced volumes and capacities and increased respiratory effort result in lower subglottal pressure, reduced phrase length, and reduced vocal intensity.
Spastic paralytic conditions:	Cerebral palsy, acquired spastic paralysis; results in increased tone of muscles of respiration and reduced range of motion, causing reduction in capacities, paradoxical respiratory effort; result is reduced ability to generate high subglottal pressures, reduced phrase length, impaired prosody secondary to inability to generate microbursts of pressure.
Ataxic conditions:	Ataxic dysarthria affecting respiration results in loss of coordination between subsystems, reduction of coordinated effort for inspiration and expiration; result may be inappropriate timing on inspiration and expiration and explosive expiratory bursts.
Muscular dystrophy and other flaccid paralytic conditions:	Loss of ability to generate high subglottal pressure, reduction in capacities, and reduced range of motion of muscles of respiration result in reduced phrase length, impaired prosody, low vocal intensity.
Huntington's disease, athetosis, and other hyperkinetic conditions:	The addition of uncontrollable motion overlaid upon voluntary contraction produces unpredictable inspiration and expiration; speech impairment may include explosive bursts, inappropriate termination or pausing of inspiration or expiration, loss of control of vocal intensity, and disrupted prosody.

Parkinson's disease and other conditions resulting in hypokinesias:	The muscular rigidity results in loss of capacities and range of motion; speech result is extremely low vocal intensity, including loss of subglottal pressure adequate to sustain phonation.
Respiratory insufficiency causing ventilator dependency:	Many diseases result in a dependence on mechanical ventilation, and the result is loss of phonation because the phonatory mechanism is bypassed via tracheostomy. Valving technology exists to circumvent this difficulty for some clients.

Phonatory Subsystem

Vocal fold paralysis:	Arises from damage to the X vagus nerve; arises from surgical procedures (surgery on thyroid), or trauma (vehicular accident); typically paralysis of adduction if lesion is extracranial, or of abductors if lesion is intracranial. Abductor paralysis results in phonation on both inhalation and exhalation (stridor), whereas adductor paralysis results in loss of ability to adduct vocal folds for phonation.
Space-occupying lesions:	Include papilloma, carcinoma, polyps. Lesions that occupy space can cause asymmetrical vibration of the vocal folds (resulting in diplophonia), reduction in fundamental frequency and range of phonation, harsh and hoarse phonation, "popping" sound on inhalation or exhalation but with little other phonatory impact (pedunculated polyps), aphonia, reduction in vocal intensity.
Spastic paralytic conditions:	Include spasmodic dysphonia and spasticity arising from cerebrovascular accident or other disease condition. Speech result is strained, harsh phonation, reduced range of intensity and fundamental frequency, dysprosody secondary to excessive and equal syllabic stress, and sometimes excessively high vocal intensity. In spasmodic dysphonia the spasticity may cause uncontrollable abduction or adduction of the vocal folds, causing loss of phonation and harsh phonatory onset.
Hormone treatment:	Use of male hormones to treat some carcinomas can result in irreversible lowering of fundamental frequency.
Vocal hyperfunction:	Functional abuse of vocal mechanism, such as that resulting from excessively loud speech, can cause vocal nodules. Attempting to speak below one's optimal fundamental frequency may result in contact ulcers, especially if more forceful speech is attempted.
Laryngectomy:	Removal of larynx because of carcinoma results in complete loss of phonation.
Flaccid paralytic conditions:	Lower motor neuron damage can result in flaccid paralysis of vocal apparatus. Direct damage to recurrent laryngeal nerve or superior laryngeal nerve results in vocal fold paralysis (see above). More generalized conditions such as muscular dystrophy result in weakened

adductory force, reduced ability to abduct vocal folds, reduced range of fundamental frequency, and reduced vocal intensity. Myasthenia gravis (a disease of the myoneural junction) presents a unique constellation of phonatory signs, in that the flaccid condition progresses as a result of exertion, with phonatory ability returning to near-baseline levels following adequate rest.

Ataxic conditions:	Conditions causing damage to the cerebellum or pontine nuclei of the brainstem result in discoordination of the phonatory act. Adduction and abduction will be poorly timed, with discoordination of phonation with other subsystems (respiration, articulation), explosive bursts of phonation, inappropriate terminations of phonation, and inadequate control of vocal intensity and fundamental frequency.
Hypokinetic conditions:	Predominantly, Parkinson's disease results in muscular rigidity. The phonatory mechanism shows a marked reduction in vocal intensity, as well as reduced range of vocal intensity and fundamental frequency.
Hyperkinetic conditions:	Huntington's disease, athetosis, dystonia, and other hyperkinesias result in unpredictable muscular contraction overlaid upon voluntary movements. In the case of the phonatory mechanism, hyperkinesias result in uncontrollable increases and decreases in vocal intensity, fluctuations in fundamental frequency, and loss of voicing during normally phonated segments.
Dyspraxic conditions:	Dyspraxia is reduction in the ability to voluntarily contract musculature in the absence of muscular weakness or paralysis, and typically with retained involuntary function. Frequent etiology is cerebrovascular accident, and the result is difficulty initiating phonation voluntarily, but with retained ability to phonate in over-learned situations, as well as normal cough and throat-clearing.
Mixed dysarthria:	Diseases such as amyotrophic lateral sclerosis or Wilson's disease result in mixed dysarthrias. The impact on phonation depends on the type of dysarthria (spastic, flaccid, ataxic, unilateral upper motor neuron, hypokinetic, hyperkinetic).
Cleft palate:	Although cleft palate does not typically directly involve the phonatory mechanism, there is very often an impact on phonation. The child with inadequate mechanical separation of the oral and nasal cavities may resort to vocal hyperfunction, perhaps in an attempt to increase vocal intensity or to increase the high-frequency energy in the acoustic phonatory source (see hyperfunction, above). In addition, the child may resort to vocal hyperfunction in an attempt to increase laryngeal control, as loss of adequate supraglottal (oral) pressure results in excessive transglottal pressure and poor laryngeal control.

Laryngeal web:	Congenital laryngeal web consists of connective tissue above, below, or at the level of the vocal folds. Webs may be life-threatening and will compromise phonation.

Articulatory Subsystem

Cleft lip and cleft palate:	Congenital defect of lip and/or palate that results in inadequate closure of bony or muscular palate in cleft palate, and alveolar, lip, and/or premaxillary suture in cleft lip. The impact on speech will be primarily on high-pressure consonants (fricatives, stops, affricates), often resulting in phonological deficiencies arising from compensatory articulations.
Submucous cleft:	Presence of fistula or cleft of the bony palate that is covered by epithelium so that it is hidden ("occult") to casual examination. The cleft will have a bluish cast to it, and will move during palpation. Speech will have a nasal quality despite no apparent communication between the oral and nasal cavities, arising from the acoustical coupling provided by the epithelial lining separating the two cavities.
Palatal insufficiency:	Insufficient muscular tissue of soft palate, or inadequate movement of soft palate arising from muscular weakness, can result in hypernasality or assimilated nasality (nasalization of phonemes that occur before or after nasal sounds).
Maxillary carcinoma:	Surgical removal of maxilla results in communication between the oral and nasal cavities that must be instrumentally corrected for production of non-nasal speech.
Flaccid paralytic conditions:	Any condition (e.g., muscular dystrophy, myasthenia gravis) that results in muscular weakness to the oral or velar muscles will result in articulatory distortion. Flaccid paralysis may result in loss of accuracy in articulatory contact, weak plosion, weak fricatives or even conversion of fricatives to plosives, hypernasality secondary to inadequate velopharyngeal valving, but with relatively normal diadochokinetic rates.
Spastic paralytic conditions:	Conditions that produce spasticity (e.g., cerebrovascular accident) will result in increased resistance to movement of the articulators. Speech accuracy and rate of speaking are reduced, and signs of spasticity characterized as "gaglike" sounds during articulation can be noted during palatal and velar articulations.
Ataxic dysarthria:	Damage to the cerebellum or nuclei and pathways serving the cerebellum can result in discoordination of the articulatory muscles, as well as loss of intersystem coordination with respiration and phonation. Articulatory inaccuracies will be characterized as inconsistent distortions, explosive articulations, errors in rate, range, and force of motion. Diadochokinesis will be defective.

Hyperkinetic conditions:	Addition of involuntary movements arising from disease states such as Huntington's disease, dystonia, or athetosis will result in inaccurate articulations characterized by distortions.
Hypokinetic conditions:	Primarily arising from Parkinson's disease, the result of progressive muscular rigidity is increasingly reduced range of motion, weak and inadequate articulations, and (paradoxically) rapid diadochokinetic rate resulting from reduced range of motion.
Mixed dysarthrias:	Arising from disease states such as hepatolenticular degeneration, amyotrophic lateral sclerosis, or multiple sclerosis, the impact on speech will be determined by type of dysarthria involved.
Dental anomalies:	Absent dentition or teeth that are off-axis can cause distortion of fricatives and other articulatory inaccuracies.
Oral myofunctional disorders:	"Tongue thrust" is a disorder that involves loss of balance of oral/pharyngeal musculature, loss of tone of muscles of mastication and lingual musculature, and increased or decreased labial musculature tone. The individual with tongue thrust may develop a low-tone, open-mouthed posture that, if uncorrected, may result in a permanently vaulted hard palate and long, narrow face. The uncorrected tongue thrust swallow includes inadequate bolus preparation and propulsion. Speech in tongue thrust is most often characterized by distorted lingual fricatives secondary to the weakened lingual musculature. Speech remediation is frequently inconsequential until the underlying oral myofunctional deficits have been remediated.
Relative macroglossia:	When the tongue is excessively large relative to the oral cavity, it is termed macroglossia. This condition is often seen in individuals with hypotonic conditions (Down syndrome). Distorted articulation may be due to the relatively large tongue or the flaccid condition.
Tongue tie:	A short lingual frenum results in the inability to make alveolar, palatal, and velar articulations. Surgical release of the frenum can improve speech in cases where it is demonstrated to be short.
Hypertrophied adenoids:	Hypertrophied adenoidal tissue may result in difficulty breathing through the nose, increased upper respiratory disease, inadequate ventilation of the middle ear by means of the Eustachian tube, habitual mouth breathing, and hyponasal speech. Depending on the individual, the result may be facial dysmorphia (mouth breathing), chronic otitis media and hearing loss (Eustachian tube dysfunction), and substitution of non-nasal consonants for nasals.

Auditory Mechanism

Inflammatory conditions of the external ear:	Otitis media externa is painful inflammation of the outer ear, especially of the external auditory meatus. Pain is particularly acute due to the tight bonding of the epithelial lining to ear cartilage.

Congenital deficiencies of the outer ear:	A number of congenital conditions exist that have an impact on external ear structures. The pinna may be congenitally absent (congenital atresia) or dysmorphic. The external auditory meatus may be congenitally absent (atresia) or narrowed (stenosis). Preauricular pits and ear tags are of no clinical significance, but signal the potential presence of genetic conditions such as branchio-oto-renal syndrome. Low-set auricles are characteristics for a number of genetic syndromes (e.g., Apert syndrome), and posteriorly rotated auricles are one component of fetal alcohol syndrome.
Inflammatory middle ear disease:	Chronic otitis media frequently arises from inadequate ventilation of the middle ear space or from bacterial infection. The result is conductive hearing loss that appears to have a significant impact on speech and language development.
Trauma to middle ear:	Disarticulation of the ossicles can occur as a result of temporal bone trauma or from high-intensity acoustic shock, such as that experienced during explosions. Fracture of the temporal bone can occur as a result of head trauma, and can result in cerebrospinal fluid otorrhea (loss of cerebrospinal fluid from the cranial space into the middle ear space), which, of course, can be a life-threatening condition considering the potential for bacterial infection of the meninges.
Neoplasm of middle ear:	Glomus jugulare tumors can be mistaken for a host of otologic conditions. If the tumor contacts the tympanic membrane, it will provide objective, pulsatile movement of the ear drum; if it contacts the ossicles, it can cause what appears to be otosclerosis. The degree of hearing impairment is typically related to the degree to which structures of the middle ear conduction mechanism are involved.
Otosclerosis:	This disease condition involves fixation of the stapes in the oval window, resulting in a conductive hearing loss.
Diseases of inner ear:	Viral or bacterial infection may cause labyrinthitis, an inflammation of the inner ear. The effects of labyrinthitis include dizziness, balance problems, and tinnitus, potentially remitting at the end of the infection course. Other problems include perilymph fistula, in which one of the cochlear membranes (typically Reissner's) is torn so that perilymph and endolymph mix, producing a relatively localized sensorineural loss. Endolymphatic hydrops is a disease characterized by increased endolymph and perilymph pressure, resulting in permanent damage to vestibular and cochlear sensing mechanisms, with symptoms ranging from tinnitus to vestibular disturbances. Head trauma can fracture the temporal bone, causing sensorineural hearing loss.

Neurological Conditions

Cerebrovascular accident:	Cerebrovascular accidents include conditions in which obstruction of blood flow results in damage to neuronal tissue. Because of the

centrality of the brain to speech function, the impact on speech can range from none to complete loss of motor, cognitive, and linguistic function.

Degenerative conditions: A number of disease conditions result in degeneration of nervous tissue. Cerebellar degeneration arises from a number of conditions, but results in loss of coordination of motor function. Frontal lobe degeneration in Huntington's disease results in loss of cognitive function, while substantia nigra degeneration in Parkinson's disease results in loss of the ability to initiate movement. Generally, the focal nature of a given lesion will define the nature of the deficit experienced, with diseases having broader impact (e.g., multiple sclerosis) showing more diverse symptomatology.

Trauma: Head trauma can have widespread impact on speech, language, and cognitive function. The degree and type of impairment depend in large part on the location of the trauma, the magnitude and type of trauma, and the speed with which treatment was implemented. Frontal lobe damage is common in vehicular trauma, and may result in memory, cognitive, motor, and expressive language deficits. Missile trauma (e.g., gunshot wounds, shrapnel) may affect any portion of the brain but will have more focal effects. Rotatory trauma can produce devastating damage to the brainstem and projection fibers of the tracts of the brain.

Glossary

-a-	Without; lack of
-ab-	Away from
Abdomen	/ˈæbdəmən/ Region of the body between the thorax and pelvis
Abdominal fixation	Process of impounding air within the lungs through inhalation and forceful vocal fold adduction which results in increased intra-abdominal pressure
Abdominal viscera	/æbˈdamənl ˈvɪsɚə/ Organs of the abdominal region
Abduction	/æbˈdʌkʃən/ To draw a structure away from midline
Absolutely refractory period	Period following depolarization of a cell membrane during which stimulation will not result in further depolarization
Acetylcholine	/əˈsitlkolin/ Neurotransmitter involved in communication between several classes of neurons and between nerve and muscle
Actin	One of two muscle proteins
Action potential (AP)	Electrical potential arising from depolarizing a cell membrane
ad-	Combining form meaning toward
Adduct	/æˈdʌkt/ To draw two structures closer together or to move toward midline
Adduction	Process of drawing two structures closer together or moving a structure toward midline
Adenoids	/ˈædnɔɪdz/ Lymphoid tissue within the nasopharynx
Adequate stimulus	Stimulation of sufficient intensity or frequency to cause a response
Adipose	/ˈædəpos/ Connective tissue impregnated with fat cells
Aditus of mastoid antrum	/æˈditəs ʌv ˈmæstɔɪd ˈæntrʌm/ Entryway to the tympanic antrum
Aeration	/ɛrēɪʃən/ The process of introducing air to a space or cavity

713

Afferent	Carrying toward a central location; generally, sensory nerve impulses
Agonists	Muscle contracted for purpose of a specific motor act (as contrasted to the antagonist)
Ala	/ˈeɪlə/ Winglike structure
-algia	Combining form meaning pain
Alpha motor neurons	Motor neurons involved in activation of the majority of skeletal musculature
Alveolar pressure	/æl ˈvilɚ/ Air pressure measured at the level of the alveolus in the lung
Alveolus	/ælvi ˈoləs/ Small cavity; as in alveolus of lung, the air sac wherein gas exchange occurs
Ambulation	Walking
Amphi-	On both sides
Amphiarthrodial	/æmfiar ˈθrodiəl/ Bony articulation in which bones are connected by cartilage
Ampulla	/ˈæmpulə/ Dilation of structure
an-	Without; lack of
Ana	Up
Anastomoses	/ænæstə ˈmosəs/ Communication between two vessels or structures
Anatomical dead space	Space within the conducting passageway of the respiratory system that is not involved in exchange of gasses
Anatomical position	Erect body, with palms, arms, and hands face forward
Anatomy	The study of structure of an organism
Aneurysm	/ˈænjɚɪzm/ Abnormal dilation or ballooning of a blood vessel (typically an artery)
angio-	/ˈændʒio/ Blood vessels
Angiology	/ændʒi ˈalədʒi/ Science dealing with blood vessels and the lymphatic system
Annular	/ˈænjulɚ/ Ringlike
Anomia	/əˈnomiə/ Inability to remember names of objects
Ansa	/ænsə/ Structure that forms a loop or arc
Antagonist	A muscle that opposes the contraction of another muscle (the agonist)
ante-	Before
Anterior	In front of; before
Anterior process of manubrium	/məˈnubriəm/ Anterior prominence of manubrium, providing point of attachment for anterior ligament of malleus
antero-	Before
Antitragus	/ænt ˈɪreɪgəs/ Region posterior and inferior to the tragus
Antrum	/ˈæntrəm/ An incompletely closed cavity
Apex	Peak; extremity
Aphasia	/əˈfeɪʒə/ Acquired language disorder, typically arising from cerebrovascular accident

Apical	Referring to the apex of a structure
apo-	Away from
Aponeurosis	/ˈæpanjɚosəs/ Sheetlike tendon
Appendicular skeleton	/ˈæpəndɪkjulɚ/ The skeleton including upper and lower extremities
Applied anatomy	The subdiscipline of anatomy concerned with diagnosis, treatment, and surgical intervention
Approximate	To bring closer together
Areolar	/ɛriˈolar/ Loose connective tissue
Arm	The upper extremity including the region from the elbow to the shoulder
arthr-	A joint
Arthrology	/arˈθralodʒi/ The study of joints
Articulation	The point of union between two structures
Articulators	In speech production, the moveable and immobile structures used to produce the sounds of speech
Articulatory system	In speech science, the system of structures involved in shaping the oral cavity for production of the sounds of speech
Ascending pathways	Sensory pathways of the nervous system
Association fibers	Neurons that transmit information between two regions of the same cerebral hemisphere
Asthenia	/əsˈθinjə/ Weakness
Astrocytes	/ˈæstrosa͞ɪts/ A form of neuroglial cell
Ataxia	Deficit in motor coordination
Atlas	The first cervical vertebra
Atmospheric pressure	Pressure of the atmosphere generated by its weight; approximately 760 mm Hg
Attrition	/əˈtrɪʃən/ Wearing away
Audition	Hearing
Auditory evoked potentials	Electrical potentials arising from auditory stimulation
Auditory tube	Eustachian tube; aerating tube connecting nasopharynx and middle ear
Auricular tubercle	/oˈrɪkjulɚ ˈtubɚkl/ Bulge on superior-posterior aspect of helix
Autonomic	Independently functioning
Autonomic nervous system	Portion of nervous system controlling involuntary bodily functions
Axial skeleton	Portion of the skeleton including the trunk, head, and neck
Axis	Imaginary line representing the point around which a body pivots
Axoaxonic synapses	/ˈæksoæk ˈsanɪk/ Synapses between two axons
Axodendritic synapses	/ˈæksoden ˈdrɪtɪk/ Synapses involving axon and dendrite

Axon	The process of a neuron that conducts information away from the soma or body
Babinski reflex	/bə'bɪnskɪ/ Dorsiflexion of the great toe and spreading of other toes upon stimulation of the ventral surface of the foot
Baroreceptors	Pressure sensors
Basal ganglia	Nuclei deep within the cerebral hemispheres, involved in movement initiation and termination, and including the caudate nucleus, lentiform nucleus, amygdala, and claustrum
Base	The lower or supporting portion of a structure
Basilar membrane	Portion of cochlear duct upon which organ of Corti is attached
Bellies	The fleshy portions of a muscle
Bernoulli effect	/bɚ'nuli/ The effect which dictates that, given a constant volume flow of air or fluid, at a point of constriction there will be a decrease in air pressure perpendicular to the flow and an increase in velocity of the flow
Best frequency	Frequency of sound stimulation to which a neuron responds most vigorously
bi-	Two
Bifurcate	/'baɪfɚkeɪt/ Two-forked; to split into two parts or channels
Bite block	A structure used experimentally or clinically to eliminate movement of the mandible during articulatory tasks
blast-	Germ
Bolus	/'boləs/ A ball or lump of masticated food ready to swallow
Boyle's law	The law stating that, given a gas of constant temperature, an increase in the volume of the chamber in which the gas is contained will cause a decrease in air pressure
brachy-	Short
brady-	Slow
Brain mapping	Procedure of identifying functional regions of the cerebral cortex by electrical stimulation during speech, reading, or other tasks
Brevis	/'brɛvəs/ Short; brief
Broca's aphasia	Aphasia characterized by loss of fluency and reduced paucity of vocabulary, usually arising from lesion to Brodmann areas 44 and 45 of the dominant cerebral hemisphere (Broca's area)
Broca's area	Brodmann areas 44 and 45 of the dominant cerebral hemisphere, responsible for motor planning for speech and components of expressive language
Brodmann areas	Regions of the cerebral hemisphere, identified by numeric characterization based upon functional and anatomical organization
Bronchi	/'brankaɪ/ The two major branches from the trachea leading to right and left lungs
Bronchial tree	/'brankijl̩/ Network of bronchi and bronchial tubes
Bronchial tube	Divisions of the respiratory tree below the level of the mainstem bronchi
Bronchioles	/'brankijl̩z/ Small divisions of bronchial tree

Buccal	/ˈbʌkl̩/ Pertaining to the cheek
Buccal cavity	Cavity lateral to the teeth, bounded by the cheek
Buildup response	Neural responses characterized by slow increase in firing rate during the initial stages of firing
Bulb	Pertaining to the brainstem
Bulbar	/ˈbəlbar/ Pertaining to the brainstem
Capillary	Minute blood vessel
capit-	/ˈkæpət/ Combining form meaning head, or toward the head end
Caput	/ˈkæpət/ The head
Caries	/ˈkɛriz/ Decay of soft or bony tissue
-carpal	Combining form meaning wrist
Cartilage	Connective tissue embedded in matrix, capable of withstanding significant compressive and tensile forces
Cartilaginous	Constructed of cartilage
Cartilaginous joints	Joint in which cartilage serves to connect two bones
Caudal	/ˈkɔd̩l/ Toward the tail or coccyx
Cavum conchae	/ˈkævəm ˈkaŋkeɪ/ Deep portion of the concha
-cele	Combining form meaning tumor
Cementum	/səˈmɛntəm/ Thin layer of bone joining tooth and alveolus
Central	Relative to the center of a structure
Central nervous system	Brain and spinal cord components
cephalo-	/ˈsɛfəlo/ Combining form meaning head, or toward the head end
Cerebrospinal fluid	/səˈribroˈspaɪnlˈfluəd/ Fluid originating in the choroid plexuses of the ventricles, and providing cushion to brain structures
Cerebrovascular system	Vascular system serving the nervous system
Cerumen	/səˈrumən/ The waxy secretion within the external auditory meatus
Channel proteins	Specialized proteins in cell membrane that allow specific ions to pass through the membrane
Characteristic frequency	Frequency of sound stimulation to which a neuron responds most vigorously
Checking action	The use of muscles of inspiration to impede the outward flow of air during respiration for speech
Chemoreceptors	/ˈkimorɪˈsɛptɚz/ Sensory organ that is sensitive to properties of specific chemicals
Chondral	/ˈkandrl̩/ Pertaining to cartilage
Chopper response	Neural responses characterized by periodic, chopped temporal pattern that is present throughout stimulation
Cilia	/ˈsɪliə/ Hairlike processes
Circum	/ˈsɚkəm/ Around

Class I malocclusion	Malocclusion in which there is normal orientation of the molars, but an abnormal orientation of the incisors
Class I occlusion	Relationship between upper and lower dental arches in which the first molar of the mandibular arch is one-half tooth advanced of the maxillary molar
Class II malocclusion	Relationship between upper and lower dental arches in which the first mandibular molars are retracted at least one tooth from the first maxillary molars
Class III malocclusion	Relationship between upper and lower dental arches in which the first mandibular molar is advanced farther than one tooth beyond the first maxillary molar
-cle	Combining form that implies something very small
Clinical eruption	Eruption of teeth into the oral cavity
Clinker	A mass of noncombustible material identified by a master engineer
cm	Centimeter
Coarticulation	The overlapping effect of one sound upon another
Cochlear aqueduct	/ˈkokliɚ ˈakwədəkt/ Small opening between the scala vestibuli and the subarachnoid space of the cranial cavity
Cochlear duct	The membranous cochlear labyrinth, housing the sensory organs of the inner ear
Cochlear microphonic	Stimulus-related auditory potential, being a direct electrical analog to the stimulus
Cochlear nucleus	Initial brainstem nucleus of the auditory pathway, found within the pons, and subdivided into anteroventral, posteroventral, and dorsal cochlear nuclei
com-	Combining form meaning with or together with
Commissural fibers	/ˈkamiʃɚl ˈfaɪbɚz/ Neural fibers that run from one location on a hemisphere to the corresponding location on the other hemisphere
Comparative anatomy	Study of homologous structures of different animals
Compressive strength	The ability to withstand crushing forces
con-	Combining form meaning with or together with
Concha	/ˈkaɴkə/ Entrance to the ear canal
Conduction aphasia	Aphasia due to lesion of the arcuate fasciculus
Conduction velocity	Rate of conduction of impulse through a neuron
Condyle	/ˈkandaɪl/ Rounded prominence of a bone
Cone of light	Bright region of tympanic membrane on inferior-anterior aspect, arising from tautness of the membrane
contra-	Combining form meaning opposite
Contracture	Permanent contraction of a muscle
Contralateral	Originating on the opposite side
Convergence	Coming together toward a common point

Convolutions	Turns; infoldings
cor-	Combining form meaning heart
Cornu	/kor ˈnu/ Horn
Coronal section	A section dividing the body into front and back halves
corp-	Combining form meaning body
Corpus	/ˈkorpəs/ Body
Cortex	Outer covering
Cough	Forceful evacuation of the respiratory passageway, including deep inhalation through widely abducted vocal folds, tensing and tight adduction of the vocal folds, and elevation of the larynx, followed by forceful expiration
Cranial	Toward the head
Cranial nerves	The 12 pairs of nerves arising from the brain
Craniostosis	/krenɪoˈstosəs/ Premature ossification of cranial sutures
Cranium	/ˈkrenɪəm/ The portion of the skull containing the brain
Crista ampularis	/ˈkristə æmpjəˈlɛrəs/ Thickened region of semicircular canal lining containing sensory cells
Crossed olivocochlear bundle	/alivoˈkokliɚ/ Portion of efferent auditory pathway, apparently integral to the processing of a signal in noise
Crown	The highest point of a structure
crur-, crus	Combining form meaning cross; leglike part
Crura anthelicis	/ˈkrɚə æntɛˈlɪkəs/ Auricle landmark produced by bifurcation of the antihelix
Crux	/krus/ Cross
cryo-	Combining form meaning cold
-cule	Combining form that implies something very small
-culum, -culus	Combining form that gives diminutive form of a noun
Cycle of respiration	Completion of both inspiration and expiration phases of respiration
Cycle of vibration	Point in a vibratory cycle at which the function begins to repeat itself
-cyte	Combining form meaning cell
Cytology	/saɪ ˈtalodʒi/ Science dealing with structure of cells
de-	Away from
Dead space air	The air within the conducting passageways that cannot be involved in gas exchange
Decibel	The logarithmic expression of the ratio of two sound pressures or powers to express acoustic level
Deciduous	/dəˈsɪdjuəs/ Shedding
Deciduous dental arch	The dental arch containing the 10 temporary teeth
Decussate	/ˈdɛkəseɪt/ To cross over
Deep	Further from the surface

Defecation	/'dɛfəkeɪʃən/ Evacuation of bowels
Deglutition	/di'glutɪʃən/ Swallowing
Dendrite	The process of a neuron that transmits information to the cell body
Dendrodendritic synapse	Synapse between two dendrites
Dentate	/'dɛnteɪt/ Referring to tooth; notched; toothlike
Dentin	/'dɛnt ɪn/ Osseous portion of the tooth
Depolarization	Neutralizing of polarity difference between two structures
Dermatome	/'dɚmətom/ Region of body innervated by a given spinal nerve
Descending pathways	Motor pathways of the central nervous system
Developmental anatomy	Study of anatomy with reference to growth and development to birth
dextro-	Right
Diffusion	Migration or mixing of one material (e.g., liquid) through another
Digestive system	The system of organs and glands involved in digestion of food and liquids
Dilate	/'daɪleɪt/ To open or expand an orifice
Dissection	The process of separating tissues of a cadaveric specimen
Distoverted	/'dɪstovɚtəd/ Tilted away from midline
Divergence	/daɪ'vɚdʒəns/ To become progressively farther apart
Dorsal	/'dorsl̩/ Pertaining to the back of the body or distal
Dorsum	/'dorsəm/ Posterior side of a structure
-dynia	Pain
dys-	Bad; with difficulty
Dysmetria	/dɪs'mɛtriə/ Deficit in control of the range of movement of a structure, such as a limb or the tongue
e-	Out from
Ear drum	The membranous separation between the outer and middle ears, responsible for initiating the mechanical impedance-matching process of the middle ear
ec-	Out of
ecto-	On the outer side; toward the surface
-ectomy	Excision
Efferent	/'ɛfərənt/ Carrying away from a central point
Elasticity	The quality of a material that causes it to return to its original position after being distended
Electrophysiology	The study of electrical phenomena associated with cellular physiology
Ellipsoid	/i'lipsɔɪd/ Shaped like a spindle
Embolism	/'ɛmbəlizm/ The obstruction of a blood vessel by an object or clot
Embolus	/'ɛmbələs/ An object within a blood vessel that has been carried by the bloodstream

Embryonic development	In humans, the stage between the second and eighth weeks of gestation
-emia	Referring to blood
En passant	/an pə'san/ In passing
Enamel	The hard outer surface of the tooth
Encephalon	/ɛn'sɛfəlɑn/ The brain
endo-	Toward the interior; within
Endocochlear potential	/ɛndo'koklɪɚ/ The constant positive potential difference between the scala media and the peripheral scalae vestibuli and tympani
Endolymph	The fluid found in the scala media
Endolymphatic duct	Duct arising from the saccule of the vestibule, terminating blindly in the petrous portion of the temporal bone
Ensiform	/'ɛnsɪform/ Swordlike
ento-	Toward the interior; within
ep-, epi-	Upon or above something else
Epimysium	/ɛpə'mɪziəm/ Sheath of connective tissue around skeletal muscle
Equilibrium	A condition of balance
Equipotentiality	Having equal electrical charge
Esophageal reflux	/ɛ'safədʒil/ Introduction of gastric juices into the pharyngeal region through the esophagus
etio-	Pertaining to cause or origin
Eustachian tube	/'justeɪʃən/ Also known as the *auditory tube*, coursing from the middle ear space to the nasopharynx; responsible for aeration of the middle ear
Eversion	/i'vɚʒən/ Turning outward
ex-	Out of, toward the surface
Expiration	Process of evacuating air from the lungs during respiration
Extension	Straightening or moving out of the flexed position
External	Toward the exterior of a body
External auditory meatus	External ear canal, terminating at the tympanic membrane
extero-	Aimed outward or nearer to exteroceptors
extra-	Outside
Eye tooth	Cuspid
Facet	A small surface
Fasciculus	/fə'sɪkjuləs/ A small bundle
Feature detectors	Neurons that respond to specific characteristics of a stimulus
Fibroblasts	Germinal cell of connective tissue
Final common pathway	The lower motor neuron serving a muscle or a muscle bundle

Fissure	/'fɪʃɚ/ A relatively deep groove
Flexion	/'flɛkʃən/ The act of bending, often upon the ventral surfaces
Foramen	/'forēɪmən/ An opening or passageway
Fossa	/'fasə/ A depression, groove, or furrow
Fovea	/'foviə/ A pit
Frenum	/'frinəm/ A small band of tissue connecting two structures, one of which is mobile
Frenulum	/'frɛnjuləm/ A small frenum; often synonymous with frenum
Frequency	Number of cycles of vibration per second
Frontal	Anterior; pertaining to the front
Frontal plane	Divides body into anterior and posterior
Function	The process or action of a structure
Functional unity	Structures that demonstrate similarities in function
Fundamental frequency	The lowest frequency of vibration of the vocal folds or of a harmonic series
Funiculus	/fə'nɪkjuləs/ Small, cordlike structure
Ganglion	/'gæŋgliən/ Mass of nerve cell bodies lying outside of the central nervous system
-gen	Producing
General somatic afferent	Sensory nerves that communicate sensory information from skin, muscles, and joints, including pain, temperature, mechanical stimulation of skin, length and tension of muscle, and movement and position of joints
General somatic efferent	Nerves providing innervation of skeletal muscle
General visceral afferent	Nerves that transmit sensory information from receptors in visceral structures, such as the digestive tract
General visceral efferent	The autonomic efferent fibers serving viscera and glands
-genic	Producing
Genu	/'dʒēɪnu/ Knee
Gingiva	/'dʒɪndʒɪvə/ Gum tissue
Glia	Support tissue of the brain
Glottal	Referring to the glottis
Glottal fry	Phonatory mode characterized by low fundamental frequency and syncopated beat
Glottis	/'glatəs/ The space between the true vocal folds
Gooseflesh, goosebumps	Autonomic skin response resulting in erection of skin papillae
Gray matter	Cell bodies of neurons
Gross anatomy	Study of the body and its parts as visible without the aid of microscopy
Gustation	/gəstēɪʃən/ Sense of taste
Gyrus	Outfolding of tissue in cerebral cortex

Habitual pitch	The perceptual correlate of vocal fundamental frequency habitually used by an individual
Hamulus	/ˈhæmjuləs/ Hook
Hard palate	The bony portion of the roof of the mouth, made up of the palatal processes of the maxillae and the horizontal plates of the palatine bones
Head	Proximal portion of a bone
Helicotrema	/ˈhɛlɪkotrimə/ Hooklike region of the cochlea, forming the minute union of the scala vestibuli and scala tympani
hemi-	Half
Hemiballism	/hɛmiˈbalɪzm/ Hyperkinetic condition involving involuntary and uncontrollable flailing of extremities of the right or left half of the body
Hemispheric specialization	The concept that one cerebral hemisphere is more highly specialized for a given task or function (e.g., language) than the other hemisphere
Hertz	Cycles per second
Heschl's gyrus	/ˈheʃlz ˈdʒaɪrəs/ Area 41 of the temporal lobe; the primary reception area for auditory sense
Hg	Mercury
Hiatus	/ˈhaɪeɪtəs/ Opening
High spontaneous rate	Auditory nerve fibers demonstrating a high rate of spontaneous discharge and low threshold of stimulation
Histogram	Display of data arrayed with reference to its frequency of occurrence
Histology	Study of tissue through microscopy
Homunculus	/ho ˈmʌnkjuləs/ Literally, "little man"; referring to the spatiotopic array of fiber distribution along the central sulcus, representing body parts served by the cortical region
Horizontal plane	Divides body or part into upper and lower portions
Hyaline cartilage	/ˈhaɪəlɪn/ Smooth cartilage covering the ends of bones at articulations
hyper-	Above; increased, or too much of something
Hyperextension	Extreme extension
Hyperpolarization	The condition wherein the threshold for depolarization is elevated, requiring increased stimulation to discharge
hypo-	Below; decreased, or too little of something
Hypotonia	/haɪpoˈtoniə/ Low muscle tone
Hypoxic	/ha ˈpaksɪk/ Oxygen deficiency
idio-	Peculiar
-ilos	Diminutive form of noun
Impedance	Resistance to flow of energy
Incisors	Anterior four teeth of dental arch
Incudostapedial joint	/ɪnkjudostəpidɪjəl/ Point of union of incus and stapes

Incus	Middle bone of ossicular chain of middle ear
Indirect system	Extrapyramidal system of central nervous system, responsible for control of background movement, equilibrium, and muscle tone
Inertia	/ɪˈnɚʃə/ The tendency for a body at rest to remain at rest, and for a body in motion to remain in motion
Inferior	The lower point; nearer the feet
Inferior colliculus	/ɪnˈfɪriɚ koˈlɪkjuləs/ Nuclear relay of brainstem apparently involved in localization of sound in space
infra-	Below
Infraverted	/ɪnˈfrəvɚtd/ In dentition, an inadequately erupted tooth
Inhibition	In nervous system function, the process of reducing the ability of a neuron to discharge through synaptic action
Inner hair cells	The inner row of hair cells of the cochlea, numbering approximately 3,500, maintaining the primary role of auditory signal transduction
Innervation	Stimulation by means of a nerve
Insertion	The relatively mobile point of attachment of a muscle
Inspiration	Inhalation; drawing air into the respiratory system
Inspiratory capacity	The maximum inspiratory volume possible after tidal expiration
Inspiratory reserve volume	The volume of air that can be inhaled after a tidal inspiration
Intensity	Magnitude of sound, expressed as the relationship between two pressures or powers
inter-	Between
Interaural intensity difference	The difference between signal intensity arriving at left and right ears of a listener
Interaural phase difference	The difference in arrival time of an auditory signal arriving at left and right ears of a listener
Interchondral	/ɪntɚ ˈkandrl̩/ The region between the cartilaginous portion of the anterior rib cage
Intercostal	Between the ribs
Internal	Within the body
intero-	Aimed inward or farther from the surface
Interoceptor	/ɪntɚoˈsɛptɚ/ Sensory receptor activated by stimuli from within the body (as opposed to exteroceptor)
Interspike interval histogram	Neural response histogram providing detail of the timing between individual responses of nerve fibers
Interstitial	/ɪntɚˈstɪʃəl/ Space between cells or organs
Intertragic incisure	/ɪntɚˈtreɪdʒɪk ɪnˈsaɪʒɚ/ Region between tragus and antitragus
Intonation	The melody of speech, provided by variation of fundamental frequency during speech

intra-	Within
Intracellular	Within the cell
Intracellular resting potential	Negative electrical potential difference between the endolymph and the surrounding fluid
Intrafusal muscle fibers	/ɪntrəˈfuzl̩/ Muscle to which the muscle spindle is attached
Intraoral	/ɪntrəˈorl̩/ Within the mouth
Intraosseous eruption	Eruption of tooth through bone
Intrapleural pressure	/ɪntrəˈplɚəl/ Pressure measured within the pleural linings of the lungs
intro-	Into
Ion	A particle carrying positive or negative charge
ipsi-	Same
Ipsilateral	Same side
iso-	Equal
Isthmus	/ˈɪsməs/ A narrow passageway between cavities
-itis	Inflammation or irritation
-ium	Diminutive form of noun
Joint	Articulation
Kinesthesia	/kɪnɛsˈθiʒə/ Including sense of range, direction, and weight
Kinocilium	/kaɪnoˈsɪliəm/ Unitary cilium found on each hair cell of vestibular mechanism
Labioverted	/ˈleɪbiovɚtd/ Tilted toward the lip
Lamina	/ˈlæmənə/ A flat membrane or layer
Laryngologist	/lɛrɪnˈgalodʒɪst/ Specialist in the study of vocal pathology
Laryngoscope	/lɛˈrɪngoskop/ Instrument of visualization of the larynx and associated structures
Lateral	Toward the side
Lateral process of manubrium	/məˈnubriəm/ Superior process of manubrium to which tympanic membrane is attached, forming the anterior and posterior malleolar folds and the pars flaccida of the tympanic membrane
Lateral semicircular canal	The more horizontally placed semicircular canal, which senses movement in the transverse plane of the body
Lateral superior olive	Nuclear aggregate of superior olivary complex involved in processing interaural intensity differences
latero-	Side
Leg	1. The lower anatomical extremity, particularly the region between the knee and ankle. 2. A device used for raising grain from ground level to the top of a bin, consisting of a continuous flexible belt with a series of metal buckets or scoops.
lepto-	Thick
Lesion	/ˈliʒən/ A region of damaged tissue or a wound

leuco-	White
Lever advantage	The benefit derived through reduction of the length of the long process of stapes relative to the manubrium malli
levo-	Left
Ligaments	Fibrous connective tissue connecting bones or cartilage
Limbic system	The central nervous system structures responsible for mediation of motivation and arousal, including the hippocampus, amygdala, dentate gyrus, cingulate gyrus, and fornix
Lingual	Referring to the tongue
Linguaverted	/ˈliŋgwəvɚtd/ Tilted toward the tongue
Lobe	A well-defined region of a structure
Localization	The process of identification of a sound source presented in free field
Loudness	The psychological correlate of sound intensity
Low spontaneous rate	Auditory nerve fibers with low rate of spontaneous discharge and relatively high threshold of stimulation
Lower motor neuron	The final common neurological pathway leading to the muscle, including the anterior horn cell of the spinal cord, nerve roots, and nerves
Lumbar puncture	Insertion of aspiration needle into subarachnoid region of spinal cord, usually below L4
Lymphoid tissue	/ˈlɪmfɔ͞ɪd/ Tissue comprising lymphatic organs, including tonsils and adenoids
macro-	Large
Macula	/ˈmækjələ/ Sensory organ of saccule and utricle
Malleus	/ˈmæliəs/ Initial bone of the ossicular chain
Manometer	Device for measuring air pressure differences
Manubrium	/məˈnubriəm/ Process of malleus forming the major attachment to the tympanic membrane
Mass	The characteristic of matter that gives it inertia
Mastication	Chewing
Maximum phonation time	The duration in seconds that an individual is capable of sustaining phonation
Meatus	/miˈe͞ɪtəs/ Passageway
Mechanoreceptors	Sensory receptors sensitive to mechanical stimulation such as pressure upon the skin
Medial	Toward the midline of the body or subpart (syn. mesial)
Medial compression	The degree of force that may be applied by the vocal folds at their point of contact
Medial geniculate body	/ˈmidiəl dʒəˈnɪkjəlɪt/ Final brainstem nucleus of auditory pathway
Medial superior olive	Nuclear aggregate of superior olivary complex involved in processing interaural time (phase) differences

Median	Middle
Mediastinal	/mɪdɪˈə stɑ̄ɪnl̩/ Referring to the middle space; in respiration, referring to the organs separating the lungs
medio-, medius	Middle
megalo-	Large
Membranous glottis	/mɛmˈbrēɪnəs ˈglatəs/ The anterior three-fifths of the vocal fold margin; the soft tissue of the vocal folds (note that the term "glottis" is loosely used here, because glottis is actually the space between the vocal folds)
Membranous labyrinth	/mɛmˈbrēɪnəs ˈlæbɪrɪnθ/ Membranous sac housed within bony labyrinth of inner ear, holding the receptor organs of hearing and vestibular sense
Meningeal infection	/məˈnɪndʒɪəl/ Infection of the meningeal linings of the brain and spinal cord
Meninges	/məˈnɪndʒiz/ The membranous linings of the brain and spinal cord
Mesencephalon	/mɛsɛnˈsɛfələn/ The midbrain
Mesial	/ˈmi zɪəl/ Toward the midline of the body or subpart (syn. medial)
Mesioverted	/misioˈvɚtd/ Tilted toward the midline
meso-	Middle
meta-	After; mounted or built upon
Metencephalon	/mɛtɛnˈsɛfələn/ Embyronic portion of brain from which cerebellum and pons originate
micro-	Small
Micron	One-thousandth of a millimeter; one-millionth of a meter
Microscopic anatomy	Study of structure of the body by means of microscopy
Minute volume	The volume of air exchanged by an organism in one minute
Mitochondria	/maɪtoˈkandriə/ Microscopic cellular structures that provide the energy source for a cell
ml	Milliliters; one-thousandth of a liter, equal to one centimeter
mm	Millimeter; one-thousandth of a meter
Modal register	/ˈmodl̩/ The vocal register used during normal conversation (i.e., that vocal register used most frequently)
Modiolus	/moˈdaɪoləs/ The structure of the bony labyrinth forming the central core of the cochlea
Molars	/ˈmolɚz/ The posterior three teeth of the mature dental arch, used for grinding
mono-	Single
Monoloud	Without variation in vocal loudness (the perception of vocal intensity)
Monopitch	Without variation in vocal pitch (the perception of frequency)
morph-	Form
Morphology	/morˈfalədʒɪ/ Study of the form of a structure without regard to function
Motor endplate	Point of contact between motor neuron and muscle fiber

Motor neurons	Neurons that innervate muscle
Motor strip	The precentral gyrus of the frontal lobe; the point at which execution of voluntary motor acts is initiated
Motor unit	The lower motor neuron and muscle fibers it innervates
Mucous	/ˈmjukəs/ Tissue that secretes mucus
Mucus	/ˈmjukəs/ Viscous fluid secreted by mucous tissue and glands
Multipolar neurons	Neurons possessing more than two processes
Muscle	An aggregation of muscle fibers with functional unity
my-	Pertaining to muscle
Myelencephalon	/ˈmaɪɛlɛnsɛfəlan/ Portion of embryonic brain giving rise to the medulla oblongata
Myelin	Fatty sheath surrounding axons of some nerves
myelo-	Pertaining to spinal cord
myo-	Pertaining to muscle
Myoelastic-aerodynamic theory	/maɪoəˈlæstɪk-ɛrodaɪˈnæmɪk/ Theory of vocal fold function that accounts for phonation through the lawful interplay of tissue mass, elasticity, and aerodynamic principles
Myology	/maɪaləd͡ʒɪ/ The study of muscles and their parts
Naris	/ˈnerɪs/ Nostril (plural, nares)
naso-	Nose
Nasopharynx	/nezoˈfɛrɪŋks/ The region of the pharynx posterior to the nasal cavity and superior to the velum
Neck	Constricted portion of a structure
neo-	New
Neologism	/niˈoləd͡ʒɪzm/ New word; in pathology, novel word coined by individual, but without meaning shared with listener
Nerve	Bundle of nerve fibers outside the central nervous system that has functional unity
Neuraxis	/nɚˈæksɪs/ The axis of the nervous system, representing the embryonic brain axis
neuro-	Nerve
Neurology	Study of the nervous system
Neuromotor dysfunction	Dysfunction in motor ability arising from lesion within the nervous system or the neuromotor junction
Neuromuscular junction	The point of contact between a muscle fiber and the nerve innervating it
Neuron	A nerve cell
Neurotransmitters	Substance that is released into synaptic cleft upon excitation of a neuron
Neutroclusion	/ˈnutrokluʒən/ Normal molar relationship between upper and lower dental arches

Nodes of Ranvier	/ˈnodz ʌv ˈranvieɪ/ Regions of myelinated fibers in which there is no myelin
Nucleus	/ˈnukliəs/ An aggregate of neuron cell bodies within the central nervous system
Oblique	Diagonal
Occlusal surface	/əˈkluzl̩/ The surfaces of teeth within opposing dental arches that make contact
Occlusion	State of being closed
oculo-	Eye
Olfaction	The sense of smell
Olivocochlear bundle	/alɪ voˈkokliɚ/ Collective term for crossed and uncrossed olivocochlear bundles, the efferent auditory nerve fibers involved in processing auditory signal in noise
-oma	Morbid condition of a part, often a tumor
Onset response	Neural response in which there is an initial burst of activity related to the onset of a stimulus, followed by silence
Optimal pitch	The perceptual characteristic representing the ideal or most efficient frequency of vibration of the vocal folds
Oral cavity	The region extending from the orifice of the mouth in the anterior, and bounded laterally by the dental arches and posteriorly by the fauces
Oral diadochokinesis	/ˈdaɪədokokɪ ˈnisɪs/ A task involving repetition of movements requiring alternating contraction of antagonists muscles associated with speech (lips, mandible, tongue)
Organ of Corti	Sensory organ of hearing within inner ear
Organelles	A specialized structure of a cell (e.g., mitochondria)
Organs	Tissue of the body with functional unity
Origin	Proximal attachment of a muscle; point of attachment of a muscle with relatively little movement
oro-	Mouth
Oropharynx	/oroˈfɛrɪŋks/ The region of the pharynx bounded posteriorly by the faucial pillars, superiorly by the velum, and inferiorly by the epiglottis
ortho	Straight
Oscillation	/asɪˈleɪʃən/ Predictably repetitive movement
-osis	Condition
osseo-	A hardened or bony part
osseous labyrinth	/asiəs/ The bony cavities of the inner ear
Osseous serial lamina	Bony plate along the surface of the modiolus, forming the separation of the scalae vestibuli and tympani
Ossicular chain	/aˈsɪkjulɚ/ Collective term for malleus, incus, and stapes
Ossified	The process of tissue turning into bone

osteo-	Bone
Osteology	Study of the structure and function of bones
Otolithic membrane	/oto'lɪθɪk/ Membranous covering over the utricular macula
Outer hair cells	Outer three rows of hair cells of the organ of Corti, numbering approximately 12,000
Oval window	The opening into the scala vestibuli to which the footplate of stapes is attached
Overbite	The vertical overlap of maxillary incisors over the mandibular incisors when molars are occluded
Overjet	Vertical overlap of maxillary incisors over mandibular incisors
pachy-	Thick
Palatine tonsils	/pælətaɪn/ Lymphoid tissue between the fauces
palato-	Palate
Palmar	/ˈpalmɚ/ Pertaining to the palm of the hand
Palpate	/ˈpælpeɪt/ To examine by means of touch
Para	Beside; partial
Pars	Part
Pars flaccida	/ˈparz ˈflæsɪdə/ A flaccid portion of the tympanic membrane in the superior region
patho-	Abnormal in some way
Pathological anatomy	Study of parts of the body with respect to the pathological entity
-pathy	Disease
Pauser response	/ˈpazɚ/ Nerve response characterized by an initial on-response followed by silence, and subsequent low-level firing rate throughout stimulation
ped-	Foot; child
-penia	Poverty
Per	Through; passing through; before
Perfusion	Migration of fluid through a barrier
Peri	Around
Pericardium	/pɛrəˈkardiəm/ The membranous sac surrounding the heart
Perilymph	/ˈpɛrəlɪmf/ Fluid of the scala vestibuli and scala tympani
Perimysium	/pɛrəˈmisiəm/ The sheath surrounding muscle bundles
Period	The time required to complete one cycle of vibration or movement
Periodic	Having predictable repetition
Peripheral	Relative to the periphery or away from
Peripheral nervous system	That portion of the nervous system including spinal and cranial nerves
Permeability	/pɚmiəˈbɪlətɪ/ The quality of penetrability

Persistent closed bite	The condition wherein supraversion of the anterior dental arch prohibits the posterior teeth from occlusion
Persistent open bite	The condition wherein the incisors of upper and lower dental arches show a vertical gap, due to malocclusion of the posterior arch that prohibits anterior contact
Pes	A footlike structure
-phage, phagia	Eating
Pharyngeal tonsil	/fɛˈrɪndʒɪəl/ The mass of lymphatic tissue within the nasopharynx; a.k.a. adenoids
Pharynx	/ˈfɛrɪŋks/ The respiratory passageway from the larynx to the oral and nasal cavities
Phase-locking	The tendency of a neuron to respond to a particular phase of an acoustic signal
-pher-	Bearing or carrying
Phonation	The voiced tone produced by the vibrating vocal folds
Phonatory system	The system including the laryngeal structures through which phonation is achieved
Photoreceptors	Sensory receptors for visual stimulation
Physiological dead space	In respiration, ventilatory capacity that is wasted; in nonpathological conditions, physiological dead space is the same as anatomical dead space
Physiology	/fɪziˈalədʒɪ/ The study of function of the body and its components
Pillar cells of Corti	Supportive cells of the organ of Corti
Pinna	/pɪnə/ Auricle, making up the readily visible portion of the outer ear
Pitch	The psychological (perceptual) correlate of frequency of vibration
Pitch range	The perceptual correlate of the range of fundamental frequency variation possible for an individual
Place Theory of Hearing	Theory of hearing stating that frequency processing of the cochlea arises primarily through differential displacement of locations along the basilar membrane and, subsequently, stimulation of the hair cells of the stimulated regions
Plantar	/ˈplæntɚ/ Pertaining to the sole of the foot
Plantar grasp reflex	Grasping by the toes upon light stimulation of the sole of the foot
-plasia	Growth
-plastic	Capable of being molded
-plasty	Molding, forming
Pleural	/ˈplɝl̩/ Pertaining to the pleurae of the lungs
Pleurisy	/plɝəsɪ/ Inflammation of the pleural linings of the lungs
Plexus	/ˈplɛksəs/ A network of nerves
poly-	Many

post-	After; behind
Postsynaptic neuron	The neuron receiving input
Posterior	Toward the rear
postero-	Behind
Potential energy	Energy that may be expended
pre-	Before; in front of
Premotor area	The region of the cerebral cortex anterior to the precentral gyrus (area 6)
Pressure	The derived measure representing force expended over an area
Primary oral apraxia	/əˈpræksiə/ Deficit in planning the nonspeech act, resulting in difficulty with imitating or producing voluntary nonspeech oral gestures, but in absence of muscular weakness or paralysis
Primary verbal apraxia	/əˈpræksiə/ Deficit in planning the speech act, resulting in inconsistent phonemic distortions and substitutions with oral groping behaviors for voluntary verbal motor acts, but in absence of muscular weakness or paralysis
Primarylike response	Neural response patterns of brainstem fibers that have characteristics similar to those of the auditory nerve
pro-	Before; in front of
Process	A prominence of an anatomical structure
Projection fibers	Neural tracts running to and from the cerebral cortex connecting it with distant locations
Pronate	/ˈproneɪt/ To place in the prone position
Prone	/ˈpron/ Body in horizontal position with face down
Proprioception	/proprioˈsɛpʃən/ The awareness of weight, posture, movement, position in space
Prosencephalon	/prasɛnˈsɛfələn/ In embryology, the forebrain, from which the telencephalon and diencephalon will arise
proto-	Primitive; simple form
Protuberance	/protubɚəns/ A bulge or prominence above a structure's surface
Proximal	/ˈpraksəml̩/ Closer to the trunk or thorax; nearer to pubic bone
Psychoacousticians	Researchers involved in study of the psychological correlate of auditory stimulus parameters
Pulse register	Glottal fry; the vocal register characterized by low fundamental frequency, with syncopated vibration of vocal folds
quadra-, quadri	Four
Quiet tidal volume	The volume of air exchanged during one cycle of quiet respiration
Radial	Pertaining to the radius bone
Ramus	/ˈreɪməs/ A branch or division
-raphy	Suturing or stitching

Rate of discharge	Of a neuron, the rate at which the neuron depolarizes
re-	Back or again; curved back
Reciprocal	Interchangeable
Reflex	Motor acts that are involuntary responses to stimulation
Reissner's membrane	/ˈraɪznɚz/ Membranous separation between scala vestibuli and scala media
Relative micrognathia	/maɪkrəˈnæθiə/ The hypoplasia of the mandible relative to the maxilla
Residual volume	In respiration, the volume of air remaining after a maximum exhalation
Resonant frequency	Frequency of stimulation to which a resonant system responds most vigorously
Resonatory system	The portion of the vocal tract through which the acoustical product of vocal fold vibration resonates (usually the oral, pharyngeal, and nasal cavities combined; sometimes referring only to the nasal cavities and nasopharynx)
Respiration	The process of exchange of gas between an organism and its environment
Respiratory physiology	The study of function in respiration
Respiratory system	The physical system involved in respiration, including the lungs, bronchial passageway, trachea, larynx, pharynx, oral, and nasal cavities
Resting lung volume	The volume of air remaining within the lungs after quiet tidal expiration (a.k.a. expiratory reserve volume)
Resting potential	Voltage potential differences that can be measured from the cochlea at rest
retro-	Backward, toward the rear
Rhinorrhea	/raɪnəˈriə/ Liquid discharge from the nose
Rhombencephalon	/rambənˈsɛfələn/ Embryonic division of the brain from which the pons, cerebellum, and medulla oblongata ultimately arise
Rima glottidis	/ˈraɪmə glaˈtidɪs/ Space between the vocal folds; glottis
Rima vestibuli	/ˈraɪmə vɛˈstɪbjuli/ The space between the false (ventricular) vocal folds
Root	The part of an organ hidden within other tissues
Rostrum	/ˈrastrəm/ A beaked or hooked structure
Round window	The opening between the scala tympani of the inner ear and the middle ear space
-rrhea	A flowing
Ruga, rugae	/ˈrugə/ /ˈrugeɪ/ Folds or creases of tissue
Saccule	The smaller of the vestibular sensory mechanisms housed within the vestibule of the inner ear
Sagittal plane	/ˈsædʒɪtəl/ Divides body or body part into right and left
Scala media	/ˈskeɪlə/ The middle space of the cochlea created by the membranous labyrinth, and containing the sensory organ of hearing
Scala tympani	/ˈtɪmpəni/ The peripheral cavity of the cochlea that communicates with the middle ear via the round window
Scala vestibuli	/ˈskeɪlə vɛˈstɪbjuli/ The peripheral cavity of the cochlea that communicates with the middle ear via the vestibule and oval window

Scaphoid fossa	/ˈskæfɔɪd ˈfasə/ The region between the helix and antihelix
scirrho-, sclero	Hard
-sclerosis	/sklɚˈosɪs/ Hardening
scolio-	Curved
Segmental	Divided into segments
Selective enhancement	Relative benefit of auditory signal arising from resonance of the auditory mechanism
Sellar	/ˈsɛlɚ/ Saddlelike
semi-	Half
Semicircular canals	Canals of the vestibular system, responsible for sensation of movement of the head in space
Sensation	Awareness of body conditions sensed
Septum	/ˈsɛptəm/ A divider
Shearing action	The bending action of the hair cells arising from the relative movement of the basilar membrane and tectorial membrane during auditory stimulation
Short association fibers	Neurons of the cerebrum connecting regions within the same hemisphere
sinistro-	Left
Sinus	A cavity or passageway
Skeletal muscle	Striated or voluntary muscle
Slow twitch	Muscle fibers displaying a slow modal response
Smooth muscle	Visceral muscle
Soft palate	The musculotendinous structure separating the oropharynx and nasopharynx; a.k.a. velum
Soma	A cell body
Somatic muscle	Skeletal muscle; striated muscle
somato-	Pertaining to the body
Somesthetic	/soməsˈθɛtɪk/ Pertaining to awareness of body sensation
Sound wave	The acoustical manifestation of physical disturbance in a medium
Spatiotopic	/speɪʃioˈtɑpɪk/ The physical array of many of the regions of the cerebral cortex which defines the specific region of the body represented (e.g., the pre- and postcentral gyri)
Special senses	Olfaction, audition, and vision
Special somatic afferent	Cranial nerves that serve the special body senses such as vision and hearing
Special visceral afferent	Cranial nerves that provide information from the special visceral senses of taste and smell
Special visceral efferent	Cranial nerves that innervate striated muscle of branchial arch origin, including the larynx, pharynx, soft palate, face, and muscles of mastication
Spectral analysis	Analysis of an acoustical signal to determine the relative contribution of individual frequency components

Speculum	/ˈspɛkjuləm/ Instrument used to examine orifices and canals
Spheroid	/ˈsfirɔ̄ɪd/ Shaped like a sphere
Spike rate	Rate of discharge of a neuron
Spinal column	The vertebral column
Spinal cord	The nerve tracts and cell bodies within the spinal column
Spinal cord segment	A segment of the spinal cord corresponding to a vertebral region
Spinal nerves	Nerves arising from the spinal cord
Spiral ligament	Region of scala media to which stria vascularis is attached
Spiral limbus	Region of scala media from which the tectorial membrane arises
Spirometer	/spa̅ɪrˈamətɚ/ Device used to measure respiratory volume
Stapedius	/stəˈpidiəs/ Muscle of middle ear that acts on the stapes
Stapes	/ˈste̅ɪpiz/ The final bone of the ossicular chain
steno-	Narrow
Stereocilia	/stɛrioˈsɪliə/ Minute cilia protruding from the surface of hair cells
Stereognosis	/ˈstɛriagnosəs/ Ability to recognize objects through tactile sensation
strepto-	Swift
Stress	In speech, the product of relative increase in fundamental frequency, vocal intensity, and duration
Stria vascularis	/ˈstriə væskjuˈlɛrɪs/ Vascularized tissue arising from the spiral ligament of the scala media
Striated	Striped
Strohbass	Glottal fry; pulse register
sub-	Under
Subglottal	/sʌbˈglatl̩/ Beneath the glottis
Subglottal pressure	Air pressure generated by the respiratory system beneath the level of the vocal folds
Sulcus	/ˈsʌlkəs/ A groove
Summating potential	A sustained, direct current (DC) shift in the endocochlear potential that occurs when the organ of Corti is stimulated by sound
sup-	Under; moderately
super-	Above; excessively
Superficial	Near to the surface
Superior	The upper point; nearer the head
Superior olivary complex	Brainstem nuclear complex primarily responsible for localization of sound in space
Supination	/supɪˈneɪʃən/ Placement in the supine position
Supine	/ˈsupa̅ɪn/ Body in horizontal position with face up
supra-	Above, upon

Supraverted	/suprə ˈvɝt ɪd/ Turning up
Surface anatomy	Study of the body and its surface markings, as related to underlying structures
Surfactant	/sɚˈfæktənt/ A chemical agent that reduces surface tension
Suture	/ˈsutʃɚ/ The demarcation of union between two structures through immobile articulation
sym-	With or together
Symphysis	/sɪmfɪsɪs/ The type of union of two structures that were separated in early development, resulting in an immobile articulation
syn-	With or together
Synapse	/ˈsɪnæps/ The junction between two communicating neurons
Synaptic cleft	The region between two communicating neurons into which neurotransmitter is released
Synaptic vesicles	/sɪˈnæptɪk ˈvɛsəklz/ The saccules within the end bouton of an axon that contain neurotransmitter substance
Synergist	/ˈsɪnɚdʒɪst/ A muscle in conjuction with another muscle to facilitate movement
Synovial fluid	/sɪnoviəl/ The fluid within a synovial joint
System	A functionally defined group of organs
Systematic anatomy	Descriptive anatomy
tachy-	Swift; fast
Tactile	Referring to the sense of touch
-tarsal	Ankle
Tectorial membrane	/tɛkˈtoriəl/ The membranous structure overlying the hair cells of the cochlea
Teleceptors	/ˈtɛlɛsɛptɚz/ Sensory receptors responsive to stimuli originating outside of the body
Telencephalon	/tɛlɛnˈsɛfəlan/ Embryonic structure from which cerebral hemispheres and rhinencephalon develop
telo-	Far from, toward the extreme
Telodendria	/tɛlodɛnˈdriə/ The terminal arborization of an axon
Tendon	/ˈtɛndən/ Connective tissue attaching muscle to bone or cartilage
Tensile strength	The quality of a material that provides resistance to destructive pulling forces
Tensor tympani	/ˈtɛnsɚ ˈtɪmpənɪ/ Middle ear muscle acting on the malleus
Teratogen	/tɛˈrætodʒən/ An agent that causes abnormal embryonic development
tetra-	Four
Thermoreceptors	Sensors responsive to temperature
Thorax	The part of the body between the diaphragm and the 7th cervical vertebra
Thrombosis	/θramˈbosɪs/ Formation of a blood clot in the vascular system
Thrombus	/ˈθrambəs/ An obstructing blood clot

Tidal volume	The volume inspired and expired during normal, quiet respiration
Tissue recoil	The property of tissue that causes it to return to its original form after distention and release
-tomy	Cutting
Tonic	Pertaining to muscular contraction
Tonotopic arrangement	/tonə'tapɪk/ The arrangement of auditory nerve fibers such that fibers innervating the apex process low-frequency information, while fibers in the basal region process high-frequency information
Torque	Rotary twisting
Torsiversion	/torsə'vɚʒən/ Rotating a tooth about its long axis
Torso	The trunk of the body
Total lung capacity	Sum of tidal volume, inspiratory reserve volume, expiratory reserve volume, and residual volume
Tracts	In the central nervous system, a bundle of nerve fibers
Tragus	/'treɪgəs/ Flaplike landmark of auricle approximating the concha
trans-	Beyond or on the other side
Transduce	To change from one form of energy to another
Transducer	Mechanism for converting energy from one form to another
Transverse	At right angles to the long axis
Traveling wave	The wavelike action of the basilar membrane arising from stimulation of the perilymph of the vestibule
Tremor	Minute, involuntary repetitive movements
tri-	Three
Triangular fossa	/'traɪæŋgjulɚ fasə/ Region between the crura anthelicis
Trifurcate	/'traɪfɚkeɪt/ To divide into three parts
Trochleariform process	/trakli'arəform 'prasɛs/ Bony outcropping of middle ear from which the tendon for the tensor tympani arises
-trophic	Related to nourishment
-trophy	Growth, usually by expanding
-tropy	Implies seeking or heading for something
Trunk	The body excluding head and limbs
Tubercle	/'tubɚkl/ A small rounded prominence on bone
Tunnel of Corti	Region of the organ of Corti produced by articulation of the rods of Corti
Turbulence	Disturbance within fluid or gas caused by irregularity in passageway
Tympanic membrane	The membranous separation between the outer and middle ears, responsible for initiating the mechanical impedance-matching process of the middle ear
Umbo	/'ʌmbo/ The most distal point of attachment of the inner tympanic membrane to one of the malleus
uni-	One

Upper extremity	The arm, the forearm, wrist, and hand
Utricle	/ˈjutrɪkl̩/ Regions of vestibule housing the otolithic organs of the vestibular system
Vascularized	/ˈvæskjulɚ͞aɪzd/ To become vascular
Vasoconstriction	/væsoˈkənstrɪkʃən/ Decrease in diameter of blood vessel
Velum	/ˈviləm/ Soft palate
Ventilation	Air inhaled per unit time
Ventral	Pertaining to the belly or anterior surface
Ventricular system	/vɛnˈtrɪkjulɚ/ System of cavities and passageways of the brain and spinal cord through which cerebrospinal fluid passes
Venules	/ˈvɛnulz/ A minute vein
Vestibule	/ˈvɛstəbjul/ Entryway
Viscera	/ˈvisɚə/ Internal organs within a cavity
Visceral	/ˈvisɚəl/ Pertaining to internal organs
Vital capacity	The total volume of air that can be inspired after a maximal expiration
Vocal fundamental frequency	Primary frequency of vibration of the vocal folds
Vocal intensity	Sound pressure level associated of a given speech production
Vocal jitter	Cycle-by-cycle variation in fundamental frequency of vibration
Voiced	Speech produced using the vibrating vocal folds
Voiceless phonemes	Phonemes produced without the use of vocal folds
Waveform	Graphic depiction of change in amplitude of vibration over time
Wet spirometer	/sp͞aɪrˈamətɚ/ Device used for measurement of respiratory volumes

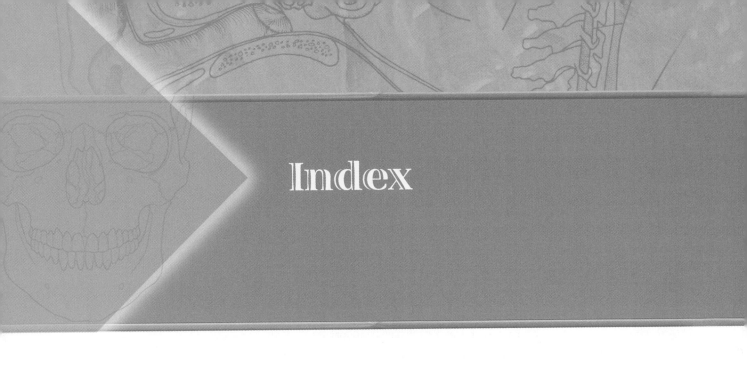

Index

A

A band, 634
Abdomen, definition, 8, 12
Abdominal aponeurosis, 103, 108–110, 111–112
Abdominal fixation, 222
Abdominal muscles of expiration, *see under* Muscles of forced expiration
Abductor paralysis, 207, 253
Absolutely refractory period (absolute refractory period), 626
Accessory cuneate nucleus, 560
Accessory muscles of inspiration, *see under* Muscles of inspiration
Accessory muscles of neck, 92–96
  see also under Muscles of inspiration
Accessory muscles of upper arm and shoulder, 96–101
  see also under Muscles of inspiration
Acetylcholine, 629, 632, 648
Acoustic reflex (stapedial reflex), 447
Actin protein, 633
Action potential (AP), 625–631
Active transport, 624–626
Adductor paralysis, 207
Adenosine triphosphate (ATP), 624, 634, 635
Adhesions, 75
Adipose tissue, 14, 15
Aditus laryngis, 169
Aditus to the mastoid antrum, 448
Afferent, definition, 25, 502
Age, effects of
  changes in oral and velar structures, 392–394
  changes in pitch and vocal fold length, 241, 242

increase in alveoli numbers with age, 132–133
lungs, age-related changes, 132–134
respiration rates as a function of age, 132, 134
respiratory volumes and capacities, 139
Air, movement through the system, 75–78
Air pressure, definition and properties, 36–38
Airway, effect of position on patency, 62, 70
Ala, 283
Alpha motor neurons, 512–513, 638
Alveolar (pulmonic) pressure (P_{al}), 141, 143–144
Alveolar ridge, 266, 267, 316, 380–381, 415
Alveoli, 35, 69–72, 132–133
Ambulation, 49
Amelogenesis imperfecta, 308
Amphiarthrodial joints, 20, 23
  see also Cartilaginous joints
Ampulla, 451, 454
Amygdaloid body (or amygdala), 539–540
Amyotrophic lateral sclerosis (ALS), 25, 151, 378, 538
Anastomoses, 544, 546
Anatesse software labs, about, 2
Anatomical dead space, 138
Anatomical position, 8, 10
Anatomical terms, 671–672 *(app)*
Anatomy, basic elements, 5–31
  definition, 6, 7
  terminology, 8–13
Aneurysm, 186, 207, 546–547, 654–655

Angiology, definition, 7
Angular gyrus, 533
Anosmia, 567
Anterior, definition, 10, 12
Anterior and middle cerebral arteries, 544
Anterior and posterior malleolar folds, 440
Anterior and posterior spinal arteries, 544
Anterior (anterior vertical, superior) semicircular canals, 451
Anterior communicating artery, 544
Anterior funiculus, 602
Anterior-posterior mode of phonation, 235
Anterior spinocerebellar tract, 602–603
Anterior spinothalamic tract, 601–602
Antihelix, 436
Antitragus, 437
Apert syndrome, 22
Aphonia, 231
Apical pleurae, 75–76
Aponeuroses, 19, 103, 108–110, 111–112, 349–350
Appendicular skeleton, 9, 12
Applied (clinical) anatomy, definition, 6
Approximation, 180
Arachnoid mater, 515, 519
Arcuate fasciculus, 538, 657
Arthrology, definition, 7, 8
Articulation, definition, 19, 263
Articulation and resonation, anatomy of, 263–355
  articulators, 267–268
  immobile articulators, *see* Alveolar ridge; Hard palate; Teeth

INSTALLING ANATESSE

1. Insert CD-ROM in CD-ROM drive on your computer.
2. Before program can be installed, you will be queried to read and agree to the Thomson Delmar Learning licensing agreement. You will not be able to continue with the installation until you click the AGREE button.
3. Installation should continue automatically and a SKULL icon will appear on the desktop.
4. If this does not happen, double-click on SETUP.EXE in the CD and follow the instructions in the installer. When done, you should have an icon for Anatesse showing on your desktop.
5. If the installer finished properly but you don't have a SKULL icon, you can run Anatesse from the Start button or create an icon.

RUNNING ANATESSE FOR THE FIRST TIME

1. Anatesse is a study guide that always gives you a grade report at the end of each lesson. Your instructor will decide whether that report is to be recorded for actual grading. If so, you should keep a floppy disk to hold your grades and turn in the disk when your instructor requests it.
2. On the first use of Anatesse, insert an empty disk in the computer's slot, then start the program. You will be asked for a name or ID; your instructor should specify a form of identification, such as last name or student number. Then you will need to enter a password. This should consist of letters and/or numbers, with no spaces or punctuation. Capitalization does not matter: if you set up your password as SNAP and later enter snap or sNaP, it will still work. Once the floppy has been registered, you can continue on to the actual lessons.
3. After the first use, simply insert the same floppy disk before starting the program; you will be asked for your password.
4. When this initial stage is over, you will see a Select Lesson list; from there you will proceed to work whichever lesson is assigned or is next.
5. If you have to leave a lesson before finishing, a Bookmark will be created on your floppy disk. The next time you start up the Select Lesson menu will indicate a Bookmark for that lesson and you will be able to start where you left off by clicking the "Start from Bookmark" button instead of the regular Start.
6. You can see your own grades by starting Anatesse and hitting the Read Grades button. (A separate Help text is available inside that action.)
7. Anatesse looks best at a screen resolution of 800 _ 600. At larger resolutions the frame expands to fill the screen, but some images will look rough. If you prefer a frame that stays the same size, switch the desktop shortcut from ANATESSE.EXE to ANATESSE2.EXE.

License Agreement for Thomson Delmar Learning

IMPORTANT! READ CAREFULLY: This End User License Agreement ("Agreement") sets forth the conditions by which Thomson Delmar Learning, a division of Thomson Learning Inc. ("Thomson") will make electronic access to the Thomson Delmar Learning-owned licensed content and associated media, software, documentation, printed materials, and electronic documentation contained in this package and/or made available to you via this product (the "Licensed Content"), available to you (the "End User"). BY CLICKING THE "I ACCEPT" BUTTON AND/OR OPENING THIS PACKAGE, YOU ACKNOWLEDGE THAT YOU HAVE READ ALL OF THE TERMS AND CONDITIONS, AND THAT YOU AGREE TO BE BOUND BY ITS TERMS, CONDITIONS, AND ALL APPLICABLE LAWS AND REGULATIONS GOVERNING THE USE OF THE LICENSED CONTENT.

1.0 SCOPE OF LICENSE

1.1 *Licensed Content.* The Licensed Content may contain portions of modifiable content ("Modifiable Content") and content which may not be modified or otherwise altered by the End User ("Non-Modifiable Content"). For purposes of this Agreement, Modifiable Content and Non-Modifiable Content may be collectively referred to herein as the "Licensed Content." All Licensed Content shall be considered Non-Modifiable Content, unless such Licensed Content is presented to the End User in a modifiable format and it is clearly indicated that modification of the Licensed Content is permitted.

1.2 Subject to the End User's compliance with the terms and conditions of this Agreement, Thomson Delmar Learning hereby grants the End User, a nontransferable, non-exclusive, limited right to access and view a single copy of the Licensed Content on a single personal computer system for noncommercial, internal, personal use only. The End User shall not (i) reproduce, copy, modify (except in the case of Modifiable Content), distribute, display, transfer, sublicense, prepare derivative work(s) based on, sell, exchange, barter or transfer, rent, lease, loan, resell, or in any other manner exploit the Licensed Content; (ii) remove, obscure, or alter any notice of Thomson Delmar Learning's intellectual property rights present on or in the Licensed Content, including, but not limited to, copyright, trademark, and/or patent notices; or (iii) disassemble, decompile, translate, reverse engineer, or otherwise reduce the Licensed Content.

2.0 TERMINATION

2.1 Thomson Delmar Learning may at any time (without prejudice to its other rights or remedies) immediately terminate this Agreement and/or suspend access to some or all of the Licensed Content, in the event that the End User does not comply with any of the terms and conditions of this Agreement. In the event of such termination by Thomson Delmar Learning, the End User shall immediately return any and all copies of the Licensed Content to Thomson Delmar Learning.

3.0 PROPRIETARY RIGHTS

3.1 The End User acknowledges that Thomson Delmar Learning owns all rights, title and interest, including, but not limited to all copyright rights therein, in and to the Licensed Content, and that the End User shall not take any action inconsistent with such ownership. The Licensed Content is protected by U.S., Canadian and other applicable copyright laws and by international treaties, including the Berne Convention and the Universal Copyright Convention. Nothing contained in this Agreement shall be construed as granting the End User any ownership rights in or to the Licensed Content.

3.2 Thomson Delmar Learning reserves the right at any time to withdraw from the Licensed Content any item or part of an item for which it no longer retains the right to publish, or which it has reasonable grounds to believe infringes copyright or is defamatory, unlawful, or otherwise objectionable.

4.0 PROTECTION AND SECURITY

4.1 The End User shall use its best efforts and take all reasonable steps to safeguard its copy of the Licensed Content to ensure that no unauthorized reproduction, publication, disclosure, modification, or distribution of the Licensed Content, in whole or in part, is made. To the extent that the End User becomes aware of any such unauthorized use of the Licensed Content, the End User shall immediately notify Thomson Delmar Learning. Notification of such violations may be made by sending an e-mail to delmarhelp@thomson.com.

5.0 MISUSE OF THE LICENSED PRODUCT

5.1 In the event that the End User uses the Licensed Content in violation of this Agreement, Thomson Delmar Learning shall have the option of electing liquidated damages, which shall include all profits generated by the End User's use of the Licensed Content plus interest computed at the maximum rate permitted by law and all legal fees and other expenses incurred by Thomson Delmar Learning in enforcing its rights, plus penalties.

6.0 FEDERAL GOVERNMENT CLIENTS

6.1 Except as expressly authorized by Thomson Delmar Learning, Federal Government clients obtain only the rights specified in this Agreement and no other rights. The Government acknowledges that (i) all software and related documentation incorporated in the Licensed Content is existing commercial computer software within the meaning of FAR 27.405(b)(2); and (2) all other data delivered in whatever form, is limited rights data within the meaning of FAR 27.401. The restrictions in this section are acceptable as consistent with the Government's need for software and other data under this Agreement.

7.0 DISCLAIMER OF WARRANTIES AND LIABILITIES

7.1 Although Thomson Delmar Learning believes the Licensed Content to be reliable, Thomson Delmar Learning does not guarantee or warrant (i) any information or materials contained in or produced by the Licensed Content, (ii) the accuracy, completeness or reliability of the Licensed Content, or (iii) that the Licensed Content is free from errors or other material defects. THE LICENSED PRODUCT IS PROVIDED "AS IS," WITHOUT ANY WARRANTY OF ANY KIND AND THOMSON DELMAR LEARNING DISCLAIMS ANY AND ALL WARRANTIES, EXPRESSED OR IMPLIED, INCLUDING, WITHOUT LIMITATION, WARRANTIES OF MERCHANTABILITY OR FITNESS FOR A PARTICULAR PURPOSE. IN NO EVENT SHALL THOMSON DELMAR LEARNING BE LIABLE FOR: INDIRECT, SPECIAL, PUNITIVE OR CONSEQUENTIAL DAMAGES INCLUDING FOR LOST PROFITS, LOST DATA, OR OTHERWISE. IN NO EVENT SHALL THOMSON DELMAR LEARNING'S AGGREGATE LIABILITY HEREUNDER, WHETHER ARISING IN CONTRACT, TORT, STRICT LIABILITY OR OTHERWISE, EXCEED THE AMOUNT OF FEES PAID BY THE END USER HEREUNDER FOR THE LICENSE OF THE LICENSED CONTENT.

8.0 GENERAL

8.1 *Entire Agreement.* This Agreement shall constitute the entire Agreement between the Parties and supercedes all prior Agreements and understandings oral or written relating to the subject matter hereof.

8.2 *Enhancements/Modifications of Licensed Content.* From time to time, and in Thomson Delmar Learning's sole discretion, Thomson Delmar Learning may advise the End User of updates, upgrades, enhancements and/or improvements to the Licensed Content, and may permit the End User to access and use, subject to the terms and conditions of this Agreement, such modifications, upon payment of prices as may be established by Thomson Delmar Learning.

8.3 *No Export.* The End User shall use the Licensed Content solely in the United States and shall not transfer or export, directly or indirectly, the Licensed Content outside the United States.

8.4 *Severability.* If any provision of this Agreement is invalid, illegal, or unenforceable under any applicable statute or rule of law, the provision shall be deemed omitted to the extent that it is invalid, illegal, or unenforceable. In such a case, the remainder of the Agreement shall be construed in a manner as to give greatest effect to the original intention of the parties hereto.

8.5 *Waiver.* The waiver of any right or failure of either party to exercise in any respect any right provided in this Agreement in any instance shall not be deemed to be a waiver of such right in the future or a waiver of any other right under this Agreement.

8.6 *Choice of Law/Venue.* This Agreement shall be interpreted, construed, and governed by and in accordance with the laws of the State of New York, applicable to contracts executed and to be wholly preformed therein, without regard to its principles governing conflicts of law. Each party agrees that any proceeding arising out of or relating to this Agreement or the breach or threatened breach of this Agreement may be commenced and prosecuted in a court in the State and County of New York. Each party consents and submits to the non-exclusive personal jurisdiction of any court in the State and County of New York in respect of any such proceeding.

8.7 *Acknowledgment.* By opening this package and/or by accessing the Licensed Content on this Web site, THE END USER ACKNOWLEDGES THAT IT HAS READ THIS AGREEMENT, UNDERSTANDS IT, AND AGREES TO BE BOUND BY ITS TERMS AND CONDITIONS. IF YOU DO NOT ACCEPT THESE TERMS AND CONDITIONS, YOU MUST NOT ACCESS THE LICENSED CONTENT AND RETURN THE LICENSED PRODUCT TO DELMAR LEARNING (WITHIN 30 CALENDAR DAYS OF THE END USER'S PURCHASE) WITH PROOF OF PAYMENT ACCEPTABLE TO THOMSON DELMAR LEARNING, FOR A CREDIT OR A REFUND. Should the End User have any questions/comments regarding this Agreement, please contact Thomson Delmar Learning at delmarhelp@thomson.com.